ROUTLEDGE HANDBOOK OF THE MEDICAL HUMANITIES

This authoritative new handbook offers a comprehensive and cutting-edge overview of the state of the medical humanities globally, showing how clinically oriented medical humanities, the critical study of medicine as a global historical and cultural phenomenon, and medicine as a force for cultural change can inform each other.

Composed of eight parts, the *Routledge Handbook of the Medical Humanities* looks at the medical humanities as:

- a network and system
- therapeutic
- provocation
- forms of resistance
- a way of reconceptualising the medical curriculum
- concerned with performance and narrative
- mediated by artists as diagnosticians of culture through public engagement.

This book describes how the medical humanities can be used in and out of clinical settings, acting as a point of resistance, redistributing medicine's capital amongst its stakeholders, embracing the complexity of medical instances, shaping medical education, promoting interdisciplinary understandings and recognising an identity for the medical humanities as a network effect. This book is an essential read for all students, scholars and practitioners with an interest in the medical humanities.

Alan Bleakley is Emeritus Professor of Medical Education and Medical Humanities at Plymouth University's Peninsula School of Medicine, UK, and has been Visiting Scholar at the Wilson Centre, University of Toronto, Canada. He is immediate past president of the Association for Medical Humanities Council.

ROUTLEDGE HANDBOOK OF THE MEDICAL HUMANITIES

Edited by Alan Bleakley

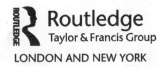

Routledge
Taylor & Francis Group

LONDON AND NEW YORK

First published 2020 by Routledge

2 Park Square, Milton Park, Abingdon, Oxon OX14 4RN
605 Third Avenue, New York, NY 10017

Routledge is an imprint of the Taylor & Francis Group, an informa business

First issued in paperback 2022

Publisher's Note

The publisher has gone to great lengths to ensure the quality of this reprint but points out that some imperfections in the original copies may be apparent.

British Library Cataloguing-in-Publication Data
A catalogue record for this book is available from the British Library

Library of Congress Cataloging-in-Publication Data
A catalog record has been requested for this book

ISBN: 978-0-815-37461-9 (hbk)
ISBN: 978-1-03-233810-1 (pbk)
DOI: 10.4324/9781351241779

Typeset in Bembo
by Swales & Willis Ltd, Exeter, Devon, UK

CONTENTS

Contents

CONTRIBUTORS

Jon Allard works as a Researcher for Cornwall Partnership NHS Foundation Trust and is an Honorary Fellow with the University of Plymouth. He has worked in a research capacity across a variety of healthcare settings and completed his PhD in 2013. This was an in-depth ethnographic study focused on micropolitics (power dynamics) on an acute mental health ward and in a hospital emergency department. He is particularly interested in qualitative research approaches and their use across complex and challenging patient care environments. Jon moved from London to Cornwall 15 years ago and surfs as much as possible.

Natalie Beausoleil is a feminist critical obesity sociologist, artist and Professor of Social Sciences and Health in the Division of Community Health and Humanities in the Faculty of Medicine at Memorial University of Newfoundland. She holds her PhD from the University of California at Los Angeles (UCLA). Her scholarship and activism focus on the social production, representation and experiences of the body and health, as well as the arts and social justice in medical education and medical humanities. She has published several peer-reviewed art pieces, articles and book chapters in Canadian and international publications.

Alan Bleakley is Emeritus Professor of Medical Education and Medical Humanities at Plymouth University Peninsula School of Medicine. He was instrumental in setting up an innovative medical humanities programme at Peninsula Medical School, Universities of Exeter and Plymouth, and has an international reputation in medical education and medical humanities. He was President of the Association for Medical Humanities 2013–2016. He has a background in zoology, cultural studies, psychology and education and has practised clinically as a psycho-dynamic psychotherapist as well as an academic. He has published over 100 peer-reviewed academic papers and book chapters and has written and/or edited 15 books. He is a widely published poet and a keen surfer.

Susan Bleakley is a visual artist and runs Special Study Units in 'how to look' for fourth-year medical students at the University of Exeter Medical School. Sue was a self-taught naïve painter before studying formally for a sculpture degree (First Class honours) from Falmouth University and an MA in Sculpture from the Royal College of Art (London). She paints as well as making sculpture, and is a trained counsellor. Her work, sold internationally, is represented by Crane

Kalman Gallery (London), Circle Contemporary Gallery (Wadebridge) and whitecourtart.com. She has a permanent exhibition of medically related artworks at the Royal Cornwall Hospital, Truro site of Exeter Medical School.

Stella Bolaki is Reader in the School of English at the University of Kent, UK. She is the author of *Illness as Many Narratives: Arts, Medicine and Culture* (2016) and has published articles in *Literature and Medicine*, *Medical Humanities*, the *Journal of Literary & Cultural Disability Studies*, *Mosaic*, *Textual Practice*, and *Symbiosis*. She is the Director of Kent's postgraduate programme in Medical Humanities. In 2016, she curated (with Egidija Čiricaitė) an exhibition of artists' books in Canterbury, 'Prescriptions,' that was part of the Wellcome Trust-funded project 'Artists' Books and the Medical Humanities.'

Gianna Bouchard is a Senior Lecturer in Theatre at the University of Birmingham. Her research focuses on contemporary theatre and performance in relation to medical science, live art, critical theory and feminist practice. She is completing a monograph titled *Performing Specimens: Contemporary Performance and Biomedical Display* for publication in 2019. She co-edited *Performance and the Medical Body* with Alex Mermikides (2016), and a special issue titled 'On Medicine' (2014) for *Performance Research* with Martin O'Brien. Her work has also been published in *Performance Research*, *Contemporary Theatre Review* and other edited collections.

Marijke Boucherie is a Dutch-speaking Belgian and has lived most of her adult life in Portugal. She has a PhD in English Literature from the University of Lisbon where she has been an Assistant Professor in the English Department. She is a Researcher at the University of Lisbon Centre for English Studies (ULICES) and participates in the programme of narrative medicine (http://narrativaemedicina.letras.ulisboa.pt). Her research has mainly focused on the Victorian Literature of Nonsense and on the ways meaning is conveyed through non-linguistic elements. Her research interests were motivated by the experience of living in a foreign country and by a life shared with a person diagnosed with autism.

Pamela Brett-Maclean is Associate Professor in the Department of Psychiatry, and Director of the Arts and Humanities in Health and Medicine (AHHM) programme, in the Faculty of Medicine and Dentistry at the University of Alberta in Edmonton, Alberta. Along with Allan Peterkin, she helped to found 'Creating Space,' the ongoing health humanities meeting organised annually in Canada; and also, more recently, the newly announced Canadian Association for Health Humanities. Pamela networks internationally across medical/health humanities communities and has been instrumental in promoting public engagement in health humanities.

Brian Brown is Professor of Health Communication at De Montfort University, Leicester, UK. The core of Professor Brown's work has focused on the interpretation of human experience across a variety of different disciplines including healthcare, philosophy, education and spirituality studies, exploring how this may be understood with a view to improving practice and with regard to theoretical development in the social sciences. Particularly, this concerns notions of governmentality and habitus from Foucauldian and Bourdieusian sociology and how the analysis of everyday experience can afford novel theoretical developments. Professor Brown has completed 12 books and around 70 refereed journal articles. His books include *Evidence-Based Health Communication* (with P. Crawford and R. Carter, 2006) and *Evidence-Based Research: Dilemmas and Debates in Health Care* (with P. Crawford and C. Hicks, 2003).

Cari Costanzo is a Cultural Anthropologist (Stanford PhD, 2005) and an Academic Advisor who co-teaches 'Reading the Body' in Stanford's 'Thinking Matters' programme. Dr Costanzo's research and writing focus on ritual, embodiment and identity formation in contemporary society, looking closely at the cultural construction of race, class, gender and sexuality. Dr Costanzo designs Ethnographic Body Mapping workshops that combine cultural awareness with artistic and contemplative practices to encourage the reframing and reclaiming of embodied experiences, enabling participants to both reflect upon and creatively share their life stories.

David Cotterrell (www.cotterrell.com) is an installation artist, academic and consultant. David works internationally and regularly collaborates with artists, activists, academics and administrators to realise art, advocacy and social research projects. His work spans galleries, architecture and the public realm and he has realised over 105 exhibitions or public artworks, 40 publications and 75 papers and public lectures in the UK, North America, Europe, Middle East and Asia. In recent years David and the Sri Lankan playwright and theatre director Ruwanthie de Chickera have been working in collaboration to develop multidisciplinary interventions within visual arts, theatre and policy. Over the past 15 years, David has led and delivered research projects for the Leverhulme Trust, Wellcome Trust, Department of Health, British Council, Arts and Humanities Research Council (AHRC), Commission for Architecture and the Built Environment (CABE) and the Royal Society for the Encouragement of the Arts (RSA). He has held academic posts within the UK since 2000. He was first awarded a personal chair in 2008, was the recipient of the Philip Leverhulme Prize for research in 2010 and was appointed Director of Research and Development at the University of Brighton in 2016. Since 2018, he has held the post of Research Professor at Sheffield Hallam University and is centrally involved in the leadership of an active and diverse research community.

Paul Crawford is the world's first Professor of Health Humanities, pioneering this new and fast-growing field. He directs the Centre for Social Futures (Institute of Mental Health) and co-directs the Health Humanities Research Priority Area at the University of Nottingham. He is a Fellow of the Royal Society of Public Health, Royal Society of Arts and the Academy of Social Sciences. His research has attracted substantial, prestigious funding from major awarding bodies and he consults globally on health humanities. His recent publications include *Health Humanities* (2015) and *The Companion to Health Humanities* (2019).

Henry A. Curtis MD, FACEP, FAAEM is a Clinical Assistant Professor in the Department of Emergency Medicine at the Stanford University School of Medicine. He serves as a member of the School of Medicine's medical humanities steering committee and as the founder and director of the section of medical humanities within the emergency department. He is fellowship trained in simulation education and has developed expertise in film education, virtual reality medical education and the medical humanities. He is currently pursuing a Master of Fine Arts degree in Directing at the Academy of Art in San Francisco, California. This craft is integrated into his medical educational offerings through industrial films to provoke challenging discussions, medical student coursework in film analysis and production, resident electives in the humanities and projects stimulating faculty sensitivity in the department. He continues to seek out gripping means of communicating valuable messages and is now exploring the best methods of delivering compelling virtual reality-based medical education.

James Dalton is a freelance director and works across new writing, participatory theatre and interdisciplinary projects informed by his artistic collaborative practice. He is currently a PhD candidate with the Department of Theatre and Performance Studies at the University of Sydney, researching healthcare as performance practice, and is a member of the Sydney Arts Health Collective.

Randi Davenport is the author of a novel, *The End of Always* (2014)—an *O Magazine* 'Ten Titles to Pick Up Now' selection that was also long-listed for the Center for Fiction's Flaherty-Dunnan First Novel Prize, selected by *Woman's Day* as a Best Book of 2014 and was a *Woman's Day* Book Club Pick—and a memoir, *The Boy Who Loved Tornadoes* (2010), which won the Great Lakes Colleges Association's Award for creative non-fiction, was a top five finalist for the Books for a Better Life Award and was nominated for the Ragan Old North State Cup Award for Non-Fiction. Her short fiction and essays have appeared in *The New York Times*, *Washington Post, Salon, Huffington Post, Ontario Review, Alaska Quarterly Review, Women's History Review, Literature/Film Quarterly* and *Victorian Literature and Culture*, among others. She earned a PhD in literature and an MA in Creative Writing—Fiction from Syracuse University, and a BA in History from William Smith College. She has been a Summer Fellow of the National Endowment for the Humanities, and a Public Fellow at the Institute of Arts and Humanities at the University of North Carolina at Chapel Hill. She has taught literature and writing and/or served in administrative positions at Hobart and William Smith Colleges, Duke University and the University of North Carolina at Chapel Hill. Randi has a son and a daughter. She lives in Chapel Hill, North Carolina. You can learn more by following her on Facebook or by visiting her website: www.randidavenport.com.

Sarah de Leeuw is an award-winning researcher and author, and an Associate Professor with the Northern Medical Program at the University of Northern British Columbia, the Faculty of Medicine at the University of British Columbia. A poet, essayist and critical geographer, she teaches health humanities and community-based scholarship while working with anti-colonial and feminist theories, combined with creative and arts-based methods, to address health inequities especially in northern and rural geographies.

Courtney Donovan is Associate Professor in the Department of Geography and Environment, San Francisco State University, California. Her specialties are: health geography, health disparities, health humanities, narrative medicine, feminist geography, political geography, visual methodologies, critical geographies of race and ethnicity and digital health. Dr Donovan's teaching specialties include: geographies of health, qualitative field methods, narrative medicine and medical humanities, ethnic communities, geographic perspectives on gender and world regional geography. She has pioneered work in the developing field of geo-humanities.

Bella Eacott is Research Manager at performance company 'Clod Ensemble,' working across public engagement and on the company's 'Performing Medicine' programme of arts-based education for healthcare professionals. This role includes designing and programming a wide range of practical workshops, talks, panel discussions, symposia and other activities in collaboration with hospitals, medical schools, university departments and cultural institutions. She studied History and Philosophy of Science at University College London, and Medical Humanities (MSc) at King's College London. Her research interests are focused on conceptions of healthcare as an embodied practice, and the ways that undergraduate and professional healthcare training can address and reflect these embodied aspects.

Quentin Eichbaum is Professor of Pathology, Microbiology and Immunology at Vanderbilt University Medical Center, Nashville, TN; and Professor of Medical Education and Administration at Vanderbilt University School of Medicine (VUSM). He is also: Director of Transfusion Medicine; Director of Vanderbilt Pathology Education Research Group; and Director of Vanderbilt Pathology Program in Global Health. He works with new medical schools in Africa (Consortium of Southern African Medical Schools—CONSAMS) and with the American Society for Clinical Pathology on pathology education and cancer diagnostic capacitation in Africa. Further, he teaches a medical humanities course at VUSM.

Eivind Engebretsen is a Professor of Medical Philosophy and the Research Director at the Faculty of Medicine, University of Oslo. His research interest is mainly concerned with the concepts of evidence and 'knowledge translation' in medicine. He is co-PI of a research group on medical humanities and knowledge translation at the Centre for Advanced Study at the Norwegian Academy of Science and Letters.

Yrjö Engeström is Professor Emeritus of Adult Education at the University of Helsinki and Professor Emeritus of Communication at the University of California, San Diego. He is Director of the Center for Research on Activity, Development and Learning (CRADLE), and serves as visiting professor at Rhodes University in South Africa and at University West in Sweden. In his work, he applies and develops cultural-historical activity theory as a framework for the study of transformations in educational settings and work activities, with a particular focus on health-care. He is known for his theory of expansive learning and for the methodology of formative interventions, including the Change Laboratory method. His most recent book is *Expertise in Transition: Expansive Learning in Medical Work* (2018).

Glenda Eoyang is the founding executive director of the Human Systems Dynamics Institute in Circle Pines, Minnesota, USA. Since 2003, Dr Eoyang has consulted with public and private institutions internationally to build adaptive capacity. She also leads a network of over 700 scholar-practitioners who apply her methods to a variety of wicked problems in diverse disciplines. She has authored many chapters, articles and books, including (with Stewart Mennin and Mary Nations) *Lead Complex Change: The Future of Health Professions Education* (2016); and with Royce Holladay, *Adaptive Action: Leveraging Uncertainty in Your Organization* (2013). Find out more about her work at www.hsdinstitute.org.

Ian Fussell has worked in Cornwall as a doctor since 1990 and is the Vice Dean of Education (Interim) at the Medical School, College of Medicine and Health, University of Exeter, where he has led and developed an exceptional and eclectic catalogue of medical humanities provision for the undergraduate medicine and surgery curriculum (including his own 'Medical School of Rock' Special Study Unit). His career includes senior NHS management and he has been a Council member, Association for Medical Humanities. His interests include the use of IT in Medical Education, Global Health and Event Medicine; and he is a trustee of Medical Education, Sanitation and Health in Ethiopia (MESHE), a charity helping to bring fresh water to rural Ethiopia. Ian is a father of four, a keen surfer and plays the guitar in a psych/punk/rock band with his son.

Kathryn E. Goldfarb is Assistant Professor of Anthropology at the University of Colorado at Boulder. She received her PhD in Anthropology at the University of Chicago. Her research considers how social inclusion and exclusion shape holistic wellbeing and embodied experience, bringing together analytical perspectives on kinship, medical anthropology and semiotics to examine how past and present social relationships are experienced in visceral, embodied terms.

Her in-progress book manuscript explores the ways that in Japan—a society often understood as 'hyper-relational'—relationships and their absence shape embodied experience and alignments towards socially normative kinship practices. A second project examines the international circulation of psychological expertise surrounding interpersonal trauma, and the communication ideologies that undergird clinicians' attempts to translate attachment therapy techniques to a Japanese context.

Mark Goldszmidt is an MD, PhD at the Schulich School of Medicine and Dentistry in London, Ontario, Canada where he is a Professor in the Division of Internal Medicine and the Associate Director of the Center for Education Research and Innovation. His work combines active clinical practice, education research and education leadership. His research focuses on the complex relationship between clinical care and clinical teaching. For instance: How do a teaching team's communication practices shape care? In what ways do different attending practices shape care and influence learning? What is the impact of organisational values on teaching teams' clinical practices?

Sophie Holloway is currently a final-year medical student at the University of Exeter. "Originally from South Wales, I moved to Exeter when I started medical school. What drew me into a career in medicine was the joy of meeting different people every day, and the unique interactions experienced as you attempt to make patients feel better. For this reason, I am keen to pursue a career in general practice. I wrote the piece in this book as part of a medical humanities project looking into the aspects of communication between a physician and patient. I hope what I have learned through writing the piece will stay with me and be carried through my career as a doctor."

Claire Hooker is Senior Lecturer, Health and Medical Humanities, Director, Bioethics Program (Sydney Health Ethics) and Co-Chair, Arts Health Network NSW/ACT. Claire's research programme is focused on exploring the uses of theatre and performance approaches to improving communication and workplace culture in healthcare situations and settings, within a broader framework of committed advocacy for the intersection between the creative arts and health. As part of the multidisciplinary 'Sydney Arts and Health Collective,' Claire has produced theatre-based workshops and a verbatim theatre work, 'Grace Under Pressure,' as ways of exploring and improving healthcare workplace culture. Prior research has focused on intersections between the philosophical (for example, the conceptual framework to understand 'empathy' and 'dignity,' how this language is used and what empathised bodies can do) and the applied (for example, how to improve risk communication where measures of risk are low, but patient or public concern is very high).

Therese (Tess) Jones is Associate Director of the Center for Bioethics and Humanities; Director of the Arts and Humanities in Healthcare Program at the University of Colorado Anschutz Medical Campus; and Associate Professor in the Department of Medicine. She received her PhD in English from the University of Colorado, Boulder, with major emphases in American literature, modern and contemporary drama and gender studies, and completed a postdoctoral fellowship over three years in medical humanities. She has published and presented extensively on HIV/AIDS and the arts; literature, film and medicine; and medical education; and is the longstanding editor of the *Journal of Medical Humanities* and lead editor for the *Health Humanities Reader* published in 2014. Her teaching includes required and elective courses in the humanities and arts for health professions students; co-directing a health humanities minor for undergraduate students at the University of Colorado Denver; and directing a graduate certificate in health humanities and ethics. She is a member of the Academy of Medical Educators.

Lisa Folkmarson Käll is Associate Professor of Theoretical Philosophy and Associate Senior Lecturer in Gender Studies at Stockholm University, Sweden. Her work brings together phenomenology with current gender research and feminist theory to inquire into questions concerning embodied subjectivity, vulnerability, bodily constitution of sexual difference and sexual identity, intersubjectivity and the relation between selfhood and otherness. She is currently completing a book project on conceptualisations of subjectivity in relation to age-related dementia. Käll is editor of *Bodies, Boundaries and Vulnerabilities: Interrogating Social, Cultural and Political Aspects of Embodiment* (2015) and *Dimensions of Pain* (Routledge, 2013) and co-editor with Kristin Zeiler of *Feminist Phenomenology and Medicine* (2014).

Monica Kidd is a family physician in Calgary, with practice and research interests in child and maternal health and global health. She is a former reporter with CBC Radio, a writer of poetry, fiction and non-fiction and an editor with the literary publishing house Pedlar Press. Her research and creative work have appeared in more than 30 journals and anthologies.

Julia Kristeva is Professor Emerita at the Université Paris Diderot. She is one of the most prominent intellectuals of our time. Several of her concepts—such as intertextuality, the semiotic and the abject—have reformed modern humanities and social science research, and in 2004 she was awarded the first Holberg Prize for her research. She is active in disability studies, reflected in her 2015 novel *The Enchanted Clock*.

Arno K. Kumagai is Professor and Vice Chair for Education at the University of Toronto Department of Medicine and Researcher at the Wilson Centre, Toronto. He holds the FM Hill Chair in Humanism Education, Women's College Hospital and University of Toronto. Arno is an experienced diabetologist with a thriving practice, and also father, spouse and medical educator; and has contributed significantly to the field of medical/health humanities. He has published widely and is a regular conference keynote speaker.

Ayelet Kuper is a Scientist and Associate Director of Faculty Affairs at the Wilson Centre, Toronto, as well as a Clinician-Scientist, Associate Professor and Co-Lead for Person-Centred Care Education in the Department of Medicine at the University of Toronto. Dr Kuper is a member of the Division of General Internal Medicine at Sunnybrook Health Sciences Centre where she attends on the inpatient Clinical Teaching Units. Her research programme focuses on the legitimacy of different forms of medical knowledge, with a particular interest in challenging taken-for-granted assumptions and in foregrounding ways of knowing that promote equity and reflexivity.

Susan Levine is an Associate Professor of Anthropology at the University of Cape Town in South Africa. Her research interests include medical and visual anthropology, and, in particular, the use of documentary film to promote dialogue, understanding and debate around issues associated with HIV/AIDS, sexuality and poverty in Sub-Saharan Africa. Susan is the author of *Children of a Bitter Harvest* (2013), about child labour in South Africa's wine industry, and the editor of *Medicine and the Politics of Knowledge* (2009) and *At the Foot of the Volcano: Reflections on Higher Education in South Africa* (2018). Dedicated to building bridges across the health sciences, the arts and the humanities, Susan is a lead educator on a Massive Open Online Course (MOOC) entitled 'Medicine and the Arts.'

Lorelei Lingard is Professor, Department of Medicine, and Director, Centre for Education Research and Innovation, Schulich School of Medicine and Dentistry, Western University, Ontario, Canada. Her collaborative research programme describes healthcare team communication patterns and explores their influence on healthcare training, team competence and patient safety. Trained as a rhetorician, Lorelei loves language: she is happiest writing at her kitchen table, and she can increasingly be found teaching others how to turn their scientific manuscripts into something people will want to read. Lorelei was 2018 recipient of the prestigious Karolinska Institutet Prize for Research in Medical Education.

Alphonso Lingis is Professor of Philosophy Emeritus at the Pennsylvania State University. Among his books published are *The Community of Those Who Have Nothing in Common*, *Abuses*, *The Imperative*, *Dangerous Emotions*, *Trust*, *The First Person Singular*, *Contact*, *Violence and Splendor*, *Irrevocable* and *The Alphonso Lingis Reader*. He is a seminal figure in contemporary phenomenological thinking and a riveting public speaker.

Paul Macneill has taught ethics, law and professionalism for many years, in the medical schools of the University of New South Wales, the University of Singapore and the University of Sydney. He is an Honorary Associate Professor in Sydney Health Ethics, University of Sydney, and the Co-ordinator of the Arts Bioethics Network within the International Association of Bioethics. He serves as a member of disciplinary committees and tribunals for the medical, and other health professional, Councils within New South Wales. Paul's publications include *Ethics and the Arts* (2014); 'Balancing bioethics by sensing the aesthetic' (*Bioethics*, 2017); 'The arts and medicine: a challenging relationship' (*Medical Humanities*, 2011); and 'Art and bioethics: shifts in understanding across genres' (*Journal of Bioethical Inquiry*, 2011). He has presented many keynote addresses on bioethics and the arts at international bioethics conferences: most recently at the World Congress of Bioethics in Edinburgh (2016). He is currently working on two books (provisionally) titled: *Philosophy and Ethics: East and West* and *The Over-Valued Idea* (a critique of ethics and post-'Enlightenment' rationality).

Robert Marshall has been a consultant pathologist at the Royal Cornwall Hospital, Truro, Cornwall, UK for 32 years, where he initiated in-service medical humanities as head of postgraduate education, also developing an in-house journal *The Remedy*, and appointing an arts co-ordinator for the hospital. He is a senior clinical lecturer at the University of Exeter Medical School, where he was involved in the design of the medical humanities aspects of the curriculum at the planning and launch of Peninsula Medical School in 2002. He continues to contribute to this curriculum. His research and publications in medical humanities have been on the relevance of Homer's *Iliad* and *Odyssey* to medical education, culminating in (with Alan Bleakley) the book *Rejuvenating Medical Education: Seeking Help from Homer* (2017). He has also developed an international portfolio, and started a project linking the University of Exeter Medical School with one in Nekemte, Ethiopia, which has developed into a charity—Medical Education, Sanitation and Health in Ethiopia (MESHE).

Maria Athina (Tina) Martimianakis is Associate Professor and Director of Medical Education Scholarship in the Department of Paediatrics, and Scientist and Associate Director International and Partnerships at the Wilson Centre, University of Toronto. Dr Martimianakis studies the material effects of discourse and is currently researching how organisational practices associated with discourses of collaboration support or hinder the capacity of interprofessional teams to practise and learn together. Her previous work has explored the relationships between discourses of the hidden curriculum and humanism, the politics and effects of knowledge stratification in pain clinics and the discourse of globalisation and its relationship to medical competency.

Cara Martin was born and raised in Toronto, Canada. She earned a biomechanical engineering degree from Queen's University in Kingston, Canada before shifting her focus to medicine. She will soon graduate from the University of Exeter Medical School and she hopes to pursue a career in emergency medicine. She lives in the southwest of England. Her interest in writing began early in her adolescence. She will continue to dabble with her writing in between her shifts after she joins the ranks of the junior doctors.

Gwinyai Masukume is a medical doctor and public health researcher with expertise in Epidemiology and Biostatistics. His main contribution has been in the area of Women's Health, including topics such as anaemia during pregnancy, male-to-female birth ratios, caesarean section and cervical cancer. He is an expert on food-related medical terms, a subject he blogs about for the Annals of Improbable Research, the organisation that awards the annual Ig Nobel Prize at Sanders Theatre, Harvard University. He is the Assistant Editor of the *WikiJournal of Medicine*.

Stewart Mennin is a Consulting Associate of the Human Systems Dynamics Institute; Adjunct Professor, Department of Medicine, The Uniformed Services University for the Health Sciences; Professor Emeritus, Department of Cell Biology and Physiology; and former Assistant Dean for Educational Development and Research, the University of New Mexico School of Medicine. Stewart was co-director of the University of New Mexico School of Medicine's innovative community-oriented, problem-based Primary Care Curriculum and Director of the Office of Program Evaluation, Education and Research and the Office of Teacher and Educational Development. He has published widely, and served as an invited consultant and teacher at more than 100 medical schools and health institutions worldwide. He wrote and developed the 'Essential Skills in Medical Education' and 'Leadership in Medical Education' courses for the International Association for Medical Education in Europe (AMEE). In 2017, Dr Mennin was given the AMEE Lifetime Achievement Award in Medical Education.

Marie Rose Moro is a Professor of Psychiatry at the Université Paris Descartes and the Director of the Maison des Adolescents (Maison de Solenn) at the Cochin Hospital. She is also the scientific director of the journal *L'autre*. Professor Moro is one of the pioneers in French ethnopsychiatry and continues to enjoy an international reputation in the field. She engages in pioneering therapeutic work with immigrant and displaced families based on principles of transcultural psychiatry, particularly the transgenerational transmission of trauma from mother to child.

Thirusha Naidu is a Lecturer in the Department of Behavioural Medicine at the Nelson R. Mandela School of Medicine at the University of KwaZulu-Natal, and head of clinical psychology at King Dinuzulu Hospital, South Africa. Thirusha's research interests include ethics in research; community, social and cultural psychology; as well as psychotherapy models, methods and training. Her PhD degree from the University of KwaZulu-Natal focused on identity, culture and context with home-based care volunteers in rural South Africa. She has published papers in the areas of health communication and critical reflective practice in clinical encounters and contexts. Thirusha is a passionate advocate for alternative methods and art forms such as poetry for presenting and understanding research data and findings.

Mary Nations is a Consulting Associate of the Human Systems Dynamics (HSD) Institute. She has taught, consulted and coached in different capacities over the last 12 years, and has co-authored many works in the HSD field. Mary helps organisations and the people in them to become more adaptable and effective in changing environments. HSD is foundational to her work in applications across sectors for a variety of organisations. Her current interests are: exploring resilience essential for health, wellbeing and opportunity in our networked, interconnected lives; and helping individuals and groups to develop the capacity to adapt in the midst of tension caused by differences, to create worthy options and possibilities for going forward together.

Crispian Neill is a Wellcome Trust Institutional Strategic Support Fund Early Career Researcher at the University of Leeds. His current research project examines the historical and current significance of olfaction among clinicians and medical students. His doctoral thesis investigated the representation of olfaction in modernist literature and aesthetics, and is currently undergoing revision prior to publication as a monograph.

Shane Neilson is a poet, critic, memoirist and physician. He was born in New Brunswick, Canada and much of his writing reflects this origin. At present he works as a family physician and is completing his PhD in English and Cultural Studies at McMaster University, Hamilton, ON, where he researches the representations of pain in Canadian literature. Shane is editor of Frog Hollow Press based out of Victoria, BC and is self-appointed 'Manifestoist Editor' at Anstruther Press of Toronto, ON. The author of several books, most recently he published *Dysphoria*, a book of poems about how mental illness is regulated. This book has just been shortlisted for a Hamilton Literary Award. In 2016 he edited *Heart on Fist*, a selected prose volume, and *Witch of the Inner Wood*, a collection of long poems by Travis Lane. In 2017 Shane won the sixth annual Walrus Poetry Prize, juried by Margaret Atwood. In 2019 he will publish *Constructive Negativity*, the first book of literary criticism on Canadian disability poetics.

Hesam Noroozi MD MPH is a physician with interests in medicine, humanity and visual art. He has worked as a physician for more than 10 years in emergency departments and other clinical settings. He regularly writes as a medical humanities columnist in a professional medical journal. As a visual artist, he has participated in many group art exhibitions and been nominated as the best cartoonist several times. Currently, he is working as a medical researcher and clinical advisor in Toronto, Canada.

Martin O'Brien is a performance artist and academic (Lecturer at Queen Mary University, London) whose work considers existence with severe chronic illness within our contemporary situation. Martin suffers from cystic fibrosis and his practice uses physical endurance, hardship and pain-based practices to challenge common representations of illness and examine what it means to be born with a life-threatening disease. Martin's work is an act of resistance to dominant notions of 'illness,' and a claim to embodied agency. He has gained a series of prestigious funding and regularly performs endurance pieces, most recently concerned with the twilight world of the zombie as Martin's 'due death date' as a CF sufferer has passed!

John Ødemark is an Associate Professor of Cultural History at the University of Oslo. He specialises in cultural translation and the history of human sciences. He is Co-Principal Investigator of a research group on medical humanities and knowledge translation at the Centre for Advanced Study at the Norwegian Academy of Science and Letters.

Seamus O'Mahony is Professor and a Consultant Gastroenterologist at Cork University Hospital. He has published extensively in the fields of endoscopy, inflammatory bowel disease and coeliac disease. For the past several years, his main academic interest has been the medical humanities. He was Associate Editor for Medical Humanities at the *Journal of the Royal College of Physicians of Edinburgh* from 2014–2017. He is a regular contributor to the *Dublin Review of Books*. His book *The Way We Die Now* was published in London in 2016 and in New York in 2017. The book won the prestigious Council Chair's Choice Award at the British Medical Association's annual book awards in 2017. His new book *Can Medicine Be Cured?* was published in February 2019.

Bahar Orang is a Resident at the University of Toronto. She holds an MA in Comparative Literature, and her first book of prose/poetry is forthcoming in spring 2020.

Gil Pena is a pathologist dedicated to surgical pathology/immunohistochemistry with an interest in the study of diagnostic processes and the epistemological and educational aspects of pathology. He is presently Professor of Anatomic Pathology, Centro Universitário de Belo Horizonte—Uni-BH, and a pathologist at Instituto Roberto Alvarenga, Belo Horizonte, MG, Brazil.

Allan Peterkin MD is a Professor in the Departments of Psychiatry and Family and Community Medicine at the University of Toronto where he heads the Programme in Health, Arts and Humanities, and serves as Humanities Faculty Lead for Undergraduate Medical Education and Post-MD Studies. He is the author/co-author of 14 books on cultural studies, human sexuality, narrative medicine, physician health and the health humanities. Titles include: *Portfolio to Go: 1000 Writing Prompts and Provocations for Clinical Learners*, *Staying Human During the Foundation Programme* (with Alan Bleakley) and *Keeping Reflection Fresh: A Practical Guide For Clinical Educators* (co-editor with Pamela Brett-Maclean). Allan has an international reputation in health humanities and has been instrumental in developing a health humanities culture in both undergraduate and postgraduate medical education in Canada, and in setting up the annual Creating Space conference and associated Canadian Association for Health Humanities. See www.health-humanities.com.

Nicole M. Piemonte PhD is the Assistant Dean for Medical Education, and an Assistant Professor, in the Department of Medical Education at Creighton University School of Medicine in Phoenix, Arizona, where she teaches and supports medical students, residents and clinical faculty. She received her PhD in Medical Humanities from the University of Texas Medical Branch where she studied continental philosophy, medical ethics, literature and medicine and medical pedagogy. She recently published a book, *Afflicted: How Vulnerability Can Heal Medical Education and Practice*, in 2018 and is currently contracted to write a second book on death and dying in the American hospital.

Radha Ramaswamy has a PhD in theatre research and received training in Theatre of the Oppressed at the Seattle-based Mandala Center for Change. In March 2011, she founded the Centre for Community Dialogue and Change (CCDC), dedicated to promoting the use of this unique methodology for teaching and learning among communities in India. Radha has pioneered the use of Forum Theatre with senior citizens, in medical humanities and in mental health. Radha has been invited to present papers and conduct workshops at national and international conferences on education and teacher training.

Ravi Ramaswamy received training in Theatre of the Oppressed in 2010, and has since been leading workshops in schools and colleges across cities in India. He is a trustee at the Centre for Community Dialogue and Change, Bangalore, a globally recognised centre for trainings in Theatre of the Oppressed. Ravi has been facilitating Theatre of the Oppressed workshops for faculty and students of several of the premier government and private medical colleges in India. Ravi brings to his theatre practice a strong commitment to social justice and human rights issues.

Steve Reid is a family physician with extensive experience in clinical practice, education and research in the field of rural health in South Africa. After 10 years in rural district hospital practice in northern KwaZulu-Natal, he directed the Centre for Health and Social Studies at the University of KwaZulu-Natal, and in 2010 he took up the Chair of Primary Health Care at the University of Cape Town. He is developing this role to support medical and health science graduates to become more relevant and appropriately skilled in Africa. He is also involved in integrating the arts and social sciences with health sciences by promoting the development of critical health and medical humanities in the African context.

William J. Robertson is a PhD candidate in Medical Anthropology with a minor in Gender and Women's Studies at the University of Arizona. His research involves questions concerning how biomedical knowledge and practice are co-constitutive with sex/gender and sexuality. His dissertation research uses HPV-related anal disease as a lens through which to examine the interplay of biomedical practices—especially technologies related to screening and treatment— and sex/gender and sexuality. His work seeks to illuminate the cultural assumptions at work in the enactment of a sexually transmitted infection that has been highly gendered in public health campaigns and medical interventions alike.

Judy Z. Segal is Professor in the Department of English Language and Literatures and in the Science and Technology Studies Graduate Program at the University of British Columbia. Her primary teaching and research are on the rhetorical elements in discourses of health and medicine. She is the author of many essays and of the monograph *Health and the Rhetoric of Medicine* (2005). Her work appears in rhetoric journals, health humanities journals, science study journals, medical journals and various essay collections. She was a founding member of the President's Advisory Committee of the Canadian Institutes of Health Research, and has been a Distinguished Scholar at the Peter Wall Institute for Advanced Studies and recipient of the Killam Teaching Prize.

Katherine Shwetz is a PhD candidate at the University of Toronto, and researches representations of contagious disease in Canadian literature. Her dissertation is at the intersection of literary criticism and the health humanities, and considers how narratives of contagion draw together a range of anxieties about embodiment, community and borders.

Delese Wear PhD is Professor of Family and Community Medicine at Northeast Ohio Medical University. She is a key figure internationally in the medical/health humanities. Delese is the author (with Lois LaCivita Nixon) of *Literary Anatomies: Women's Bodies and Health in Literature* (1994) and *Privilege in the Medical Academy: A Feminist Examines Gender, Race, and Power* (1997), and the editor of *Women in Medical Education: An Anthology of Experience* (1996) and (with Janet Bickel) *Educating for Professionalism: Creating a Climate of Humanism in Medical Education* (2001). In addition, she is an associate editor of the collection *On Doctoring*, a literary anthology distributed each year to every medical student in the United States. She was editor of the *Journal of Medical Humanities* from 1997 to 2004.

Caroline Wellbery is Professor of Family Medicine at Georgetown University School of Medicine, and Associate Deputy Editor of *American Family Physician*. Her longstanding interest in medical humanities began with her graduate studies in Comparative Literature at Stanford University. Her humanities work is represented on the website 'Interacting with the Arts in Medicine' (mdarts.georgetown.edu). She has published on art observation, medical uncertainty and cognitive biases, the health effects of climate change and human interest topics in national and international journals, including *Academic Medicine*, *BMJ*, *The Lancet*, *JAMA*, the *New England Journal of Medicine* and *American Family Physician*.

Leonard White is a neuroscientist and educator at Duke University where he serves across the university teaching brain science and administering educational programmes. Dr White's research interests encompass the evolution and development of functional neural circuits in the cerebral cortex and the impact of sensory experience and neurological disease on brain structure and function. He is co-author and co-editor of a leading textbook on neuroscience and a digital atlas of the human brain and spinal cord; he also teaches 'Medical Neuroscience,' a free online course taken by people worldwide.

Cynthia R. Whitehead is Director and Scientist at the Wilson Centre Faculty of Medicine, University of Toronto at University Health Network, and has been appointed as BMO Financial Group Chair in Health Professions Research at University Health Network for a five-year term from January 2016. She is also an Associate Professor in the Department of Family and Community Medicine at the University of Toronto, and the Vice-President of Education, Women's College Hospital. She has, historically, held many education leadership positions in medical education at the University of Toronto. Dr Whitehead obtained her PhD from the University of Toronto and MD from McMaster University. Her programme of research as a Wilson Centre Scientist focuses on deconstructing 'truths' of health professions education to expand our understandings of possibilities for change. Some of Dr Whitehead's specific content areas of research interest include globalisation of medical education, outcomes-based education, interprofessional education and the history of medical education. Dr Whitehead has been involved in teaching, curriculum design, curriculum evaluation and educational administration. Internationally, she has provided education consultations and worked collaboratively with educators in multiple countries in Africa, Asia, South America, North America and Europe.

Suzy Willson is the co-founder and Artistic Director of theatre company 'Clod Ensemble' and creator of their 'Performing Medicine' programme. She is Honorary Professor at Barts and the London School of Medicine and Dentistry at Queen Mary University. Suzy has been pioneering the use of arts in healthcare education for over 20 years, working with a range of medical schools, higher education institutions and NHS Trusts, as well as curating public events about health and medicine with leading cultural venues across the UK. Suzy is a regular contributor to journals and books on both performance and medicine—with articles in *The Guardian*, *The Lancet*, *Performance Research* and edited collections, and appearances on radio and TV. With Clod

Ensemble she has directed over 20 productions—several of them drawing on medical themes including *An Anatomie in Four Quarters* and *Under Glass* (both commissioned by Sadler's Wells), and *Placebo*.

Michael Wilson is Professor of Drama and Dean in the School of Arts, English and Drama at Loughborough University, UK. His main research interests lie broadly within the field of popular and vernacular performance and over the past 10 years he has led numerous projects that explore the application of storytelling to a variety of social and policy contexts, especially around environmental policy, health, education and social justice. He has been a member of the Advisory Boards for the Digital Economy Programme (Research Councils UK, led by the Engineering and Physical Sciences Research Council), Connected Communities (AHRC) and Digital Transformations (AHRC). He is also Chair of the Arts and Humanities Panel for the British Council's Newton Fund programme.

Anita Wohlmann is Assistant Professor of Literature and Narrative Medicine at the University of Southern Denmark, Odense. She is also the project leader of 'Body and Metaphor: Narrative-Based Metaphor Analysis in Medical Humanities,' funded by the German Research Foundation (2017–2020). Her academic background is in American literature and film studies, and her research focuses on metaphors, age and ageing, narrative medicine, gender, illness, disability and seriality.

Jefferson Wong is an advocate of patients' basic rights. He believes that all patients should not only be treated with kindness, care and compassion, but also with respect, dignity, empathy and equity. His exposures to the healthcare systems and medical practices in Hong Kong and England have given him insight into the vulnerability of patients and the potential dehumanising nature of medicine. He aspires to make changes in the way medicine is practised in Hong Kong, especially by revolutionising and eliminating such dehumanising processes when he practises medicine there in the future.

Kristin Zeiler is Professor at the Department of Thematic Studies: Technology and Social Change, Linköping University, Sweden. Her research examines the philosophical, ethical and sociocultural aspects of medical practices, often from phenomenological, hermeneutical or combined empirical and philosophical perspectives. She is currently leading a research programme on the existential, ethical and sociomaterial aspects of medical screening (VR 2017–2023). Previous work of hers has examined death definition pluralism, norms about bodies and their implications for healthcare practices, bodily donation and surrogate motherhood as practices of bodily sharing, intercorporeal personhood in dementia care and bodily relational autonomy, as some examples.

INTRODUCTION

The medical humanities: a mixed weather front on a global scale

Alan Bleakley

The humanities are implicit in medicine, where democracy must be built

In *Democracy in America* Alexis de Tocqueville (1835–40; 2003) links the development of democracy with that of the humanities, where "Poetry, eloquence, memory, the beauty of wit, the fires of imagination, the depths of thought (are) . . . turned to the advantage of democracy." The arts and humanities can flourish under autocracies and theocracies, but their purpose in such political contexts is to celebrate ideologues, and not to act as media for resistance or critique. There is no better account of such resistance that I know than Peter Weiss' (2005) novel *The Aesthetics of Resistance*. A group of young socialists growing up in pre-WWII Nazi Germany are part of the underground resistance movement. They meet in galleries and museums to study art, honing their humanitarian beliefs through discussions about relationships between aesthetics and the politics of resistance. Weiss shows how art can be sterile until mobilised as a form of social resistance embodying justice, equality and tolerance of difference. This offers an important critique of medical humanities 'lite'—oriented to mere diversion or embellishment, as supplement or complement to medical studies. Such a version of medical humanities serves to reinforce a tradition of hierarchy and oppression in medical culture that educates for insensibility (as denial of aesthetics) and insensitivity (as denial of politics), rather than serving to challenge and change that tradition for the better. Weiss seeks a deeper and more challenging seam for art's purposes—also one that is ultimately more nourishing.

Despite the public face of healthcare as collaborative, team-based and patient-centred, medicine, stained by its history, retains undemocratic and paternalistic authority structures as the norm, reproduced through both undergraduate and postgraduate education (Crowe, Clarke and Brugha 2017). The major challenge for medical culture now is surely the slow movement to authentic democracy, where, for example, longstanding evidence from organisational psychology studies shows that improving democratic relationships in healthcare teams leads to improvements in patient health outcomes, patient safety and practitioner work satisfaction (Borrill undated). The art of medicine and the humanity of democracy are one and the same, but this identification has been frustrated by medical education's commitment to functional approaches embodied particularly in learning professional communication through simulation, and in reducing complex clinical learning to menus of instrumental competencies.

1

Medicine and the humanities are inevitably yoked where the maturation of medicine must shadow the maturation of democracy (necessarily a work in progress, or a 'democracy to come'). This involves making tolerance of ambiguity a primary and explicit aim of medical education. A medicine that has not matured either politically or aesthetically (the primary values arenas for the medical humanities) is trapped in what Immanuel Kant (1784) described as a "self-imposed immaturity." In his seminal 1784 essay 'Answering the Question: What Is Enlightenment?' Kant argues that an enlightened, humane culture must show critical, reflective thinking in the presence of repressive ideology and unjustified opinion.

'Humanists' had to be created. The rise of humanism, civility and sensibility in Europe after the Renaissance was not a straightforward public awakening to the virtues of the arts and humanities such as literature and history (Barker-Benfield 1992). As Marilynne Robinson (2017) notes: "To put books into English, the vulgar tongue, the language of the masses, was once radical." Forgetting that once all doctors would be educated in the Classics, modern languages and science, contemporary medical education has now spent the better part of half a century wringing its hands over whether or not medical students should explore literature as they listen to patients' stories; or visual art as they learn anatomy or look at MRI images; or drama and performance as they attempt to simultaneously impress their seniors and engage with patients on a ward round; or music as they learn to percuss a patient's body; or iambic pentameter as they listen to a heartbeat; or song as they recite the standard 'case.' Further, how will medical students make sense of the conundrum that they are simultaneously educated for both sensibility (such as close noticing in anatomy learning and clinical diagnosis) and insensibility (shutting down the 'natural' reactions of aversion and disgust to cadavers, pus, open wounds, vomit, and so forth)?

Strangely, it seems hard for medicine to admit that science is not only political (knowledge is power), but also intrinsically aesthetic, where a good rule of thumb is that appreciation precedes explanation: the body is sculptural; chemical formulae are elegant; a pathological specimen may be painterly; and so forth. The aesthetic is inherently challenging as it approaches the sublime, and medical students learn to tolerate the ambiguity that pathology may be for them at once fascinating and repulsive, while for their patients entails suffering. The humanities then are integral to medicine and there is no need to imagine that we must tack them on as added extras. 'Dig where you stand' may be a good piece of advice for medical students who ask: 'where will I find a use for the medical humanities?' Perhaps the hardest challenge for medical humanities in moving beyond the mild—even milksop—status of 'soft supplement' to medical studies is to realise *through medical pedagogy* that the aesthetic (*what* and *how* we appreciate and value, and how we educate for sensibility) is deeply tied to the political. The aesthetic, like the political, is capital unevenly distributed in medical culture and poorly re-distributed through medical pedagogies. The aesthetic and political are necessarily intertwined and inter-dependent, where the labour of sensing (fundamental to doctoring) has been commodified and is subject to inequalities of distribution. Meanwhile, the worthless capital of insensibility is freely distributed amongst medical neophytes. While 'the medical humanities' is an inadequate collective term for a disparate set of approaches, for the moment let us imagine that 'the medical humanities' provide the primary media through which inequalities of distribution of aesthetic capital in medical education can be articulated and addressed.

Those privileged doctors from the past, mentioned above, who had 'rounded' educations, did not necessarily subscribe to democratic structures (especially in medicine), or to social justice principles or dissenting activism (see Chapters 5 and 6); and their 'arts' and 'humanities' were almost certainly 'high' and not 'popular.' These days, we would like medical students to be able to empathise with their patients through an understanding that much of the lay knowledge patients have about their medical conditions is gained through the Internet and television medical soap operas with follow-up advice lines (see Chapter 21). Medical students are more likely to play in an indie rock band than a string quartet, and enjoy slam poetry more than reading Coleridge. They should know the language of popular culture to better treat the wide mix of the populace. Which brings us back to social justice, and the relationships between politics, ethics and aesthetics that characterise the 'medical humanities' and/or 'health humanities' (see Chapter 39).

Professional expertise such as stitching a wound, knowing how the immune system works, prescribing a drug or breaking bad news is sterile until applied in an actual clinical encounter to another's flesh, blood, mind and personality that in turn are products of their cultural circumstances. We do not need to conjure a magical humanities potion to enliven a moribund, or fix a misguided, medicine. Rather, we need to articulate how medicine, healthcare and the arts and humanities are co-implied, and then extend translations such that they generate benefit for doctors, healthcare professionals, patients and communities alike (see Chapters 2, 3 and 22) on a global scale.

As I write this, I realise that although this text promises a 'global' input, it is far from inclusive—even constrained by a form of imperialism—as it reflects a cosmopolitan Western outlook (clear exceptions are Chapters 23, 28, 34 and 35). For example, where Rabie E. Abdel-Halim and Khaled M. AlKattan (2012) describe the first forays into the medical humanities in a medical school in Saudi Arabia, this is centred on restoring Islamic spiritual elements to a positivist and materialist medicine. The introduction of the medical humanities here marks a withdrawal from an imperialism of secular Western medicine. Ian Fussell and Robert Marshall (Chapter 35) echo these concerns in their ethically sensitive accounts of initiating a medical humanities programme in a medical school in Ethiopia, twinned with a UK school. They tread softly on Ethiopian soil, but are nevertheless disturbed by both local political unrest on the one hand, and an unsettling example of how the local medical students view gender ethics on the other. In the latter scenario, a dramatised rape scene engenders laughter on the part of the local medical school and University community, where visiting medical students and tutors from the UK are surprised, even horrified, at this response.

Steve Reid and Susan Levine, from South Africa (Chapter 34), make the claim that:

> Medical humanities in the 'global north' appear to be largely text-based and disembodied, embedded in ethics, history, philosophy and English literature. By contrast, the 'global south' expression of medical humanities could be seen as more interdisciplinary and embodied, rooted in the arts such as oral narrative, song, dance and movement rather than exclusively in text.

While they provide no evidence for this claim, it is thought provoking, and offers quite a different way of conceiving development in medical humanities than the debate surrounding separation of academic, University department-based studies of medical culture from studies grounded in the clinical encounter and applied to medical education (Bleakley 2015; Whitehead and Woods 2016). How clumsy this all feels! Yet it matters—especially for funding of research. In the UK certainly, while medical humanities research funding is generally thin on the ground, it is easier to obtain through University-based humanities departments than through medical schools.

Bone-tired, on skeletal resourcing, but muscling through—can the medical humanities help?

In a recent *New York Times* article, Lisa Pryor (2017), an Australian junior doctor, discusses work stress and high suicide prevalence amongst fellow doctors. This is a global phenomenon (Alosaimi et al. 2018). She notes that studying medicine involves an almost inhuman commitment, where medical students and doctors are aware that they are entering a hugely demanding profession that will consume their lives. Paradoxically, medical culture itself does little to alleviate such stress, for example in providing appropriate workforce conditions (including adequate remuneration for the most junior doctors) or psychological support for novices (Peterkin and Bleakley 2017). Historically, medical culture has cultivated a quasi-militaristic devotion to perfectionism and personality 'grit' that can be read as dysfunctional (Marshall and Bleakley 2017). 'Grit,' widely in use for some time as a metaphor outside of medicine and healthcare (John Wayne's *True Grit* dates from 1969), is—at the time of writing—flourishing in medicine, although it promises, like many metaphors, to become overused, tired or indeed exhausted of life.

Metaphor is unavoidable and pervasive in medical language and praxis (Bleakley 2017), despite Susan Sontag's (1978) famous plea for the abolition of metaphors that stigmatise patients—in any case an impossibility, for we cannot cleanse medicine of metaphor. But we can change the metaphors that shape medical thinking and practice for the better, as Chapters 12–17 show; particularly highlighting the artful use of metaphor and rhetoric, as Anita Wohlmann shows in her celebration of medicine's aesthetic (Chapter 12), and Judy Z. Segal (Chapter 15) in her wry account of ageism. A good metaphor for this book is that medical humanities afford the grit that makes the pearl of 'deep' clinical practice—innovative, rounded, considerate, humble and, above all, reflexive or self-critically knowing. Alan Bleakley's chapter (11) shows how medicine's historical legacy of hubris has kept such 'tender' sentiments at arm's length.

Rachel Clarke's (2017) auto-ethnography of working in England's National Health Service (NHS) as a junior doctor mirrors Lisa Pryor's account, noting how certain ingrained structural constraints within medicine, such as masculine-based (heroic), hierarchical structures; poor preparation for the transition from medical student to doctor; the absorption of medicine into party political ideology; and the expectations of exhausting hospital shifts without adequate human and technical resources, again point to self-generated symptoms in medical culture that compromise patient care and safety. Medicine shoots itself in the foot, or self-harms, and needs to go on the couch for therapy and subsequent intervention. It is bad enough that medicine has to bear the burden of structural pressures—such as lack of resources, fear of litigation, over-determined management and ideologically motivated interference from politicians—without adding the extra burden of a self-imposed set of symptoms that hinder work. An example of this is doctors (properly) complaining of being bone-tired through overwork at the same time as medicine has, historically, celebrated punishing work schedules where, again, you must develop heroic 'grit,' or 'resilience,' in the face of adversity ('if you can't stand the heat, get out of the kitchen') (Marshall and Bleakley 2017). The medical humanities can articulate such historical habits, sharply interrogate them and offer practical alternatives.

Lisa Pryor's account suggests that stress levels could be reduced if medicine and medical education encouraged doctors' self-care and provided better networks of professional support (see Chapters 40 and 41); structural factors such as under-resourcing within health services were addressed; and socialisation into medicine did not seek to produce high-achieving individuals who beat themselves up if there is any sign of weakness or failure, in Pryor's (2017) words: "The unrelenting, unforgiving culture of medicine that weighs its junior members down with debt and duty." In summary, Pryor (ibid.) suggests that:

> We need to let go of our shiny doctor selves and accept the vulnerability, doubt and imperfection within, rather than try to obliterate it. We need to find kindness for ourselves, our medical and nursing colleagues, and our patients because sometimes that is the only thing that makes this path bearable. We need a medical culture that sees humanity as a precondition for being a good doctor, not an obstacle.

Rachel Clarke's (2017) account above echoes this. These contemporary pleas both imply a need for injecting what is in effect a 'lost' humanity into medicine, reinforcing the traditional rationale for the medical humanities—that they primarily educate for empathy in the face of evidence that medical students show increasing empathy decline and cynicism from Year 3 onwards (Neumann et al. 2011). But such an equation is not straightforward—first, 'empathy' itself is a modern term concealing as much as it reveals (Marshall and Bleakley 2017), a notion both critically and imaginatively explored by the visual artist David Cotterrell (Chapter 18). Second, there is debate around a distinction between 'cognitive empathy' (understanding somebody else's position) and 'affective empathy' (feeling for somebody else) (Smith, Norman and Decety 2017), and which kind medicine needs. And third, that arts and humanities automatically and transparently educate for either kind of empathy is problematic—what kind of empathy, for example, is generated by early 20th-century Italian Fascist artists and writers such as Marinetti and other 'Futurists,' who show contempt for the 'weak'? Caroline Wellbery engages deeply with the troubling term 'empathy' in Chapter 37, suggesting that we must shift from locating empathy 'in' individuals to seeing empathy as a socially generated phenomenon; while Claire Hooker and James Dalton echo this in Chapter 19 in the context of medical students' 'impression management.' 'Empathy' can be an overbearing form of governance rather than a natural human concern. Indeed, I have argued with colleagues (Petersen et al. 2008) that, handled insensitively, the 'medical humanities' in medical education can also act as a potentially repressive form of governance through the imperative to 'be humane!,' problematising the naïve view that the 'medical humanities' are automatically liberating (from the chains of reductive science or the deadening effects of an instrumental clinical practice).

Hard-nosed biomedical scientists and sceptical clinicians continue to demand evidence that the medical humanities have a positive effect on clinical practice beyond a 'feelgood' factor (Kumagai 2018). A recent large-scale North American study shows that active interest and involvement in the arts and humanities on the part of medical students does indeed correlate with increased empathy, tolerance for ambiguity, emotional intelligence, self-efficacy and prevention of burnout, suggesting that concern and active care for patients goes hand in hand with active self-concern and care (Mangione et al. 2018). More, those students who show most interest and involvement in the arts and humanities are also more spatially aware—a key attribute for diagnosis and many hands-on clinical skills. Mangione and colleagues' artfully designed study suggests that incorporation of medical humanities into the undergraduate medicine curriculum is a necessity and not just a luxury.

The medical humanities grew out of bioethics, and this flame continues to burn brightly, where medical education addresses values shaping practices (see Chapter 33). There has been a turn in interest from the context-based ethics of specific patient care to 'professionalism.' What is it to be a *concerned* and *politicised* medical student and doctor embracing issues of social justice, as explored by Arno Kumagai and Thirusha Naidu in Chapter 6? For example, affirmative action should be expected from doctors to counter social injustice, while doctors can also become surrogate family members, for example in supporting patients with dementia (see Chapter 29). Such professionals take pride in thinking through the consequences of their actions. This offers a new ground for identity construction of the doctor as 'medical citizen' (Bleakley, Bligh and Browne 2011), aware that reducing historical, cultural and social determinants of health to the biochemical or the neurological offers a potentially fatal misreading of symptom presentation (see Kathryn E. Goldfarb's Chapter 28). Such reductionism is not simply an 'alternative fact' but a rhetorical gesture (Chapters 11–18 and 28 in particular address such rhetorical moves).

Breaking down traditional hierarchies in the democratising of healthcare is a major part of the social justice agenda in healthcare education. As well as empowering patients, doctors need creative spaces in which they can express their vulnerabilities and humanity, and where the 'professional' persona can be temporarily suspended and treated as a symptom, rather than encouraged as part of the armoury of impression management (McGaghie 2018) (see Chapter 40 where doctors are empowered by 'medicine watchers' or medical education researchers). The safe, creative space for reflection is also a critical space, where doctors can gain distance from the common rhetorical activities of their own profession. This is what supervision is supposed to do, where supervision in psychiatry or psychotherapy is considered to be an essential aspect of continuing education. But why is this not universal for doctors? A recent North American survey showed that the highest self-reported burnout rate (60%) is amongst Emergency medicine doctors, with the lowest in Psychiatry (40%) (Parks 2017).

Paul Crawford and Brian Brown (Chapter 39) remind us that health humanities must not fall foul of self-interest in attending to the needs of only doctors and healthcare professionals. We must also look beyond patients to engage with the normally silent (or 'silenced'?) voices of carers. The medical humanities do, of course, have a long history of public engagement (Chapter 22), and this includes representations of medicine as 'edutainment,' such as TV medi-soaps (Chapter 21).

Networks, border crossings, translations

A new, critical, wave of scholars has misgivings with the idealistic tone that informs the work of medical humanities as a 'humanising' medium—a common, albeit simplistic, reading. Despite the turn to social justice issues such as equality and equity, critics ask 'what "humanising" are we talking about, and in whose image?' For example, is 'humanising' gendered? Further, if we are to mobilise the arts and humanities as 'humanising' media, we should remember that one of the key purposes of the arts and humanities is to create (often extreme) disquiet through subversion, inversion and diversion of mainstream or conventional taste (pundits in medical humanities scholarship and research appear to agree on one thing—that a key pedagogic outcome of medical humanities interest and intervention is 'tolerance of ambiguity'). Tess Jones and Delese Wear (Chapter 5) remind us that the arts and humanities applied to healthcare education and practice demand the involvement of artists and humanities scholars as experts, and we must not accept that hobbyists (such as interested clinicians) can provide such expertise.

The arts can disrupt pieties and offer provocations such as seeing value in symptoms and celebrating risk over regulation, as explored by Martin O'Brien and Gianna Bouchard (Chapter 24), Stella Bolaki (Chapter 20) and Alphonso Lingis (Chapter 27) in particular. Here, work of 'humanising' is problematic. Martin O'Brien and Gianna Bouchard ask what we can learn from a post-human, traumatised culture of the walking dead, a zombie culture of, for example, those with terminal illnesses who are still young, advertising premature death sentences, and going against the grain of standard ideals of 'health' and 'wellbeing' promoted by medicine and healthcare. Martin himself has cystic fibrosis. He has decided that the only authentic way to live his illness is to perform it, as deeply and fully as possible. This ironic celebration embraces homoeroticism and pain. In what sense might pain be a 'humanising' medium? See also Marijke Boucherie's (Chapter 38) sensitive account of how family members may collectively perform dynamic 'symptoms,' describing life with a son diagnosed as autistic whose difference should be celebrated and not negatively medicalised, as stigma.

Stella Bolaki (Chapter 20), writing about artists' books and representations of illness, notes a shift away from interest in conventional narrative forms in 'first wave' medical humanities towards disruptive, experimental forms in 'second wave' medical humanities. Such textual disruptions can be literary. Sara Wasson, at Lancaster University, UK, has archived alternative representations of chronic pain to conventional narrative telling, where episodic and intense pain experiences are captured in 'flash fiction' that evades conventional structures of plot and characterisation (http://wp.lancs.ac.uk/translatingpain). Such fictional forms are far more representative of how patients 'tell' their stories in consultations than conventional narratives—as episodic, jagged, disjointed, uneven and sometimes dissimulating.

Stella Bolaki's chapter opens an important new door of inquiry in the medical/ health humanities, where texts are embodied, or literally 'matter,' as 'artists' books.' These are constructions—stitched, glued, nailed, encased—where symptoms are transposed as embodied metaphor through cultural, material objects. Bolaki describes how makers of books may use their artefacts (demanding thinking otherwise about symptoms) as interlocutory media in consultations with doctors. The very act of sharing 'reading' of the artists' books shapes the consultation as 'close' and dialogical. A paradox emerges that the 'object' of the book provides the frame for resisting objectification of the patient as the book is treated as animated, acting as a beautiful illustrative example of the power of the 'object' in expanding an activity system, as explored by Yrjö Engeström's exposition of how activity theory can lead to a rich understanding of medical work in Chapter 3.

Quentin Eichbaum, Gil Pena, Leonard White and Gwinyai Masukume (Chapter 32) offer a clear demonstration of how—in activity theory terms—the 'object' of pathology (the patient's tissue) is 'performed' and re-materialised. Eichbaum and colleagues remind us that, paradoxically, the most 'objective' of medicine's scientific specialities—pathology—is an art. The medical humanities may, indeed, be most at home in the house of histopathology. But do medical students get to hear this?

Whatever medical work's gifts to humankind, and there are many, the medical humanities offer an important constructive critical foil. Medicine's historical hubris or inflation (Chapter 11), still vigorously cultivated in some quarters such as patriarchal surgical culture, disguises the reality of the crooked timber of medical practice, where contradictions abound. Five are listed below, each of which is critically addressed by current medical humanities research and practice. First, ambiguity, and not certainty, pervades medical work (a necessary symptom to carry, as Yrjö Engeström explores in Chapter 3, where 'ambiguity' is described as 'contradiction'). Claire Hooker and James Dalton (Chapter 19) remind us that living with ambiguity while suspending intolerance is to inhabit the subjunctive mode—"the 'what if' that opens the door to *poiesis*." This is a critical insight and provocation. Is the primary function of the medical humanities to shift language—thinking and imagination embodied in voice, performativity and activity—from the indicative to the subjunctive? The former mean and pinched, even if advertising clarity; the latter flourishing and promising.

Second, dissimulation is central not only to the *performance* of medicine (see again Chapter 19), but also to the education of patients through mass media representations of medicine, such as TV medi-soaps, that distort the realities of, for example, day-to-day emergency medicine, as Henry Curtis, an emergency doctor himself, explores in Chapter 21. Third, medicine has to 'grow up and get with it' as far as social awareness is concerned—ridding itself of blind spots about engaging with thorny issues of social justice, including explicit and tacit homophobia (see William J. Robertson's Chapter 8), to embrace 'responsibility' (see Tess Jones and Delese Wear's Chapter 5). Fourth, medical culture must develop psychological maturity in shifting from 'anality' (compulsive control) to 'genitality' or jouissance (authentic collaboration and celebration); or, a shift from fascination with hierarchy to embrace democratic habits exercised as collectivism (Chapter 3), as argued at the beginning of this Introduction. Fifth, and finally, doctors remain vulnerable psychologically but cannot find ways in their culture to properly admit or express such wounds (Chapter 40).

'Humanising' medical and broader healthcare interventions, however, may be a laudable aim in the face of an often patently dehumanising medicine including the objectification of patients (while medical culture, in turn, can be objectified and vilified, as Katherine Shwetz, in Chapter 17, shows through her close reading and exposure of the illogic of public anti-vaccination narratives embodied as online text). As Alan Bleakley notes in Chapter 11, the 'body as machine' has been one of medicine's primary objectifying and dehumanising metaphors since its introduction by Vesalius in the 16th century. Such dominant metaphors are not readily shrugged off even as they ossify or become 'dead' metaphors. Rather, they become dead weight, historical burdens. Ideals of 'humanising' are readily compromised by such a history of instrumentalism in medicine. For example, the transition from multi- to interdisciplinary teamwork is often modelled on linear, mechanical process as the fitting together of a jigsaw. But healthcare is not like this—it is often raw, ragged, undisciplined and unpredictable because it encompasses fluid meetings of a number of fuzzy, open, complex, adaptive systems (or the 'attractors' within such systems), as explored by Stewart Mennin, Glenda Eoyang and Mary Nations in Chapter 4. The move from appreciating and developing healthcare interventions as linear structures (treated as engineering problems to be fixed instrumentally) to complex, adaptive systems (where the key issue is translation across fluid systems) means that we must re-think descriptors such as 'inter-' to encompass the messy realities of actual clinical process. Medical education's—albeit slow—turn to systems theory draws on the leading edge of complexity *science* rather than the medical *humanities*, but it is precisely this kind of science, which celebrates uncertainty and fuzzy logic's 'degrees of truth,' that can also claim to be an art, avoiding neat solutions.

It is a scandal that medical education has for so long ignored social learning pedagogies such as Cultural-Historical Activity Theory (Chapter 3), grounded in principles of democratising learning, where the 'inter-' is the primary unit of analysis; and in complexity. The medical humanities are not limited to drawing just on arts and humanities, but also on radical pedagogies that are artful and cultured and that above all embrace politics of identity and resistance (Barone 2000; Pinar 2012). Such 'curriculum reconceptualisation' pedagogies are currently, and sadly, largely ignored in medical education circles, where quick fixes are preferred to complexity, unpredictable translations and boundary crossings between cultures such as medical and surgical specialties and entanglements. Radical shifts are needed in our medical-pedagogical thinking. For example, drawing on Caroline Wellbery's (Chapter 37) notion of empathy as a social phenomenon (not 'socially constructed,' but collaboratively enriched), we would stop 'teaching' empathy as a 'social skill' lodged in individuals. Rather, 'empathy' would be envisaged as one amongst many circulating objects in an expanding activity system (Chapter 3), or an actor doing the work of translation within an opportunistic network. Medical students would come to see 'empathy' not so much as something inside people to be cultivated, but as an emergent property of a dynamic, complex, adaptive system (Chapter 4); and as opportunistic (Chapter 18). Attention would shift from 'training' empathy to setting up the conditions of possibility for the expansion of an activity system or engagement with complex systems, the reflexive understanding of which is set out eloquently by Stewart Mennin, Glenda Eoyang and Mary Nations in Chapter 4. Make no mistake—these chapters provide powerful blueprints for a medical pedagogy revolution. But again, their implementation requires high tolerance for ambiguity or entanglement.

The descriptor 'entanglement' (Barad 2007) has been co-opted by a number of researchers and commentators in the 'critical' medical humanities as an alternative to the neat solution of 'integration' of factors perceived as oppositional pairs (Fitzgerald and Callard 2016). Julia Kristeva and colleagues (Chapter 2) prefer the term 'translational,' where entanglements are apprehended in terms of research findings sedimenting rapidly in embodied, collaborative living.

'Quantum entanglement' in physics describes pairs or groups of particles interacting in such a way that they are *implicated* in each other's being—that is, each particle cannot be described independently of its relationship to another particle. Isn't this another way of talking about the complex project we call 'democracy'? However we see it, democracy, as Jacques Derrida (2005) sets out most fully in *Rogues: Two Essays on Reason*, is an 'horizon' project, always a work in progress as "the democracy to come." Democracy is an art and not an end-game engineering problem. Democracy demands reflexive critical thinking of the kind initiated by the Frankfurt School (Theodor Adorno, Walter Benjamin, et al.) who worked in the face of the rise of Fascism during the interwar period and laid out principles for living where aesthetics and politics coincide (Weiss 2005). 'Entanglement' carries its own shadow—as a noun, it can mean a barrier, a form of stasis. A 'translational' medical humanities (Chapter 2) is entangled in the complexities of tolerance of difference and subscription to what Jacques Derrida called *différance* (deferral of meaning). Here, competing values, appreciative living and keeping 'closure' (as fixed opinions) at arm's length are valued, eschewing an instrumental approach where the medical humanities merely act as a salve. An *inquiring* medical humanities raises issues rather than solves problems, again illustrated beautifully by Martin O'Brien and Gianna Bouchard in Chapter 24 as they interrogate conventional notions of 'health' and 'wellbeing'; and by Judy Z. Segal's sardonic interrogation of the rhetoric of ageing and ageism (Chapter 15) in a climate in which we are living longer, but our latter years must face the prejudices generated out of the veneration of youth.

As a rhetorical tactic, in 'first wave' medical humanities biomedical sciences have been placed in opposition to the arts and humanities, framing a need for integration. This echoes the tired 'two cultures' debate (Snow 1959), reflected in the once-influential model of 'contrary imaginations' of convergent (science-oriented) and divergent (arts and humanities-oriented) personality types (Hudson 1975), conveniently ignoring 'bivergence.' Moreover, there is a morality at work where the sciences are vilified and the humanities celebrated. Actually, science and arts/humanities imply and inform one another, and this in turn is sometimes engaged with ethics. For example, where a pathologist looks at a slide of cancerous tissue, it may look beautiful (or sublime)—the pathologist has a subjective aesthetic response to the objective presentation of another's suffering, as explored by Quentin Eichbaum, Gil Pena, Leonard White and Gwinyai Masukume in Chapter 32.

Where a pathologist, dermatologist or radiologist (the 'visual' specialties in medicine) looks at a specimen, a rash or multiple images from a scan, the doctor 'looks' in a culturally determined way that is quite different from the way that a visual artist may be taught to 'look' (Bleakley et al. 2003). Moreover, how such images are prepared and presented, and how judgements are then made about the images, are historically conditioned 'artful' practices (Daston and Galison 2007). Spaces of suffering—and 'beyond suffering'—such as the mortuary also afford aesthetic worth, as Susan Bleakley's (Chapter 26) photographs show. While a functional space for pathologists and mortuary workers, the morgue is chillingly beautiful and expressive where Bleakley captures the footprints of its workers in white, hanging aprons that look like ghosts and neatly ordered rubber boots.

While the medical humanities may operate by bringing disciplines together to work around a common topic, Fitzgerald and Callard (2016: 42) argue that the primary yield here is to expose and explore not only how phenomena are co-implicated in particular sets of relations—material, human and conceptual—but also how such relations themselves constitute the very phenomena studied; then, "the medical humanities does (sic) not need to break down boundaries, but rather to understand how practices of making, breaking and shifting boundaries *constitute* illness and healing." 'Boundaries' between things and activities are not to be understood as impediments to be dissolved in acts of integration, but as necessary *products* and *producers* of performances. 'Boundaries' become actors in their own rights/rites. A 'boundary crossing' can be seen to be an activity not of dissolving the boundary, but rather of bringing it in to play as an actor in exposing the scripts that form it (see Yrjö Engeström's Chapter 3). Boundaries are paradoxical 'de-territorialised territories' where maximum complexity exists at the edge of chaos. A medical humanities-oriented medical education can prepare for life in this exacting zone, drawing on complexity science.

Hannele Kerosuo (Kerosuo and Engeström 2003; Kerosuo 2004) calls 'boundary crossing' and 'boundary encounters' "tool creation," where roles and identities are re-negotiated through redistribution of labour capital and associated emotional capital. Annemarie Mol's (2002) *Body Multiple: Ontology in Medical Practice* in particular addresses boundary crossings from a socio-material perspective, where artefacts perform as boundary indicators and actors, inscribing and often empowering those who work with such artefacts (human tissue samples, for example). A different form of boundary crossing is particularly well documented in the visual artist Ai Wei Wei's (2017) film *Human Flow*, about the global refugee crises, and in the writer William T. Vollmann's (2009) *Imperial* (including an accompanying book of photographs) concerning issues centred on the movement of persons across the Mexico/USA border. In both cases, persons are disidentified, disempowered and disenfranchised, repeating a common theme in doctor–patient encounters and a primary topic for the medical humanities' gaze. Here, one side of the fence is empowered while the other side is hollowed out.

Borders appear in response to such persons' presence to obstruct their flow and to inscribe them as 'liminal' or living a 'bare life' (Agamben 1995), the equivalent of city outcasts or the banished in ancient Greece, marked as 'ostracised.' With the current refugee crisis, liminality is often a result of fleeing conflict; where, in Vollmann's (2009) description of border cross-ings from Mexico to the USA, there is a desire to re-inscribe identity with the lure of escaping from poverty that also promises better access to healthcare. The liminality and 'bare life' of such populations extends globally as a product of limited access to healthcare or exacerbated health disparities. We must then develop responsible and responsive medical humanities that specialise in border crossings as a redistribution of the capital of dignity. But, entangled with such con-cerns is the new phenomenon of 'alternative truth' drawn on by a disenfranchised population to argue cases that have no basis in 'fact' or evidence from research. In Chapter 17, Katherine Shwetz shows how web-based blogs can empower and form an 'attractor' for parents who (mis)perceive their children as suffering from illnesses ascribed to vaccinations. Narratives of anti-vaccination form around a limited number of circulating common themes that advertise Art Frank's (1995) model of illness narratives as 'chaotic'—troubled, turbulent, unsettling and, above all, denying simple explanation. It is then understandable at a metaphorical level that such entangled, boundary-bouncing, chaos narratives should be lassoed and roped in, or brought under control, by reductive fictions.

Border activities (a necessary product of entanglement and the interpenetration of dynamic complex systems, activity systems or expanding networks) are a key topic for study through the medical humanities where they are reproduced in the flow of persons in and out of hospitals and primary care surgeries. As 'patients' rather than 'persons,' they are variously labelled through diagnoses, sometimes stigmatising; and enter and exit across hospital borders with varying degrees of identity change (parodied by Jefferson Wong in Chapter 10). Such human flow—necessarily related to embodiment in space and place—is a rich field of inquiry for the newly emerging field of geohumanities applied to medicine (see Chapter 7 by Courtney Donovan and Sarah de Leeuw, and Chapter 30 by Cari Costanzo); and is also tied to identity structures. We know that higher incidences of disease and earlier mortality follow poverty. William Vollmann's (2007) ethnography *Poor People*, however, shows that poverty and impoverishment can be different, and are necessarily relative to culture and context. Impoverishment is a standard, historical form of teaching by humiliation in medicine, reinforced by 'pimping.' Forms of knowledge and power are distributed spatially in medicine and medical education through structures maintaining inequality and reinforcing insensibility. For example, formal settings such as operating theatres and wards are used to amplify students' impoverished knowledge and skill to keep the most junior in their places on the hierarchy, and to harden borders, where informal settings such as corridors—as soft borders—can enhance redistribution of medical capital, particularly sensory and emotional capital (Bleakley 2015). The geographies of emotional teaching and learning in medical education offer a nascent area of study best addressed through the medical humanities where politics and aesthetics are bedfellows.

In Chapter 29, Kristin Zeiler and Lisa Folkmarson Käll frame the key medical border as 'memory,' where the onset of dementia promises permanent exile and identity de-construction, a refugee from a life now dis-membered rather than re-membered. Dementia is of course one of our biggest global health concerns. In Chapter 13 Shane Neilson shows how metaphor can act as both border patrol and translational medium for border crossings; where Anita Wohlmann in Chapter 12 focuses on the use of metaphors to patrol and police a cultural border between genders as represented in scientific texts.

Returning to 'entanglement,' within the 'second wave' medical humanities community (Whitehead and Woods 2016), this metaphor has already taken on the status that the rhetorician Kenneth Burke called a 'God-term,' concealing as much as it reveals. However, other powerful models can be employed to analyse the work of the medical humanities, such as Actor Network Theory (Latour 2005) and Cultural-Historical Activity Theory (Engeström 2008, 2018) (see Chapter 3). These approaches focus on what factors cause a network or an activity system (a relationship between persons, ideas and artefacts) to be initiated and to expand, or to be compromised (fail to get off the ground, stall, crystallise or collapse). Where networks expand or develop, translations occur between artefacts, ideas and persons through the work of mediators. *Medical humanities interventions comprise sets of mediators.* Important, or high-profile, mediators are metaphors used rhetorically (Chapters 11–18).

Where the network fails to initiate or expand, an intermediary rather than a mediator is at work. Intermediaries merely reproduce the status quo or degrade the situation through lack of translation or mis-translation. There will be plenty of examples of the introduction of medical/ health humanities interventions and research in which the intervention has not moved beyond the status of intermediary to that of mediator, and here the intervention has no effect or even a deleterious effect. In medical education, this is the medical humanities intervention as "dose effect," eloquently described by Jeff Bishop (2008). As Paul Macneill (2011, 2014) suggests, there is no straightforward connection between studying the humanities and consequent ethical and caring human interaction (see Chapter 33). Where the medical humanities act as mediators, their effects can often be described by what Yrjö Engeström (2008, 2018) has termed 'knotworking'— temporary, loose associations or 'coming together' for the purposes of achieving a goal, completing a task or widening a network.

Deleuze and Guattari (1988) distinguish between 'striation'—such as lines of latitude and longitude and 'territorialisation,' such as castle walls and national borders—and a de-territorialised world, a body-without-organs, an undifferentiated state. The former is settled, the latter nomadic. As a work in progress and a fluid or dynamic system, the 'medical humanities' are perhaps best appreciated as largely un-striated or nomadic, refusing territorial boundaries. But in an academic climate where circumscribed territory through disciplines is jealously maintained (and its research projects are more readily funded), this becomes the default position, making the medical humanities as an authentic inter-discipline, trans-discipline or circum-discipline (Bleakley 2014) harder to attain.

Alternatively, the medical humanities can offer a set of 'attractors' to organise otherwise undifferentiated dynamic, complex connections across activities—a medium for temporary 'knotworking.' The clinical encounter, with its 'handovers,' has been a primary site of investigation but has not been central to the interests of 'second wave' medical humanities. Here, focus may be on issues such as power relations in the shaping of policy (see Kathryn E. Goldfarb's Chapter 28); the rhetorical power of narratives around population health issues such as vaccination (Katherine Shwetz's Chapter 17); rhetoric around 'ageism' (Judy Z. Segal's Chapter 15); historical, cross-cultural and gendered notions of 'the body' (Chapters 27–31); and constructions of illness in an age of personalised medicine. Of less interest to the new wave of medical humanities academics are first-hand 'experiences' of illness and their traditional accounts in narrative forms, although these bloom in the popular press and in print—unless such accounts advertise a bigger identity politics phenomenon such as 'women's writing' embedded in feminist studies, 'queer writing' embedded in queer studies (see Chapter 8) or accounts of disability embedded in 'disability studies' (Jones, Wear and Friedman 2014).

Surfing the waves of the medical humanities

A dominant narrative across medical humanities communities describes the recent emergence of a 'second wave,' 'critical' medical humanities in response to the limitations of a more pragmatic 'first wave.' Again, the first wave was focused largely on the 'primal scene' of the clinical encounter and its grounding in medical education, sited largely in academic centres in medical schools. It tended to avoid discussions about the cultural constructions of medicine, and was explicitly 'integrative' and 'applied,' aiming to heal a perceived split between biomedical sciences and arts and humanities, where the arts and humanities could offer a supplement to core science education. The second wave draws on critical thinking and critical theory to explore how cultural constructions of medicine generate knowledge and identity serving favoured stakeholders, including how medicine is represented in popular culture and what rhetorical devices are used in that context. Research is generally situated in University departments but is inter- or trans-disciplinary and rejects models of neat 'integration' for messy 'entanglements.' Scholars usually have backgrounds in the humanities, such as history or literature, and, while not focused on clinical scenarios or clinical applications of their work, they have interests in cultural constructions of 'health' and 'illness,' and the cultural and historical production and shaping of 'medicine' and 'medical expertise.'

The University of Liverpool's Centre for the Humanities and Social Sciences of Health, Medicine and Technology (www.liverpool.ac.uk/humanities-social-sciences-health-medicine-technology) sums up a 'second wave' 'critical' medical humanities as follows:

> The Critical Medical Humanities is an emerging area in Medical Humanities research. It encompasses scholarly work in the humanities and social sciences that is concerned with the critical examination of how issues around, and knowledges of, health, illness, wellbeing and medicine are constituted, represented and governed at various levels (historical, political, economic, socio-cultural). To do this, the Critical Medical Humanities engages with critical theory and radical social movements to explore new methods and ways of knowing which decentre medical expertise, as well as open up opportunities for critical collaborations with the medical and life sciences.

The medical humanities in this guise have served to reassemble once discrete, discipline-based research into topic-based, trans-disciplinary inquiries such as 'the life of breath' (Macnaughton and Carel 2016). Such radical de-territorialising again presents a challenge to University structures based on traditional, territorial subject departments linked to discipline-based research funding. A key development here that cuts across disciplines is the interest in 'big data,' through access to digitalised information. The challenge is how to utilise large chunks of data across disciplines, sources, interests and aims (TOON 2016). The field has already identified gender bias, advertised in language such as 'big data' and 'big questions' (bigger is better—whatever happened to 'small is beautiful'?); and 'text mining,' implying muscular work. The etymology of 'big' (a Middle English word) relates to 'strong' and 'mighty.'

Despite the trend to relegate the clinical encounter as a site for study, in this Handbook such encounters are central to a critical appreciation and an understanding of medicine. Patient encounters are rapidly changing in character and style, where the medical humanities can help to make meaning of such changes. The 'primal scene' of the clinical encounter is no longer sharply defined. For example, consultations now vary in terms of the primary medium, where standard face-to-face meetings are being augmented by telephone and online encounters; virtual self-help groups; phone-in helplines tied to specific television programmes (medi-soaps and reality TV) (see Chapter 21); team-based acute and emergency admissions; surgical treatment where the pre-surgical consultation is with an anaesthetist and nurse focusing upon consent and safety; nurse- and pharmacist-led chronic care; and so forth. Indeed, palliative care has in some ways now become a consultation as patients are asked to set out what would be a 'good death' for them. Indeed, the most popular 'primal scene' now is probably the virtual encounter between the public and Google as a search engine gateway to medical information sites.

The medical humanities—once strongly resisted by sceptics in medicine, including anatomists and biomedical scientists; then accepted only as a handmaiden to medicine—have developed to provide fundamental critiques of issues such as medicalisation of symptoms (especially in mental health, with its habitual framing of symptoms as 'normal' or 'pathological') (see Seamus O'Mahony's commentary on the lasting influence of Ivan Illich's critique of medicalisation in Chapter 9). Part of the turn in contemporary medical humanities has been to cast a diagnostic eye over the symptoms of medical culture itself. The new, 'critical,' medical humanities now offer, for example, sophisticated, organised resistance to perceived injustices in medical care, as well as education for tolerance of ambiguity (or careful suspension of judgement). Just as the medical humanities have asked medicine to turn an interrogative eye to its own practices, so now the medical humanities must themselves become reflexive—turning a critical eye to some of their own claims and practices, and avoiding the inflations of hyper-intellectualism (and then losing touch with practical applications to healthcare) by advertising some humility.

Certainly in the UK the centre of gravity (and associated research) for the medical humanities has now shifted from medical schools to the Academy, where funding opportunities for research are more plentiful (although still restricted, as cross-disciplinary activities, rather than 'pure' intra-disciplinary research, are still treated with some reserve, even suspicion). Much of what is now researched under the banner 'medical humanities' is not immediately applicable to medical education, clinical practice or improvement of patient care and safety. The sophisticated, but sometimes insular, literature that is produced in the Academy fails to appeal to jobbing clinicians who question its applicability and resist its intellectual demands (see Chapters 5 and 22). In summary, the rift between the biomedical sciences and the arts/humanities has now been overshadowed by a rift between clinically relevant medical humanities mainly sited in medical schools with 'face value' translational research agendas, and academic medical humanities sited in Universities with 'widening the knowledge base' agendas, also embracing identity constructions of 'inter/trans-disciplinary researchers' that we might characterise as 'entanglers.'

The narrative of the development of a more theoretically sophisticated 'second wave' medical humanities that eschews translation into clinical applications and has outstripped the 'first wave' should, however, be questioned. It is too neat and is not based on rigorous archive-based historical research. For example, a key assumption that the medical humanities were birthed in medical education is itself misguided. The medical humanities in the UK, for example, have their origins in post-WWII Art Therapy, and then medical ethics (Bleakley 2015). Ideas and practices developed here were grafted on to medical education much later. Second, the absence of critical reflexivity in 'first wave' medical humanities has been overstated, challenging the idea that a second wave of medical humanities has introduced a 'critical' element to a previously naïve outlook; and has also failed to critically address its own biases and deficiencies. 'Critical' is effectively a superfluous descriptor in the 'critical medical humanities.'

New horizons for the medical humanities

Julia Kristeva, Marie Rose Moro, John Ødemark and Eivind Engebretsen (Chapter 2) replace the metaphor of 'entanglement' with that of 'translation' for a new vision of the work of the medical humanities. Drawing on Homer's *Iliad* and *Odyssey* to 'think otherwise' about medicine and medical education, Robert Marshall and Alan Bleakley (2017, particularly Chapter 4) offer a case study illustrating the facilitative work of the medical humanities in an interdisciplinary translation across the Classics and medical pedagogies. They make comparisons between issues of translation in Homeric studies and in medical encounters between patients and doctors, where what is lost in translation proves to be as important as what is gained.

Kristeva and colleagues (Chapter 2) bemoan the separation of 'objective' science and 'subjective' humanities—a legacy of modernist oppositional thinking—where science and objectivity can be seen as culturally produced objects, while culture can readily constitute objective pathology, or shape the body (not just the literal effects of poverty, air pollution, dirty water and road traffic accidents, but also the longstanding traces of child bullying or the noxious effects of a manufactured ideal body image underpinning eating disorders). This extends to an ethical dilemma—the 'humanities' must not be seen as the sustenance brought in to feed a malnourished science, for the humanities themselves are in need of forms of reparation, and culture itself can be malevolent, producing embodied symptoms (obesity, anxiety and so forth). Freud of course reminded us—in *Civilisation and Its Discontents*—that the price we pay for culture is everyday neurosis produced by repression of basic desire.

Second wave, 'critical' medical humanities follow social constructionist orthodoxy in promoting multiple, complex and sophisticated examples of how science 'facts' are historically and socially produced, manipulated and framed. Kristeva and colleagues remind us that culture is not just an idea or set of values that forms what is taken for perception and fact, but is a set of material objects and practice embodiments. Culture is materially productive, and has "pathological and healing powers" (Kristeva et al., Chapter 2), chiming with Marx's view that: "The mode of production of material life conditions the social, political and intellectual life process in general." The culture of medicine, which can be seen as part of a bourgeois 'ideological apparatus,' is surely productive of 'normalised' bodies and statistically average 'population health' as an embodied *translational* phenomenon.

While, for Kristeva and colleagues, 'translation' can do new work "in the interdisciplinary space of the medical humanities" (Chapter 2), this still leaves us with the knotty issue of defining what the 'medical humanities' are. Perhaps the medical humanities resist definition, where circumscribing the object opens the door to those who judge value only in measurement, literalising what can remain in imagination and unconscious, as the tacit dimension (Polanyi 1966), or as a medium for activity. After all, in medical education, we are happy to engage with the notion of a tacit, or an implicate, order in the form of 'illness scripts'—memorised and inter-weaving pieces of biochemical, physiological, genetic and anatomical knowledge that form the basis for Type 1 clinical reasoning, the surface expression of which is 'pattern recognition' or the "blink of an eye" diagnosis, to borrow Abraham Verghese's phrase (1999: 299). While the diagnosis may be in the patient's story, the latter is fleshed out by means of invoking illness scripts. Further, where illness scripts can remain restricted to scientific information, it is the medical humanities that can bring such information to complex embodiment.

Kristeva and colleagues (Chapter 2) then draw an important conclusion, worth quoting in full:

> we do not consider the humanities as a critical and potentially liberating perspective that can be applied *to* medicine as an object in need of repairment. Medical humanities should not be construed as a humanistic perspective *on* medicine. *They should rather be seen as a cross-disciplinary and cross-cultural space for translation and bidirectional critical interrogation of medicine and the humanities across the nature–culture divide.* On the one hand, this implies breaking with the culture–nature dichotomy and considering both the humanities and medicine as bio-cultural practices. On the other hand, it also implies understanding *that boundary work requires boundaries*, and that incommensurability between various partial disciplinary perspectives can, will and should emerge.

This surely constitutes not just a shift in metaphor from 'second wave' medical humanities of 'entanglement' to a specific form of 'translation,' but also a fresh way of conceiving the medical humanities. Not a bundle of disciplines, but the space in which interdisciplinary work is made possible, echoing Mikhail Bakhtin's notion of the 'dialogical.' Such a view also resonates deeply with Yrjö Engeström's (Chapter 3) model of "transformative expertise" in medicine as one of 'boundary crossing' in which pursuit of risky "possibility knowledge" (what we might know and value) is valued over regression to the safety of "stability knowledge" (what we already know and value) where boundaries are strictly maintained. Where Kristeva and colleagues discuss a role for *humanities* in medical education and practice, Engeström's emphasis on an imagination of practice prescribes a role for the *arts*. Rather than considering the arts as a bundle of techniques and expertise across media, we might think of the arts too as collectively constituting 'a space for translation.' The arts constitute a mindset and an approach, a way of 'thinking otherwise,' as well as material products.

The arts, then, are surely not just for decoration or embellishment, but afford the primary media for critical interrogation of culture and nature alike, exposing and exploring the value of disruptions and contradictions. The arts educate for tolerance of ambiguity. Yrjö Engeström further shows how contradictions provide the engine for expansion of activity, and how learning theory must embrace contradiction as a resource. Here, I use contradiction not in the philosophical sense of a *logic* of contradiction, or either/or thinking, but rather as both/and thinking. Where Immanuel Kant noted: "Out of the crooked timber of humanity, no straight thing was ever made," medicine and its associated pedagogies (formalised as 'medical education') must account for, and then address, the crooked timber of medicine—not to straighten it out, but to engage with its contradictions as potential 'both/and' resources.

A basic contradiction haunts modern medicine. This was introduced earlier not as a problem to be solved, but as an emergent property of a complex system to be imaginatively addressed.

Medical pedagogies promise an acute education of sensibility essential to close noticing of patients (and their test results) as a basis for gaining clinical acumen, yet such pedagogies persistently educate for insensibility. This begins with the paradox of the longstanding tradition of learning anatomy through human cadaver dissection. Here, medical students must learn to assimilate, accommodate to, displace, deny or project their natural disgust, distaste and embarrassment—not only in the visual and tactile presence of a naked dead person, but also in the presence of an overwhelming odour of formaldehyde used to preserve the cadaver.

Managing the contradiction of keeping the senses open in order to gaze into the corpse, and simultaneously toning the senses down to prevent nausea and/or being overwhelmed by the stink of formaldehyde, is of course the sensory and affective basis to forming the identity of a 'trainee doctor' through the traditional ritual of cadaver dissection. Education of sensibility and insensibility go hand in hand as a both/and contradiction. Here, the medical humanities can help, as medical education evolves. For example, we know that disgust in the presence of smells is historically and culturally conditioned, so working with a perfumer who has knowledge of the cultural history of smells can bring an illuminating perspective to the occasion of the formative anatomy lesson. Meanwhile, students can read Patrick Süskind's (2010) novel *Perfume: The Story of a Murderer* that famously brings together literary suspense and a history of smells.

In medical schools where dissection and prosection have been replaced by other methods of learning anatomy (especially where the option of attending a post-mortem provides both a better learning setting for 'seeing into the body' and some of the ritual associated with gaining an identity within medical culture), the arts and humanities can, and do, play a central role. Surface and living anatomy invite drawing from observing artists' models, and interacting with actors and performance artists; computer modelling of the body invites input from graphic artists; learning the arts of auscultation, palpation and percussion—to gain a depth perspective on the body—cries out for input from musicians, sound artists, pianists, drummers, tabla players (fingertip experts); while visual artists can work side by side with radiologists in discussing how one 'looks' and 'sees' with 'disciplined' senses. Case notes and reports on what is perceived are illuminated by study of narrative forms. Meanwhile, medical history and sociology can provide accounts of how the medical gaze has evolved from 'seeing into some corpses' (Foucault's (1989) classic account of the birth of modern medicine) to contemporary accounts of a distributed gaze informed by diagnostic imaging technologies such as MRI and CT scanning.

Use of plastination models can be amplified through critical study of Gunther von Hagens' 'Bodyworlds' exhibitions. (In a controversial televised autopsy carried out by von Hagens, a pathologist gave a running commentary on the anatomy being explored, while an anatomy illustrator produced live drawings. At a medical humanities conference that I ran, the same pathologist and illustrator gave a talk, where students and faculty were able to join a debate with them about the educational and ethical issues raised by von Hagens' work, illustrating the value of medical humanities engagement.)

Importantly, beyond these discipline-specific approaches are the interdisciplinary issues of how learning is interconnected (crossing boundaries while respecting the meanings of boundaries), and provides a critical framework for understanding the body in context without resorting to simplistic divisions of the 'normal' and the 'pathological' (Canguilhem 1978). This returns us to the issues of 'translation' and 'possibility knowledge' reviewed earlier. It also reminds us, again, of the cultural production of 'objectivity' in science as well as the bodily fact of culture. Canguilhem shows how the birth of modern biology was not an accumulation of facts about nature but an ideological imperative deeply connected to both political and economic discourses. The 'normal' can be reconfigured from the statistical mean, median or mode to frequencies—of a range of shifting and pulsating attractors within a complex, dynamic system.

The discussion above has vacillated between subjects (such as medical students and patients) and how their subjectivities and identities are traditionally formed (e.g. initiation through the ritual of cadaver dissection), and the artefacts with which they interact (scalpels, anatomy laboratory), or the process of objectifying (turning donated corpses into anatomical objects; turning patients into disease categories). But the processes of educating for insensibility—a de-sensitising and an-aesthetising—can be accounted for by switching attention from subject and object to the abject. Discussion of the abject in medical education reveals how the medical humanities can meaningfully engage medical students.

Indeed, the encounter with the abject in medical education may well form the sensibility of a writer as artist, rather than educate for insensibility in protecting the medical student and would-be doctor, as scientists, from sensory overload. The writer J.G. Ballard initially trained as a medical student but left after two years, yet learning anatomy made a deep, sensual impression, where:

> The cadavers, greenish-yellow with formaldehyde, lay naked on their backs, their skins covered with scars and contusions, and seemed barely human, as if they had just been taken down from a Grünewald Crucifixion. Several students in my group dropped out, unable to cope with the sight of their first dead bodies . . . I still think that my two years of anatomy were among the most important of my life, and helped to frame a large part of my imagination.
>
> *(in Boyd 2017)*

In contrast, a young English doctor relates how, while studying anatomy through cadaver dissection, she dreamed that she ate the flesh of the corpse she was dissecting (Sinclair 1997). A psychiatrist reports "repeated nightmares about dissections" 40 years after the experience:

> I am one of those who almost gave up medicine because of the corpses! [. . .] I still clearly remember this dream. The corpses were after me. I would jump through windows, run, go up the stairs, and they were after me. They wanted to get me. I had this dream many times, I had been deeply shocked.
>
> *(Godeau 2017)*

Emmanuelle Godeau (ibid.) further reports a story concerning "Thomas Platter, a middle-age Dutch medical student who went around France and Europe with his brother during his medical studies" some 500 years ago. After "a week of dissection" Platter "wrote in his diary that he had dreamt he had eaten human flesh and had woken up in the middle of the night to vomit." Here is the return of the repressed—Freud's dictum that the repressed returns in a distorted form. What is denied, put aside, pushed under, ignored, forced into forgetfulness will come back, but as a distortion, and bite, depress or disappoint. And so with organisations and cultures, as well as individuals—as medicine represses what it does not wish to face, or face up to in a clean manner, so this comes to haunt medicine as symptoms. We can include medicine as part of Kant's "crooked timber of humanity" and suggest that, like all institutions, medicine displays typically unaddressed symptoms.

Where medicine's job is to cure symptoms, both somatic and psychological, it is notoriously poor at accounting for its own crooked timber. This must be left to auto-ethnographers— doctors in the role of social anthropologists such as Emmanuelle Godeau, or the American surgeon-writer Richard Selzer; "medicine watchers" (Thomas 1983) such as sociologists studying medical culture, including Barney Glaser, Anselm Strauss and Simon Sinclair; and

17

performance artists, such as Martin O'Brien (Chapter 24), who fundamentally questions Utilitarian definitions of 'health,' and ORLAN (www.orlan.eu), whose work comments critically on issues of the feminine body and radical aesthetic surgery. Once in the territory of the 'medicine watchers' it is easy to see the value of the medical humanities, where the primary gift to medicine is to critically address its symptoms, taking the Sisyphean burden of such a task off the already strained backs of jobbing doctors, to return it to them with interest as an educational provocation.

Fred Hafferty's (1991) *Into the Valley: Death and the Socialization of Medical Students* catalogues 'cadaver stories' from the period when medical training was largely a male domain and part of that faux dominion was to actively disenfranchise women students. Featured amongst such stories were tales of male students cutting the penis of a cadaver to put it in another cadaver's vagina, setting out to shock female students. These historical occasions provide a backdrop for current discussions of the feminising of medicine in the realm of the #MeToo movement. Emmanuelle Godeau (2017), introduced earlier, a medical doctor with a PhD in social anthropology, studied more recent learning of anatomy through cadaver dissection for her doctoral thesis, interviewing 100 medical students and doctors from France, Switzerland, Italy and the USA. She concluded that "the ordeal of dissection" has little value for learning anatomy in comparison with its importance as a rite of passage, where:

> Behind the doors of the anatomy lab, the ordeal of dissection separates forever those who will become doctors from those who will not, those who have managed to control their senses from those who did not succeed, those who have overcome the horror of death from those who have not been confronted with it and never will be, at least not as a doctor.

Yet medical schools worldwide continue to teach anatomy through cadaveric dissection (CD), particularly in Africa and the USA (Memon 2018). As noted, claims that CD is the best way to learn anatomy have been challenged, where plastinated, plastic and virtual models combined with radiological images—and with an emphasis on surface and living anatomy—have in some medical schools come to entirely displace CD (MacLachlan et al. 2004; Godeau 2017). In such schools, there is often an option to attend an autopsy or to intercalate to study for an anatomy degree where CD is an option. Access to plastinated bodies offers a spectacular alternative to Michel Foucault's (1989) "open up a few corpses."

That CD may not be the best way to learn anatomy again confirms that dissection affords "a different role: a rite of passage and creating an *esprit de corps* for the profession" (Godeau 2017). But the rite of passage—a means of socialising (and 'professionalising') into an identity construction (first as 'medical student,' then as 'trainee doctor')—does have specific utility, albeit in one sense counterproductive or leading to unintended consequences. Again, medical students must learn to overcome disgust and repulsion, as, down the line, they will face the necessary insults of spurting arterial blood, bodily fluids and excrement, suppurating and open wounds, bad odours and so forth; and, most importantly, impending death and corpses (where disgust is generally ousted by shock). Again, a medical education is fundamentally contradictory— while students are taught a specific sharpening of sensibility (Notice! The clinical gaze! The physical examination! Clinical judgement!) requiring close noticing, they are simultaneously dulled, de-sensitised, an-aesthetised or educated into insensibility as a form of protection against sensory insult while gaining emotional distance. Emmanuelle Godeau (ibid.) calls this "the *professionalization* of the senses, opened by the paradigmatic experience of dissection" (my emphasis). Such an education of insensibility is a necessary defence, but, like all defence mechanisms, it can be overdetermined.

Lining the nostrils with Vicks VapoRub, or using a perfumed handkerchief or scarf, is a first step to insensibility as it masks the smell of the formaldehyde that 'fixes' the cadaver. Once, as a means of disguising the smell of formalin (the aqueous version of formaldehyde), smoking while dissecting was common. The formaldehyde itself offers an insult to the senses. Medicine then, traditionally, begins with the contradiction of the interjection of the abject between subject (medical student and cadaver treated as dead human) and object (cadaver treated as anatomical specimen and learning resource). The cadaver is neither subject nor object, but the dis-gusting abject, suspended between life and decay. 'Abjection' literally means 'cast off' and so includes all that is considered foreign or 'other.'

An unnatural fascination with disease is of course the calling card of the medical student, both vocational impetus and burden. In *Powers of Horror* Julia Kristeva (1980) describes the effect of encountering the abject as: "Unflaggingly, like an inescapable boomerang, a vortex of summons and repulsion places the one haunted by it literally beside himself," where "abjection is above all ambiguity." Throughout this book, we find examples confirming that a primary role for the medical humanities is education for tolerating ambiguity, and that the pursuit of democracy in particular demands such tolerance. The physician and writer Danielle Ofri (2018), noting that "Like many doctors and nurses, I became politically active for the first time during the summer of 2017, when Congress tried to repeal the Affordable Care Act," argues that doctors should 'prescribe' democracy, for social justice is a necessary condition for public health. But Ofri misses the opportunity to reflect on the health of medical culture itself that refuses democracy and persists with hierarchical and authoritarian structures. Intolerance of ambiguity is the primary signifier of the authoritarian personality and culture.

Julia Kristeva (1980) makes an important connection: "To each ego its object, to each superego its abject." This should be catalogued amongst medicine's famous body of aphorisms. Medicine's necessary fascination with the abject is intimately linked with its historical legacy of hubris. The brain surgeon Henry Marsh (in Wakefield 2017) says: "I often think I became a brain surgeon to justify my own sense of self-importance," where "The funny thing about medical hubris is that nemesis is visited on the patients rather than the surgeon." This is not funny, but regrettable. Doctors, particularly surgeons, have traditionally been socialised to swell not only the ego, but also the superego, claiming the moral high ground over 'other' healthcare colleagues. Central to this swelling of the superego (medicine's martial law) is the fantastic aspiration of dominion over death (see Chapter 11).

The abject, and its associated emotional states of disgust and revulsion, acts in the space between developing sensibility for close noticing and insensibility as defence and cloak. In an early hospital placement as a medical student, Danielle Ofri (2018: 9) recalls an encounter with a homeless patient:

> Gingerly, I took several steps towards her. As I grew closer, a pungent odor enveloped me, the fetid smell of an unwashed body and moldering clothes . . . a roach emerged from a fold in her threadbare sweater . . . I knew that I had to swallow it all back . . . This is what I'd signed on for . . . (but) the rancid smell of this patient undid me.

In her fieldwork, Emmanuelle Godeau (2017) noted:

> In the corridors of the lab, I saw a worried male student trying to make a female student smell his neck just after his first dissection. This smell is the first characteristic of the corpse. He or she who breathes it becomes impregnated with it: "I have a friend who, afterwards, always smelt his hands . . . ." Smell is the first evidence of the transformation of the students.

The abject includes all that human society wishes to contain, be rid of or cast out, and yet must integrate: general pollution and 'waste'; and bodily fluids and waste: shit, piss, snot, sputum, phlegm, menstrual blood, semen, pus, sweat and blood. A major function of religion has been to set out rules of purification that prevent supposed pollution. Medicine follows this same route, priest becoming doctor. Medicine's encounter with the abject is so fundamental that it is never formally articulated as such in medical education, despite the common ritual of giving thanks to those who have donated their bodies to the anatomy laboratory. It is rather acted out through medical socialisation in well-known rituals, beginning again with learning anatomy through dissection. Medical students (in the UK fresh from school, at age 18) encounter human cadavers embalmed in formalin, the aqueous version of formaldehyde that is essentially a poison.

The production of insensibility as a necessary but paradoxical consequence of educating for sensibility and sensitivity in medical education is then a key area for engagement through the medical humanities. The primary issue revolves around the balance between the care and safety of patients and the self-care and community safety of medical students and doctors. Again, too much insensibility can lead to a dulling of clinical acumen and poor self-care, while too much sensibility can lead to overload and burnout. Doctors typically are insensible about medical error, refusing and rationalising actual and potential incidence. As a 'compulsory mis-education' (to borrow Paul Goodman's description) of insensibility proceeds, so medical students begin to defend themselves against sensory overload (stemming from the 'primal scene' of facing the abject, such as the disgusting). This feeds in to the well-documented development of empathy decline and cynicism, where the love of medicine can outpace the love for patients. As the physician and educator Tom Inui (2003) says: "(medical) students learn that medicine is a profession in which you say one thing and do another, *a profession of cynics*." Henry Marsh (in Adams 2017) says of doctors and surgeons, we "have a very complicated relationship with patients . . . as soon as we have any interaction with patients, we start lying. We have to. There is nothing more frightening for a patient than an anxious or doubtful doctor." Meanwhile, as the writer Dennis Johnson (1992: 9) suggests: "it's always been my tendency to lie to doctors, as if good health consisted only of the ability to fool them."

The compulsory mis-education of sensibility of medical students is further exacerbated by how sensibility capital is distributed. By sensibility capital I mean what is considered worth noticing, and who is privileged to notice and appreciate—or "the politics of aesthetics" (Rancière 2006), discussed early in this Introduction. In an effort to educate the sensibilities of medical students and junior doctors, better senior doctors teach through distributing sensibility capital that they have gained through experience, as expertise. But often, as a result of poor pedagogical understanding and technique, or as a regression to infantile forms of control and exercise of authority, sensibility capital is not distributed fairly or is even withheld. This complex of a controlling (sometimes bullying) medical pedagogy can be challenged by the medical humanities where they act as a form of 'adult play' in which medical education is reconfigured as opportunity rather than control. Pedagogies of control refuse jouissance or 'deep effervescence' in the lives of medical students and junior doctors. Such pedagogies and their practice consequences are grounded in traditions of patriarchy and machismo, bolstered by the (now 'dead') primary shaping metaphor of 'medicine as war' (see Chapter 11). And so our young, vital, animated 'real-life' medical students globally, in most medical schools, engage with dead bodies and dead metaphors as formal introductions to their chosen profession, in a culture dogged by a dying ethic of patriarchy.

Properly, but slowly, times are changing—for example, in gender equality in medicine. Yet a cautionary tale from Japan tells of the difficulties that women in medicine still suffer. In the 1980s in Japan women constituted only around 8% of medical school intake and today this has only risen to 21% against a background of a global 60% of women now entering medical schools. However, a prominent Japanese medical school has recently been exposed as systematically rigging its entrance exams against female applicants for more than a decade (McCurry 2018). The school was forced to publicly apologise for this behaviour and now enjoys a properly gender-democratic entrance process.

Summary of the work of the medical humanities

Here, in summary, are some roles and identities for the broad and complex field of the medical humanities—with an emphasis upon clinical application—that the chapters of this Handbook address:

1   *The medical humanities bring an aesthetic dimension to medicine, warning against cultivating insensibility.*
    To talk of medicine as both science and art often seems hollow to contemporary medical students who no longer read Anton Chekhov or William Osler (and who generally don't bother either with Richard Selzer, Abraham Verghese or Gabriel Weston; nor do they read historically important humanist biologists such as Julian Huxley and Adolf Portmann). The arts and the sciences have been separated out in these students' formal education to such a degree that most medical students have lost touch with the methods and purposes of the arts and humanities. The medical humanities can, and should, bring aesthetics back into medicine especially to remind us that biomedical science itself is intrinsically aesthetic. 'Aesthetics' literally means 'sense impression' or using the senses—sensibility—in 'close noticing,' and this is surely where medical practice (as diagnostic acumen) starts. An insensible medicine (one that sets out to dull or an-aesthetise) seems ridiculous, and yet, a paradoxically cultivated insensibility is surely medicine's most prominent symptom as a self-inflicted wound, a self-harming (advertised in symptoms such as doctors' poor self-care; objectifying patients; cynicism; and tolerating numbing hospital environments).
    An example of the medical humanities countering insensibility and insensitivity in medicine is the restoration of lyricism to clinical work. Normally, clinical work is recounted as epic, tragic or dark comic, avoiding the lyrical genre as a 'soft' medicine of care. Lyricism operates as a counter to bluntness such as the persistent use of monological rather than dialogical communication (common in surgical settings where the tone and climate are set by the most senior surgeon). Where lyricism is repressed, there tends to be bitterness and recrimination rather than celebration of work. Finding the poetry in medicine, or employing a poetic imagination, is an important task for doctors. As both doctor and poet, William Carlos Williams, said in the poem 'Asphodel, That Greeny Flower': "It is difficult to get the news from poems yet men die miserably every day for lack of what is found there." Williams suggests that poetry is not just luxury but indispensable. Doctors without a cultivated imagination (achieved through education of sensibility) are merely technicians.
    The medical humanities can challenge the dominance of literalism and instrumentality, the main strategies used to cultivate insensibility. One of medicine's key flaws and symptoms is objectification of patients, treating them as machines or engineering problems. This is a symptom of the denial of the power of metaphor to shape medicine. The medical humanities can expose and address this flaw. A parallel issue is medicine's refusal of the subjunctive mood and narrative tension in language, preferring the certainty of the indicative ('this is') rather than the ambiguity of the subjunctive mood ('this might be') and modal auxiliaries for the verb: 'might,' 'could,' 'possibly,' and 'maybe.' The indicative mood (and

illocutionary language) is gendered male and draws on oppositional categories leading to hierarchy. A more feminine language (*écriture féminine*) draws on subjunctivising and per-locutionary speech acts that inscribe through tenderness and succour (what Hélène Cixous (1975) calls "writing with mother's milk").

The medical humanities challenge poor self-care or a cultivated insensibility amongst doctors, perceived as a by-product of the historical legacy of hubris. A key role for the medical humanities, as we have seen, is to challenge a range of insensibilities that blunt medicine. Doctors have the highest rates of suicide, suicidal ideation, burnout and alcohol and substance abuse across the professions, yet research—discussed earlier—indicates that medical students who show the greatest involvement with the arts and humanities also show less tendency to anxiety and burnout, or show better self-care. Blunted doctors may also be inappropriately and unthinkingly blunt with patients and colleagues.

The view from the medical humanities questions the value of high levels of simulation and dissimulation in medical education. A self-imposed symptom in medical education, and a key form of educating for insensibility, is wholesale and uncritical adoption of learning through simulation. This is understandable and necessary where invasive clinical skills such as suturing or intimate examinations cannot be conducted on patients without prior preparation, but learning through simulation makes no sense in non-technical areas such as communication. A culture of simulation can educate students for dissimulation or 'faking it,' accepting that a false consciousness is necessary as a defence against being overwhelmed by a demanding job, and is a common way for medical students to get by on clinical placements. Medical humanities can illuminate these phenomena, particularly through knowledge of impression management, 'imposter syndrome,' performance studies and academic interests in simulation and the simulacrum in culture.

Replacing hands-on physical examination (auscultation, palpation and percussion) with cold technologies in medical education adds to insensibility (and probably insensitivity) in medicine. Appropriate intimate contact with patients signals warmth and connection, a staple of good practice, but this is being eroded. Once again, an aesthetic medicine is hands-on, sense-based. This is not to deny the immense value of technological progress in medicine, but to warn against such technologies freezing out humanity and intimacy.

2   *The medical humanities bring a political dimension to medicine.*

Medicine holds two kinds of capital: the 'technical' (clinical skills and knowledge) and the 'non-technical' (values, sensibility, communication) (an arbitrary division that serves as an heuristic). Technical knowledge is held by experts (senior doctors) and re-distributed amongst the community of medical staff according to hierarchy. Non-technical knowledge capital, such as sensibility capital, is thinner on the ground amongst seniors and is treated in the same way as technical capital, where it is re-distributed according to the desires of senior doctors. A politicised medicine challenges these modes of distribution of capital, pointing out that non-technical capital, such as communication capabilities and sensibility, may be higher amongst medical students or juniors, as it is characteristically flattened throughout a career. Such capital must be recognised and fairly distributed—an issue of power and resistance. (Interested readers are referred to the body of work of Jacques Rancière as a touchstone in this area.)

A non-reflexive medicine (common) does not think through the values that inform its own practice. The primary issue here is that medicine would do better work if the culture was more fully democratised. Aesthetics plus politics provides a powerful framework for inquiry into medicine and medical education. For example, a body of research—noted earlier—shows that better teamwork leads to better patient care and safety and to greater staff satisfaction. The democratising of medicine must happen somewhere and it certainly is not happening generally through medical education. The humanities, however, offer a democratising impetus and medium. The medical humanities can act as a politicising and consciousness-raising medium to challenge structural problems in medicine caused by ideological interests; for example, how does medicine square its 'open-door' policy of non-discrimination at the point of treatment with its own discriminatory, archaic hierarchical systems? Is the failure to democratise (although signs are there, such as patient-centredness and inter-professional teamwork) not just a historical hangover but also a defence against losing perceived status?

In the politicising of medicine, the medical humanities can act as provocation for 'thinking otherwise' about the primary purposes of medicine; for example, is medicine's purpose to treat the effects of sedentary lifestyles, poor diet, inequalities and conflict; or should medicine be at the front end as a preventive intervention, acting ideologically in the interests of democracy and social justice? Where the medical humanities are reflexive, they can critically address medical education as a form of Western imperialism. The medical humanities can also promote the redistribution of the capital of medicine amongst its stakeholders, particularly the public; and those who bring debate about, and representations of, medicine to the public through engagement, such as artists. This includes addressing issues of equality, diversity and social justice. Capital, as noted above, is not just economic or skill- and knowledge-based, but includes sensibility capital or how judgements are made about the 'worth' of things and how the senses are central to such judgements and not independent of cultural shaping. The ways in which we see and feel, and the things that we pay particular attention to, are not shaped 'naturally' but culturally. The rules for such judgements are made and held by an elite. This ownership and subsequent uses of sensory capital, where perceived as unjust, can be resisted. This is a key part of the wider democratising of medicine.

3   *The medical humanities can act as therapy addressing medicine's most pressing symptoms.*

The medical humanities can afford a psychodynamic therapy addressing medicine's symptoms such as inflation or hubris, masculinism and heroism, refusal to acknowledge vulnerability, low tolerance of ambiguity, fear of failure and techniques of de-sensualising medical students and doctors (education into insensibility). These symptoms are reflected in perseverative and defensive behaviours of doctors such as overdiagnosis and ordering too many tests as a defence against potential failure (a fear of failure), and in poor self-care. We should, however, 'think otherwise' about medicine's self-induced symptoms. One of the tenets of psychoanalysis is that symptoms serve a purpose, such as defending a fragile ego in a hostile and disturbing environment. Medicine's symptoms too are ingrained—they have a long history, have gained deep traction and search for new modes of expression. For example, a classic defence mechanism in medicine in the face of extreme sensuality (pressing bodies, bodily fluids, intimate examinations, body interiors, wounds, florid behaviours, witnesses to births and deaths) is to close down or de-sensitise; this is both an an-aesthetising and a de-sensualisation, sometimes dressed up as 'professionalism.' In medical education, as noted above, there has been a turn to learning through simulation. On the one hand, this makes sense in a climate of increasing regard for patient safety—thus medical students do not practise suturing on patients. However, this also acts as a defence against the intimacies and over-sensuality of real body contacts that may be overwhelming. The deadening effect of working with models in simulation conditions as a basis for learning clinical skills can be read as a new defence mechanism in the tradition of deadening and exhausting work schedules, and working in numbing environments such as hospitals.

Smell may be the most undervalued of the senses, but excising it completely from learning clinical skills is a pedagogic error.

4   *The medical humanities can help us to 'think otherwise' about 'health' and 'illness.'*

In the wake of the arts therapy movement, the application of the arts in particular to medicine has by-passed one of the most important functions of art (especially the avant-garde) in culture—to upset and interrogate habits and conventions. More radical arts, such as body modification performance art, ask fundamental questions about categories of 'illness' and 'health,' where what medicine takes as symptoms are turned into expressive qualities. Such approaches reject the Utilitarian philosophy that has shaped Western thinking about ideals of 'health' and 'happiness.'

5   *The medical humanities expose and explore surprising origins of medical phenomena.*

The bread and butter content of medical humanities—such as the history of medicine, narrative medicine and narrative bioethics—exposes the unexpected and generates unique perspectives on taken-for-granted conditions. Research in the sciences is often replication of original research. Innovations are relatively thin on the ground. In the arts and humanities, there is perhaps more pressure for innovation and surprise. The main criterion for success of a PhD thesis is to make an 'original' contribution to the literature. As a benchmark, think how radical Michel Foucault's contribution to the medical humanities has been in tracing the historical conditions for the emergence and formation of 'governmentality' phenomena such as 'madness' and 'sexual abnormalities.' Or, reflect on how Anselm Strauss and Barney Glaser exposed how end-of-life care in the 1960s, governed by doctors, engaged in tactics of deception in an atmosphere of secrecy to prevent dying cancer patients from knowing their prognoses. This blocked the open grief of families as well as deceiving patients. Or, where bioethics case studies had attained a kind of 'truth' status, think what a radical turn it was to treat such case studies as 'fictions,' or narratives drawing on a variety of rhetorical techniques to persuade readers into the authenticity of the accounts (Chambers 1999).

6   *The medical humanities promote public engagement with medicine.*

Public engagement with medicine has traditionally been about passive education rather than interaction where lay input can shape medicine. Clearly such input is welcome in the shape of patients who are experts in their own illnesses and have collaborated with others to employ social media and form information channels such as interactive blogs (see for example http://e-patients.net/about-e-patientsnet). Patients also write best-selling auto-ethnographies. The major interface for public engagement with medicine continues to be medical television soap operas with phone-in help lines. Finally, the 'health' of a culture has long been diagnosed and debated by artists, as 'diagnosticians' of the relative health of that culture.

7   *The medical humanities introduce a variety of methods and methodologies.*

The turn to the arts and humanities to shape medical education and to better understand constructions of medical culture has brought with it a wealth of research and inquiry techniques that were previously only used in arts and humanities research. An example is the use of reflexive video-based ethnography, where practitioners can retrospectively watch themselves at work and analyse elements of that work with, or as, researchers. (I pioneered such video ethnography on hospital wards and in operating theatres in the UK.) Use of such research media immediately opens the door to collaboration with arts practitioners—for example, medical students' and doctors' work can be explored as performance; the behaviour of surgical teams can be explored for the use of non-verbal behaviour as a rhetorical strategy to persuade others into behaving in certain ways.

Conceptual frames, methodologies and methods of inquiry

To extend point 7 above, this Handbook is not structured around distinctions between theory and practice, rhetoric and research, or methodologies and methods. I did not set out in any way to format the book according to groupings of different approaches to research or data gathering. Chapters are not grouped under a classification scheme in which 'modes of inquiry,' 'forms of practice' and 'theoretical orientations' are separated. Parts include a variety of approaches to research, data gathering and speculation, including explicitly rhetorical and creative writing. In light of this lack of a front-loaded structure reflecting research approaches, the Handbook instead includes an important concluding chapter (42) by Maria Athina (Tina) Martimianakis, Ayelet Kuper and Cynthia Whitehead—from the Wilson Centre, Toronto—that makes sense of the variety of approaches to research across the Handbook's chapters. I am grateful to these three femusketeers for taking on this complex task, providing a partner overview to this Introduction. Drawing on Bourdieu, they describe the medical humanities as an emergent 'field' that is still 'organising,' affording an opportunity, and not a threat, for innovation in research. Importantly, they point to the opportunity for interactional and transactional activity across arts, humanities, social sciences, medicine and medical sciences in negotiating knowledge, identities and modes of inquiry:

> When a field—such as the medical humanities—is organising, the potential for partial uptake of methodological traditions affords exciting opportunities to scholars who are freed to introduce new (or perhaps just different) approaches of inquiry to support the socio-political operations of the developing knowledge base. 'New' or 'different' of course do not automatically equate with 'better,' and—not surprisingly—the issue of who is authorised to judge quality is a topic explicitly and implicitly reflected in this book.

Finally, throughout the Handbook, I celebrate the 'Persian flaw.' Where rug makers traditionally celebrate the human as a flawed being ('crooked timber of humanity') by incorporating a flaw in the rug design, so I celebrate the appearance throughout these chapters of contradictions that are neither swept under the carpet nor straightened through deception, but rather act as springboards for further thinking and action. Such contradictions are the breeding grounds for ideas and interventions that we call, for want of better terms, the medical and health humanities.

References

Abdel-Halim RE, AlKattan KM. Introducing medical humanities in the medical curriculum in Saudi Arabia: A pedagogical experiment. *Urology Annals.* 2012; 4: 73–9.

Adams T. Henry Marsh: The mind–matter problem is not a problem for me, mind is matter. Neuroscience: *The Observer,* Sunday 16 July 2017. Available at: www.theguardian.com/science/2017/jul/16/henry-marsh-mind-matter-not-a-problem-interview-neurosurgeon-admissions. Last accessed: 23 May 2018.

Agamben G. 1995. *Homo Sacer: Sovereign Power and Bare Life.* Stanford, CA: Stanford University Press.

Ai Wei Wei. 2017. *Human Flow.* (Film).

Alosaimi FD, Alawad HS, Alamri AK, et al. Patterns and determinants of stress among consultant physicians working in Saudi Arabia. *Advances in Medical Education and Practice.* 2018; 9: 165–74.

Barad K. 2007. *Meeting the Universe Halfway: Quantum Physics and the Entanglement of Matter.* Durham, NC: Duke University Press.

Barker-Benfield GJ. 1992. *The Culture of Sensibility: Sex and Society in Eighteenth-Century Britain.* Chicago, IL: University of Chicago Press.

Barone T. 2000. *Aesthetics, Politics, and Educational Inquiry: Essays and Examples.* New York, NY: Peter Lang Publishing Inc.

Bishop J. Rejecting medical humanism: Medical humanities and the metaphysics of medicine. *Journal of Medical Humanities.* 2008; 29: 15–25.

Bleakley A. 2014. *Patient-Centred Medicine in Transition: The Heart of the Matter.* London: Routledge.

Bleakley A. 2015. *Medical Humanities and Medical Education: How the medical Humanities Can Shape Better Doctors.* London: Routledge.

Bleakley A. 2017. *Thinking with Metaphors in Medicine: The State of the Art.* London: Routledge.

Bleakley A, Bligh J, Browne J. 2011. *Medical Education for the Future: Identity, Power and Location.* Dordrecht: Springer.

Bleakley A, Farrow R, Gould D, Marshall R. Making sense of clinical reasoning: Judgement and the evidence of the senses. *Medical Education.* 2003; 37: 544–52.

Borrill CS. (Undated). The effectiveness of health care teams in the National Health Service: Report. Available at: http://ctrtraining.co.uk/documents/TheEffectivenessofHealthCareTeamsintheNHS_004.pdf. Last accessed: 23 May 2018.

Boyd W. A matter of life and death: William Boyd on the rise of the surgeon memoir. *The Guardian,* 6 May 2017. Available at: www.theguardian.com/books/2017/may/06/surgeon-writer-life-hands-william-boyd. Last accessed: 8 November 2018.

Canguilhem G. 1978. *The Normal and the Pathological.* New York, NY: Zone Books.

Chambers T. 1999. *The Fiction of Bioethics: Cases as Literary Texts.* London: Routledge.

Cixous H. 1975. *Coming to Writing and Other Essays.* Cambridge, MA: Harvard University Press.

Clarke R. 2017. *Your Life in My Hands.* London: Metro Books.

Crowe S, Clarke N, Brugha R. 'You do not cross them': Hierarchy and emotion in doctors' narratives of power relations in specialist training. *Social Science and Medicine.* 2017; 186: 70–7.

Daston L, Galison P. 2007. *Objectivity.* New York, NY: Zone Books.

Deleuze, G, Guattari F. 1988. *A Thousand Plateaus: Capitalism and Schizophrenia.* London: Athlone.

Derrida J. 2005. *Rogues: Two Essays on Reason.* Stanford, CA: Stanford University Press.

de Tocqueville A. 1835–40; 2003. *Democracy in America and Two Essays on America.* London: Penguin Books.

Engeström Y. 2008. *From Teams to Knots: Activity-Theoretical Studies of Learning at Work.* Cambridge: Cambridge University Press.

Engeström Y. 2018. *Expertise in Transition: Expansive Learning in Medical Work.* Cambridge: Cambridge University Press.

Fitzgerald D, Callard F. 2016. Entangling the medical humanities. In: A Whitehead and A Woods (eds.) *The Edinburgh Companion to the Critical Medical Humanities.* Edinburgh: Edinburgh University Press, 35–49.

Foucault M. 1989. *The Birth of the Clinic: An Archaeology of Medical Perception.* London: Routledge.

Frank A. 1995. *The Wounded Storyteller: Body, Illness and Ethics.* Chicago, IL: University of Chicago Press.

Godeau E. 2017. Dissecting cadavers: Learning anatomy or a rite of passage? *Hektoen International: A Journal of Medical Humanities.* 2009; 1: 5. Available at: http://hekint.org/2017/01/22/dissecting-cadavers-learning-anatomy-or-a-rite-of-passage. Last accessed: 11 November 2018.

Hafferty F. 1991. *Into the Valley: Death and the Socialization of Medical Students.* New Haven, CT: Yale University Press.

Hudson L 1975. *Contrary Imaginations: A Psychological Study of the English Schoolboy.* Harmondsworth: Penguin.

Illich I. 1975. *Medical Nemesis: The Expropriation of Health.* New York, NY: Pantheon Books.

Inui TS. 2003. A flag in the wind: Educating for professionalism in medicine. Association of American Medical Colleges. Available at: https://members.aamc.org/eweb/upload/A%20Flag%20in%20the%20Wind%20Report.pdf. Last accessed: 11 November 2018.

Johnson D. 1992. *Jesus' Son: Stories.* New York, NY: Farrar, Straus & Giroux.

Jones T, Wear D, Friedman L (eds.) 2014. *Health Humanities Reader.* New Brunswick, NJ: Rutgers University Press.

Kant I. Answering the question: What is enlightenment? 1784. Philosophical Explorations. Full text. Available at: http://braungardt.trialectics.com/philosophy/early-modern-philosophy-16th-18th-century-europe/kant/enlightenment. Last accessed: 23 May 2018.

Kerosuo H, Engeström Y. Boundary crossing and learning in creation of new work practice. *Journal of Workplace Learning.* 2003; 15: 345–51.

Kerosuo H. Examining boundaries in health care: Outline of a method for studying organizational boundaries in interaction. *Outlines: Critical Practice Studies.* 2004; 6: 35–60.

Kristeva J. 1980. *Powers of Horror.* New York, NY: Columbia University Press.

Kumagai AK. Beyond 'Dr. Feel-Good': A role for the humanities in medical education. *Academic Medicine.* 2018; 92: 1659–60.

Lacan J. 2007. *Écrits: A Selection.* Ed. A Sheridan. London: Tavistock.

Latour B. 2005. *Reassembling the Social: An Introduction to Actor Network Theory.* Oxford: Oxford University Press.

MacLachlan J, Bligh J, Bradley P, Searle J. Teaching anatomy without cadavers. *Medical Education.* 2004; 38: 418–24.

Macnaughton J, Carel H. 2016. Breathing and breathlessness in clinic and culture: Using critical medical humanities to bridge an epistemic gap. In: A Whitehead and A Woods (eds.) *The Edinburgh Companion to the Critical Medical Humanities.* Edinburgh: Edinburgh University Press, 294–309.

Macneill PU. The arts and medicine: A challenging relationship. *Medical Humanities.* 2011; 37: 85–90.

Macneill P (ed.). 2014. *Ethics and the Arts.* Dordrecht: Springer.

Mangione S, Chakraborti C, Staltari G, et al. Medical students' exposure to the humanities correlates with positive personal qualities and reduced burnout: A multi-institutional U.S. survey. *Journal of General Internal Medicine.* 2018; 33: 628–34.

Marshall R, Bleakley A. 2017. *Rejuvenating Medical Education: Seeking Help from Homer.* Newcastle: Cambridge Scholars Publishing.

McCurry J. 2018. Tokyo medical school admits changing results to exclude women: University manipulated test scores for more than a decade to ensure more men became doctors. *The Guardian,* 8 August 2018. Available at: www.theguardian.com/world/2018/aug/08/tokyo-medical-school-admits-changing-results-to-exclude-women. Last accessed: 8 November 2018.

McGaghie WC. Evaluation apprehension and impression management in clinical medical education. *Academic Medicine.* 2018; 93: 685–86.

Memon I. Cadaver dissection is obsolete in medical training! A misinterpreted notion. *Medical Principles and Practice.* 2018; 27: 201–10.

Mol A. 2002. *Body Multiple: Ontology in Medical Practice.* Durham, NC: Duke University Press.

Neumann M, Edelhäuser F, Tauschel D, et al. Empathy decline and its reasons: A systematic review of studies with medical students and residents. *Academic Medicine.* 2011; 86: 996–1009.

Ofri D. 2018. *What Doctors Feel: How Emotions Affect the Practice of Medicine.* Boston, MA: Beacon Press.

Parks T. 2017. Report reveals severity of burnout by specialty. *AMA Wire.* Available at: https://wire.ama-assn.org/life-career/report-reveals-severity-burnout-specialty. Last accessed: 29 May 2018.

Peterkin A, Bleakley A. 2017. *Staying Human During the Foundation Programme and Beyond: How to Thrive After Medical School.* Baton Rouge, FL: CRC Press.

Petersen A, Bleakley A, Brömer R, Marshall R. The medical humanities today: Humane health care or tool of governance? *Journal of Medical Humanities.* 2008; 29: 1–4.

Pinar W. 2012. *What Is Curriculum Theory?* London: Routledge.

Polanyi M. 1966. *The Tacit Dimension.* Chicago, IL: University of Chicago Press.

Pryor L. Doctors are human too. *New York Times,* 21 April 2017. Available at: www.nytimes.com/2017/04/21/opinion/doctors-are-human-too.html. Last accessed: 29 May 2018.

Rancière J. 2006. *The Politics of Aesthetics.* London: Continuum.

Robinson M. What are we doing here? *The New York Review of Books,* 9 November 2017. Available at: www.nybooks.com/articles/2017/11/09/what-are-we-doing-here. Last accessed: 29 May 2018.

Sinclair S. 1997. *Making Doctors: An Institutional Apprenticeship.* Oxford: Berg.

Smith KE, Norman GJ, Decety J. The complexity of empathy during medical school training: Evidence for positive changes. *Medical Education.* 2017; 51: 1146–59.

Snow CP. 1959. *The Two Cultures.* Cambridge: Cambridge University Press.

Sontag S. 1978. *Illness as Metaphor.* New York, NY: Farrar, Straus and Giroux.

Strauss A, Glaser B. 1967. *The Discovery of Grounded Theory: Strategies for Qualitative Research.* Piscataway, NJ: Transaction Publishers.

Süskind P. 2010. *Perfume: The Story of a Murderer.* London: Penguin Books.

The University of Liverpool's Centre for the Humanities and Social Sciences of Health, Medicine and Technology. Available at: www.liverpool.ac.uk/humanities-social-sciences-health-medicine-technology/themes/critical-medical-humanities. Last accessed: 29 May 2018.

Thomas L. 1983. *The Youngest Science: Notes of a Medicine-Watcher.* New York, NY: Viking Press.

TOON. 2016. Big data and the 7 V's. Available at: https://websitetoon.com/2016/09/08/big-data-7-vs. Last accessed: 29 May 2018.

Verghese A. 1999. *The Tennis Partner.* London: Vintage.

Vollmann WT. 2007. *Poor People*. New York, NY: Harper Perennial.

Vollmann WT. 2009. *Imperial*. New York, NY: Viking Books.

Wakefield M. Henry Marsh: How doctors can become monsters. *The Spectator*, 6 May 2017. Available at: www.spectator.co.uk/2017/05/henry-marsh-how-doctors-can-become-monsters. Last accessed: 8 November 2018.

Weiss P. 2005. *The Aesthetics of Resistance, Vol. 1*. Durham, NC: Duke University Press.

Whitehead A, Woods A (eds.) 2016. *The Edinburgh Companion to the Critical Medical Humanities*. Edinburgh: Edinburgh University Press.

Wikipedia (https://en.wikipedia.org/wiki/Medical_humanities).

PART I

Medical humanities as networks, systems and translations

1

A DOSE OF EMPATHY FROM MY SYRIAN DOCTOR

Randi Davenport

A woman with a debilitating disease finds hope in a man who's come from a war-ravaged country.

He lifted his glasses and let them rest on his forehead before taking hold of my right leg. "Pull me closer," he said.

I pulled.

"Push me away."

I pushed.

I thought: This is the game lovers play. Pull me closer, push me away, each action holding the promise of a specific outcome: If I push you away, you will come after me. If I pull you closer, you will let me in. But he wasn't my lover. He was my doctor.

And then I felt my leg give way, a sensation of water running downhill. I came back to myself. To the blue-white light of the exam room. The crinkly sound of the paper on the table. The feeling of his hand on my skin as again he told me to pull him closer. To push him away. The sensation of weakness once more, this time in my left leg.

He made no comment, but I saw the studied flatness of his expression. I looked down at the shrunken muscles in my feet, at my paralysed toes. And then I looked up at him. He reached into his lab coat, pulled out his reflex hammer and took aim at my knee. My leg jumped, the spasm of a too-brisk response.

"You are fine," he said, his words inflected by the Syrian accent that gave me so much comfort. "Trust me."

I tried to trust him, but I wasn't fine and we both knew it. My motor neurons were failing. They had been failing for two decades, slowly, in a sleepy subterranean wave.

I knew I was lucky. Motor neuron disease is incurable and most people who have it die within a year or two, maybe five. But I was still alive. Soldiering on.

So when my doctor said I was fine, he meant he had discovered nothing new and alarming during this exam. I was holding steady. I wasn't fine but I wasn't dying, either.

We met every three months. The regularity of these appointments, and the close monitoring that the schedule suggested, should have terrified me. Instead, it made me feel safe. As time passed, I realised it wasn't just the monitoring that brought me comfort but the doctor himself.

I liked the way he wore his hair cut short, so I could see the contours of his skull. I liked the shape of his hands and the patient way he answered my questions. And if I hesitated, not wanting

31

to talk about embarrassing symptoms, he would soften his voice and give me a mild look. "Tell me," he'd say, and I'd tell him.

One night I dreamed of him standing in the middle of a wasteland, a world exploded by war, his sleeve pushed back so I could read the watch on his wrist. The dial read 10 minutes to 8. In the dream I thought, "Oh thank God. I still have time." But when I woke up, I felt only terror. "Time's running out," I thought.

I sent my doctor an email and he responded right away. "Do not worry," he wrote. "You are fine." I felt the force of his words, the shelter of his certainty.

It's axiomatic to say that patients with serious illnesses fall in love with their doctors, seeing them as points of light in an otherwise dismal sky. But I knew this wasn't love. It was desperation, a finger-hold on a cliff before the fall.

I wasn't in love with him, but I had come to depend on him. I was accustomed to taking care of myself and I had let him take care of me. I let him see that I was scared. And when I let him see my fear, I had to see it, too. My own fragility. The stuff I couldn't just power through.

Despite this, he gave me hope. This was the ammunition that fuelled my fight.

"Pull me closer," he said each time we met. "Push me away."

I asked about his family in Syria.

"You don't want to hear this," he said, as formal and as courteous as ever. But eventually he told me about his reckless nephews. His brother-in-law with cancer. His mother and sisters who remained there, watching daily for things that could fall from the sky: bombs, pieces of aircraft, the flotsam of war.

Inadvertently, I winced and turned away. When I looked at him once more, he was watching me recoil from things unknown.

"You are fine," he said, and smiled.

Not long after, three Muslim students were shot in our town, killed when they answered a knock at their apartment door. In San Bernardino, Calif., a newly married couple, their toddler at her grandmother's house, opened fire in a room full of county office workers. And all the news was about shooters from ISIS, Muslims and the threat they posed to the American way of life.

At my next appointment, I could tell my doctor was preoccupied.

"What's wrong?" I asked softly.

"It is nothing," he said. He wouldn't look at me.

I thought about the way he had come to America and chosen to work at a big state teaching hospital so he could help poor people. How he had come here to be safe and to offer safety. I had never seen him look as defeated as he did now.

"Tell me," I said.

He hesitated and then he said he was afraid for his wife and children. He would be fine, but he worried about them. "People are crazy," he said. And then he began to talk about leaving America, maybe moving to Dubai.

"You will break my heart," I said. I thought I was joking, but a minute later I was weeping.

I understood why he wanted to leave. But I also knew that if I was still alive, it was because of him. His bravery mattered when mine faltered. His mantra, "You are fine. You are fine," cut through my doubt when it seemed there was no light.

How many effects of warfare are invisible, revealed only in human trembling, that shivering language of fear? The twitching, failing muscle. The bullet in the air. Each equivalent to the other, it turns out, when the coming damage is unknown, but certain.

I wanted him to be safe. The same thing he wanted for me. And I knew I was helpless to procure that safety for him, because some people are, indeed, crazy. And he was just as helpless when it came to halting the march of my illness.

I said his name and he turned to face me.

"I am with you," he said, as if I had asked him for something, his voice fierce again. His face filled with resolve. "I am not going anywhere."

"You're O.K. too," I replied, wiping my eyes, knowing my words were futile but needing to say something anyway. "Nothing's going to happen," I said, even though I could not possibly know if he would be all right. Even so, I barrelled on. "Your family will be all right. You'll be all right."

He smiled gently and shook his head. And then I realised something: He had never once tried to reassure me about the future in that way, with false hope. He had only ever spoken about the present, telling me what he knew to be true. I was still fine. I was not yet headed for a quick death. And that was what had given me comfort.

"You are fine," I offered softly, thinking that, for at least this moment, he was. But as soon as I said this, he flicked his glance away and did not reply.

I did not blame him for ducking the conversation the way you would dodge a downpour of rain. We could hear nothing of war in that cool place, where the only sounds came from the elevators rising and falling. There were no bullets flying. No audible dying off of this neuron or the next. These things are silent until they are upon us, and by then it is too late.

So we sat without speaking, together in the dark night of that bright room. But if he had taught me anything, it was that comfort resides in the rituals of care, the steady application of optimism, the shivering light of faith in the fact that I was still okay.

And so I thought: What can I offer when the only thing I have is hope? And then: You can be his patient. You can let him take care of you.

Almost as soon as I thought this, he reached into his lab coat for his hammer. "Go like this," he said, cupping his fingers so that one hand hooked into the other. When I did, he told me to pull. Then he hit my knee with the hammer and resumed his exam.

Reprinted with permission of *The New York Times*. First published 14 April 2017 in the series 'Modern Love.'

2

THE CULTURAL CROSSINGS OF CARE

A call for translational medical humanities

Julia Kristeva, Marie Rose Moro, John Ødemark, and Eivind Engebretsen

Introduction

Modern medicine is confronted with cultural crossings in various forms: The migration wave in Europe has imposed a new awareness of the cultural dimensions of both physical and psychological therapy (Napier et al. 2014). Religious and ideological radicalisation has raised related questions about how to draw the line between pathology and conviction, and how to deal with cultural and religious discontent, also in clinical settings (Kristeva 2016). *The Lancet Commission on Culture and Health* (Napier et al. 2014: 1607) provided important insights into the cultural dimensions of health and wellbeing; most radically, it pointed out that "the distinction between the objectivity of science and the subjectivity of culture" is "itself a social fact." When the Lancet commission aims to create awareness about the "effect *of* cultural systems of values *on* health outcomes," however, it implicitly reinforces the ontological divide that caused the problem in the first place.

We believe that the medical humanities should play a vital role in a more radical rethinking of the divide between science and the humanities. But we also maintain that this endeavour calls for a fundamental rethinking of the medical humanities themselves. Such a rethinking should address the grounding assumptions about what the humanities are, as well as how they can interact with biomedicine in research, in the production and use of evidence, and in the practical art of care. Drawing upon the seminal work of Julia Kristeva (2003, 2011, 2012, 2013, 2016), we will argue that the medical humanities should fully acknowledge the pathological and healing powers of culture, and approach the human body as a complex bio-cultural fact. Consequently, cultural dimensions should no longer be construed as mere subjective aspects of medical care, but as being constituent of, and 'hard' factors behind, sickness and healing. A key element in such a project is the development of a new notion of 'translation' in the interdisciplinary space of the medical humanities.

Cura and the chronotopy of care

We will begin to tackle the challenges facing the medical humanities by way of a reading of a myth attributed to the Roman mythographer Hyginus (1960). The protagonist of the myth, the goddess Cura (Care), is traditionally associated with creativity and care, but also with concern and anxiety. Our reading of the myth of Cura draws upon and expands Kristeva's use of the tale in *Hatred and Forgiveness* (2012). Here, Kristeva uses the fable to reflect on the creation of man as a being belonging to different ontological domains and temporal orders. According to Hyginus' anthropogony, Cura crosses a river and on the other side bends down to the earth to pick up a clump of clay. From the clay she shapes a being that will become man. Jove, the celestial god of lightning and thunder, comes along, and Cura asks him to give life to the artefact she has produced. Jove complies, and gives the gift of *spirit* to the shape formed by Cura. But now a quarrel erupts over the name of the new creation. Should it be named after Cura who gave it form or after the male celestial god who gave it spirit? At this stage Tellus, the god of earth, intervenes and claims Cura's creation, arguing that he provided the material from which it was formed in the first place. Saturn, the god of time, settles the matter through *an act of naming*, and by *dividing* and *temporalising* the possession of the various parts that comprise man: Jove is offered man's soul and Tellus his body, after man's death, while Cura will possess the creation in its lifetime, since she made it. Saturn names the new being *homo* because it was originally shaped out of *humus*. According to the myth and the Latin pun that sums up its moral, then, human life as a composite assembly of spiritual (Jove) and material (Tellus) elements is held together by Cura's temporal care.

The myth of Cura has been subject to various literary elaborations and philosophical elucidations, and it has also been read in the context of the medical humanities (Heidegger 1962; Reich 1995; Kleinman and Van Der Geest 2009; Svenaeus 2011). Characteristic of Kristeva's reading, however, is her use of the myth to question the fundamental conceptual distinctions that underpin modern medicine and the medical humanities. Moreover, this reading illuminates what we here will refer to as the chronotopic organisation of care (i.e., its simultaneous temporal and spatial aspects) (Bakhtin 1981). We use this Bakhtinian coinage to draw attention to the manner in which medical research and the practical art of care are assigned not only to separate ontological domains (nature and culture), but also to different *temporal zones*: The first to the universal stasis and Platonic non-time of biomedical evidence, which should apply generally, to all instances; the second to the mundane, intertextual co-creation of meaning in encounters between medical practitioners and patients, which takes place in the singular, biographical time and life-context of individuals.

In Kristeva's rendering, Jove's intervention and Saturn's introduction of the name of man separates *homo* as a *creation* (a state of being) from the continuous process of *creativity* (coming into being), represented by Cura, the initial forming agent and female artist behind the human species. A whole series of binary oppositions, ontological conflicts and wounds, are brought into being by this separation. In a medical context, the binary structure is reflected in a demarcation between *health* as a condition with illness as its deviation, and *healing* as an ongoing process unfolding through time.

Kristeva (2012: 154) uses what she calls the "circumscribed act" of the male gods as an allegory for the cultural distinction between *health* as a "definitive state," and *healing* and *caring* as a durative "process with twists and turns in time." Thus, the myth can be read as an allegory of how health is objectified into a condition of full being (a definitive state) outside time, while illness is conceived as the privation (*steresis*) of a state of health and wellbeing considered as the origin and the norm. By the same token, *cure*—understood as a definitive act recreating a "definitive state" (i.e., health)—is distinguished from *Cura* or what Kristeva refers to as the "durative idea of care." Similarly, medical science concerned with cure (with nature or *physis*, with states of health or illness outside human time) is separated from the humanities concerned with the liminal period between birth and death. In this binary scheme, cure and care, health and healing, medical science and the medical humanities are assigned to different chronotopic zones.

On the one side of this binary structure is the transcendent and universal knowledge, the 'gold standard' in the terminology of evidence-based medicine; on the other, the messy temporal space in which humans live, and where sickness and healing actually occur simultaneously.

To be sure, our intention is not to use the myth to create some kind of alternative 'scientific model' or as 'evidence' of a universal truth of the structure of human existence. Rather, our aim is to use the tale as a yardstick against which certain instituted 'deep structures' of modern medical epistemology and ontology can be measured. By suggesting that Man lives her life in a continuous curative passage from birth to death in which health and sickness alternate, the myth represents a challenge to the binary understanding of sickness and health inherent in modern medicine. A related challenge also becomes evident from this reading: *Biomedicine is in constant need of 'repair,' and it is as an instrument of repairment that the medical humanities are usually conceived.* Even in its most radical versions, the medical humanities are reduced to a soft, 'subjective', and cultural supplement to a stable body of 'objective' biomedical and scientific knowledge, suturing *without challenging* the binary understanding of nature and culture inherent in biomedical thinking.

As Kristeva points out, remedies for the splits between biographical and biological life, *bios* and *zoe*, soul and body, are often found in pharmaceuticals, or in the production of ideal images of 'good living' and model narratives about 'successful patients' ('the integrated disabled person,' the 'empowered' or 'health-literate' patient, and so on) (Kristeva 2012: 157). Through these remedies, the biographical life of the patient is supposed to be reshaped in the image of normative ideal types of biological and healthy life. The subjectivity of the patient is *re-duced*—'led back' into static notions of 'normal' and 'good living.' As a result, the psychic life of the patient is seen as healed only when it disappears, i.e., when subjectivity corresponds with the general norm of 'human life' (Kristeva 2013: 222).

In research and theory, biomedicine also attempts to 'bridge the gap' between *bios* and *zoe* through so-called 'knowledge translation' from general conditions or states of health from the laboratory, a space constructed to be, ideally, outside the cultural time of the living, and back into the singular biography and life-context of the individual patient (Engebretsen, Sandset, and Ødemark 2017). Actually, in addition to 'knowledge translation,' a whole range of prominent medical practices, such as 'health literacy' and 'individualised care' can be seen as 'soft' cultural supplements that aim at reincorporating the individual patient, biographical time, and a 'subjective' perspective in medicine by turning 'cure' into 'care.' All these soft supplements rest upon a distinction between nature and culture, hard and soft science. In accordance with the logic of the supplement, however, these practices also have an implicit potential for undermining the oppositions (Derrida 2016).

Boundary work across the nature–culture divide

Aspects of our approach are related to the so-called 'second wave' of the medical humanities (often referred to as 'critical medical humanities'). Fully in line with this critical agenda, we intend to go beyond the three Es that have been seen as characteristic of the first wave: 'ethics,' 'education,' and 'experience,' to emphasise a fourth E, namely 'entanglement.' Medical humanities, as researchers of the 'second wave' and we understand it, are "deeply and irretrievably *entangled* in the vital, corporeal and physiological commitments of biomedicine" (Fitzgerald and Callard 2016: 35–6). In contrast to the 'second wave,' however, we also insist that tackling this entanglement requires more than the mere application of perspectives *from* the humanities *on* medicine and health care with the aim of fostering more "holistic understandings of the interaction between health, illness and disease" (Hurwitz and Dakin 2009).

The lesson we should learn from Cura is that the humanities, as much as the sciences, are a consequence of the nature–culture divide. The humanities are themselves a product of epistemological and ontological divisions that underpin the current organisation of knowledge, and in this epistemic apparatus they are inscribed on the cultural side of the nature–culture divide. Hence, neither biomedicine nor the humanities can offer 'wholeness' (as 'romantic' and/or holistic notions of medical humanities often assume they can). Accordingly, we do not consider the humanities as a critical and potentially liberating perspective that can be applied *to* medicine as an object in need of repairment. Medical humanities should not be construed as a humanistic perspective *on* medicine. *They should rather be seen as a cross-disciplinary and cross-cultural space for translation and bidirectional critical interrogation of medicine and the humanities across the nature–culture divide.* On the one hand, this implies breaking with the culture–nature dichotomy and considering both the humanities and medicine as bio-cultural practices. On the other hand, it also implies understanding *that boundary work requires boundaries*, and that incommensurability between various partial disciplinary perspectives can, will, and should emerge. Such a bidirectional and translational approach to the medical humanities suggests that the humanities are not only to be considered as a kind of meta-knowledge representing a critical or communicative 'add-on' to the 'pure' biomedical knowledge that is believed to concern and intervene in, health issues 'more directly' at a 'basic' biomedical level. The humanities also address 'hard factors' behind sickness and healing. This does not imply that biomedical approaches should be *reduced* to social or cultural factors considering culture as the real and 'hidden' reason behind the 'construction' of biomedical facts. Rather, cultural aspects of health and illness can never be clearly separated from, and are always intimately intermingled with, their biological 'other.' (A simple case in point is how human living interferes with biological life by provoking resistance against antibiotics or by influencing the spread of malaria and other mosquito-borne diseases through the growth of human settlements.)

What we should maintain from the outset, however, is that biomedicine is not only culturally produced, but that the humanities are also materially productive; they create bodies and physical conditions. Like Cura in Hyginus' tale, cultures create different kinds of bodies and realities with medical implications: cultural discontent can produce pathologies, but increased understanding and analysis of the body as a complex bio-cultural fact can also be a potential source of healing.

The healing powers of translation: the case of Souad

Over the last three years, Kristeva and Moro have explored the pathological and healing powers of culture through their seminar on the 'Need to Believe' aimed at various professionals in the health sector who deal with cross-cultural discontent among adolescents. This seminar explores how health professionals should deal with the 'ideality disorder' of adolescents that follows from an absolute and unsatisfied need for an assimilative investment in an ideal otherness. Our secularised society offers no rites of initiation for these youngsters and they are therefore exposed to 'a traumatic symbolic void' with potential pathological implications.

In *Interpréter le mal radical*, Kristeva (2016) refers to the case of Souad, a teenage girl from a Muslim family who suffered from severe anorexia, "a slow suicide addressed to her family and to the world" that subsequently metamorphosed into radicalisation:

> Souad walled herself up in silence and didn't get off the internet where, with her unknown accomplices, she exchanged furious emails against her family of 'apostates, worse than unbelievers,' and prepared her voyage 'over there,' in order to become the mistress of polygamous combatants, the mother of prolific martyrs or a kamikaze herself.

Souad was at first reticent about psychotherapy, but when confronted with the multicultural psychotherapeutic team, her attitude gradually changed. She started to find pleasure in narrating her life and in expressing her destructive urges and sufferings. Thus, she gradually began to reconnect with the French language. Together with other teenagers supported by the team, she started to attend writing and theatre workshops and to read Arabic poetry translated into French. The translations of the Arabic texts constituted a kind of 'third space' or an 'in-betweenness' in the encounter between the two cultures from which new and hybrid meanings arose. Language, theatre, and poetry now began to fill the 'symbolic void' and undid the nihilism. Roland Barthes (1989) wrote that if you find meaning in the plenitude of a language, "the divine vacuum can no longer threaten." In the case of Souad, her new cultural, symbolic, and linguistic attachments represented a lot more than a soft cultural supplement to her biomedical treatment. Her reinvestment in "the plenitude of a language" became a major creative and healing agency. Through the use and sharing of meaning and the pleasures of language, through conversation, theatre, and poetry, Souad started to re-establish ties to the world and to her own body. Hence, a process of creativity and healing was initiated that encompassed both body and soul.

Towards a translational medical humanities

To further develop and instantiate the reflections above, we are launching a global 'think-tank' on medical humanities where we will invite medical researchers and professionals, humanists, and social scientists to participate. The following fundamental issues will be discussed:

1   A new programme for the medical humanities should involve a radical concern with cultural dimensions of health as more than a 'subjective' dimension outside the 'real' of medical science. We will explore the notion that *all* clinical encounters should be considered as cultural encounters in the sense that they involve translation between health as a biomedical phenomenon and healing as lived experience. Hence, our assumption is that the cultural crossings of care are not an exception but the norm. Given this, every clinical encounter should involve a simultaneous interrogation of the patient's *and* the doctor's co-construction of new and shared meanings which can create realities with medical consequences, not 'mere' symbols of 'real' medical issues (Sturm, Baubet, and Moro 2010). It was precisely such a co-construction of shared meanings—'a hybrid space'—that was achieved successfully in the case of Souad through an act of translation between Arabic and French language. This co-creation *'over here'* in terms of a linguistic and symbolic 'in-betweenness' addressed her anorexia and her desire to go *'over there'*—into the language of ISIL, and the land of biological death.

2   A new programme also implies a deconstruction of the difference between hard and soft science. As shown in the case of Souad, cultural, symbolic, and linguistic attachments have medical and bodily implications. The humanities have creative and healing agency; they are not only instruments of care but also of cure. This materially performative aspect of the humanities as part of the medical humanities constellation needs closer attention and further theorisation. At the same time, the need for, and use of, soft supplements in biomedicine should be further explored both historically and ethnographically. This includes both the study of the adaptation of metaphors and concepts from the human sciences (for instance, 'translation,' 'literacy,' and 'empowerment') into medical discourse, and the implications of these transfers. Added to this is the translation of such practices to so-called 'global health' contexts, i.e., different cultural localities around the world. On another level, we

should also constantly keep in mind the material, biological, and ecological conditions on which cultural interpretations and translations are based. In the singular case of Souad, her anorexia and her subsequent health improvements also constitute a biomedical point of reference—a kind of inner limit—against which the legitimacy, relevance, and success of the different cultural exchanges with the team and the translations between languages must be assessed.

3   The deconstruction suggested above also presupposes a radical questioning of the medical cultures behind the production and construal of evidence in medicine. As observed, the dominant evidence-based approach in modern medicine runs the risk of exalting biology into an 'essential Being' and a normative stasis that turns the sick into persons who "lack [. . .] certain biological aptitudes" (Kristeva 2013: 227). Based on this understanding of disease as a lack of full being (*steresis*), sickness and difference are reduced to *general* 'categories of difference' where social and biological 'deviants' are seen as different in the same way, i.e., as deviants from a social and/or biological standard. Left alone, without being interrupted by a sense for the singularity of the individual case and its life-context, biomedical discourse "blends all disabled people together without taking into consideration the specificity of their sufferings and exclusions" (Kristeva 2012: 36). As an alternative to the epistemology of universal categories re-ducing difference to the same, the medical humanities should consequently contribute to a "singularised" approach to medicine (Engebretsen 2016). A singularised approach, however, is also different from merely considering the individual as a bearer of social/cultural meanings by mobilising 'patients' preferences' in clinical decisions. The singularised approach and the possibility for symbolic reinvestment and sharing offered to Souad, for instance, are not equal to a rational choice between different treatment options. Nor is this the same as reducing the individual to biology by using the "individual's genetic profile to guide decisions made in regard to the prevention, diagnosis, and treatment of disease" (McMullan 2014: 4). On the contrary, a singularised approach is contradictory to any reductionism—psychological, cultural, or biological. Most radically, it implies acknowledging that *evidence* itself is fundamentally singular; it is always evidence *for* a *particular* decision with reference to a general category in a concrete situation. Thus, general categories are also essential in evidence-based decisions—and the notion of the singular, as Hegel underscored at the outset of the *Phenomenology*, is already itself a general notion. Knowledge about universal categories and generalised pathologies is thus needed both to identify the singular case *as* singular (i.e., as distinct from a general category) and to create a linguistic, co-created place for transactions and translations between patients and medical specialists. Such general knowledge frames evidence-based decisions made locally, with reference to the particular patient, but should not be mistaken as evidence *per se*. Rather than an act of application, evidence-basing should be considered as a process of *differentiation*—it is the process of teasing out the *differences* between the singular case and the various referential spaces (laboratories, mice models, trials, systematic reviews, etc.) in which knowledge about a treatment is produced. Evidence *is* this difference between the specific and the general and not the application of a norm.

By beginning to tackle such radical questions, our 'think-tank' aims to be the impetus for a fundamental revisioning of the role of the medical humanities in relation to medical *and* humanistic research and practice. In this new intellectual and practical space, the medical humanities should be seen as a cross-disciplinary and cross-cultural space for translation and bidirectional critical interrogation of both biomedicine (simplistic reductions of life to biology) and the humanities (simplistic reductions of suffering and health injustice to cultural relativism).

Acknowledgement

This chapter builds on, and expands, an argument first presented in a paper published in the *BMJ Medical Humanities* (Kristeva et al. 2018).

References

Bakhtin M. 1981. *Forms of time and of the chronotope in the novel, in the dialogical imagination: Four essays.* Austin, TX: University of Texas Press.

Barthes R. 1989. *Sades, fourier, loyola.* Berkeley, CA: University of California Press.

Derrida J. 2016. *Of grammatology.* Baltimore, MD: JHU Press.

Engebretsen E. 2016. The medical concept of evidence and the irreducible singularity of being. Keynote speech at the Kristeva Circle in Stockholm. Available at: www.kristeva.fr/eivind-engebretsen-the-medical-concept-of-evidence.html. Last accessed: 31 March 2018.

Engebretsen E, Sandset TJ, Ødemark J. Expanding the knowledge translation metaphor. *Health Research Policy and Systems.* 2017; 15: 19.

Fitzgerald D, Callard F. 2016. Entangling the medical humanities. In: A. Whitehead, A. Woods (eds.) *The Edinburgh Companion to the Critical Medical Humanities.* Edinburgh: Edinburgh University Press, 35–49.

Heidegger M. 1962. *Being and time.* New York, NY: Harper.

Hurwitz B, Dakin P. Welcome developments in UK medical humanities. *Journal of the Royal Society of Medicine.* 2009; 102: 84–5.

Hyginus, Fabulae 200–277. 1960. *The myths of hyginus, publications in humanistic studies*, no. 34. Lawrence, MO: University of Kansas Press.

Kleinman A, Van Der Geest S. 'Care' in health care. Remaking the moral world of medicine. *Medische Antropologie.* 2009; 21: 159–68.

Kristeva J. 2003. *Lettre au président de la république sur les citoyens en situation de handicap: à l'usage de ceux qui le sont et de ceux qui ne le sont pas.* Paris: Fayard.

Kristeva J. 2011. *This incredible need to believe.* New York, NY: Columbia University Press.

Kristeva J. 2012. *Hatred and forgiveness.* New York, NY: Columbia University Press.

Kristeva J. A tragedy and a dream: Disability revisited. *Irish Theological Quarterly.* 2013; 78: 219–30.

Kristeva J. 2016. Interpréter le mal radical ('Interpreting Radical Evil'). *L'Infini.* Available at: http://www.kristeva.fr/le-mal-radical.html. Last accessed: 31 March 2018.

Kristeva, J, Moro, MR, Ødemark, J, Engebretsen, E. Cultural crossings of care: An appeal to the medical humanities. *BMJ Medical Humanities.* 2018; 44: 55–8.

McMullan D. What is personalized medicine? *Genome.* 2014: 32–9. Available at: http://genomemag.com/what-is-personalized-medicine. Last accessed: 31 March 2018.

Napier AD, Ancarno C, Butler B, et al. *The Lancet commissions: Culture and health. The Lancet.* 2014; 384: 1607–39.

Reich W. 1995. *Classic article: History of the notion of care.* New York, NY: Simon and Schuster.

Sturm G, Baubet T, Moro MR. Culture, trauma, and subjectivity: The French ethnopsychoanalytic approach. *Traumatology.* 2010; 16: 27–38.

Svenaeus F. Illness as unhomelike being-in-the-world: Heidegger and the phenomenology of medicine. *Medicine, Health Care and Philosophy.* 2011; 14: 333–43.

3

MEDICAL WORK IN TRANSITION

Towards collaborative and transformative expertise

Yrjö Engeström

This chapter is dedicated to the memory of my sister Anne Piira (1947–2018).

Introduction

Forces and demands from multiple directions mould medical work and expertise. A foundational change is going on in the overall object of medicine: the growth of chronic illnesses that bundle together into complex forms of multi-morbidity (DeVol et al. 2007; Bodenheimer, Chen and Bennett, 2009; Afshar et al. 2015; Milani and Lavie 2015; Moffat and Mercer 2015; Pefoyo et al. 2015). Whereas this would seem to require longer time perspectives as well as broader collaborative and interdisciplinary approaches from practitioners and their organisations, two other forces are often experienced as pulling in quite different, if not conflicting, directions. The rules of medicine are increasingly penetrated by market-oriented business calculations and managerialism that tend to favour rapid turnover and relatively short-term profits (Pollock 2004; Giaimo 2009; Hunter 2013; Beck and Melo 2014; Gilbert, Clarke and Leaver 2014). And the instruments of medicine are increasingly framed in terms of rationalisation and standardisation, again notions that tend to favour relatively linear and pre-packaged processes and procedures rather than horizontally co-constructed care trajectories and long-term impact (Timmermans and Berg 2010; Martin et al. 2017). Thus, we may tentatively identify systemic contradictions between the major force of change in the object on the one hand and the dominant tendencies in the rules and instruments on the other. These contradictions are marked with double-headed arrows in Figure 3.1. The components of community and division of labour in Figure 3.1 are left open, with question marks indicating widespread uncertainty in the search for optimal organisation of health care services.

In this chapter, I will argue that this contradictory state of affairs calls for deliberate and persistent efforts to redefine medical expertise so that practitioners, their organisations and society at large may begin to see and pursue expansive ways out of the seemingly uncontrollable situation. My argument is not aimed at proposing specific policies and models of health care. My aim is to chart a zone of proximal development for building the kind of medical expertise that will allow the creation and implementation of robust emancipatory solutions, not as policy dictates from above but as evolving practices generated and appropriated from below.

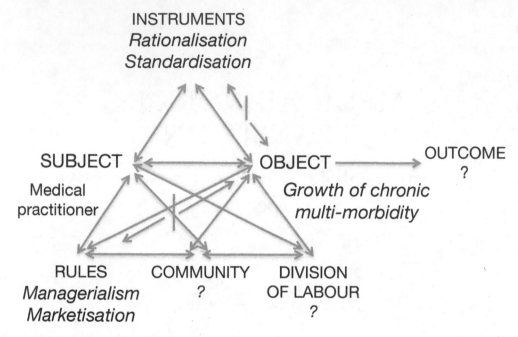

Figure 3.1 Forces and contradictions of change in medical work and expertise

To construct a zone of proximal development for medical work and expertise, we need to depict a field of identifiable historical types of this activity. In Figure 3.2, the vertical dimension represents movement from individual expertise towards collective expertise; the horizontal dimension represents movement from learning for stability towards learning for change. The historical starting point in the lower-left quadrant is professional craft medicine conducted by an individual expert and strongly bound to the expectation of stability. The two dominant forms of medical work today (in the upper-left and lower-right quadrants, respectively) are hierarchically organised medicine and market-driven medicine.

Various relatively weakly conceptualised forms of collaborative community are emerging in the upper-right quadrant, as if through the cracks that open up between and within the two dominant types (Engeström et al. 2010). Movement from one type to another is not linear or automatic. There are clashes, retreats and detours, and all four types continue to influence medical practice today. Yet I argue that the emerging collaborative and transformative expertise is a real historical possibility and an avenue towards expansive resolution of the contradictions summarised in Figure 3.1.

Moving towards collaborative and transformative expertise can be facilitated by means of appropriate conceptual instruments. Such instruments should pave the way for theoretical understanding and practical construction of new forms of expert work. They may be seen as spearheads into the zone of proximal development of medical expertise. I suggest three such spearheads: (1) object-oriented and contradiction-driven activity systems as locus of expertise, (2) knotworking as emerging forms of collaborative expertise and (3) expansive learning as emerging modes of transformative expertise. In the next sections of this chapter, I will examine each of these spearheads in turn.

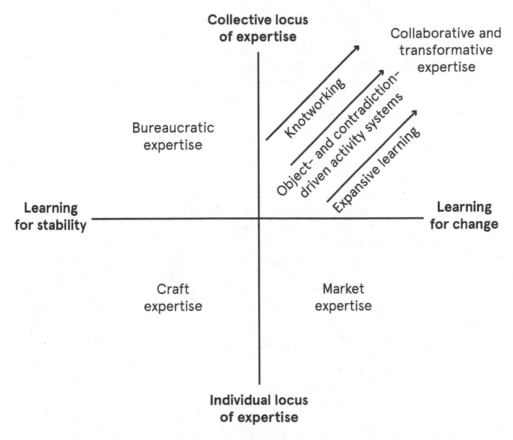

Figure 3.2   The zone of proximal development of medical expertise (Engeström 2018: 256)

Much of the empirical and interventionist research I have conducted in different arenas of medical practice over some 30 years is brought together in my book *Expertise in Transition: Expansive Learning in Medical Work* (Engeström 2018). Taking a step forward from that body of research, in this chapter I will illuminate the three spearheads by briefly reviewing recent activity-theoretical studies published by others, pertinent to each of the spearheads in turn. I will further concretise the spearheads by discussing findings obtained by my own research group in a series of studies on home care in the city of Helsinki. Although home care is not at the core of traditional medicine, I will show that it is relevant for the emergence of new forms of collaborative and transformative expertise. New patterns of activity often take shape in the margins of a complex field of activities, such as health care.

Expertise as object-oriented activity systems

In activity theory, a collective, artefact-mediated and object-oriented activity system, seen in its network relations to other activity systems, is taken as the prime unit of analysis. Goal-directed individual and group actions and action clusters, as well as automatic operations, are relatively independent but subordinate units of analysis, eventually understandable only when interpreted against the background of entire activity systems. Activity systems realise and reproduce themselves by generating actions and operations. Figure 3.1 above is built on a general model of the structure of an activity system (Engeström 2015: 63).

The object of activity is always under construction, interpreted and moulded by the actors involved in the activity. Object-oriented actions are, explicitly or implicitly, characterised by ambiguity, surprise, interpretation, sense making and potential for change. There are multiple mediations in an activity system. Instruments mediate the subject and the object, or the actor and the environment, including material tools as well as signs, symbols and representations of various kinds. The less visible social mediators of activity—rules, community and division of labour—are depicted at the bottom of the model. Between the components of the system, there are continuous transitions and transformations. The activity system incessantly reconstructs itself.

Contradictions are the prime source of change and development in activity systems. Contradictions are not the same as problems or conflicts. Contradictions are historically accumulating structural tensions within and between activity systems. An activity system is constantly working through tensions and contradictions within and between its elements. Contradictions cannot be directly observed. They must be inferred from historical analysis and from empirical analysis of their mundane manifestations, such as dilemmas, conflicts and double binds (Engeström and Sannino 2011). Thus, the identification of contradictions in activity systems is always a working hypothesis, to be tested and elaborated on. Expertise resides in object-oriented collective activity systems mediated by cultural instruments and cannot be meaningfully reduced to individual competency. Expertise is inherently heterogeneous and increasingly dependent on crossing boundaries, generating hybrids and forming alliances across contexts and domains.

In medical work, a natural starting point for an activity-theoretical analysis of expertise is to examine the interplay of the activity system of the physician and the activity system of the patient. The constellation becomes more complex when we analyse the interplay between the activity systems of a primary care health centre, a hospital and a patient, for example. An activity-theoretical framework for the study of expertise implies a shift in emphasis from what goes on inside the head of the subject to what goes on in the object. Therefore, the study of expertise should re-focus on the objects of expert work. A *trajectory of care* that transcends institutional and professional boundaries is a promising way to conceptualise and operationalise the object of medical work.

Several studies of medical activity systems, their objects and their contradictions have been published in the past 10 years or so. De Feijter et al. (2011) analysed the experiences of final-year undergraduate medical students concerning patient safety. They found that the simultaneous occurrence of two activities, namely learning to be a doctor and delivering safe patient care, generated contradictions that could be approached as potential learning opportunities. Focusing on contradictions in the object of the activity, Greig, Entwistle and Beech (2012) published an ethnographic study of primary health care teams responding to a policy aim of reducing inappropriate hospital admissions of older people by the "best practice" of rapid response teams. Teodorczuk et al. (2015: 757) analysed what they called "practice gaps" in hospital care of dementia and delirium. They found that "the primary object of activity in relation to managing successfully the confused older patient is improving the care of the confused patient through learning about the patient," and identified a number of systemic contradictions behind the practice gaps.

In recent years my own research group has conducted a series of longitudinal intervention studies on the home care of elderly clients with multiple illnesses in the city of Helsinki (Nummijoki and Engeström 2010; Engeström, Nummijoki and Sannino 2012; Engeström, Kajamaa and Nummijoki 2015; Nummijoki, Engeström and Sannino 2018). We focused our work on the implementation of the *Mobility Agreement*, a new practice and artefact aimed at facilitating the physical mobility of elderly clients by means of regular exercises embedded in everyday chores at home. On the basis of our studies, we modelled the activity systems of the client and the caregiver, as well as their mobility-related contradictions, as depicted in Figure 3.3.

The tension between the need for safety and the craving for autonomy, or more concretely between a fear of falling and a desire for movement, is a persistent primary contradiction in the life activities of frail, elderly home care clients. Correspondingly, the primary contradiction in the activity of home care workers appears as tensions between the desire to stick to the prescribed standard tasks of hygiene, nutrition and medication and the desire to respond to the client's needs in a more proactive way, activating the client by working *with* rather than doing chores *for* him or her. These primary contradictions are depicted within the objects of the respective activity systems in Figure 3.3. Put together, they can be translated into the persistent institutional contradiction between the immediate cost efficiency and long-term effectiveness of home care. In Figure 3.3, the Mobility Agreement appears as a new instrument that aggravates the latent primary contradictions, generating secondary contradictions between the new instrument and old rules and division of labour in the two interacting activity systems. These secondary contradictions are marked with lightning-shaped, double-headed arrows in Figure 3.3.

Expertise as knotworking

The notion of 'knot' refers to rapidly pulsating, distributed and partially improvised orchestration of collaborative performance between otherwise loosely connected actors and activity systems. In other words, knotworking is characterised by a pulsating movement of tying, untying and retying together otherwise separate threads of activity. The tying and dissolution of a knot of collaborative work is not reducible to any specific individual or fixed organisational entity as the centre of control. The centre does not hold. The locus of initiative changes from moment to moment within a knotworking sequence. Thus, knotworking cannot be adequately analysed from the point of view of an assumed centre of coordination and control, or as an additive sum of the separate perspectives of individuals or institutions contributing to it. The unstable knot itself needs to be made the focus of analysis.

Primarily due to the emergence of new types of objects, expert work is undergoing a historical transformation from various forms of craft, standardised mass production and mass customisation towards co-configuration, the interactional core of which is negotiated knotworking (Engeström 2008). In health care, this transition is driven by the increasing prevalence and importance of chronic illnesses and co-morbidity, the appearance of multiple simultaneous illnesses in a patient.

Knotworking is a concept in the making. It needs to be made concrete by enacting it. Knotworking cannot be easily formalised and stabilised with the help of rules and regulations. The very idea of knotworking is based on the dialectics of improvisation and long-term planning. In a divided terrain of multiple activity systems, knotworking is facilitated by certain conditions. First of all, the potentially shared object and the consequences of its fragmentation need to be made visible and analysable. Knotworking can only be accomplished by focusing on and expanding the object. In health care this means, above all, making the patient's care experiences visible. This is a demanding condition as critical visibilisation may threaten the dominant rhetorics of competence, quality and responsible professionalism.

Therefore, a second condition is needed, namely the establishment of relatively safe spaces and times of collective reflection, debate and analysis. These may take the shape of relatively permanent "trading zones" between organisational units and professional groups (Gorman 2010),

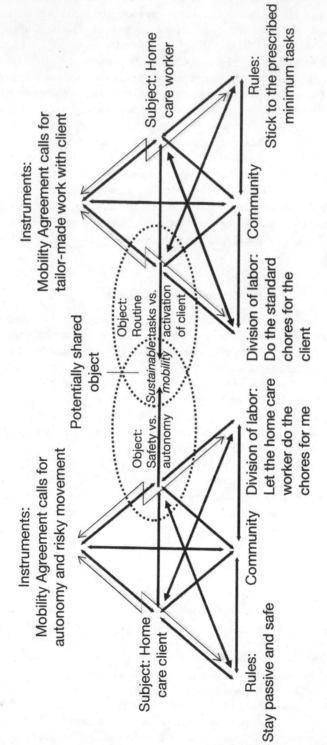

Figure 3.3 The activity systems and mobility-related contradictions of home care encounters (Nummijoki, Engeström and Sannino, 2018: 230)

or more intensive "microcosms" for practising knotworking, such as the Change Laboratory interventions (Sannino, Engeström and Lemos 2016). The purpose of such spaces is *not* to reach full agreement or unanimity:

> At root, the relevant aspect of exchange is this: what an object means to me when I give it to you may very well not be what you, as the recipient, understand that object to connote. What matters is coordination, *not* a full fledged agreement about signification.
>
> *(Galison 2010: 35)*

To reach coordination, the participants need to negotiate. To negotiate successfully, they need a minimal common language. This is the third condition of knotworking. A common language between different kinds of expertise and different positions can emerge out of an interplay between a conceptual framework such as the activity-theoretical apparatus used in this chapter *and* the specific repertoires of the participating domains or traditions of expertise.

Varpio et al. (2008: S79) used the lens of knotworking in their analysis of the role of interprofessional communication in medical errors. The authors pointed out that when rotating members of interprofessional teams share patient information across multiple communication tools, confusion or errors generated in communication tools can easily become sources of latent medical errors:

> To avoid the generation of such errors [. . .] professionals must take more complexity into account. They need to consider the distributed knots of activity involved in the patient's care and construct solutions that extend across multiple knots of team membership and activity.

Bleakley (2013, 2014) published careful in-depth analyses of the potentials and limitations of knotworking in the changing landscape of 'liquid' health care. He concluded that knotworking is contrasted with networking "not to oppose the two but to draw a distinction between forms of work that actively strive for stability and forms that show high tolerance of ambiguity and high levels of improvization where conditions demand this" (Bleakley 2013: 25).

Informed by activity theory and the idea of knotworking, Lingard et al. (2012) conducted an ethnographic study of teamwork in a solid organ transplant unit in a tertiary care hospital. Focusing on detailed analysis of the care of one patient, Mr Hearn, the authors concluded:

> The fluidity of roles, and the shifting and overlapping of the locus of authority are among the factors that create complexity and give rise to the need for extensive knotworking in the Mr Hearn case. Although the fluidity and overlap in roles create conflict among the team, this conflict is not 'avoidable' per se; it is the sine qua non of collaboration and knotworking strategies allow the team to work through the conflict productively.
>
> *(ibid.: 876)*

Larsen et al. (2017) used the concept of knotworking in their analysis of the role of learning goals in clinical education. They found that learning goals are potentially powerful tools to mediate interactions between students, supervisors and patients, and to reconcile contradictions that arose when the desired outcomes of student skill development, grading and patient care were not aligned. However, for new collaborations to take place, both students and supervisors had to engage with the goals, and the necessary patients needed to be present.

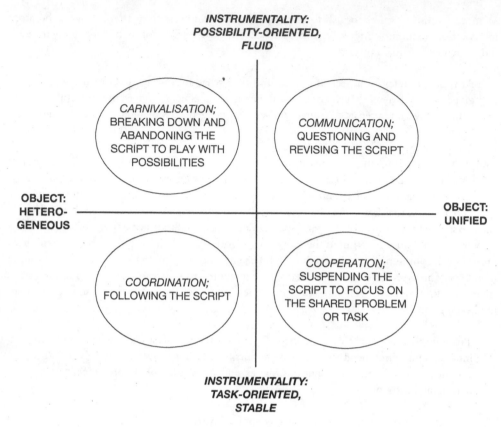

Figure 3.4 Types of collaboration in knotworking encounters (Engeström et al. 2015: 108)

In our own work on home care encounters, we have further developed the concept of knotworking by identifying four qualitatively different modes of collaboration that may occur within knotworking efforts, namely coordination, cooperation, communication and carnivalisation (Figure 3.4). In **coordination**, each participant typically has his or her own object; thus the object is heterogeneous to begin with, but the prescribed script followed by the participants conceals the heterogeneity. In **cooperation**, the participants cohere around a shared object, temporarily abandoning or going beyond the prescribed script—but the effort is limited to relatively well-bounded tasks or problems. In **communication**, the participants, focusing on a shared object, engage in questioning and revising the entire script of their collaboration. In **carnivalisation**, as the script falls apart, the concealed or suspended heterogeneity of objects becomes visible and is playfully developed by means of some open-ended and fluid instrumentality, such as photography and pictures in the home care encounters we analysed (Engeström et al. 2015; Kajamaa and Lahtinen 2016).

Expertise as expansive learning

The theory of expansive learning is aimed at understanding and fostering learning processes that go beyond the information given and generate new solutions, models and concepts for the activity in which the learning occurs (Engeström 2015; see also Engeström and Sannino 2010). In this sense, expansive learning is "learning what is not yet there" (Engeström 2016).

Expansive learning follows the dialectical movement of ascending from the abstract to the concrete. This is a movement of grasping the essence of an object by tracing and reproducing the logic of its development—its historical formation through the emergence and resolution of its inner contradictions. A new theoretical idea or concept is initially produced in the form of an abstract, simple explanatory relationship, a 'germ cell.' This initial abstraction is, step-by-step, enriched and transformed into a concrete system of multiple, constantly developing manifestations. In an expansive learning cycle, the initial simple idea is transformed into a complex object, into a new form of practice. At the same time, the cycle produces a new theoretical concept—theoretically grasped practice—concrete in systemic richness and multiplicity of manifestations.

In this framework, abstract refers to partial, separated from the concrete whole. In empirical thinking based on comparisons and classifications, abstractions capture arbitrary, only formally interconnected properties. In dialectical-theoretical thinking, based on ascending from the abstract to the concrete, an abstraction captures the smallest and simplest, genetically primary unit of the whole functionally interconnected system.

The expansive cycle begins with individual subjects questioning the accepted practice, and it gradually expands into a collective movement or institution. The cycle consists of expansive learning actions. In an ideal-typical expansive learning cycle, the following seven learning actions (Table 3.1) may be identified:

The expansive transformation of the object of medical work proceeds in multiple dimensions. In the socio-spatial dimension, it typically means shifting the focus from an individual patient's specific symptom or illness towards the complex webs of life and care of the patient. In the temporal dimension, it means moving the focus from the singular care episode or visit towards a longitudinal trajectory of illness and care. A trajectory encompasses both the object's movement in time, and the interconnections and actions in space, between the participating activity systems that make the movement happen. In other words, the concept of trajectory is spatio-temporal to begin with. The two foundational dimensions of space and time need to be complemented with two additional dimensions of expansion: the moral-ideological and the systemic-developmental. When a patient's entire care trajectory is taken as the object, physicians

Table 3.1 The key seven learning actions in an ideal-typical expansive learning cycle

1	**Questioning**, criticising, or rejecting some aspects of the accepted practice and existing wisdom.
2	**Analysing** the situation. Analysis involves mental, discursive or practical transformation of the situation to find out causes or explanatory mechanisms. One type of analysis is historical-genetic; it seeks to explain the situation by tracing its origins and evolution. Another type of analysis is actual-empirical; it seeks to explain the situation by constructing a picture of its inner systemic relations.
3	**Modelling** the newly found explanatory relationship through some publicly observable and transmittable medium. This involves constructing an explicit, simplified model of the new idea that explains and offers a solution to the problematic situation.
4	**Examining** the model—running, operating and experimenting on it to fully grasp its dynamics, potential and limitations.
5	**Implementing** the model by means of practical applications, enrichments and conceptual extensions.
6	**Reflecting** on, and evaluating, the process.
7	**Consolidating** and generalising the outcomes into a new and stable form of practice.

and nurses from different specialties, levels and organisations of medicine begin to interfere with each other. Fixed hierarchies and turf boundaries are shaken. Power and responsibility need to be re-negotiated and re-defined. Similarly, far-reaching consequences of mundane care-related decisions are made visible. When daily work routines are negotiated and debated, their systemic-developmental reasons and implications are articulated.

Expansive learning is two-faced. On the one hand, it is a conceptual framework for describing and analysing unusually radical processes of collective learning in which patterns of practices are qualitatively changed as new theoretical concepts are created and implemented. On the other hand, it is a conceptual toolkit for intentional formative interventions aimed at revealing potentials for such radical learning and reorganisation of practices. The *Change Laboratory* (Engeström 2011; Sannino, Engeström and Lemos 2016) is a well-known formative intervention method that my research group has used in multiple health care settings.

Bleakley (2006) introduced the notion of expansive learning to the community of medical education scholars. O'Keefe et al. (2016) used the framework of expansive learning to examine and assess extended collective learning efforts in a dental clinic, a community aged care facility and a rural hospital. The authors found that two of the three sites could not develop a successful implementation plan for their ideas. The expansive learning actions of modelling and testing new solutions were not achieved and the participants were unable, collectively, to reassess and reinterpret the object of their activities.

Skipper, Musaeus and Nœhr (2016) conducted a Change Laboratory intervention aimed at analysing and redesigning the outpatient clinic in a paediatric department of a hospital. The study was a collaborative effort with the doctors of the department, motivated by a perceived failure to integrate the activities of the outpatient clinic, patient care and training of residents. The ultimate goal of the intervention was to create improved care for patients through resident learning and development. The Change Laboratory sessions resulted in a joint action plan for the outpatient clinic structured around three themes: (1). Before: Preparation, expectations and introduction; (2). During: Structural context and resources; and (3). After: Follow-up and feedback. The authors pointed out that the participating doctors must be motivated to uncover inherent contradictions in their medical activity systems of which care and learning are both part.

In our research on home care, we conducted a Change Laboratory intervention among the home care managers of the city of Helsinki, aimed at generating a service palette that could facilitate movement towards more proactive and collaborative care practices (Engeström and Sannino 2011). A key new component in the service palette was the Mobility Agreement mentioned earlier. We applied the theory of expansive learning in ascending from the abstract to the concrete in compact mini-cycles of learning that took place in home care encounters. Here, the new Mobility Agreement was introduced and implemented in practice.

In a detailed analysis of the expansive mini-cycle of an elderly patient called 'Anne' we identified *standing up from the chair* as the germ cell of sustainable mobility for the elderly home care client (Figure 3.5). This is both a simple physical movement and a verbalised idea. Such an expansive germ cell is an internally contradictory unity of opposites; in this case, a contradictory unity of safety and autonomy, or fear of falling and need to move.

In the case of Anne, the discovery and conscious implementation of the germ cell led to multiple trails of enrichment and expansion in the life of the client, ranging from improved posture to regular walks, purposeful setting of the table in a way that required repeated standing up from the chair and even teaching one's relatives to conduct mobility exercises (Figure 3.6). Such trails signify ascending to the concrete and the stabilisation of a lived concept of sustainable mobility.

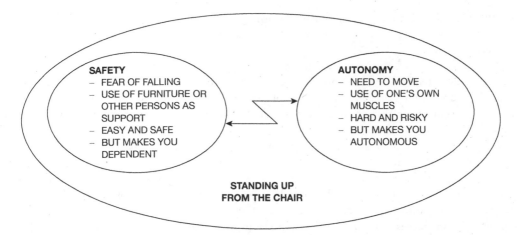

Figure 3.5 Standing up from the chair as the germ cell of sustainable mobility (Engeström, Nummijoki and Sannino 2012: 293)

We observed also a number of home care encounters in which expansive learning was blocked or did not take place. To understand these encounters, we needed to analyse both the learning cycle of the client and the learning cycle of the home care nurse in the interplay.

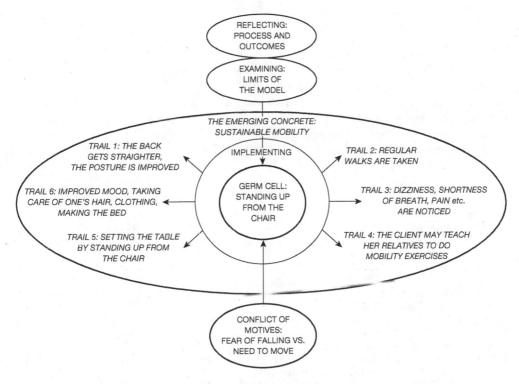

Figure 3.6 Ascending from the abstract to the concrete in the formation of the concept of sustainable physical mobility in home care for the elderly (Engeström, Nummijoki and Sannino, 2012: 304)

This led to the identification of defensive learning actions and cycles that could be analysed by translating the expansive learning actions into their opposites (Nummijoki, Engeström and Sannino 2018).

The fact that both the home care nurse and the elderly client may engage either in a predominantly defensive, or a predominantly expansive, learning cycle should alert us to the fact that in many learning processes it is not at all simple to determine who is teaching, leading or guiding whom. Even though home care encounters have an in-built asymmetry between the potentially powerful practitioner and potentially powerless elderly client, when the learning challenge requires reorientation from both parties, the power relations seem to become much more open-ended and mutable. For example, we saw instances of the client pushing or pulling the practitioner into expansive learning actions in spite of the overall defensive orientation of the latter. This study indicates that more research is needed to deepen our understanding of the dynamics of interacting cycles of learning in multi-learner settings. Expertise is not the sole property of the professional practitioner; it resides in collaborative forms of activity in which lay clients and patients play indispensable roles.

Conclusion

Collaborative and transformative expertise emerges through mundane daily decisions and actions taken by practitioners and their patients and clients. Such a transformation involves facing difficult contradictions and building coalitions from the ground up. It is a process of traversing a collective zone of proximal development, with few ready-made signposts and lots of uncertainties and struggles.

I began this chapter by pointing out crucial contradictions in today's medical work (Figure 3.1). The arguments presented above indicate that we need to generate powerful alternatives to the instruments and rules currently dominating the field of medicine. Instruments of rationalisation and standardisation are not enough and can become outright destructive. We need to complement them with instrumentalities such as negotiated agreements and representations of illness and care that allow competent dialogue across divides between specialties and between professionals and patients. Similarly, the rules of managerialism and marketisation need to be complemented, if not replaced, with rules of common good, participation and reciprocity.

References

Afshar S, Roderick PJ, Kowal P, et al. Multimorbidity and the inequalities of global ageing: A cross-sectional study of 28 countries using the World Health Surveys. *BMC Public Health*. 2015; 15: 776.

Beck M, Melo S. 2014. *Quality management and managerialism in healthcare: A critical historical survey*. New York, NY: Springer.

Bleakley A. Broadening conceptions of learning in medical education: The message from teamworking. *Medical Education*, 2006; 40: 150–7.

Bleakley A. Working in "teams" in an era of "liquid" healthcare: What is the use of theory? *Journal of Interprofessional Care*. 2013; 27: 18–26.

Bleakley A. 2014. *Patient-centred medicine in transition: The heart of the matter*. New York, NY: Springer.

Bodenheimer T, Chen E, Bennett HD. Confronting the growing burden of chronic disease: Can the US health care workforce do the job? *Health Affairs*. 2009; 28: 64–74.

DeVol R, Bedroussian A, Charuworn A, et al. 2007. *An unhealthy America: The economic burden of chronic disease*. Santa Monica, CA: The Milken Institute.

Engeström Y. 2008. *From teams to knots: Activity-theoretical studies of collaboration and learning at work*. Cambridge: Cambridge University Press.

Engeström Y. From design experiments to formative interventions. *Theory and Psychology*. 2011; 21: 598–628.

Engeström Y. 2015. *Learning by expanding: An activity-theoretical approach to developmental research*. 2nd edition. Cambridge: Cambridge University Press.

Engeström Y. 2016. *Studies in expansive learning: Learning what is not yet there*. Cambridge: Cambridge University Press.

Engeström Y. 2018. *Expertise in transition: Expansive learning in medical work*. Cambridge: Cambridge University Press.

Engeström Y, Kajamaa A, Kerosuo H, Laurila P. 2010. Process enhancement versus community building: Transcending the dichotomy through expansive learning. In: K Yamazumi (ed.) *Activity theory and fostering learning: Developmental interventions in education and work*. Osaka: Center for Human Activity Theory, Kansai University, 1–28.

Engeström Y, Kajamaa A, Lahtinen P, Sannino A. Toward a grammar of collaboration. *Mind, Culture, and Activity*. 2015; 22: 92–111.

Engeström Y, Kajamaa A, Nummijoki J. Double stimulation in everyday work: Critical encounters between home care workers and their elderly clients. *Learning, Culture and Social Interaction*. 2015; 4: 48–61.

Engeström, Y, Nummijoki J, Sannino A. Embodied germ cell at work: Building an expansive concept of physical mobility in home care. *Mind, Culture, and Activity*. 2012; 19: 287–309.

Engeström Y, Sannino A. Studies of expansive learning: Foundations, findings and future challenges. *Educational Research Review*. 2010; 5: 1–24.

Engeström Y, Sannino A. Discursive manifestations of contradictions in organizational change efforts: A methodological framework. *Journal of Organizational Change Management*. 2011; 24: 368–87.

de Feijter JM, de Grave WS, Dornan T, et al. Students' perceptions of patient safety during the transition from undergraduate to postgraduate training: An activity theory analysis. *Advances in Health Sciences Education*. 2011; 16: 347–58.

Galison P. 2010. Trading with the enemy. In: ME Gorman (ed.) *Trading zones and interactional expertise: Creating new kinds of collaboration*. Cambridge, MA: MIT Press, 25–52.

Giaimo S. 2009. *Markets and medicine: The politics of health care reform in Britain, Germany, and the United States*. Ann Arbor, MI: University of Michigan Press.

Gilbert BJ, Clarke E, Leaver L. Morality and markets in the NHS. *International Journal of Health Policy and Management*. 2014; 3: 371.

Gorman ME. (ed.) 2010. *Trading zones and interactional expertise: Creating new kinds of collaboration*. Cambridge. MA: MIT Press.

Greig G, Entwistle VA, Beech N. Addressing complex healthcare problems in diverse settings: Insights from activity theory. *Social Science & Medicine*. 2012; 74: 305–12.

Hunter DJ. 2013, 2nd ed. From tribalism to corporatism: The continuing managerial challenge to medical dominance. In: D Kelleher, J Gabe, G Williams (eds.) *Challenging medicine*. London: Routledge, 35–57.

Kajamaa A, Lahtinen P. Carnivalization as a new mode of collaboration. *Journal of Workplace Learning*. 2016; 28: 188–205.

Larsen DP, Wesevich A, Lichtenfeld J, et al. Tying knots: An activity theory analysis of student learning goals in clinical education. *Medical Education*. 2017; 51: 687–98.

Lingard L, McDougall A, Levstik M, et al. Representing complexity well: A story about teamwork, with implications for how we teach collaboration. *Medical Education*. 2012; 46: 869–77.

Martin GP, Kocman D, Stephens T, et al. Pathways to professionalism? Quality improvement, care pathways, and the interplay of standardisation and clinical autonomy. *Sociology of Health and Illness*. 2017; 39: 1314–29.

Milani RV, Lavie CJ. Health care 2020: Reengineering health care delivery to combat chronic disease. *The American Journal of Medicine*. 2015; 128: 337–43.

Moffat K, Mercer SW. Challenges of managing people with multimorbidity in today's healthcare systems. *BMC Family Practice*. 2015; 16: 129.

Nummijoki J, Engeström Y. 2010. Towards co-configuration in home care of the elderly. In: H Daniels, A Edwards, Y Engeström, et al. (eds.) *Activity theory in practice: Promoting learning across boundaries and agencies*. London: Routledge, 49–71.

Nummijoki J, Engeström Y, Sannino A. (2018). Defensive and expansive cycles of learning: A study of home care encounters. *Journal of the Learning Sciences*. 2018; 27: 224–64.

O'Keefe M, Wade V, McAllister S, et al. Improving management of student clinical placements: Insights from activity theory. *BMC Medical Education*. 2016; 16: 219.

Pefoyo AJK., Bronskill SE, Gruneir A, et al. The increasing burden and complexity of multimorbidity. *BMC Public Health*. 2015; 15: 415.

Pollock AM. NHS plc: The privatisation of our health care. *BMJ*. 2004; 329: 862.

Sannino A, Engeström Y, Lemos M. Formative interventions for expansive learning and transformative agency. *Journal of the Learning Sciences*. 2016; 25: 599–633.

Skipper M, Musaeus P, Nœhr SB. The paediatric Change Laboratory: Optimising postgraduate learning in the outpatient clinic. *BMC Medical Education*. 2016; 16: 42.

Teodorczuk A, Mukaetova-Ladinska E, Corbett S, Welfare M. Deconstructing dementia and delirium hospital practice: Using cultural historical activity theory to inform education approaches. *Advances in Health Sciences Education*. 2015; 20: 745–64.

Timmermans S, Berg M. 2010. *The gold standard: The challenge of evidence-based medicine and standardization in health care*. Philadelphia, PA: Temple University Press.

Varpio L, Hall P, Lingard L, Schryer CF. Interprofessional communication and medical error: A reframing of research questions and approaches. *Academic Medicine*. 2008; 83: S76–S81.

4

HEALTH, HEALTH CARE, AND HEALTH EDUCATION

Problems, paradigms, and patterns

Stewart Mennin, Glenda Eoyang, and
Mary Nations

It is being involved with a phenomenon, being intimately engaged to it, courting it, as it were, that after much perplexity and embarrassment we come upon insight— upon a way of seeing the phenomenon from within. Insight is accompanied by a sense of surprise. What has been closed is suddenly disclosed. It entails genuine perception, seeing anew . . . Paradoxically, insight is knowledge at first sight.

(Heschel 1962)

Introduction

It seems paradoxical that with practically unlimited access to data, information, high-speed connectivity, and advanced technology that the challenges of contemporary medicine and society are fundamentally about understanding complex human relationships—how to live together in peace and harmony, how to work together for the common good, and how to preserve and prosper in, and with, the environment: "We live in a planetary era: all human beings, wherever they may be, are embarked on a common adventure. They should recognize themselves in their common humanity and recognize the cultural diversity inherent in everything human" (Morin 2001: 21).

A very human experience in medicine is illustrated by a true story shared by Professor Ruy Souza, a neurologist and medical educator at the Federal University of Roraima, in Boa Vista, at the most northern tip of Brazil near Venezuela and Guiana:

". . . and my patient died happy and cured"

My Yanomami patient had his first seizure in the middle of a festival in his village in northern Brazil, near the border with Venezuela. He was immediately separated from his family. The tribe knew the risks that certain neurological diseases could bring to the community. A few years ago an outbreak of meningococcal meningitis had devastating effects on the village. Moreover, as a member of an extremely ancient nomadic Indian society that survives by hunting and gathering natural resources

(continued)

(continued)

in the rainforest, the situation could bring serious risks to families. The case evolved into a *status epilepticus*, and my patient had to be transferred to a tertiary hospital, where the diagnosis was quick: glioblastoma multiforme, a highly aggressive tumor that occupied much of the right cerebral hemisphere, totally beyond therapeutic possibilities. After a palliative treatment, the patient experienced significant improvement. His movements partially returned and he could now communicate with the healthcare team with the help of a translator. However, in the second week of hospitalization, the patient was isolated in what appeared to be a severe depression; a psychiatric evaluation diagnosed psychotic depression. He refused to eat and talk with members of the staff. He even refused to return to his community. It was necessary to initiate parenteral nutrition.

After 3 weeks, with the help of an anthropologist, it was suggested that we try a consultation with an Indian medicine man. Arriving at the hospital, the healer wanted to talk to me before seeing the patient. He was concerned whether the disease was transmissible and the possible risks to other members of the village. After being assured about the safety of the situation for the others members of the tribe, he performed a religious ritual at the bedside, and declared the patient cured. The result was dramatic. My patient began to interact with everyone, quickly recovered his nutritional status and then asked to return to his tribe. When asked why he did not express his wish to return to his tribe earlier, he told me that it was because now he was feeling healed. With the help of an indigenous agency, he returned to his tribe.

After a few months, I found the medicine man and asked how my former patient was. He told me that the patient returned and was able to reintegrate into his community, and after 4 months he died. When I said I was sorry, the healer said, "You shouldn't be, because he died happy and cured!" (Petroni Mennin 2016).

This case illustrates the link between medicine, culture, the humanities,[1] and health:

> Health is, therefore, seen as a resource for everyday life, not the objective of living. Health is a positive concept emphasizing social and personal resources, as well as physical capacities. Therefore, health promotion is not just the responsibility of the health sector but goes beyond healthy life-styles to well-being.
>
> *(Ottawa Charter for Health Promotion 1986)*

Wellbeing for Dr Souza's patient came from a coherence and a wholeness which was more accessible to him from the medicine man than from the modern biomedical model of medicine (Capra 1982; Engel 1995).

Medicine/health and the humanities have always been interconnected. It's as if they are fraternal twins, inseparable in their beginnings and then, over time, they drifted apart on a sea of scientific and technological progress, becoming estranged from one another. Today, feedback from patients, students, and a handful of artists, alternative healers, and physicians, among others, has rekindled an interest in reuniting the humanities, health, and health care (Bleakley 2006, 2010; Bleakley, Bligh, and Browne 2011). The humanities and health are each an expression of the whole of the human experience grounded in observation, sense-making, and action. Observation, sense-making, and action involve a continuous flow (Csikszentmihalyi 1996) and exchange of information, collecting and sorting through data, and looking for patterns.

The present chapter uses practical examples and theory together to show the link between medicine, humanities, and health. The authors argue that contemporary medical practice—and the education for that practice—are experiencing a paradigm shift. The paradigm is shifting from health as the absence of disease and as problems with known explanations and solutions, to health and education for practice as complex patterns in complex adaptive systems (CAS), not solvable in the traditional sense of having a known solution. The authors examine and question underlying assumptions about problems and patterns. They argue that solvable problems and complex health patterns arise by completely different mechanisms. The Containers/Differences/ Exchanges (CDE) model for self-organisation in human systems is presented to clarify both theoretical and practical approaches to complex patterns through the lens of Human Systems Dynamics (HSD), a field of study at the intersection of systems thinking, effective practice, and social and complexity sciences (see: www.hsdinstitute.org). It supports both description and explanation of patterns in CAS, how they form, how they are influenced, and how they change. Finally, Adaptive Action is presented as a practical and disciplined method by which to take informed action in CAS. Illustrative examples are presented throughout the chapter

The nature of patterns

We perceive the world as dynamical patterns. They are everywhere and they come in all shapes and sizes, for example: the weather, health, information technology, relationships, a functional team, family, work, education, public health, safe driving, people crossing the street, and so forth. Patterns are the foundational and functional unit with which, and from which, we infer meaning. They are how we 'know' ourselves and the world we cohabit (Rosch, 1999).

Patterns can be defined as "similarities, differences, and connections that have meaning across space and time" (Eoyang and Holladay 2013). A pattern is generated by the dynamical (complex) interaction and interdependence of its parts. Similarly, patterns organise themselves into systems (Bertalanffy 1973; Dooley, 1996; Cilliers 1998; Eoyang 2001; Eoyang and Holladay 2013). It is the pattern of the whole that we perceive first and with which we connect. Subsequently, we become aware of and name patterns as concepts and analogies (Thelen and Smith 1994; Rosch 1999; Tschacher and Haken 2007; Hofstadter and Sander 2013). The HSD Institute recognises patterns that occur in both predictable and unpredictable complex situations as "similarities, differences and the connections they make in a system over time and across space" (Eoyang and Holladay 2013), where:

> Similarities give coherence and meaning . . . differences generate tension in the present and connections from the past set conditions for future transformations of the pattern. These three conditions (similarities, differences and connections), and their relationships to one another, set the stage for meaning making and help us to articulate reality in a way that is conscious and can be shared.
>
> *(ibid.: 43)*

It thus becomes essential to understand and explain both predictable and unpredictable patterns in ways that we understand as both true and useful—in ways that help us to stay relevant as we engage with a rapidly changing environment and to learn to take informed action within the uncertain health challenges we face today.

Learners, teachers, clinicians, patients, and artists seek patterns that enable understanding. They seek a degree of control and would like to be able to predict what will happen. Prediction, replication, control, and reliability depend on clear measurable boundaries: differences and similarities with relatively strong stable connections. Examples include measuring blood pressure, setting a simple fracture, and one-best-answer multiple-choice questions. These patterns have few variables that make a difference, have known and knowable answers, and, when problems arise, it is clear what needs to be done. There are likely to be few surprises or complications. There are a finite and knowable number of possibilities and thus such patterns are said to be 'low dimensional' (Table 4.1).

On the other hand, there are patterns that follow a different set of rules. They can't be replicated or predicted, don't have known solutions, and can't be controlled. There are many interacting parts and many levels of organisation. Such patterns occur in systems that are bounded, yet open and sensitive to outside influences. In human systems, success looks different to different people. Examples include small-group problem-based learning (Mennin 2007), chronic illness, preventive medicine, community health services, and existing health disparities (Sweeney and Griffiths 2002; Holt 2004; Kernick 2004; Sweeney 2006). Each pattern and system is unique, like Dr Souza's patient, so no evidence-based practice will be relevant every time. Because of massive interdependencies and unintended consequences, best practices in one place may be worse than nothing in another place or time. In these situations, a different set of tools is needed; tools that function well in CAS. They include the tools, models and methods from the HSD Institute.

Traditional problems: the whole equals the sum of its parts

For at least a century, we have acted as if the uncollected major fragments of our knowledge, which we call disciplines, could by themselves give understanding of the emergent ideas that come from putting the concepts and results together. It is much as if we try to understand and teach the geography of the 48 contiguous states of the United States by handing out maps of the 48 states, but never took the trouble to assemble a map of the country.

(Kline 1995)

Most encounters between health professionals, patients, and learners begin with a problem: a chief complaint. Initially, there is a perception by the physician of the whole problem pattern followed by a systematic and detailed search for the parts, key factors, and root causes to identify the normal and abnormal and to facilitate appropriate treatment. Diagnosis, clinical reasoning, and the treatment of problems are based on the recognition of, and search for, the whole and the parts. Tradition teaches us that the parts add together to form the whole (Figure 4.1) that is linked to established categories of diseases. Medical students learn to recognise and name patterns such as 'redness,' 'swelling,' and 'pain' as 'inflammation.' The dosage of medicines in each pill and vial must be predictable, replicable, and precise. Medical practice is divided into many parts, as specialties and subspecialties. The basic sciences are separated into disciplines, each with its own textbook. Valid and reliable 'high-stakes' medical licensing examinations, although different every year, are derived from, and fit within, a defined set of known objectives and competencies. Scientific evidence, to be valid, must be replicable and successfully pass rigorous peer review. Traditionally, integration in both medical education and medical practice has been understood as a linear sequence of connections (vertical and horizontal), or steps and stages in close proximity that are added to, and into, other segments to make a whole (Harden 2000; Kern, Thomas, and Hughes 2009; Mennin 2016b). For example, community-based medical education is often added into, rather than woven throughout, an existing curriculum (Mennin and Petroni-Mennin 2006).

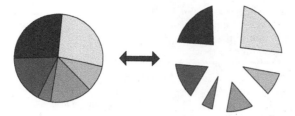

Figure 4.1 The whole is equal to the sum of its parts

The above examples are simple and complicated problems (Glouberman and Zimmerman 2002):

> You have seen them and solved them before. You know the parts and how they are related. You can see the whole thing at the same time. You can work on it bit-by-bit. You know what a solution looks like, and everyone agrees what the problem is. You control the process and the outcomes. These problems are simple. Other problems are complicated. You may have seen the problem before, but it takes special expertise to understand the parts and how they fit together. You can break the problem up into parts, solve each one separately, and then put them all back together for the 'big fix.' These problems are complicated. Simple and complicated problems require time and expertise to solve, but, if you work at it long enough and know enough, you will be able to find an answer.
>
> *(Mennin, Eoyang, and Nations 2018: 19)*

Paradigms: shift happens

Some patterns remain stable for decades, even centuries, like the concept and theory of germs and the Cartesian logic of reductionism. They are the accepted norm: a paradigm. Paradigms are "universally recognized scientific achievements that for a time provide model problems and solutions to a community of practitioners" (Kuhn 1962: x). The foundational paradigm of both the scientific method and modern medicine is that the whole is equal to the sum of its parts, and that cause and effect are directly proportional (Doll Jr 1993; Ludmerer 1999; Holt 2004; Sweeney 2006; Groopman 2007; Sturmberg and Martin 2013).

Nevertheless, over time conditions change and paradigms shift (Kuhn 1962):

> A paradigm shift takes place when one fundamental worldview is superseded by another . . . Two symptoms precede the emergence of a new paradigm. The first is that accepted models become increasingly complicated as they are expanded, distorted, and adjusted to accommodate new data.
>
> *(Eoyang and Holladay 2013: 111)*

For example, between 1996 and 2005 the Canadian Royal College of Physicians and Surgeons established a broad framework of seven complex abilities—or competencies—the goal of which was to enhance physician training: medical expert, communicator, collaborator, leader, health advocate, scholar, and professional (Frank 2005). Other countries have published similar statements. Over the past eighteen years there has been a series of revisions and a proliferation of detailed subcategories for each of the original abilities (Frank 2005; Frank, Snell, and Sherbino 2015). Competencies are

Table 4.1 Descriptors and characteristics of problems in linear logic and reductionism in which the whole equals the sum of its parts; and patterns that arise by nonlinear mechanisms and are understood via pattern logic; where the whole is greater than, and different from, the sum of its parts. The table is explained further in the text

Problems *The whole equals the sum of the parts. Problem logic*	Patterns *The whole is greater than, and different from, the sum of the parts. Pattern logic*
Solutions are known, few variables, future is predictable. There are right answers. Clear expectations set and evaluated, control is possible.	Solutions are not known or predictable. Uncertainty, emergent surprise. Control is not possible. The future is spontaneous, unpredictable.
Linear (proportional) cause and effect. Causes have known effects.	Nonlinear cause and effect. Causality is by self-organisation.
Closed, well-defined boundaries.	Fuzzy, permeable, open boundaries.
Hierarchical, top-down organisation.	Bottom-up organisation.
Measures look for central tendency, Equilibrium. Avoid outliers, minimise variance, seek balance, Gaussian statistics fits.	Inverse square law, Pareto distribution. Variability and diversity contribute to pattern formation. System far from equilibrium, dynamic systems analysis.
Few variables, low dimensional.	Many variables, high dimensional.
Expertise works well.	Inquiry works well.
Seek answers.	Ask questions, be in inquiry.
Can be scaled up, transferred, expanded.	Is at scale, scale free, self-similar patterns appear in all scales.
Success is clearly defined and measured. Competencies, objectives.	Many different definitions and measures of success.
Change is incremental, additive, step by step.	Change is irregular, episodic, comes in cascades, spurts. Self-organisation.
Behaviours are interactive.	Behaviours are interactive and interdependent.
Many similarities, few differences, high degree of agreement and certainty.	Few similarities, many differences, low degree of certainty and agreement.
Tight connections, limited ability to sense and respond to changes in conditions and environment.	Loose connections, highly responsive and sensitive to changes in conditions.

measurable performance criteria for medical students and postgraduate physicians (Frank, Mungroo et al. 2010; Frank, Snell et al. 2010). Subdividing broad frameworks, behaviours, and competencies into smaller pieces, each measured separately, reduces complex behaviour patterns into linear fragments that, when measured individually, cannot be added back together to make the whole. Another example has to do with entrustable professional activities (EPAs), the extent to which clinical supervisors can trust postgraduate trainees to conduct medical examinations and procedures without direct supervision (ten Cate 2005). The EPAs were initially broad statements of complex patterns of trust that have subsequently been subdivided into multiple milestones and competencies (Swing et al. 2013).

The second symptom of an impending paradigm shift is an increased frequency of surprises and anomalies of data that older models cannot explain adequately. One observes that creativity flourishes, multiple new perspectives appear, and potential models compete for adherents as new hypotheses arise and are tested. Medicine and medical education have become increasingly complex in ways that defy explanation through reductionism and linear logic. Examples include: social accountability (Boelen and Heck 2005; Boelen, Dharamsi, and Gibbs 2012);

competency-based medical education (McGaghie et al. 1978; Harden 1999; Frank 2005; Frank et al. 2010; Frank et al. 2015); small-group problem-based learning (Arrow, McGrath, and Berdahl 2000; Mennin 2007); professionalism (Stern 2006; Stern and Papadakis 2006); ethics (Eckles et al. 2005); relationship-centred patient care (Suchman 2006); longitudinal integrated clinical clerkships (Worley et al. 2000); entrustable professional activities (ten Cate 2005); assessment as education rather than psychometrics (Schuwirth and Van der Vleuten 2011); and developmental programme evaluation (Patton 2011), to name a few. All of these complex patterns are anomalies because they arose and exist in a paradigm of linear cause and effect and reductionism that can describe, but cannot explain, how they work. Interactions among medical practitioners and educators have become more open, more diverse, and more inter-dependent, making it difficult to suspend disbelief and sustain the illusion of prediction and control fostered by the previous limited paradigm. The number of these anomalies has been accumulating for decades.

Complex patterns: the whole is greater than, and different from, the sum of its parts

Consider three different working groups: a curriculum committee with representatives from different departments and varied interests in a medical school; a small group of learners work-ing on a problem- or team-based learning challenge; and an interdisciplinary clinical team tasked with caring for terminally ill patients. Shared interests at multiple levels hold together each of these groups and the individuals in them. They are part of the medical school, mem-bers of the health professions, members of professional societies, and so on. The individual members of each group are unique and their differences are a potential source of learning, understanding, and action. The quality of their exchanges and communications determines critical aspects of the group-wide pattern that emerges from the individual behaviours. It's not possible to predict what will happen, but when it does it is generally recognisable by the members of the group. The dynamics of these groups fit the definition of a complex adaptive system (CAS), as a "collection of agents (people, groups, ideas) that interact so that system-wide patterns emerge, and those patterns subsequently act on and influence the interactions among the agents" (Dooley 1996: 69).

Collaboration among learners in small groups, and teamwork among physicians in cardiol-ogy, mental health (Arrow and Henry 2010), and emergency medicine (Guastello 2010), is essential for successful health care. Teaching is also part of a CAS (Davis and Sumara 2006; Davis 2008; Davis, Sumara, and Luce-Kapler 2008). Also recognised as CAS are: primary care and health systems (McDaniel and Driebe, 2001; Sweeney and Griffiths 2002; Holt 2004; Sweeney 2006; Sturmberg and Martin 2009; Sturmberg and Martin 2013), medical education (Mennin 2010), and nursing (Lindberg, Nash, and Lindberg 2008; Davidson, Ray, and Turkel 2011). The number and diversity of agents in a CAS may be very large and the interactions among the agents may be nonlinear with many short feedback loops. This makes it impossible to identify a root cause or a key factor in CAS. For similar reasons, there is a high degree of uncertainty and prediction, and control is not possible. Sensitivity, responsiveness, and uncertainty create conditions for rapid response and continuous adjustment, key features, for example, of the nerv-ous system and social behaviour in families. Characteristics of CAS are listed in Table 4.1 and illustrated in Figure 4.2. The geometric shapes at the bottom of Figure 4.2 represent different agents that interact in interdependent ways (dotted lines), and over time create system-wide patterns (ovals at top) (Eoyang and Holladay 2013). The differences (tensions) among the agents generate a potential for change.

Complex Adaptive System (CAS)

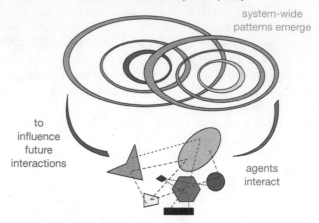

Figure 4.2 Different agents (shapes at bottom) interact (dotted lines) in nonlinear, interdependent exchanges to create system-wide patterns (ovals above). System-wide patterns that have emerged spontaneously then influence the agents

A short vignette will serve to illustrate the differences between problems that work with linear logic and reductionism (those that have solutions, where the whole equals the sum of its parts), and those that are complex patterns (the whole is greater than the sum of its parts), exhibiting self-organisation and that do not have known solutions.

Jack's dead and the boys have gone

Some years ago, our practice nurse asked me to see Mrs. B, an 85-year-old widow who, as I recall, at the time of consultation had been registered as a patient with me for about 15 years. I knew her well. Her husband, a pleasant chap who had been a builder, had died five years previously. Mrs. B was pretty much estranged from her two grown-up sons, who were recurrent petty criminals, both serving prison sentences at the time of the consultation. The list below shows the conditions from which Mrs. B suffered, and her test results, which the nurse wanted me to review with her.

Mrs. B's comorbidity:

Diabetes

Hypertension

Osteoarthritis

Macular degeneration

Hallus valgus

Mrs. B's test results:

Glycosylated haemoglobin   9.7%

Blood pressure	180/96 mmHg
Total cholesterol	8.0 mmol/l
Body mass index	29 kg/m^2

. . . When we met, at the practice nurse's request, I rehearsed the abundant evidence supporting interventions to lower her blood pressure, to improve the control of her diabetes and to reduce her lipid levels. I remember even thinking where the reference for this all lay (with a resumé in *Clinical Evidence*). I confess to feeling just a shade confident as I explained the abnormalities and how we could 'help' to reduce her risk. After a few moments I stopped—resting my case, as a barrister might say.

Mrs. B remained silent for a moment or two. Then she said, 'Well, Jack's dead and the boys have gone' . . . At the simplest level, one can say that the consultation, at the point when Mrs. B made this contribution, moved from being doctor-centered to patient-centered. It moved, one could say, from the biomedical domain to the biographical domain, or from clinical, evidence-based medicine to a consultation predicated on narrative-based evidence. But the shift was profound. When the consultation moved from its biomedical phase, it shed its parameters of P-values, absolute risk and numbers needed to treat. These were replaced by the parameters of the biographical phase of the consultation—led by Mrs. B. Here, despair, hopelessness, regret, guilt perhaps, and defeat were the parameters. Physical parameters had been replaced by metaphysical ones—two intellectual worlds seemed to have collided . . . It is clear that when Mrs. B offered her contribution, the consultation took off in another direction. Up until that point, a fairly straightforward consultation was proceeding, drawing on scientific evidence gleaned from good clinical trials, many of them randomized and controlled, in the great tradition of scientific medicine. The remainder of the consultation, led by Mrs. B, had nothing to do with that way of thinking, and arose from her lived experience (Sweeney 2006: 3–4).

The physician remembered Mrs B and reviewed her recent data in advance of their meeting. A clear and familiar pattern (diagnoses) fit the details of Mrs B's data. Preparing his thoughts and treatment plan for Mrs B was a familiar pattern from previous experience and from the literature (best practice). This was, at first, a complicated problem with known and knowable solutions. But after Mrs B said: "Jack's dead and the boys have gone," the tension (differences) increased notably and the situation became uncertain. It was in no longer in equilibrium and in fact had moved far away from equilibrium.

Self-organisation in human systems

No one was directing what happened with Mrs B during the consultation, nor was anything imposed by outside forces. The tension was within Mrs B and the factor that made a difference was how she was feeling when the physician paused. At that moment, the inner tension could no longer be contained. It had reached a critical state such that a very small stimulus, like a pause by the physician, resulted in a very large change (nonlinear). This highly sensitive critical state is called "self-organised criticality" (Bak 1996). It is the maximal tension the system can hold before there is a spontaneous release of the accumulated tension derived from an expression of differences. Consequently, a new system-wide pattern emerges spontaneously. This is "self-organisation" (Goldstein 1994; Liebovitch 2006). Self-organisation is the process whereby existing patterns emerge, pivot, and change in CAS (Goldstein 1994; Kauffman 1995; Cilliers 1998). There is no arbitrary unit of identity in self-organisation, like a psychological self. Self in self-organisation refers to the internal exchange of differences among agents within the boundaries of the system. When the tension is released, a structure emerges such that it is a better fit (less constrained) in the existing conditions compared to the previous structure (Prigogine and Stengers 1997).

An important distinction between closed systems that obey simple linear logic and reductionism, and open systems that are self-organising, is that, in the former, differences among agents create tension that moves the system towards equilibrium; whereas, in the latter, differences among agents in a CAS create tensions that shift the system far away from equilibrium towards a new emergent order that fits well with the current conditions (Table 4.1, Figure 4.2). Eventually, as the tension in a far from equilibrium CAS changes, the pattern becomes unsustainable and highly sensitive to small perturbations. Instability and sensitivity have high survival value in human systems. We wouldn't last long if our nervous and immune systems took a long time to sense and react to perturbations in the environment. Individuals in social gatherings are acutely aware of very small nonverbal and verbal stimuli. Such sensitivity serves to reduce tensions and maintain cohesion among group members. Health professionals and teachers have to be aware of and sensitive to differences in culture, gender, age, geographic origin, race, education, and economic status as they all affect the quality of the doctor–patient and teacher–learner relationship.

The World Health Organization (WHO) describes 'health' as a CAS. Health is the extent to which an individual or group is able to realise aspirations and satisfy needs, and to change or cope with the environment (Ottawa Charter for Health Promotion 1986). This statement of health assumes a flexible and adaptive capacity to function and for patterns to fit well within a changing environment. 'Fit for function,' then, refers to this emergent pattern as an outcome of self-organisation. Fit for function is the only reasonable measure of success in a CAS. 'Excellent enough' is a synonym for 'fit for function' and may be more acceptable in assessment of learners and evaluation of curricula, programmes, and institutions.

Medicine and medical education deal with CAS all the time. However, up until now, there has not been a useful way to both describe and explain how 'fit for function' works in the present tense. As we continue to learn more about how patterns emerge in CAS, it may well be time for health practitioners, health systems, and educators for the health professions to explore further the conditions necessary to account for uncertainty and variance in complex human systems. A paradigm shift that embraces both CAS and linear causal systems can promote a more sophisticated view of integration and health as emergent properties that are fit for function in teaching, learning, assessment, curriculum, and evaluation (Mennin 2016a, 2016b). Causality is radically different in a CAS than in systems that are predictable and controllable. For that reason, a new set of tools is required to support problem definition, analysis, and solution in CASs. HSD has developed a toolbox that supports professional action in a CAS. The key tools are: the CDE Model, Pattern Logic, and Adaptive Action. We will briefly introduce those tools here.

The CDE Model

There were many factors at play between the Yanomami tribe, the medicine man, Dr Souza, and his patient. The same is true in Mrs B's story. How is it possible to understand such complexity and to what extent is it possible to influence the speed, direction, and outcome of what happens (Eoyang 2001, 2004; Eoyang and Holladay 2013)? The CDE Model provides a theoretically sound and practical explanation of CAS dynamics. Three interdependent conditions—Containers (C); Differences (D); and Exchanges (E)—make it possible to identify patterns in the workplace, explore and understand how they are shaped and governed, and take wise action to shift them (Eoyang 2001; Eoyang and Holladay 2013).

The container (C) functions to hold the agents together close enough and long enough so that, under the right conditions, they will interact and form new patterns. The containers in Figure 4.3 are the large semicircles open to the outside environment at the top. There are multiple containers in the story of the Yanomami man: his spiritual beliefs and those of the medicine man, the rainforest environment, the tribe, the family, the hospital, and Dr Souza's office. The container includes a set of shared beliefs, values, culture, rules, or laws. It can be physical like a classroom, a clinical skills examination, or a community clinic; or it can be an agenda that brings members of a curriculum committee together, or a clinical department or a community. Similarities in the moment hold the agents together to engage and share differences. In CAS, there are too many differences to account for all of them.

Difference (D) in the CDE Model refers to the differences that make a difference, the ones with the potential to shift the patterns through self-organisation, for example Mrs B's statement "Jack's dead and the boys are gone." The pause after the physician explained his plan to Mrs B set the conditions that helped to shift the path, speed, and outcome of the consultation. Each situation is unique and the difference that makes a difference will be context specific. The small geometric shapes at the bottom of Figure 4.3 represent different agents.

Exchange (E) refers to connections and the flow of information, energy, and other resources generating changes in the system. The dashed lines among the geometric figures represent exchange in Figure 4.3. Exchange can be: dialogue, feedback, observation, conversation, collaboration, shared meaning, communication, and more.

The significance of the CDE Model is that it provides a way to work with CAS across multiple levels of organisations and in specific contexts. It provides a unified way to perceive, understand (explain), and take informed action to influence the path, speed, and outcome

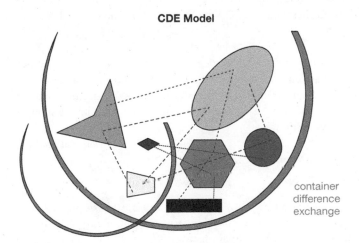

CDE Model

container
difference
exchange

Figure 4.3 Different (D) parts (agents, pieces) are held in proximity in a container (C), open to the outside. Agents interact, and they exchange. Dotted lines represent nonlinear, interdependent exchanges (E) among the parts

of self-organising patterns in CAS. While there are many other models of complexity, they are primarily descriptive, rather than providing guidance in choosing informed action (Stacy 2001; Zimmerman, Lindberg, and Plsek 2001; Gunderson and Holling 2002; Cooperrider and Whitney 2005; Scharmer 2009; Snowden 2010; Lipmanowicz and McCandless 2013). It is important to point out that while it's possible to anticipate a pattern change by influencing one or more of its conditions (CDE), it's not possible to predict or control exactly what the change will be, or what its consequences will be.

Pattern Logic

The CDE Model can help us understand and to take action in challenging issues in health professions practice and education today. Imagine: two different clinical practices, hospitals, or medical schools merge and change the container (C). The number of differences (D) in the new system increases dramatically. Effective communication (E) among people decreases as it's more difficult to know where to go for what is needed. There is confusion about new group structures (C) and leadership (C, D, and E). Another challenge could be a government's response to a shortage of health professionals resulting in a mandate to all medical schools to increase class size (increased D) without an increase in resources. Students complain that there are not enough teachers (E) and access to supervised learning time with clinicians is insufficient (D, E). Or, perhaps there have been sudden changes in the rules (C) governing access to health care in a country. Inequities in access to health care (C, D, and E) are exacerbated. A decrease in health quality among a particular population occurs (C) and the health of the local workforce (and consequently the economic wellbeing of families) is at risk. Local emergency rooms experience an increase in non-emergency visits (D) that further constrains and stresses limited resources in the local health system (C and E).

The open, high-dimension, nonlinear nature of a CAS requires a different paradigm: Pattern Logic. Pattern Logic is the use and study of disciplined reasoning based on the conditions for self-organising (CDE) (Eoyang 2016). It builds the capacity to respond with Adaptive Action and helps to identify the existing constraints on one or more of the CDE conditions. Pattern Logic makes different options for action accessible. It takes advantage of the interdependence of the CDE Model and therefore it is only necessary to shift one of the three conditions to influence the other two:

> The CDE Model provides a way to recognize and name the conditions of CAS, but intentional action requires more than just recognition. Conscious influence over self-organizing patterns requires an intentional process for seeing, understanding, and influencing the conditions that shape change in complex adaptive systems. We call that process Adaptive Action.
>
> *(Eoyang and Holladay 2013: 27)*

Adaptive Action

Dr Souza, his patient, the medicine man, Mrs B, and her physician each sought information about what was going on. Each understood the situation differently, each made different meaning, and each understood different options. In each case, an informed action was taken in the face of uncertainty and there was no way to know what would happen.

Adaptive Action is a method of disciplined informed action in iterative cycles in situations without known solutions where changes are unpredictable (Eoyang and Holladay 2013).

It consists of three simple questions—What? So What?, and Now What?—that set the conditions (CDE) that promote both understanding and shift patterns. Adaptive Action promotes making sense and seeing different options, especially when information is overwhelming or incomplete (Figure 4.4, Table 4.2).

1   **What?** 'What' is an opportunity to collect data and to describe what is happening; to describe what you see. Describe what you want. Describe the current patterns, conditions, and situation that have emerged in the system.
2   **So What?** 'So what' is a question that helps to make meaning of what is perceived, identifying the conditions that shape the world as it is experienced. 'So what' deals with the implications of the current state and possible options for action to shift the conditions and release tensions that are held in the system.
3   **Now What?** 'Now what' is the action taken to influence and bring about new patterns fit for function as conditions change. It is the choice to take one action now and to continue to observe what happens next and then move into a new 'What?'

Iterative cycles of Adaptive Action in CAS help to promote movement of the system to the edge of self-organisation as 'self-organised criticality' (Bak 1996). The three Adaptive Action questions unfold into many other useful questions, depending on the circumstances (Table 4.2). The end of each Adaptive Action cycle results in real-world action, which shifts the system and creates the question 'What changed?', then moving into the next cycle of Adaptive Action (Eoyang and Holladay 2013).

What has been closed is disclosed

Medicine and medical education are CASs in which the whole is greater than the sum of its parts and where reductionistic scientific explanations are insufficient. Self-organisation is the mechanism whereby complex patterns are formed and influenced. Attending to conditions that form and inform them—as containers (C), differences (D), and exchanges (E) (the CDE Model)—can influence complex patterns. Pattern Logic identifies, names, and promotes conditions to modify constraints and shift patterns in the system. Adaptive Action is a disciplined way to engage with and take action in complex health issues. A paradigm shift is happening in medicine and medical

Adaptive Action

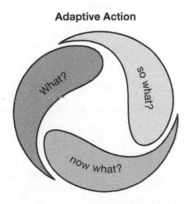

Figure 4.4   Adaptive Action consists of iterative cycles of three questions: What? So What? Now What?

Table 4.2 Some Adaptive Action questions

What?	So What?	Now What?
What do you observe?	So what does it mean to you? To your group? To others?	Now what will you do to change the conditions and create a new situation?
What is familiar?	So what are the conflicts or tensions in the current situation?	Now what are my options for action?
What is different?	So what are the conflicts or tensions between parts of the system?	Now what are the pros and cons of each?
What surprises you?	So what would be better?	Now what is feasible? Fast? Promising?
What are the data?	So what does success look like?	Now what support is there?
What does research say?	So what is the appetite for change?	Now what resistance is there likely to be?
What do people say?	So what are the risks? Benefits?	Now what are my important questions?
What suggests a finite problem? An infinite problem?	So what are our options for action?	Now what should I communicate? To whom? How?
What has changed? Stayed the same?	So what are the tensions to drive the next change?	Now what can I do to amplify or dampen the tensions to instigate change?
What holds the agents together?	So what are the foundations for coherence and collaboration?	Now what can I do to create or reinforce connections in the system?
What differences are emerging or disappearing?	So what are differences that make a difference and what focus is there on those?	Now what can we do to shift focus towards differences that make a difference?
What are the current forms of exchange? How strong are they?	So what methods are used to share information or other resources?	Now what pathways for sharing or trading would be useful?
What is the pattern of the past?	So what are the containers, differences, and exchanges that are common and familiar?	Now what can I do to strengthen or change those?
What desires are therefore patterns in the future?	So what are the hopes and dreams of the people in the system?	Now what will set conditions for those dreams to be fulfilled?
What questions do you have?	So what has surprised or troubled you?	Now what additional information will you seek?

education in which the education of future health practitioners is beginning to recognise that linear causality and reductionism are important in specific situations for problems that have known and knowable solutions. However, most of today's complex challenges and tomorrow's surprises require a paradigm shift to Pattern Logic and Adaptive Action.

It is time to reunite the wholeness of the humanities with the complexities of the health professions. It is time to engage Pattern Logic and Adaptive Action as the fundamental processes of learning, healing, and being human.

Acknowledgements

The experience, insight, and knowledge of Royce Holladay permeate this work and, although not an author, her imprint and influence are gratefully acknowledged. We thank Regina Helena Petroni Mennin for her invaluable and thoughtful critique and for keeping it grounded in practical applications.

Note

1 "Humanities—learning concerned with human culture, especially literature, history, art, music and philosophy." *Online Oxford Dictionary*. https://en.oxforddictionaries.com/definition/humanity.

References

Arrow H, Henry KB. Using complexity to promote group learning in healthcare. *Journal of Evaluation in Clinical Practice*. 2010; 16: 861–66.

Arrow H, McGrath JE, Berdahl JL. 2000. *Small groups as complex adaptive systems: Formation, coordination, development, and adaptation*. Thousand Oaks, CA: Sage.

Bak P. 1996. *How nature works: The science of self-organized criticality*. New York, NY: Springer-Verlag.

Bertalanffy LV. 1973. *General system theory: Foundations, development, applications*. New York, NY: G. Braziller.

Bleakley A. Broadening conceptions of learning in medical education: The message from team working. *Medical Education*. 2006; 40: 150–57.

Bleakley A. Blunting Occam's razor: Aligning medical education with studies of complexity. *Journal of Evaluation in Clinical Practice*. 2010; 16: 849–55.

Bleakley A, Bligh J, Browne J. 2011. *Medical education for the future: Identity, power and location*. Dordrecht: Springer.

Boelen C, Heck JE. 2005. *Defining and measuring the social accountability of medical schools*. Geneva: World Health Organization.

Boelen C, Dharamsi S, Gibbs T. The social accountability of medical schools and its indicators. *Education for Health*. 2012; 25: 180–94.

Capra F. 1982. *The turning point: Science, society, and the rising culture*. Toronto: Bantam Books.

Cilliers P. 1998. *Complexity and postmodernism: Understanding complex systems*. London: Routledge.

Cooperrider D, Whitney D. 2005. *Appreciative inquiry: A positive revolution in change*. San Francisco, CA: Berrett-Koehler.

Csikszentmihalyi M. 1996. *Creativity: Flow and the psychology of discovery and invention*. New York, NY: Harper.

Davidson AW, Ray MA, Turkel MC (eds.) 2011. *Nursing, caring, and complexity science: For human–environment well-being*. New York, NY: Springer.

Davis B. 2008. Complexity and education: vital simultaneities. In: M Mason (ed.) *Complexity theory and the philosophy of education*. Oxford: John Wiley & Sons, 46–62.

Davis B, Sumara D. 2006. *Complexity and education: Inquiries into learning, teaching, and research*. Mahwah, NJ: Lawrence Erlbaum Associates.

Davis B, Sumara D, Luce-Kapler R. 2008 (2nd ed). *Engaging minds: Changing teaching in complex times*. New York, NY: Routledge.

Doll Jr WE. 1993. *A post-modern perspective on curriculum*. New York, NY: Teachers College Press.

Dooley K. A nominal definition of complex adaptive systems. *The Chaos Network*. 1996; 8: 2–3.

Eckles RE, Meslin EM, Gaffney M, Helft PR. Medical ethics education: Where are we? Where should we be going? A review. *Academic Medicine*. 2005; 80: 1143–52.

Engel C. Medical education in the 21st century: The need for a capability approach. *Capability*. 1995; 1: 23–30.

Eoyang G. 2001. *Conditions for self-organizing in human systems*. Montpelier, VT: The Union Institute and University.

Eoyang G. Conditions for self-organizing in human systems. *Futurics*. 2004; 28: 1–67.

Eoyang GH. 2016. Pattern Logic. Available at: www.hsdinstitute.org/resources/pattern-logic-blog.html. Last accessed: 28 October 2018.

Eoyang GH, Holladay R. 2013. *Adaptive Action: Leveraging uncertainty in your organization*. Stanford, CA: Stanford University Press.

Frank JR. 2005. The CanMEDS 2005 physician competency framework. Better standards. Better physicians. Better care. Ottawa: The Royal College of physicians and surgeons of Canada.

Frank JR, Snell L, Sherbino J (eds.) 2015. *CanMEDS 2015 Physician Competency Framework*. Ottawa: Royal College of Physicians and Surgeons of Canada.

Frank JR, Mungroo R, Ahmad Y, Wang M, De Ross S, Horsley T. Toward a definition of competency-based education in medicine: A systematic review of published definitions. *Medical Teacher*. 2010; 32: 631–37.

Frank JR, Snell LS, Ten Cate O, et al. Competency-based medical education: Theory to practice. *Medical Teacher*. 2010; 32: 638–45.

Glouberman S, Zimmerman B. 2002. *Complicated and complex systems: What would successful reform of Medicare look like?* (Vol. 8): Commission on the Future of Health Care in Canada.

Goldstein JA. 1994. *The unshackled organization: Facing the challenge of unpredictability through spontaneous reorganization*. Portland, OR: Productivity Press.

Groopman J. 2007. *How doctors think*. Boston, MA: Houghton Mifflin.

Guastello SJ. Self-organization and leadership emergence in emergency response teams. *Nonlinear Dynamics, Psychology, and Life Sciences Psychology, and Life Sciences*. 2010; 14: 179–204.

Gunderson LH, Holling CS. 2002. *Panarchy: Understanding transformations in human and natural systems*. Washington, DC: Island Press.

Harden RM. AMEE Guide no 14: Outcome-based education. Part one—an introduction to outcome-based education. *Medical Teacher*. 1999; 21: 7–14.

Harden RM. The integration ladder: A tool for curriculum planning and evaluation. *Medical Education*. 2000; 34: 551–57.

Heschel JA. 1962. *The prophets*. Philadelphia, PA: The Jewish Publication Society.

Hofstadter D, Sander E. 2013. *Surfaces and essences: Analogy as the fuel and fire of thinking*. New York, NY: Basic Books.

Holt TA (ed.) 2004. *Complexity for clinicians*. Oxford: Radcliffe.

Kauffman S. 1995. *At home the in universe: The search for laws of self-organization and complexity*. New York, NY: Oxford University Press.

Kern DE, Thomas PA, Hughes MT (eds.) 2009. *Curriculum development for medical education*. Baltimore, MD: The Johns Hopkins University Press.

Kernick D (ed.) 2004. *Complexity and health care organization: A view from the street*. Oxford: Radcliffe Medical Press.

Kline SJ. 1995. *Conceptual foundations for multidisciplinary thinking*. Stanford, CA: Stanford University Press.

Kuhn TS. 1962. *The structure of scientific revolutions*. Chicago, IL: University of Chicago Press.

Liebovitch LS. 2006. What is 'self-organization'? *Emerging*. Available at: http://walt.ccs.fau.edu. Last accessed: 28 October 2018.

Lindberg C, Nash S, Lindberg C (eds.) 2008. *On the edge: Nursing in the age of complexity*. Medford, NJ: Plexus Press.

Lipmanowicz H, McCandless K. 2013. Liberating structures: Innovating by including and unleashing everyone. *E&Y Performance*. 2010; 2: 6–19.

Ludmerer KM. 1999. *Time to heal: American medical education from the turn of the century to the era of managed care*. Oxford: Oxford University Press.

McDaniel RR, Driebe DJ. 2001. Complexity science and health care management. In: MD Fottler et al. (eds.) *Advances in health care management* (Vol. 2). Amsterdam: Elsevier Science, 11–36.

McGaghie WC, Miller GE, Sajid AW, Telder TV. 1978. *Competency-based curriculum development in medical education*. Available at: http://whqlibdoc.who.int/php/WHO_PHP_68.pdf. Last accessed: 28 October 2018.

Mennin S. Small-group problem-based learning as a complex adaptive system. *Teaching and Teacher Education*. 2007; 23: 303–13.

Mennin S. Self-organization, integration and curriculum in the complex world of medical education. *Medical Education*. 2010; 44: 20–30.

Mennin S. 2016a. How can learning be made more effective in medical education? In: KA Bin Abdulrahman et al. (eds.) *Routledge international handbook of medical education*. London: Routledge, 207–20.

Mennin S. 2016b. Integration of the sciences basic to medicine and the whole of the curriculum. In: KA Bin Abdulrahman et al. (eds.) *Routledge international handbook of medical education*. London: Routledge, 171–87.

Mennin S, Eoyang G, Nations M. 2018. *Lead complex change: Innovate, assess, and sustain.* Circle Pines, MN: Human Systems Dynamics Institute.

Mennin S., Petroni-Mennin R. Community-based medical education. *The Clinical Teacher.* 2006; 3: 90–96.

Morin E. 2001. *Seven complex lessons in education for the future.* Paris: UNESCO.

Ottawa Charter for Health Promotion (1986). Retrieved from: www.betterhealth.vic.gov.au/bhcv2/bhcarticles.nsf/pages/Ottawa_Charter_for_Health_Promotion. Last accessed: 28 October 2018.

Patton MQ. 2011. *Developmental evaluation: Applying complexity concepts to enhance innovation and use.* New York, NY: The Guilford Press.

Petroni Mennin RH. 2016. Benefits and challenges associated with introducing, managing, integrating and sustaining community-based medical education. In: KA Bin Abdulrahman et al. (eds.), *Routledge international handbook of medical education.* London: Routledge, 157–70.

Prigogine I, Stengers I. 1997. *The end of certainty: Time, chaos, and the new laws of nature.* New York, NY: The Free Press.

Rosch E. Reclaiming cognition. *Journal of Consciousness Studies.* 1999: 6: 61–77.

Scharmer CO. 2009. *Theory U: Leading from the future as it emerges.* San Francisco, CA: Berrett-Koehler.

Schuwirth LWT, Van der Vleuten, CPM. Programmatic assessment: From assessment of learning to assessment for learning. *Medical Teacher.* 2011; 33: 478–85.

Snowden D. (2010). The Cynefin Framework. Available at: www.youtube.com/watch?v=N7oz366X0-8&list=PL5CB210886A3E51AE&index=1&feature=plpp_video. Last accessed: 28 October 2018.

Stacy RD. 2001. *Complex responsive processes in organizations: Learning and knowledge creation.* London: Routledge.

Stern DT (ed.) 2006. *Measuring medical professionalism.* Oxford: Oxford University Press.

Stern DT, Papadakis M. The developing physician: Becoming a professional. *The New England Journal of Medicine.* 2006; 355: 1794–99.

Sturmberg JP, Martin A (eds.) 2013. *Handbook of systems and complexity in health.* New York, NY: Springer.

Sturmberg JP, Martin CM. Complexity and health: Yesterday's traditions, tomorrow's future. *Journal of Evaluation in Clinical Practice.* 2009; 15: 543–48.

Suchman AL. A new theoretical foundation for relationship-centered care: Complex responsive processes of relating. *Journal of General Internal Medicine.* 2006; 21: S40–S44.

Sweeney K. 2006. *Complexity in primary care: Understanding its value.* Oxford: Radcliffe.

Sweeney K, Griffiths F (eds.) (2002). *Complexity and health care: An introduction.* Abingdon: Radcliffe Medical Press.

Swing SR, Beeson MS, Carraccio C, et al. Educational milestone development in the first 7 specialties to enter the next accreditation system. *Journal of Graduate Medical Education.* 2013; 5: 98–106.

ten Cate O. Entrustability of professional activities and competency-based training. *Medical Education.* 2005; 39: 1176–77.

Thelen E, Smith L. 1994. *A dynamic systems approach to the development of cognition and action.* Cambridge, MA: MIT Press.

Tschacher W, Haken H. Intentionality in non-equilibrium systems? The functional aspects of self-organized pattern formation. *New Ideas in Psychology.* 2007; 25: 1–15.

Worley P, Silagy C, Prideaux D, et al. (2000). The parallel rural community curriculum: An integrated clinical curriculum-based in rural general practice. *Medical Education.* 2000; 34: 558–65.

Zimmerman B, Lindberg C, Plsek P. 2001. *Edgeware: Insights from complexity science for health care leaders.* Irving, TX: VHA.

PART II

Democratising medicine

The medical humanities as forms of resistance

5

THE STATE OF THE UNION

Rigour and responsibility in US health humanities

Therese Jones and Delese Wear

> Learning is not attained by chance; it must be sought for with ardor and attended
> to with diligence.
>
> *(Abigail-Adams, wife of John Adams (second US President)*
> *and mother of John Quincy Adams (sixth US President))*[1]

We begin, as directed by Professor Vivian Bearing's mentor in Margaret Edson's play *Wit*, with a text—the opening sentence of a recently published article in the *Journal of the American Medical Association*'s feature 'The Arts and Medicine':[2]

> We—an internist specializing in palliative care . . . and a medical anthropologist . . . —
> recently spent a year training surgery interns in the use of narrative medicine techniques
> to influence their development as compassionate surgeons.
>
> *(Kirkland and Craig 2018: 1532)*

As scholars and educators ourselves in the health humanities, we deeply respect and appreciate the creative and thoughtful work of colleagues in the field, and it is not our intention to disparage anyone in this chapter. However, the above sentence illustrates three specific and enduring challenges regarding the arts and humanities in medical education. There is the question of expertise: who teaches? There is the question of content and methodology: what is taught and how? And finally, there is the question of evaluation: what are the goals, and how are they met?

In this chapter, we address all three of these challenges, but we devote more time and words to the first section, which addresses expertise. We believe that content, methodology, objectives and evaluation flow from the qualification and experience of the teacher or teachers.

Expertise: who teaches?

"We—an internist specializing in palliative care . . . and a medical anthropologist . . ."

Well over a decade ago, one of our colleagues, a literary and film scholar, casually mentioned to an emergency medicine physician at the same institution that the position for director of the medical humanities programme there had just been posted. The physician responded with interest: "I might apply for that." Our colleague was taken aback: "How can you do that? You're not a humanities person." She immediately countered, "I read books. I can teach literature," to which he replied, "Oh, I watch *ER*. I guess I can do an appendectomy."

There are many such anecdotes in the field of health humanities, which seemingly rest on the assumption that if one has made some study of literature or art history, for example, then one is qualified to teach a text or interpret a painting. This assumption is further propelled by the fact that medical education and clinical practice uniquely qualify physicians to teach the arts and humanities in those settings because it is, after all, their domain. Moreover, the thinking is that the relevant sense making of texts and images arises more from a physician's experience—real and memorable—and less from a humanities scholar and educator's expertise.

In their discussion, 'Exploring the Surgical Gaze Through Literature and Art,' the co-authors cited above announce their disciplinary identities; however, they do not provide any information about additional education in narratology, or literary theory and criticism, despite the fact that they are, in their words, "using narrative medicine techniques." Yet, in clinical settings, there are rigid and recognisable spheres of practice where a nurse can do one thing but not another—such as delivering medications but never prescribing them—or where a doctor can do a bowel resection but would never empty a bedpan. Thus, such disregard for the qualifications to teach narrative medicine may be notable but, we would argue, is actually commonplace and rarely challenged when dealing with the arts and humanities. Where clinical expertise and disciplinary knowledge unquestionably matter in healthcare education and practice (you wouldn't seek out a historian or a physical therapist if you needed a hysterectomy), when it comes to the arts and humanities, expertise and credentialing seem to matter very little or not at all.

Analysing the long-standing tension between the arts and the sciences, Catherine Belling (2017) quotes molecular biologist P.J.G. Butler, who claims that scientists are simply better educated than those in the humanities. His evidence is his enjoyment of discussions with colleagues about music, theatre and the visual arts. Belling (ibid.: 22) argues that simply "consuming (enjoying, appreciating, criticizing) an imaginative work does not require an understanding of how it works." She illustrates her point with two imaginary conversations: the first between two scientists, both of whom have seen a recent production of *Macbeth*. They chat about the play, exchanging thoughtful and well-supported opinions, applauding the special effects and wondering about parallels with contemporary politics. Similarly, a painter and a poet, both of whom have recently undergone routine screening mammograms, talk together about that experience, making observations and comparing notes about the probability of false positives and unnecessary biopsies.

The first conversation is, as Belling (ibid.) aptly and brilliantly exemplifies, the equivalent of Dr Butler's engagement with the arts and humanities; he simply disregards the fact there is more to interpreting *Macbeth* than reading, viewing and considering it. The two scientists do not need to "understand prosody, dramatic form, the evolution of English orthography, the political context of the play's first performance, or the history of its production." In contrast, the poet and painter are under no illusion about their ignorance of "the physics of ionizing radiation or the pathology visualization needed to generate the conclusion that their breast tissue looks normal." While it may not occur to the scientists that there is a whole lot that they neither notice nor apprehend, they are satisfied with simply discussing the experience, evaluating its quality and exploring its meaning to the end of "the social processing of a cultural object." However, there is and should be a distinct and profound difference between the "social processing of a cultural object," whether it be Will Shakespeare or Judy Chicago, and a deep understanding and recognisable expertise in the theories and methods of the humanities disciplines.

Moreover, confounding the question of authority—who teaches the health humanities?—is the question of purpose: why are they being taught at all? Here again, there have been and continue to be very different and distinct viewpoints, one of which is best illustrated by the American Association of Medical College's stated opinion in a 2017 report on the arts and humanities, where health humanities potentially provide "fundamental lessons in professionalism, ethical discernment, and communication with patients," leading to greater joy, more empathy and better care. However, from the outset of the enterprise, leaders in the health humanities have had a very different perspective. For example, one of the earliest rationales for the emergent field of the humanities in medical education included the prescription for a bright line drawn between the clinical performance of medicine and the critical work of the humanities, between an enterprise dedicated to the inculcation of human values and an enterprise dedicated to the exploration of human values. In the 1971 proceedings of the first session of the Institute on Human Values in Medicine, K. Danner Clouser (1979: 50) warned about appropriation and distraction: "The humanities should remain academic disciplines and not get caught in the role of specialists on bedside manners and professional etiquette. Basically ours is an academic role even in the medical school." A decade later, Anne Hudson Jones (1984: 32) returned to the already controversial notion that studying the humanities makes one more humane: "This expectation makes me very uncomfortable. This expectation is a burden . . . for all of the humanities."

There is, then, a long-standing tension between the instrumental justification for the humanities in medicine, which ostensibly enables and promotes more caring professionals and better caring practices—what physician and philosopher Jeffrey Bishop (2008: 17) deems the "dose effect" of the humanities—and the intellectual practice of the humanities. As literary theorist Jonathan Culler (2005: 38) notes, it is not at all surprising that the *human* in the *humanities* leads us astray because "our language proposes a strong link not just between the humanities and the human being but between *humanistic* thinking and even *humane* behavior." Peter Brooks (2014) also elaborates on the confusion that humanities scholars and educators, in any academic setting, are somehow engaged in moral education, that they are teaching humanity. He writes:

> Studying the humanities may—or may not—makes us more humane. It's important that the humanities affirm what they can do, the kind of ethics they promote in their practices of interpretation, while making it clear that they are not directly in the virtue business.

However, it's not only senior humanities scholars like Culler and Brooks who challenge the expectation that exposure to and exploration of the arts and humanities will instil certain virtues and values most memorably captured with the acronym created by the Gold Foundation for Humanism in Medicine: integrity, excellence, compassion, altruism, respect, empathy and service (I.E.C.A.R.E.S.). More than any other organisation, Gold has effectively reinforced the connection of humanistic healthcare with the integration and deployment of the arts and humanities in US medical education.[3] In an opinion for *in-Training: The agora of the medical student community*, Steven Lange (2016) writes of his and his classmates' experience with lectures and small groups with humanities content that are "touted as a panacea to medicine's current evils: lack of physician empathy, inadequate patient care, dependence on technology, *et cetera*." Such curricula, Lange notes, assume that "humanities, the field proper, possesses a humanism that can be extracted and added to the biologism of medical science." In fact, Lange argues, the 'dose effect' approach contradicts the very nature of humanism—the theory that upholds the human being as the end-in-itself and as the supreme value—by objectifying it:

That some are willing to believe that medicine needs nothing more than another class . . . does not humanize it, but . . . further subjugates it to the Western model of scientific and evidence-based thinking that is based in the assessment of outcomes. The scientific legitimization of the humanities betrays the purpose of instilling humanism in medicine, and makes humanism another area of study — alas, a Wednesday morning lecture.

If the understanding of, and from, the humanities in medical education and clinical practice is primarily that of an instrument to foster compassion and empathy; tolerate ambiguity; inculcate virtues and values; and perform normative behaviours, and what David Doukas and Rebecca Volpe (2018) of the Project to Rebalance and Integrate Medical Education call "comportment," then no real expertise *is* necessary—just time, motivation, enthusiasm and good posture. Anybody, including a molecular biologist, internist or anthropologist, can do it.

Content and methodology: what is taught and how?

". . . spent a year training surgery interns in the use of narrative medicine techniques . . ."

On an April afternoon, two black men walked into a Philadelphia Starbucks, sat down and waited to meet a colleague. They asked to use the bathroom but were refused, as they hadn't purchased anything. They were then asked to leave but declined. The manager called the police, and the men were arrested "on suspicion of trespassing." Over eight million viewers watched the video on Twitter. The men were released from custody without being charged, the manager was fired and the company announced a shutdown of all US stores for a mandatory half-day training of its 175,000 employees. Kevin Johnson, Starbucks CEO, issued the following public statement: "Closing our stores for racial bias training is just one step in a journey that requires dedication from every level of our company and partnerships in our local communities" (Fitzpatrick 2018). Both the incident and the corporate response provoked outrage in light of the historical and contemporary legacy of racism in the US, especially given the recent killing of unarmed black boys and men by police officers. A half-day 'training' would not only seem to be inadequate but also disingenuous given the complexity around the issues of race and ethnicity in America. Moreover, do we know if such interventions make any difference in attitudes and behaviours at all?

When the co-authors of the above-cited text use the word 'training,' they are speaking the native language of the medical setting. Their learners are surgery residents, often called 'trainees,' who are in the process of being 'trained,' systematically instilled with the knowledge and skills of their chosen specialty. In this particular setting, there is an emphasis on the utilitarian merits of a given text or image rather than on the cultural, aesthetic, intellectual and political elements of it. Words such as 'train,' 'use' and 'technique' stand in contrast to *processes* such as 'education,' 'exploration' and 'interpretation.' The co-authors state an end point, "the use of narrative medicine techniques," one that is presumably achievable and demonstrable.

However, the complex and subtle materials that they use—a painting, a poem—only muddle the implicit precision of 'training' and intentional specificity of 'techniques.' In the body of the article, the co-authors must ultimately resort to more imprecise and nebulous descriptors of content and methodology such as 'difficulty,' 'trouble,' 'suffering' and 'limits.' They seem to be at cross-purposes: one can interpret a painting or a poem, but by their very nature, these works are unmanageable and unruly. Simply asking surgery residents to respond to a question about a painting such as: "What do you see?" or about a poem, such as: "What do you think?"

is neither training nor educating. The response to such questions in a humanities classroom would be more questions: What does the painting or poem mean? How can you make an argument for its meanings? What are the specific elements in the painting or images in the poem to support them?

Peter Brooks (2008) writes about the intense intellectual and moral energy in trying to get those interpretations right: "Participating fully in such a process, one comes away with an understanding that there is an ethics of reading," and, we would add, viewing a work of art. It is not then a matter of "Anything goes!" or "What do you feel?" but a matter of proof that is as rigorous as science. Thus, teaching humanities disciplines with increasing complexity involves a fuller engagement with whatever text is under study—a film, a painting or Mary Shelley's *Frankenstein*. This kind of critical practice alerts learners to language in ways that they may not have recognised: the words that health professionals and patients use when attempting to understand one another, the plots of the stories patients tell, the themes and tones of various narratives, the pervasive but unspoken issues around power in healthcare settings, the layers of complexity in seemingly uncomplicated decisions and routine procedures, and the unspoken worldviews and values informed by cultural practices and religious beliefs.

In contrast to the connotations of hierarchical authority and transferrable skills captured in the phrase 'training surgical interns' is an approach that offers both teachers and learners the opportunity to examine critically the nature of their personal beliefs and values, and the beliefs and values embedded in the learning environment and institutional policies and procedures. This approach requires that both teachers and learners step out of their respective comfort zones to raise difficult and complex issues and disturb their reliance on a biomedical approach to healthcare—in other words, pursuing a "pedagogy of discomfort" (Boler 1999).

Evaluation: what are the goals, and how are they met?

". . . to influence their development as compassionate surgeons."

Several years ago, an eminent physician-poet visited a medical school to speak, read and provide wit and wisdom in support of that institution's nascent humanities programme. During one informal discussion among many about content, methodology and assessment, the question arose as to whether what happens in humanities classrooms makes any difference at all in the lives of physicians. The eminent physician-poet responded with a passion, marked by a fierce belief that such activities along with much in medical education represented an act of faith.

The co-authors cited above seem to be counting on that self-same act of faith in their explicitly stated goal of influencing the development of compassionate physicians through the arts and humanities—specifically, narrative medicine. Their endeavour rests on the assumption that exposure to painting and poetry will be both professionally and culturally transformative by taking surgical residents "from their conventional training in operating rooms and hospital wards into a space where they could grow in proficiency in perspective-training and build their tolerance for ambiguity" (Kirkland and Craig 2018: 1532). The belief that humanities content and inquiry are the major site—perhaps the exclusive site—at which humanistic virtues and values such as compassion, empathy and altruism are developed, instilled and encouraged in surgery residents as well as medical students remains a long-standing and misguided supposition. Again, we return to Clouser (1979: 50) who noted, 40 years ago, that this not only "robs humanities of its true calling, but it absolves other departments of a responsibility that should be shared by all. To compartmentalize the responsibility for humanizing is to confuse virtue and knowledge."

A commitment to developing compassion and fostering empathy should be the concern of the basic medical sciences, bedside teaching and conventional activities such as rounds in operating rooms and hospital wards.

Were there a blood test to quantify compassion, humanities scholars and educators might hypothesise that our students' titres would increase steadily through engagement with literature and art. But, in the absence of such an objective measure, how can we be sure? To be clear, we are not advocating for the familiar and reductionist methods of the dominant paradigm in medical education, those measuring competencies and outcomes. In 'Sharper Instruments: On Defending the Humanities in Undergraduate Medical Education,' Catherine Belling (2010) writes about how the very lack of precise definition of terms in what constitutes 'humanities' presents significant obstacles to their study in medical settings. Any coursework that purports to improve the doctor–patient relationship, the professional development of students or the resilience of working professionals is often thrown into the bucket of the arts and humanities along with narrative medicine, literature, visual arts, history, bioethics, communication and even global health.

There are, however, strategies that can inform us about some of the critical hoped-for effects of humanities inquiry—such as the discomfort noted above that some materials can provoke, as well as the implications of cultural and sociopolitical contexts in which texts and images are embedded. These include open and candid dialogue, honest written reflections and critical and close readings in written format. Narrative and textual analysis of students' writing is also an option. Finally, there are the tried-and-true traditional course evaluations. None of these is pro-vided by the co-authors of this article with the exception of some description about discussing imaginative works and about sharing written responses to them.

Perhaps because of the limitations of the 'Arts in Medicine' feature, readers are left wonder-ing not only about the specifics of the experience but also what learners took away from it. For example, there are no sample discussion questions; no descriptions of areas of focus, introductions of linguistic or aesthetic vocabularies, or explorations of various interpretive frames. There is no substantive evaluation report from participants. We would argue that it is highly unlikely that the development and deployment of a basic or clinical sciences educational activity, course or curriculum would ever be published in a medical journal without any data regarding outcomes and assessments. Essentially, the co-authors offer readers an enactment of what Belling describes as the social processing of a cultural object. An enriching experience, to be sure, but arguably not one that they can demonstrate "enlarge[s] . . . our capacity to provide compassionate care."

That is not to say that humanities inquiry in healthcare has no potential to make a positive difference in the way it is practised. But this cannot occur without a self-conscious critique of what we read, say, do and write. We want to overthrow any notion that the health humanities are sites of the 'culture club' or 'self-care,' that we are cultural overseers and that our disciplines hold the key to turning healthcare into practices that are caring, fair and accessible to everyone. We want to confront the fact that in our classes and certainly elsewhere in medical education, there is evidence of domination and oppression. We want to develop what Patti Lather (1990: 13) once called "the skills of self-critique, of a reflexivity which will keep us from becoming impositional and reifiers ourselves."

Conclusion

The Association of American Medical Colleges (AAMC) is a not-for-profit organisation ded-icated to medical education, patient care and scientific research whose members include all accredited US and Canadian medical schools, over 400 teaching hospitals and health systems and over 80 academic societies. The association serves nearly 175,000 faculty members, 89,000 medical students and 129,000 residents. In summer 2017, AAMC leadership convened a 'thought forum,' bringing together active scholars, educators, clinicians and administrators to understand the current landscape of the arts and humanities in medical education and to create parity with the biosciences and social sciences.[4]

A summary report was published in the *AAMCNews* under the headline 'Focusing on Arts, Humanities to Develop Well-Rounded Physicians' with the following lede: "Learning about history, visual and performing arts, and literature can help physicians develop empathy and professionalism—skills that will lead to deeper connections with patients." Beneath is an image of a white male, in profile, focusing on a canvas as he prepares to daub paint on a figure in the foreground. The caption reads: 'Penn State College of Medicine student . . . creates a copy of a Van Gogh painting based on a partner's description. The class emphasizes the importance of open-ended communication in medicine.' Notwithstanding the visual reification of what has been traditionally the most acceptable and appropriate representation of a future doctor—the white male—the image also reinforces how unnecessary it is to provide even the semblance of a logical argument or a measure of statistical support for a connection between this student's crude imitation of a famous artist and his improved communication skills with future patients.

The article goes on to describe some of the courses and activities offered to US medical students in the arts and humanities and includes a graph that proudly reports the 119 institutions that require such educational work. However, not included are any criteria to specify what these institutions identify as arts and humanities education: a semester-long elective in the history of medicine? a visit to the local art museum? a workshop on improvisational theatre? shadowing the hospital ethics committee? We simply do not know, and while we do not have specific data ourselves, we do have anecdotal knowledge that many medical schools identify content that spans communication skills, professional development, clinical ethics decision-making, cultural competency training and health disparities as arts and humanities.

Such imprecision would never occur in scientific disciplines and only strengthens the long-standing belief that the arts and humanities can be taught by anyone, can foster virtues and values and cannot be effectively evaluated. However, scholars and educators in the humanities whose primary appointments are in health sciences centres and medical schools find themselves often and understandably conflicted. That the AAMC leadership came out as a staunch and public supporter of the arts and humanities in medical education is crucial—and affirming. However, we are still the Other, we are still vulnerable and we are—consciously or unwittingly—still in danger of being complicit in claiming a causal relationship between good doctoring and humanities inquiry, and in framing our intentions and outcomes within the real or imagined boundaries of science with its ordered, privileged language when we employ words such as 'training,' 'skills,' 'practices,' 'interventions' and 'competencies.' For Lange (2016), the humanities in his medical school experience simply instrumentalise doctors just as medicine instrumentalises patients: "Narrative competence is no longer a quality of a humanistic doctor, but a quantifiable asset of his or her efficiency."

Artist and activist Audre Lorde once warned that the master's tools will never dismantle the master's house. While instrumentalising the arts and humanities may secure our faculty positions and increase our popularity on curriculum committees, we must continue to support and advance the expertise of our colleagues; to develop and implement rigorous courses for our students; and to critique and challenge the checklist mentality of our institutional leaders as they push pedagogies *du jour* like 'narrative,' 'reflection,' 'resilience' and 'self-care' under the catchy catch-all of 'the arts and humanities.'

Notes

1 *The Adams Papers*,Volume 3. Letter from Abigail Adams to John Quincy Adams dated 20 March 1780. Archived and published online by the Massachusetts Historical Society. www.masshist.org/publications/apde2/view?id=ADMS-04-03-02-0240.
2 *The Journal of the American Medical Association (JAMA)* is a leading peer-reviewed medical journal with an extremely broad readership. It is published 48 times per year by the American Medical Association and includes original research, reviews and editorials, while the journal's impact is 44.405. *JAMA* is widely read by clinicians, researchers and educators across a variety of specialties and disciplines.
3 The Arnold P. Gold Foundation's overarching goal is to provide compassionate, collaborative and scientifically excellent care and to support clinicians throughout their career, so 'the humanistic passion' that motivates them at the beginning of their education is sustained. The Gold Foundation supports a wide-ranging number of grants and programmes, including the White Coat Ceremony for matriculating medical students in the United States, and is one of the most important sources for the inclusion and use of the word 'humanism' to define and describe what are considered to be important and desirable values and behaviours of medical professionals: www.gold-foundation.org.
4 See the American Association of Medical Colleges website at www.aamc.org.

References

Belling C. Arts, Sciences, Humanities: Triangulating the Two Cultures. *Journal of Literature and Science.* 2017; 10: 19–25.

Belling C. Sharper Instruments: On Defending the Humanities in Undergraduate Medical Education. *Academic Medicine.* 2010; 85: 938–40.

Bishop J. Rejecting Medical Humanism: Medical Humanities and the Metaphysics of Medicine. *Journal of Medical Humanities.* 2008; 29: 15–25.

Boler M. 1999. *Feeling Power: Emotions and Education.* New York, NY: Routledge.

Brooks P. The Ethics of Reading. *The Chronicle of Higher Education* (8 February 2008). Available at: www.chronicle.com/article/The-Ethics-of-Reading/20323. Last accessed: 22 May 2018.

Brooks P. Misunderstanding the Humanities. *The Chronicle of Higher Education* (15 December 2014). Available at: www.chronicle.com/article/Misunderstanding-the/150785 Last accessed: 22 May 2018.

Clouser KD. 1979. Humanities and the Medical School. In: LL Hunt (ed.) *Proceedings of the First Session, Institute on Human Values in Medicine.* Philadelphia, PA: Society for Health and Human Values, 47–80.

Culler J. In Need of a Name? *New Literary History.* 2005; 36: 37–42.

Doukas DJ, Volpe RL. Why Pull the Arrow When You Cannot See the Target? Framing Professionalism Goals in Medical Education. *Academic Medicine* (24 April 2018). Available at: www.researchgate.net/publication/324763386_Why_Pull_the_Arrow_When_You_Cannot_See_the_Target_Framing_Professionalism_Goals_in_Medical_Education. Last accessed: 7 May 2019.

Fitzpatrick A. Starbucks is Closing Thousands of Stories for Racial Bias Training. *Time* (17 April 2018). Available at: http://time.com/5243608/starbucks-closing-racial-bias. Last accessed: 22 May 2018.

Jones AH. 1984. Reflections, Projections, and the Future of Literature-and-Medicine. In: D Wear, M Kohn, S Stocker (eds.) *Literature and Medicine: A Claim for a Discipline.* Rootstown, OH: Northeastern Ohio Universities College of Medicine, 29–40.

Kirkland KB, Craig SR. Exploring the Surgical Gaze Through Literature and Art. *Journal of the American Medical Association.* 2018; 319: 1532–34.

Lange S. Is Medical Humanism a Humanism? *in-Training: The agora of the medical student community* (10 January 2016). Available at: http://in-training.org/medical-humanism-humanism-10202. Last accessed: 12 May 2018.

Lather P. 1990. *Getting Smart: Feminist Research and Pedagogy within the Postmodern.* New York, NY: Routledge.

Mann S. Focusing on Arts, Humanities to Develop Well-Rounded Physicians. *AAMCNEWS* (15 August 2017). Available at: https://news.aamc.org/medical-education/article/focusing-arts-humanities-well-rounded-physicians. Last accessed: 12 May 2018.

6

THE CUTTING EDGE

Health humanities for equity and social justice

Arno K. Kumagai and Thirusha Naidu

Introduction

Self-inflicted wounds: the problem with the health humanities

The health humanities are often regarded as a type of intellectual and emotional balm, a salve that may be spread liberally, not only over the injuries from disease but over the dehumanising wounds *caused by* health care. Those wounds are inflicted by implicit biases, stigmatisation, inequities in treatment, unequal access to services, the impersonal conveyor belt-like character of patient care—and by the brutalising influences of training in the health professions. In contrast, the health humanities have been viewed as a way to get back in touch with our emotional selves, our humanity, to rekindle our sense of purpose and idealism in serving others. The humanities—the creative visual arts, literature, music, philosophy, sociology, anthropology, and history—have been advocated as a means of teaching empathy and communication and observation skills, increasing self-reflection and reflective practice, and enhancing the wellbeing of health professionals. While these goals are all laudable, the predominance of biomedical, technico-rational ways of knowing in health professions education and health care has frustrated their realisation.

Furthermore, even the most passionate proponents of these humanistic approaches often unwittingly contribute to weakening their own positions through self-inflicted wounds. In an effort to introduce the health humanities into the education of health professionals, there often is no overall conceptual objective other than some vague, even pious, notion of 'feels good,' 'self-reflection,' and 'getting in touch with our inner healers.' Even the language that one hears from the most passionate proponents tends to belie the value of their proposals: 'soft,' 'touchy-feely' subjects in contrast to the 'hard' clinical and biomedical sciences; the defensive, almost apologetic arguments for inclusion of the humanities in the curriculum, the lack of conceptual rigour in the design of activities, and the lack of critical questioning of methods to determine how the effectiveness of such activities may be measured. Together, the challenges of legitimacy and these self-inflicted wounds ensure the banishment of the health humanities to what Catherine Belling (2010) terms "the decorative edges of the curriculum."

In contrast to many of the goals mentioned above, we propose that the health humanities play an essential role in the education of health professionals, particularly in the areas of equity and social justice, in two ways: first, by introducing a critical lens through which processes, values, and practices of health professions education and health care itself may be viewed; and second, by opening up spaces for reflection, dialogue, and action in addressing social injustice and oppression. Levy and Sidel (2006) define equity in health as "the absence of systematic disparities in health (or in the major social determinants of health) between social groups that have different levels of underlying social advantage or disadvantage." Health equity as a remedy to social injustice emanating from inequity has been defined as the elimination of health disparities. Health equity comprises aspirational principle and vision, shaping practices as the action needed for current structural change to occur (Stone 2013). This view has been debated in global perspectives of justice and health with a recent preference for Amartya Sen's (2005) pragmatic slant towards justice in terms of capabilities, further refined by Martha Nussbaum (2011). Sen asserts that good health must include an evaluation of the freedom a person may have to function. Beauchamp and Childress (2008) add that the allocation of goods and services, rationing, and setting priorities must also be considered (Hatchett et al. 2015).

The lack of education to address disparities in health care has been acknowledged as a deficit in medical education, where physicians have been reported to show a "lack of knowledge and skills in working with socio-economically disadvantaged patients" (Hudon et al. 2016: 2). Teaching in this area has traditionally focused on content material covering the 'social determinants of health.' In this approach, students learn lists of social characteristics (e.g., race/ethnicity, gender, socioeconomic class, immigration status, etc.) as a way to explain 'naturally' occurring causes of disparities in health care and outcomes, instead of prompting learners towards action and activism to address root causes (Sharma et al. 2018). More recently, the impetus has been for "wider adoption of the materials and methods of social medicine which studies the health of collective groups of people along with the power relationships between those groups and the institutions that impact their health" (Hixon et al. 2013: 162).

An examination of social justice and equity in health humanities necessitates reference to the concept of 'structural violence.' Structural violence refers to injustice and inequities "embedded in ubiquitous social structures and normalized by stable institutions and regular experience" (Winter and Leighton 2001: 99). These social structures, composed of social relations and political, religious, or cultural (including medical) arrangements, are 'violent' because they subjugate people and communities, restrict their agency, choices, and freedom, waste their talents, knowledge, and skills, and debase their dignity and humanity. They violate. In doing so, they perpetuate discrimination and oppression by causing, illness, injury, suffering, and death. There has been substantial writing on structural violence and the politics of blame (Berns 2001; Parker and Aggleton 2003; Farmer 2004; Castro and Farmer 2005; Farmer et al. 2006). What is needed, however, is an exploration of how educators may prompt relatively privileged health professions students and practitioners to reflect deeply on the social injustice and inequities created by structural violence (Farmer 2003; Rylko-Bauer and Farmer 2016).

Also missing is discussion of a means to guard against abstraction, i.e., to prevent teaching for social justice and equity from becoming an intellectual exercise confined to the classroom with no real-world effects or outcomes. We call for exploring these constructs in meaningful ways through embodied practices—interactions in the learning environment—that stimulate a provocative positioning and interrogative stance. Embodied practices entail patterns of ongoing interaction between an organism and its physical and cultural environments, where understanding is deeply embodied. Human interpretation and reasoning rely on sensory, motor, and affective patterns and processes to shape understanding of, and engagement with, the world (Johnson 2015). These ways espouse not just dialogues on equity and justice but engagement through action, participation, activism, and advocacy through a pedagogy that is based on disruption, distraction, destabilisation, and discord to understand the interrupting effects of dis-ease on human health and flourishing.

Here, dis-ease represents a state of discomfort, disequilibrium, or instability that may precede and/or cause the manifestation of ill health. It is the intersection between a patient's subjective experience of ill health (illness) and the medical establishment's hegemonically based descriptions of ill health as 'disease' or 'disorder' (Wilkinson 2017). Structural dis-ease may be a harbinger of structural violence provoking disease and illness. For example, forced migration usually affects the most vulnerable in a nation: the stress and suffering provoke destabilisation of health in individuals and groups, thus creating disease and illness. This dis-ease—and the resultant illness—accompanies people into new contexts and perpetuates their vulnerability and disadvantage.

The effects of structural violence have been referred to as "social suffering," the lived experience of distress and injustice that lays bare the inextricable links between personal and societal problems (Kleinman 2000). Frank (1995) refers to a "pedagogy of suffering" in which patients' narratives make their suffering evident and visible, while teaching occurs through exposure to these experiences. He refers to the humanities in medicine as a "sociology of witnessing," where the unmasking and witnessing of suffering create discord, disruption, and dis-ease, compelling the witness to account for, or to acknowledge, the patient's active role and participation in the illness context or drama. Otherwise, the patient is merely a silent enduring body, or worse, a system or organ being acted on by an imbalance of social forces (structural violence), in addition to the physiological imbalances leading to disease manifestation. In the view of post-colonial philosopher Gayathri Spivak (Spivak and Morris 2010), this would be an instance of the subaltern (marginalised or subjugated people) attempting to raise her voice while remaining unheard because of a lack of a context in which her voice may be perceived. Sharma (2018: 1), building on Spivak's assertions, considers that "the positioning of the patient as 'subaltern' can provide channels of resistance against traditional power asymmetries." We contend that for the 'subalterns' (i.e., subjugated and oppressed voices/patients) to be heard in the context of medicine, disruption, discord, and distraction must be included in the fabric of medical thought and practice. Where it concerns health professions education, this must occur in the very weaving of this fabric itself.

Equity and social justice lose their rigour if they are static concepts, both idealised and idolised; or aspirations to be achieved over time rather than tangible, pressing concerns. As social constructs, equity and social justice are in danger of being abstracted away from actual suffering and the power structures (within the medicine and health care establishments) that produce such suffering. This engagement must extend from verbal dialogue to include embodied dialogical engagement in corporeal (patients' and doctors' physical bodies) and institutional spaces (health professions schools and related health contexts). An example from medical education is Rachel Prentice's examination of how surgical training as a structured environment prepares students for the embodied lessons taught by a surgeon (Prentice 2007). While patients enter and leave the contexts of medicine, medical professionals are consistently present and have their thoughts, ideas, and identities shaped by the context. In the absence of disruption and reflection, they will perpetuate the structures that create social inequities and injustice within the establishment.

Disruption of such habits can cause gaps to create a context for the subaltern's voice to be heard. Spivak demands that those in power establish these kinds of contexts. Patients have been lulled into social control through unconscious collusion with the power structures in the medical establishment via "governmentality" (Foucault 1991). The relationship between patients (as subjects) and hospitals and medical establishments—including medical schools—(as institutions) perhaps most tangibly represents the Foucauldian view of biopolitics, the extension of state or sovereign power over both the physical and political bodies of a population. A Foucauldian perspective of governmentality accounts for how people unwittingly concede and subject themselves to be acted on as 'patients' (an identity position), although the exercise of sovereign power does invite resistance:

> Human technologies involve the calculated organization of human forces and capacities. Relations of hierarchy, from age to educational qualifications and accreditation, locate individuals in chains of allegiance and dependency, empowering some to direct others and obliging others to comply. Mechanisms of reformation and therapy provide the means whereby self-regulatory techniques may be reshaped according to the principles of psychological theory. As networks form, as relays, translations and connections couple political aspirations with modes of action upon persons, technologies of subjectivity are established that enable strategies of power to infiltrate the interstices of the human soul.
>
> *(Rose 1999: 8)*

In medicine, patients' voices are typically silenced. Their position of powerlessness is intensified where patients carry the mantle of other silenced identities such as poverty, gender, race, or class. Equity is severely threatened because they are not only silenced but also invisible. Their issues do not exist because they do not have a space in the context. Their voices resonate at a different pitch so they are not heard, and they reflect light at a different wavelength so they are invisible where their light is not reflected. Equity and social justice in the health humanities should aim to foster and teach health professionals how to bend and shape contexts to catch the invisible wavelengths of light and vibrate at frequencies that allow silent voices to be heard. We advocate for teaching for equity and social justice. Health professions education for social justice and equity must take an accountability and advocacy perspective. It does so by engaging concepts and approaches drawn from disciplines in the humanities and social sciences, such as philosophy, critical theory, literature, poetry, the visual and performance arts, sociology, anthropology, and history, while looking at health, illness, health care, and the education of health professionals (pedagogy) in new and generative ways. We propose that the critical health humanities may in part achieve these goals by fostering the development of a critical consciousness of self, others, and the world. This praxis combines both content and critical pedagogy, using numerous techniques and concepts explored in depth below.

Critical consciousness: the object of learning in critical humanities

Instead of a body of knowledge of critical humanities—a 'Critical Canon' of sorts—that one learns, we would argue that the object of knowledge and the goal of learning in this field are not as much content as ways of knowing and acting in the world. This orientation may be termed 'critical consciousness' and represents an awareness of Self, Other, and the World, as well as an awareness of social injustice and a commitment to act to address injustice.

Critical consciousness, or *conscientizaçao*, is a concept originally developed by the Brazilian educational theorist Paulo Freire (1993) to describe a way of learning to perceive ('to read'), and act on, educational, social, economic, political, and historical contradictions that lead to oppression and suffering. It posits that human beings are conscious, reflective, social beings who are capable of interacting with fellow human beings to address inequities and injustices in the world. This approach is not only epistemological but also existential and embodied: it is both thought and action in the world.

As a form of thinking, teaching, learning, and being, critical consciousness is distinct from the notion of 'critical thinking,' to which educators devote innumerable hours of thought and effort. Critical thinking is analytical and evaluative; it involves abstraction and attempts to assess facts and phenomena as objectively as possible. The individual who engages in critical thinking uses the Cartesian *res cogitans*—the 'mental substance'—that exists separately from being. Critical thinking may be done by oneself alone in a room—it is 'monological'; that is, the meaning and product of thought may be the outcome of a single individual, disconnected from others and the world (Burbules and Berk 1999). In medicine, one may engage in critical thinking regarding a differential diagnosis, diagnostic strategy, and treatment plan of a patient without regard to the social context in which illness and its consequences play out—without consideration of the ethical, societal, historical, political, and structural issues that have resulted in a given patient presenting for care at a given time in a given set of circumstances. Issues of privilege, power, equity, or justice do not enter into the picture; they are often considered as separate, or not considered at all. In contrast, critical consciousness addresses these social and societal issues in the context of illness and medical care. Critical consciousness demands answers to the question 'why?'; not only why does a specific disease process result in these clinical findings and sequelae, but also why have social forces resulted in an individual being unable to flourish in health and wellness at a given time and a given place?

The point here is not that critical consciousness is 'better' than critical thinking. Critical thinking itself is an essential activity in medicine; alone, however, it is insufficient to deliver care with excellence, compassion, and justice (Kumagai and Lypson 2009). Critical consciousness connects differential diagnoses to societal and structural inequities and links diagnostic strategies and treatment plans with human needs and contexts. Its emphasis on both understanding and action ties identification of inequities into the social determinants of health to address such inequities and to support the social contract and consequent accountability underlying health care (Sharma, Pinto, and Kumagai 2018). From an epistemological point of view, in contrast to critical thinking, which takes an instrumental approach to understanding abnormal processes to discover effective interventions, critical consciousness is fundamentally *emancipatory*: it addresses interests and action with human social needs in order to alleviate suffering and oppression (Kumagai 2013). But here too is an ethical challenge: who decides on who shall be 'emancipated,' for what reasons, and what form the 'emancipation' shall take can all constitute a form of imperialism, a 'violence,' conscious governmentality, or an imposed religiosity.

The power of stories

Narratives—'stories' in the broadest sense—may play a crucially important role in the development of critical consciousness, in the ability, as Freire (1993: 39) describes it, "to see the world unveiled." Whether through literature, the visual arts, music, song, or oral traditions, stories have the ability to create an affective link between individuals of different backgrounds, identities, life experiences, and even time periods; and to imagine the world through another's eyes (Kumagai 2008). This may be particularly important in stories from individuals whose views are traditionally silenced in a process that the writer bell hooks (1994) calls "coming to voice." In *Borderlands/La Frontera*, the Chicana writer Gloria Anzaldúa (2012) speaks of a capacity, which she terms *la facultad*, that allows individuals from marginalised groups to see beyond superficial appearances: "to see the deep structures below the surface" that oppress and dominate the lives of individuals without power. These stories have the capacity to stimulate shifts in perspective and create allies in struggle.

There are, however, risks to narratives. Although stories have great power to transform perspectives and values, not all stories and the ways they are told are 'good.' As the feminist writer Megan Boler (1999) points out, the suffering and oppression of silenced groups may be appropriated—often unwittingly—by privileged individuals or groups, who upon hearing the stories conclude that they 'now get it,' i.e., they understand the experience even though it is not one that they have had themselves. This returns us to our earlier warning about 'emancipation' as potentially colonising rather than liberating. In this sense, instead of fostering empathy and forging allies, the appropriation of stories can replicate existing power hierarchies and result in 're-victimisation' of those who are the subjects of the stories themselves. Boler talks of two types of narratives: "spectating," in which the listener, while moved by the story, leaves the story unchanged; and "bearing witness," in which the listener acknowledges responsibility for addressing suffering and is prompted to act. There is thus a moral dimension to storytelling itself, where stories become instruments to sharpen one's moral vision towards justice and humanistic care.

Narrative disruption

An element of stories that plays an essential role in the development of critical consciousness is the power to disrupt: to produce discomfort in order to prompt reflection on self, others, and the world, prompting 'thinking otherwise.' Boler's concept of "the pedagogy of discomfort" is useful in this context. She argues that in contrast to "spectating," where individuals consider the lives of others living under conditions of injustice and oppression from a privileged distance—a "gaping distance between self and other"—a pedagogy of discomfort prompts the individual to engage in an act of "witnessing" in which she recognises historical responsibilities and individual agency as well as the possibility of taking action for change. Here,

> The aim of discomfort is for each person, myself included, to explore beliefs and value; to examine when visual 'habits' and emotional selectivity have become rigid and immune to flexibility; and to identify when and how our habits harm ourselves and others.
>
> *(Boler 1999: 186)*

A pedagogy of discomfort recognises complexity and prevents us from letting ourselves off the hook for moral responsibility and challenges. If done skilfully, a nuanced approach to speaking about justice and injustice can move beyond questions of guilt and innocence and may instead invite students "to leave the familiar shores of learned beliefs and habits and swim further out into the 'foreign' and risky depths of the sea of ethical and moral differences" (ibid.: 181). This approach recalls Paulo Freire's (1993) idea of "reading the world," i.e., to lift the veil of naturalness behind dehumanising conditions to understand the complex relationships of power, privilege, and oppression that operate underneath. For Freire, this type of learning-through-contradiction often takes the form of a *ruptura*—a break—from the past: "[T]here is no creativity without *ruptura*, without a break from the old, without conflict in which you have to make a decision. I would say there is no human existence without *ruptura*" (Horton and Freire 1991: 38).

Shielding learners from confrontation and controversy through attempts to remain 'neutral' or 'objective' in fact tends to reinforce both individual preconceived ideas and the status quo and to perpetuate existing hierarchies of power, by-passing resistance. In this setting, one may talk about race without speaking about racism, gender without speaking about sexism, homosexuality without speaking about homophobia (Kumagai and Lypson 2009; Sharma and Kuper 2016). One may also diligently list all of the 'social determinants of health' as factors that explain why the health status of a given patient is poor without attempting to understand or address the larger societal or structural issues that prevent health and wellness (Sharma, Pinto, and Kumagai 2018). Deliberate attempts to shake up complacent assumptions and beliefs—in which implicit biases and dehumanising ways of labelling and thinking lurk—can force reflection and new ways of thinking and being.

On the other hand, exposure of learners to uncomfortable things—either in an attempt to disrupt thinking or as an intrinsic part of the learning to care for the ill, the injured, the distraught, or the dying—can provoke more than produce discomfort. Depending on the learner's background, lived experiences, identities, or life situation, teaching and learning about subjects of societal and social significance, such as bigotry, violence, abuse, suffering, suicide, and loss, may not remain as abstract subjects of an educational curriculum, but instead become sources of profound personal distress. For example, any lecture to a health professions class on domestic violence or sexual assault will invariably expose individuals who are actual survivors in the audience. In this sense, use of literature, stories, art, or movies to teach about socially relevant issues can 'cut close to the bone' and provoke distress in ways that are neither predictable nor desired (Kumagai et al. 2017). Rather than attempting to avoid such trauma—which is arguably unavoidable in medicine—by making the teaching of such subjects as sterile and abstract as possible, institutions must demonstrate sensitivity, creativity, and foresight in addressing these risks as part of a fundamental educational responsibility to learners and their needs.

Questioning postcolonialism and neocolonialism in decolonising medical education

Another way in which the humanities act as the 'sharp edge' of education is by questioning concepts, practices, and motivations that are taken for granted as 'inspirational' and well meaning (Bleakley, Bligh, and Browne 2011). An example of this trend is the rapid development of global medical education as a discipline in the West. This often is characterised by two related approaches: first, in what has been described as neocolonialism in medical education (Bleakley et al. 2008), where Western medical educators work to 'correct' perceived underdevelopment in non-Western global contexts through the introduction of 'more advanced' forms of Western medicine (i.e., 'the West is best' approach). Second, where concepts deemed 'universal' in Western medical education, such as teaching and assessment methods, communication styles, and even notions of empathy and reflection, are introduced in an unmodified and non-critical form into non-Western health environments (Nguyen et al. 2009; Naidu and Kumagai 2016). The unfortunate end result that accompanies much self-congratulation on the part of educators is but a newer form of intellectual or educational imperialism.

Bleakley, Bligh, and Browne (2011) address this 'postcolonial' dilemma in medical education by noting that knowledge may be culturally legitimated in spaces left by withdrawing colonising nations. They warn that Westerners must be cautious about exporting a homogenised brand of Western medical education that may thwart locally adaptive practices, while research funding for medicine is unfairly skewed towards research that investigates medical conditions dominant in the West. Referring to these trends as "imperialism through the back door," Bleakley and colleagues recommend a reflexive approach suggesting that Western medical educators develop new ways of reflecting on what they are doing when they advocate for the spread of Western curricula, approaches, and teaching technology.

We add that a postcolonial view using this lens would also ask medical educators in the global South (developing countries/the Third World, etc.) to cultivate—in research, education, and practice—resistance to the unreflective adoption of Western pedagogies: curricula approaches and teaching technologies. The latter is perhaps a more challenging prospect because it requires resistance to the insidious forces of empire bolstered by economic (capitalism), linguistic (global dominance of colonisers' languages, e.g., French, Spanish, English), and cultural (Western music, art, and literature) factors (Roy 2004). It requires colonised peoples to reject or at least externalise conceptions of themselves as 'the other' in their own eyes (Said 2003). This form of resistance might already be emerging in medical education and research through what Homi Bhabha (2004) refers to as "mimicry" or "sly civility." Here, colonised peoples consciously but ironically simulate the actions, views, and philosophies of the colonisers for the purpose of gaining access to colonial spoils. This may be characterised by researchers from the global South participating in global collaborative projects and changing ideas from within. Increasing numbers of students from the developing world enter Western medical schools subverting Western ideas imposed on them from within the colonisers' worlds and institutions. As these researchers and students become more empowered, so their resistant identities may emerge and develop leading to heretofore hidden traditional health practices gaining recognition.

The largest medical research funding sources tend to originate in the West with funding calls generally requiring developing country researchers to collaborate with Western researchers. Often, such calls specify that lead investigators be Westerners, creating skewed partnerships in research and global medical education that favour Western researchers and students and Western ideas and practices (Bleakley, Brice, and Bligh 2008; Karle et al. 2008; Adams et al. 2016). In addition, many global health programmes offer medical students paid or funded experiences in developing health contexts and access to 'data' gathering or observation opportunities in developing countries that established local researchers would take years to access for lack of funding and resources (Nguyen et al. 2009; Adams et al. 2016). In such instances, students need to be enlightened about how their experiences and observations may be come across as intrusion or 'gawking' in the eyes of local people (Conrad et al. 2006; Ackerman 2010; Abedini et al. 2012), echoing 'othering' and emphasising of difference by Western ways of seeing (Said 2003). In these contexts, students might begin to see their Western mentor-researchers not as the great white hopes or saviours who descend to discover what the true nature of local medical and health issues is, but people, who, by virtue of racial, class, political, and economic privilege, are able to impose their neocolonial will on people—communities and nations who have yet to shed the yokes of the original colonisers.

There is no social justice and equity without reflexivity: how does who I am influence what I see and how others see me?

As neo-colonisers, Western medical researchers can build lucrative careers and celebrity status in their disciplines globally, in what might be called the 'appropriation of data' in a colonising setting that controls access to medical data, health trends, and funding for research. A social justice and equity perspective would demand that Western researchers and their students assume an accountability by taking a reflexive stance to consider how their positions of privilege afford them access to power and status (Finnegan et al. 2017). They would be obliged to confront how people in non-Western contexts are subtly cajoled or even coerced to compromise and relinquish their cultural knowledge, ideas, bodies, and lives for the sake of 'global' medical research. Perhaps this may be tempered by teaching reflexivity, so that health profession students may interrogate their own perspectives as well as the social structures (socio-cultural, historical, and economic) by which their gazes, lenses, positionalities, and perspectives are shaped. This could in part entail:

first, equipping health professions schools with the tools and technology to deliver this imperative; second, addressing the mismatch between the skills taught in most schools and those needed to improve fragile health systems and finally ensuring that health professions schools that strive to eliminate health inequities should 'walk the walk,' adopting progressive practices to institutionalize equity.

(Drobac and Morse 2016: 702)

Again, this behests the challenge to confront silence and invisibility from within social structures that do not yet possess method or means to perceive what needs to be seen or heard (Spivak and Morris 2010). While concepts of individual justice focus on an individual's rights and obligations within an organised state, the tenets of social justice expand these rights and obligations to include the responsibilities of society to its members and its members' responsibilities to each other (Hixon et al. 2013).

Putting the health humanities under a critical gaze

While the health humanities may be engaged productively in health professions education, this should be scrutinised critically. For example, a popular means of introducing the arts into medical education is planned activities around a visit to art museums (Bardes et al. 2001; Dolev et al. 2001; Reilly et al. 2005; Kirklin et al. 2007; Gaufberg and Williams 2011). The goals of such activities range from sharpening observational skills and clinical reasoning to improving health care professionals' wellness and compassion. Although such activities probably meet most, if not all, of their stated objectives, they also run the risk of reinforcing existing and traditional power hierarchies through an unquestioned approach to the arts. In the same manner that an uncritical reliance on the Western literary canon as educational material in the health humanities may reinforce traditional notions of art and aesthetics, a lack of care and thoughtfulness in introducing art into education may restrict one's perspectives and questioning to certain culturally sanctioned "ways of seeing" (Berger 1972), instead of prompting learners to question or critique societal values and norms.

Making strange

Expanding on the theme of disruption, the health humanities can play an additional role in health professions education: that of 'making strange.' One of the most powerful functions of modern art is to distort perception of common things, events, people, and things in order to prompt a 're-imagining' of them. Although the idea of 'making strange' has been used in art and literature for millennia—from the satires of the Greeks and Romans to the surrealist vision of René Magritte—the conceptual articulation of this phenomenon was first made by the Russian Formalist Victor Shklovsky (Shklovsky and Sher 1991). Shklovsky maintains that habituation in thought naturally leads to what he called "automatic thinking" in which objects, places, events, and individuals "fade away" and become inaccessible in their uniqueness to consciousness. Art functions to renew awareness of these things by distorting perception so that they are viewed afresh. He calls this process "estrangement" (*ostranenie*):

> [I]n order to return sensation to our limbs, in order to make us feel objects, to make a stone feel stony, man has been given the tool of art. The purpose of art, then, is to lead us to a knowledge of a thing through the organ of sight instead of through recognition. By 'estranging' objects and complicating form, the device of art makes perception long and laborious.

(ibid.: 6)

Inspired by Shklovsky's theories, the German playwright Bertolt Brecht (1964) employed the concept of the "alienation" or "A-effect" in his sociopolitical dramas to disrupt audience identification with the protagonists and to lay bare the actual mechanics of the staging and production. In doing so, the drama creates a sense of alienation in the audience and forces them to question the seeming naturalness of conditions in the play—and by extension, in modern society. Unlike Shklovsky, Brecht attributes this seeming naturalness not to the automaticity of human perception, but to the distorting forces of capitalist economies (ibid.; Kumagai and Wear 2013). Literature, film, poetry, painting, and sculpture—from Kafka's *Metamorphosis* to the paintings of Frida Kahlo and Francis Bacon, to short videos on YouTube—can be used in medical education to 'make strange' seemingly natural ways of looking at patients, doctors, and the practice of medicine in order to renew our vision of health care in 'rehumanised' forms (ibid.).

Towards a dialogical approach to teaching for social justice

So how do we create this cutting edge for the health humanities? We propose that it involves not only different content and approaches, but also different ways of communicating and interacting as teachers and learners. Much attention has been paid to the transfer of new biomedical knowledge and the fostering of critical thinking skills; however, how do we teach for critical consciousness and action to address inequities and injustice in the world? We propose that the answer to this question lies in the praxis of 'dialogue' (Kumagai and Naidu 2015; Kumagai et al. 2018).

Discussions, which are driven chiefly by cognitive processes, often involve methods of argumentation or persuasion. They rely on analysis of data, claims of authority, and hierarchies of expertise. Above all, discussions are goal-oriented: the interlocutors aim to arrive at an answer in the form of the approach most rigorously based on evidence, the most probable outcome, the consensus view. In contrast, dialogues engage the participant's whole person: backgrounds, identities, lived experiences, values, feelings, and perspectives. This type of engagement is open and exploratory and depends on relationships of trust and mutual respect. It also relies on confidence in the process of authentic inquiry, regardless of the outcome. Dialogues open up perspectives and invite new approaches; they end not with a solution or a specific answer, but with additional questions and possibilities of knowing, understanding, and being (ibid.).

Importantly, dialogues have the potential to disrupt or even reverse hierarchical authority. For example, when speaking of personal experiences of marginalisation, discrimination, or bigotry, authority may shift to those individuals who otherwise have little power, whose opinion carries little weight. In a process of what bell hooks (1994: 148) calls "coming to voice," normally silenced perspectives are given voice and authority within the dialogical space; such exchanges have the potential of becoming a polyglossal mixture of voices (Bakhtin and Emerson 1984) that adds to the rich complexity and nuances of human experiences in health professions education and practice. In a broader sense, dialogue also has the potential to up-end traditional educational practices:

> Through dialogue, the teacher-of-the-students and the students-of-the-teacher cease to exist and a new term emerges: teacher-student with student-teachers. The teacher is no longer merely the-one-who-teaches, but one who is himself taught in dialogue with the students, who in turn while being taught also teach. They become jointly responsible for a process in which all grow.
>
> *(Freire 1993: 80)*

Dialogues may be prompted by questions, paradoxes, problem-posing, or stories. Arthur Frank's (2010) concept of telling stories without endings is relevant here: by presenting an ethical dilemma without providing a clear solution, the learner is prompted to engage in critical self-reflection in order to arrive at her own approach and resolution (Macleod et al. 2018; Naidu 2018). Stories such as Dagoberto Gilb's (2010) *Please Thank You*, about the thoughts of a Mexican American middle-aged man after suffering a stroke, can lend a provocative start to a dialogue about implicit bias, identity, and illness. A group reading or enactment of William Carlos Williams' (1984) *A Face of Stone*, as part of a Medical Readers' Theatre (Savitt 2002) activity, can embody issues of objectification, bigotry, and a subtle transformation of the doctor's perception of the patient from object—a 'face of stone'—to a sentient, vulnerable human being. Zimbabwean writer Tsitsi Dangarembga's (1988) *Nervous Conditions* can highlight how colonisation impacts on marginalised intersectional identities to produce illness. Literature, art, music, and poetry can serve to launch transformative dialogical interactions and explorations of the human and ethical dimensions of health and illness. By creating a space in which differences in identity, backgrounds, values, perspectives, and lived experiences may interact, dialogue contributes to a democratising of education and a ground from which critical consciousness of self, others, and the world may arise.

In summary, the health humanities offer not only the content and the values but also the pedagogical approaches that can enrich the ways in which health professionals address issues of social inequity and injustice. The health humanities represent in effect the whetstone on which critical reflection and humanism may be sharpened as critical and powerful instruments of care. We believe in Paulo Freire's (1993) notion of "teaching as the practice of freedom," and posit that health humanities provide essential means to achieve the practice of medicine with excellence, compassion, and, above all, justice.

Coda

Spivak speaks
Spivak speaks . . .
Silver shod and silver tongued
to a distant audience.
Sounding a warning
that the time has come
for the subaltern who cannot speak,
to be martyred on
the paradoxical pyre of democracy.
Committing Sati
to come to the terrible conclusion
Cui bono?
Spivak speaks . . .
Practice norms theory.
Curriculum theorises.
Theory must learn from practice,
monumentalised in norming.
Foucault's political. Canguilhem's polemical.
In class continuous academic priority
The mass era regains
Skeumorphistic
The subaltern gapes as if to speak
But still, is silent.

Mimesis of voice
in quiet.
Spivak speaks . . .
National connectivity
is not a revolution when
all can call the spirits
from the vast deep.
But who amongst these,
by telling truth,
can shame the devil.
Belief is the smallest speck of reason.
Crazed knowledge management
fires epistemological machinery.
Imagination creates
cause for pause.
In the multi-faced collective
we cannot bring the subaltern to citizenship.
In a mixed crowd of the poor,
curriculum is strangled
by its own umbilical cord.
Spivak speaks . . .
"It's easy for me to say.
I don't care about anything . . .
I might die tonight"
Thirusha Naidu
> *(After a seminar by Prof Gayatri Spivak:*
> *'Curriculum Transformation in Higher*
> *Education in Asia and Africa:*
> *A Reality Check.' Durban. Monday,*
> *7 August 2017)*

Acknowledgements

AK Kumagai acknowledges the FM Hill Foundation of Women's College Hospital for support of his work and Drs L Richardson, A Kuper, S Khan, B Jackson, and S Rizack for many helpful discussions.

References

Abedini NC, Gruppen LD, Kolars JC, Kumagai AK. Understanding the effects of short-term international service learning trips on medical students. *Academic Medicine*. 2012; 87: 820–28.

Ackerman LK. The ethics of short-term international health electives in developing countries. *Annals of Behavioral Science and Medical Education*. 2010; 16: 40–43.

Adams LV, Wagner CM, Nutt CT, Binagwaho A. The future of global health education: training for equity in global health. *BMC Medical Education*. 2016; 16: 296.

Anzaldúa G. 2012. *Borderlands/La Frontera*. San Francisco, CA: Aunt Lute Books.

Bakhtin MM, Emerson C. 1984. *Problems of Dostoevsky's poetics*. Minneapolis, MN: University of Minnesota Press.

Bardes CL, Gillers D, Herman AE. Learning to look: developing clinical observational skills at an art museum. *Medical Education.* 2001; 35: 1157–61.

Beauchamp TL, Childress JF. 2008 (6th ed.). *Principles of biomedical ethics.* Oxford: Oxford University Press.

Belling C. Commentary: sharper instruments—on defending the humanities in undergraduate medical education. *Academic Medicine.* 2010; 85: 938–40.

Berger J. 1972. *Ways of seeing.* Harmondsworth: Penguin.

Berns N. Degendering the problem and gendering the blame: political discourse on women and violence. *Gender and Society.* 2001; 15: 262.

Bhabha HK. 2004. *The location of culture.* London: Routledge.

Bleakley A, Bligh J, Browne J. 2011. *Medical education for the future: Identity, power and location.* Dordrecht: Springer.

Bleakley A, Brice J, Bligh J. Thinking the post-colonial in medical education. *Medical Education.* 2008; 42: 266–70.

Boler M. 1999. *Feeling power: Emotions and education.* New York, NY: Routledge.

Brecht B. 1964. The modern theatre is the epic theatre. In: *Brecht on Theatre: The Development of an Aesthetic.* New York, NY: Hill and Wang Methuen, 33–42.

Burbules NC, Berk R. 1999. Critical thinking and critical pedagogy: Relations, differences, and limits. In: *Critical theories in education: Changing terrains of knowledge and politics.* New York, NY: Routledge.

Castro A, Farmer P. Understanding and addressing AIDS-related stigma: from anthropological theory to clinical practice in Haiti. *American Journal of Public Health.* 2005; 95: 53.

Conrad CJ, Kahn MJ, D'eSalvo KB, Hamm LL. Student clinical experiences in Africa: who are we helping? *Virtual Mentor: American Medical Association Journal of Ethics.* 2006; 8: 855–58.

Dangarembga T. 1988. *Nervous conditions.* London: Women's Press.

Dolev JC, Friedlaender LK, Braverman IM. Use of fine art to enhance visual diagnostic skills. *JAMA.* 2001; 286: 1020–21.

Drobac P, Morse M. Medical education and global health equity. *Virtual Mentor: American Medical Association Journal of Ethics.* 2016; 8: 855–58.

Farmer P. 2003. *Pathologies of power: Health, human rights, and the new war on the poor.* Berkeley, CA: University of California Press.

Farmer P. An anthropology of structural violence. *Current Anthropology.* 2004; 45: 305–25.

Farmer PE, Nizeye B, Stulac S, Keshavjee S. Structural violence and clinical medicine. *PLoS Medicine.* 2006; 3: 1686.

Finnegan A, Morse M, Nadas M, Westerhaus M. Where we fall down: Tensions in teaching social medicine and global health. *Annals of Global Health.* 2017; 83: 347–55.

Foucault M. 1991. Governmentality. In: *The Foucault effect: Studies in governmentality—With two lectures by and an interview with Michel Foucault.* Chicago, IL: University of Chicago Press, 307.

Frank AW. 1995. *The wounded storyteller: Body, illness, and ethics.* Chicago, IL: University of Chicago Press.

Frank AW. 2010. *Letting stories breathe: A socio-narratology.* Chicago, IL: University of Chicago Press.

Freire P. 1993. *Pedagogy of the oppressed.* New York, NY: Continuum.

Gaufberg E, Williams R. Reflection in a museum setting: The personal responses tour. *The Journal of Graduate Medical Education.* 2011; 3: 546–49.

Gilb D. Please, thank you. *Harper's Magazine.* June 2010; 65–70.

Hatchett L, Elster N, Wasson K, et al. Integrating social justice for health professional education: Self-reflection, advocacy, and collaborative learning. *Online Journal of Health Ethics.* 2015; 11. Available at: https://aquila.usm.edu/ojhe/vol11/iss1/4. Last accessed: 26 July 2018.

Hixon A, Yamada Y, Farmer P, Maskarinec G. Social justice: the heart of medical education. *Social Medicine.* 2013; 7: 161–68.

hooks b. 1994. *Teaching to transgress: Education as the practice of freedom* New York, NY: Routledge.

Horton M, Freire P. 1991. *We make the road by walking: Conversations on education and social change.* Philadelphia, PA: Temple University Press.

Hudon C, Loignon C, Grabovschi C, et al. Medical education for equity in health: a participatory action research involving persons living in poverty and healthcare professionals. *BMC Medical Education.* 2016; 16: 106.

Johnson M. Embodied understanding. *Frontiers in Psychology.* 2015; 29 June; 6.

Karle H, Christensen L, Gordon D, Nystrup J. 2008. Neo-colonialism versus sound globalization policy in medical education. *Medical Education.* 42: 956–58.

Kirklin D, Duncan J, McBride S, et al. A cluster design controlled trial of arts-based observational skills training in primary care. *Medical Education*. 2007; 41: 395–401.

Kleinman A. 2000. The violences of everyday life: The multiple forms and dynamics of social violence. In: *Violence and subjectivity*. Berkeley, CA: University of California Press, 379.

Kumagai AK. A conceptual framework for use of illness narratives in medical education. *Academic Medicine*. 2008; 83: 653–58.

Kumagai AK. From competencies to human interests: ways of knowing and understanding in medical education. *Academic Medicine*. 2013; 89: 978–83.

Kumagai AK, Jackson B, Razack S. Cutting close to the bone: Student trauma, free speech, and institutional responsibility in medical education. *Academic Medicine*. 2017; 92: 318–23.

Kumagai AK, Lypson ML. Beyond cultural competence: critical consciousness, social justice, and multicultural education. *Academic Medicine*. 2009; 84: 82–87.

Kumagai AK, Naidu T. Reflection, dialogue, and the possibilities of space. *Academic Medicine*. 2015; 90: 283–88.

Kumagai AK, Richardson L, Khan S, Kuper A. Dialogues on the threshold: Dialogical learning for humanism and justice. *Academic Medicine*. 2018; 93: 1778–83.

Kumagai AK, Wear D. Making strange: a role for the humanities in medical education. *Academic Medicine*. 2013; 89: 973–77.

Levy BS, Sidel VW. 2006. *Social injustice and public health*. Oxford: Oxford University Press.

Macleod CI, Marx J, Mnyaka P, Treharne GJ. 2018. *The Palgrave handbook of ethics in critical research*. London: Palgrave Macmillan.

Naidu T. 2018. Not my science. In: CI Macleod et al. (eds.) *The Palgrave handbook of ethics in critical research*. London: Palgrave Macmillan, v–vi.

Naidu T, Kumagai AK. Troubling muddy waters: Problematizing reflective practice in global medical education. *Academic Medicine*. 2016; 91: 317–21.

Nguyen P-M, Elliott JG, Terlouw C, Pilot A. Neocolonialism in education: cooperative learning in an Asian context. *Comparative Education*. 2009; 45: 109.

Nussbaum MC. 2011. *Creating capabilities: The human development approach*. Cambridge, MA: Harvard University Press.

Parker R, Aggleton P. HIV and AIDS-related stigma and discrimination: a conceptual framework and implications for action. *Social Science & Medicine*. 2003; 57: 13–24.

Prentice R. Drilling surgeons: the social lessons of embodied surgical learning. *Science Technology & Human Values*. 2007; 32: 534–55.

Reilly JM, Ring J, Duke L. Visual thinking strategies: a new role for art in medical education. *Family Medicine*. 2005; 37: 250–52.

Rose NS. 1999. *Governing the soul: The shaping of the private self*. New York, NY: Free Association Books.

Roy A. 2004. *An ordinary person's guide to empire*. Cambridge, MA: South End Press.

Rylko-Bauer B, Farmer P. 2016. Structural violence, poverty, and social suffering. In: *The Oxford handbook of the social science of poverty*. New York, NY: Oxford University Press.

Said EW. 2003. *Orientalism*. New York, NY: Vintage Books.

Savitt TL. 2002. *Medical readers' theater: A guide and scripts*. Iowa City, IA: University of Iowa Press.

Sen A. Human rights and capabilities. *Journal of Human Development*. 2005; 6: 151–66.

Sharma M. 'Can the patient speak?': postcolonialism and patient involvement in undergraduate and postgraduate medical education. *Medical Education*. 2018; 52: 471–79.

Sharma M, Kuper A. The elephant in the room: talking race in medical education. *Advances in Health Sciences Education*. 2016; 22: 761–64.

Sharma M, Pinto AD, Kumagai AK. Teaching the social determinants of health: A path to equity or a road to nowhere? *Academic Medicine*. 2018; 93: 25–30.

Shklovsky V, Sher B. 1991. *Theory of prose*. Elmwood Park, IL: Dalkey Archive Press.

Spivak GC, Morris RC. 2010. *Can the subaltern speak? Reflections on the history of an idea*. New York, NY: Columbia University Press.

Stone J. 2013. Health equity: concepts and ethics. (Panel on Health Equity). American Society for Bioethics and Humanities Annual Meeting.

Wilkinson SR. The need for a dis-ease model for medicine: illness, sickness, disease, disorder and predicament. *International Journal of Clinical Neurosciences and Mental Health*. 2017; 4: 2–5.

Williams WC. 1984. A face of stone. In: *The doctor stories*. New York, NY: New Directions.

Winter D, Leighton D. 2001. Structural violence. In: *Peace, conflict, and violence: Peace psychology for the 21st century*. Upper Saddle River, NJ: Prentice Hall.

7

GEOGRAPHY AS ENGAGED MEDICAL-HEALTH-HUMANITIES

Courtney Donovan and Sarah de Leeuw

Introduction

Just as work in medical-health-humanities grows, there is increasing discussion about the ways in which the field can more fully engage with critical social questions and problems. Recent work emphasises the importance of addressing health experiences and perspectives of marginalised and often unrecognised populations (Wear and Aultman 2005; Green 2011; Garden 2015; Viney et al. 2015; Fioretti et al. 2016; McLaughlin 2017). In addition to identifying the ways in which the arts and humanities give voice to diverse perspectives and provide insights into experiences of social exclusion, scholars and practitioners are interested in expanding the application of medical-health-humanities work in medical and healthcare education and patient engagement. Coming out of this literature is a greater drive towards understanding and addressing the role of structural and social factors in health and healthcare experiences (Banner 2016).

Despite these important discussions in critical medical-health-humanities, often missing from the scholarship is recognition of *geography* as both a complex theoretical concept and as a key physical or material location in health inequities. Many scholars reference geography—often understood as a passive space in which action unfolds—as a component of access to, and reliance on, health care services in creative works. Geography thus conceptualised is often minimised to features of a landscape or mentioned narrowly in terms of healthcare access (Hollin and Giraud 2017). Absent from these discussions is an understanding that geography is an active, multifaceted concept and a field of study that elaborates the complexity of everyday interactions giving rise to health disparities and shaping determinants of health experiences. Understood this way, a geographic lens is especially useful for looking at the ways in which micro-aggressions operate and form the basis of discrimination and biases enacted by medical institutions as well as individuals, including health professionals and patients (Brown and Pickerill 2009; Schwartz 2014; Fleras 2016). Moreover, geography can be used to critically theorise how micro-aggressions contribute to and perpetuate health disparities through and in space and place. Creative works can capture and convey how health disparities and geography can work overtly in concert, particularly in expressions of blatant biases and prejudices. However, in most cases, the arts and humanities help to show that health disparities result from subtle engagements and inactions that are situated in diverse geographies. We contend that in order for true change to come out of medical-health-humanities practice, geography must be given greater attention as an integral component of everyday situations of health and healthcare. A focus on the interplay of geography and micro-aggressions is especially important as critical medical-health-humanities scholarship and practice aim to become more engaged in addressing social justice issues.

To illustrate our point, we consider the relationship of place to micro-aggressions in creative works about health and health care experiences. To offer context, we provide an overview of *place* as a conceptual and theoretical tool and discuss its importance within the field of health geography. We also address how place offers insights into the nuances of everyday micro-aggressions. We then address how place is presented in creative health narratives. As a starting point, we consider the representation and function of place in Eileen Pollack's short story 'Milk.' In particular, we focus on ways in which Pollack describes activities in the place of a hospital room to communicate differences in care provided to two new mothers. Pollack's short story deftly explores how a specific and socioculturally produced place (the hospital room) provides detailed insights into how hospital staff members deal with women coming from different socioeconomic backgrounds; and emphasises ways in which places of care are structured by discourses and political ideologies. Understanding and harnessing the power of place, we argue, ultimately allows humanities and arts to gain criticality and applicability within social and health care justice.

Medical-health-humanities as approaches to capturing overlooked experiences

The themes of inequality and social marginalisation are at the forefront of numerous works in the humanities and arts (Manning 1997; Pollack 2008). Focusing on individuals as well as communities, different creative pieces help to provide insight into both myriad circumstances that contribute to marginalisation and the human experience of that marginalisation. In different formats, artists ask us—as readers, listeners and viewers—to engage with scenarios in which we immediately confront experiences like social isolation, pain and fear. Such works shed light on, and allow for a sympathetic symbiotic relationship with, the context of everyday events and scenarios that provide settings for everyday health experiences that might otherwise be beyond a lived gaze. Creative- and humanities-informed works also motivate researchers to address health-related issues that have bearing on patient health but may not always take place in medical settings.

Out of efforts to move a medical-health-humanities imaginary away from just clinical encounters, recent scholarly work aims to open up possibilities for critical consideration of the social, cultural and political economic contexts that give rise to inequality in the first place (Viney et al. 2015; Banner 2016; Whitehead and Woods 2016). The integration of newer theoretical frameworks and consideration of race, class, gender, ability and disability have situated medical-health-humanities scholarship in new sites and experiences of health, medicine and illness. This widening focus has resulted in a more rigorous field in which contributors assert pedagogical and research agendas that challenge entrenched biases in the field of medicine and other health-related disciplines. Banner (2016), for instance, has argued that a focus on structural competency (rather than narrative competency) offers opportunities to provide more thorough training of medical students on structural racism. Writing on disability in medical humanities, Garden (2015) identifies that a disability studies perspective enables medical humanities to go beyond narrow definitions and approaches that tend to medicalise disability.

These newer critical themes and approaches have been key in helping to re-articulate the role of the humanities and arts in transforming healthcare in general and medicine in particular. At the heart of these recent expansions are efforts at creating a more socially and politically engaged medical-health-humanities. In particular, scholars have expressed interest in using observations from the arts and humanities to address issues that include inequalities. By situating medical-health-humanities within a more critical frame, scholars have created a greater impetus for developing more innovative approaches to addressing issues in research, practice and the classroom. As an existing focus of pedagogical work, practitioners emphasise approaches that take students out of the classroom and into the communities they study (Donohoe and Danielson 2004; Tsai 2008). Advocates argue for the importance of designing curricula that specifically rely on collaborative partnerships with institutions and individuals engaged in community work. They contend that by linking medical-health-humanities students with groups directly engaged in enacting social change, such students develop a much stronger awareness of factors contributing to health disparities; students also develop deeper commitments to communities that are most affected by barriers to care. Direct action work within underserviced communities has also been identified as an approach that can promote trust between certain patient populations who have historically been mistreated by medicine and public health. By preparing students with critical approaches and frameworks, students can better understand the circumstances that lead to health disparities, including conventional roles and biases of medical institutions.

Research and teaching strategies focusing on medical institutions offer a starting point for reflection on aspects of healthcare and medicine that may typically be under-examined within medical-health-humanities scholarship. One particular area that has not been given ample attention, however, is the significance of geography. For the most part, medical-health-humanities work has offered rather simplistic explanations of the concept of geography and how it operates in health and health care (Hollin and Giraud 2017). We contend that geography, especially the concept of *place*, needs to be given more consideration in discussions about marginalised communities. This is especially true if researchers, educators and practitioners want to deepen understandings about health inequities and inequalities. In the section that follows, we offer a brief explanation of how relationships between geography and health are framed from within the field of health geography; and we provide a brief overview of how health geographers approach broader issues of health inequities. We then give particular attention to the ways in which geographers address the relevance of place in unequal access to, and use of, health care. Finally, to illustrate place's particular relevance in and as medical settings, we offer a brief geographic analysis of Eileen Pollack's short story 'Milk.' We hope this discussion will do two things: first, prompt further discussion in medical-health-humanities work on the complexity of mobilising geographical perspectives in studies of health, illness, healthcare and medicine; second, demonstrate how a geographical lens can contribute to an ever more engaged medical-health-humanities.

Place and micro-aggressions in geographies of health

Health geography scholarship focuses on understanding the complex and spatialised nature of health experiences for groups and individuals who often tend to be sidelined. Health geographers examine how diverse social, cultural, historical and political economic factors—as they are expressed in and through place and space—give rise to social exclusion and inequality, which often contribute to differences in health access and health status (Holdsworth and Robinson 2013; Jewitt and Ryley 2014; Makki and van Vuuren 2017). Health geography is replete with works that address the significance of socioeconomic status, race and ethnicity, and disability, in addition to other variables, that may ultimately have a negative effect on the health choices and outcomes of diverse populations (Jewitt and Ryley 2014; Holt 2017; Sziarto 2017). In an effort to better understand how these factors may inform health, geographers consider the role of geography in creating barriers to care and complicating health access. Numerous studies reflect on the particular importance of place in creating and perpetuating health inequalities and inequities (Loyd 2009; Pearce et al. 2012; Donovan 2014; Baker and Beagan 2016).

The work of health geographers, then, has been to demonstrate and document how place is a flexible concept and an active ontological force that must be integrated with other critical social concepts to understand processes leading to health inequalities. For instance, health geographers demonstrate how place is useful for understanding the ways in which micro-aggressions may inform health experiences in medical settings (Smith and Easterlow 2005; Loyd 2009). Below, we offer a brief overview of how health geographers approach the concept of place in their work. We then consider how place relates to micro-aggressions, offering insight into factors and processes that give rise to health disparities and preventable health issues.

At the outset, place is a flexible concept identifying the personal associations and meanings that individuals attribute to specific locations (Gatrell and Elliott 2009). Place can conjure a number of physical and material sites or locations—including the home, and/or settings where individuals receive care, including hospitals and health clinics. 'Places' range in scale and size, from a hospital room to an entire hospital building, and refer to both physical and discursive 'spaces,' within which 'places' are nested. Place is rarely static for a geographer; instead, it is mobile, active, transformative and forceful. Place gives concrete meaning to the abstraction of space. Geographers acknowledge that the connotations of place are often linked to the names and labels used to describe them. In some cases, meanings attributed to place may be rooted in personal experiences, including a childhood experience (Donovan 2014). For instance, a negative experience in a single and specific hospital room at a young age may explain why someone later in life is reluctant to visit others in a hospital or to seek care from a hospital or even to be suspicious of all hospitals in general. Individual experiences and perceptions in settings like hospital rooms are often hard to disentangle from broader social factors and processes. Meanings and associations in places are reflections of broader political ideologies and discourses that interplay with natural and historical factors and ultimately inform the actions and experiences of individuals as well as groups. Places like a hospital room therefore offer insights into assumptions over equity, justice and prevailing views concerning patients and people seeking medical care.

To interrogate the interrelationship of place with social attitudes and practices that may inform health equity, geographers draw from interdisciplinary concepts and frameworks. From work that focuses on race, for instance, health geographers explore the ways in which everyday racism and micro-aggressions structure places of care and inform health experiences (Smith and Easterlow 2005; Loyd 2009). The concept of 'everyday racism' encompasses subtle forms of normalised bias that are perpetuated discursively and materially in mainstream institutions. Micro-aggressions manifest in three main ways: first, by way of more conscious micro-assaults, which are explicit racist acts that intend to cause harm; second, as micro-insults, which are unconscious forms of communication that belittle or demean individuals; and third, as micro-invalidations, in which the thoughts and feelings of a person of colour are minimised or disregarded. The language and actions of micro-aggressions are a critical factor in shaping relationships, experiences and meanings associated with particular health settings. Moreover, micro-aggressions are a significant factor in shaping health choices and outcomes.

In the next section, we address the importance of geography in medical-health-humanities by demonstrating ways in which micro-aggressions unfold within places of care. Using Eileen Pollack's short story 'Milk,' we focus on how micro-aggressions form the basis of interactions in a hospital room where two new mothers are recovering. Pollack specifically presents a small glimpse into subtle and more overt examples of micro-aggressions that may be enacted by health care professionals. She offers the opportunity to reflect on how exchanges, movements and inactions situated in one place can contribute to preventable health outcomes.

Unpacking the relationship of inequality and geography in 'Milk'

A consideration of geographic concepts such as 'place' can offer useful insights for understanding how structural conditions of inequality and entrenched biases manifest in everyday settings. The formal places traditionally associated with health and healthcare are good starting points for evaluating both the subtle and apparent ways that injustices take shape in these settings, and ultimately inform patient experiences. Looking at these settings in particular can help to illustrate prejudices that may not be readily visible, but play a significant role in patients' attitudes towards health and healthcare. There are numerous creative works that help to illustrate the nuances and potential consequences of inequality in healthcare settings. Eileen Pollack's short story 'Milk' is an example that shows specifically how, based on their subjectivities, two new mothers sharing a hospital room may receive distinct medical care and support immediately after childbirth. Pollack emphasises how micro-aggressions in particular motivate the provision of incompetent care given to an African American mother, resulting in negative health outcomes.

Although written as a fictional account, Pollack has explained that 'Milk' is based on actual observations she made of the treatment of an African American hospital roommate after she had given birth to her own son. According to Pollack, the final published version of 'Milk' is toned down from the events she observed, because friends did not believe details presented in the original draft (Short 2009). Just as Pollack observed specific interactions between nurses, other hospital staff and her roommate, Pollack recounts in 'Milk' from the perspective of a white mother who witnesses exchanges between hospital staff and a black mother from her hospital bed. Presenting the story through the eyes of a white woman, Pollack helps to call attention to the ways in which bias informs the actions of hospital staff along with the casual thoughts of a seemingly neutral onlooker. Her aim is to offer a glimpse into how bias contributes to micro-aggressions that operate in the context of everyday scenarios.

'Milk' critically highlights the ways in which discrimination and biases in the form of micro-aggressions manifest in places, and create the basis for health disparities. Pollack relies on spatial interactions and other forms of engagement within the hospital room to emphasise different dimensions of micro-aggressions. Pollack specifically emphasises distinct interactions and exchanges between hospital staff and the two mothers to show how micro-aggressions underlie non-verbal forms of communication, which result in negligent treatment. She lays out these distinctions from the opening paragraph, in which she discusses nurses hovering attentively over the white mother. To emphasise the constant buzz of attention surrounding Bea, Pollack (2008: 111) first asks, "How many nurses cared for her needs?" She then enumerates examples of the ways in which four different nurses engage physically with her body and seek to resolve her discomfort.

The description of the bustle of nurses around Bea's hospital bed stands in stark contrast to the initial description of her roommate, Coreen, who is at first hidden behind a heavy drawn curtain. Her presence on the other side of the curtain is only made apparent through intermittent sounds from a television programme, and when Coreen apparently struggles to put a diaper on her baby. By late afternoon, none of the nurses who helped out Bea have come to check on Coreen or to provide her assistance. When one nurse later brings Bea's son to her and coaches her to nurse, there is no equivalent help offered to Coreen. If not for the sounds coming from Coreen's side of the hospital, one would assume Bea is the sole occupant of the hospital room.

The distinctly different treatments of Bea and Coreen in the hospital room help to offer insight into the ways in which a single place of care may function or be experienced in dissimilar ways. Based on Bea's thoughts and her interactions with the nurses, the hospital room seems to take on meaning as a place of care and respite. The nurses attend to her needs and help her navigate being a new mother. They gently apologise when they need to wake Bea and engage with her in casual, friendly dialogue. When Bea is on her own she is able to relax—made evident when she remarks on the pleasant flavour of food brought to her, and when she daydreams while looking out the hospital window. Told through Bea's observations, Coreen's experience of the hospital room is distinctly as a place of isolation. In the few instances when the nurses and medical staff check on Coreen, there is no physical touch or friendly casual dialogue. Instead, hospital staff members maintain a distance. At no time does any hospital staff member approach to physically evaluate Coreen or her son.

The discrepancy in how Bea and Coreen are treated is reinforced in different conversations between the two women and the hospital staff—for example, when a young statistician comes to the hospital room to ask the mothers questions about their pregnancies. Speaking first with Bea she states, rhetorically: "I'm sure that you had the sense not to smoke or use drugs while you were pregnant" (2008: 116). Yet, we learn early on from Bea that she had not intended to become pregnant. She reflects: "She hadn't conceived him on purpose. She had slept with a man without taking precautions, like any ignorant schoolgirl" (ibid.: 111). When the statistician speaks with Coreen, she pointedly asks: "Now try to think hard. Did you use alcohol, or smoke or take any drugs at all—heroin, cocaine, or even marijuana—while your child was inside you?" (ibid.: 117).

The exchange between the statistician and Coreen provides a glimpse into numerous other conversations that transpire between her and hospital staff members, punctuated by micro-insults and micro-invalidations. In addition to making the assumption that Coreen engaged in risky behaviour during her pregnancy, the statistician incorrectly guesses that Coreen is unemployed and that she is an immigrant. The statistician in turn challenges Coreen's knowledge of basic information. At another moment, when Coreen is clearly ill, Bea calls a nurse for assistance. The nurse who responds fails to check on Coreen and dismisses Bea's concern: "she's just being melodramatic" (ibid.: 119). When Coreen repeatedly expresses concern over her son's health, nurses and doctors alike dismiss her. Unaware of the distant interaction between the nurses and Coreen, a paediatrician bristles at her suggestion that something is wrong: "I'll look into it. But I'm sure if the nurses had seen anything amiss, I would have been notified" (ibid.: 122).

Pollack conveys in 'Milk' that the micro-aggressions undergirding spatial interactions and aloof engagements between hospital staff and Coreen are not isolated. Coreen references an earlier instance in which micro-aggressions led to her receiving negligent treatment. Pollack emphasises that routine micro-insults and micro-invalidations in the hospital and other places of care are the primary reasons Coreen and her son are forced to receive emergency medical care. Even as Bea listens and observes some of the clear exchanges and inactions that provide evidence of careless care, she is unable to recognise the different forms of verbal and non-verbal communication in the hospital room that ultimately contribute to Coreen developing sepsis and her son dying.

Conclusion

Existing medical-health-humanities work has tended to minimise or overlook the importance of geography in health experiences and outcomes. By drawing from the insights and contributions of arts and humanities, medical-health-humanities scholarship and practice can identify the nuanced ways that geography plays a critical role in creating and perpetuating actual barriers to care. Creative works therefore present an opportunity to consider the ways in which geography is implicated in preventable health differences. Our evaluation of 'Milk' offers a starting point for critically considering future ways in which a more 'engaged' medical-health-humanities can incorporate and celebrate geography.

As we show, Pollack's short story helps to demonstrate the ways in which micro-aggressions inform spatial interactions, exchanges and inactions that form the basis of treatment and experiences in places of care. Subtle and overt forms of communication and social engagement work together and play a role in shaping barriers to equitable care. Creative works, like short stories, are compelling tools for giving attention to these everyday dynamics that might otherwise go unnoticed. They allow for closer evaluation of interactions in health settings, which in turn offers the possibility for recognition of how micro-aggressions manifest, and how they can lead to changes in patient–provider relations, and to potential health improvements for populations that tend to be socially marginalised.

While solely focusing on a hospital room, Pollack's short story also helps to point to how micro-aggressions perpetuated in single places of care are often not isolated events. Instead, racial biases that structure the health experiences of people of colour in particular health settings are linked to, and reinforced by, other geographies of health and healthcare. We contend that recognising the concatenated nature of health inequalities is a critical component in producing social and structural changes to health systems. 'Milk' helps to illustrate these often-overlooked relationships between places of care that present barriers to equitable health outcomes, where geography becomes a possible conceptual and pedagogical tool in expanding arts- and humanities-informed conversations with health inequities. Mobilised through and in creative practice, place is recognised as conjoined with, and inextricable from, marginalisation. Geography and health are activated, readable through fiction and set up to be acted upon by those of us who hope for positive and radical social change.

References

Baker K, Beagan B. 'Unlike Vancouver . . . here there's nothing': imagined geographies of idealized health care for LBGTQ women. *Gender, Place, and Culture.* 2016; 23: 927–40.

Banner O. Structural racism and the practices of reading in the medical humanities. *Literature and Medicine.* 2016; 34: 25–52.

Brown G, Pickerill J. Space for emotion in spaces of activism. *Emotion, Space, and Society.* 2009; 2: 24–35.

Donohoe M, Danielson S. A community-based approach to the medical humanities. *Medical Education.* 2004; 38: 204–17.

Donovan C. Graphic pathogeographies. *Journal of Medical Humanities.* 2014; 35: 273–300.

Fioretti C, Mazzocco K, Riva S, et al. Research studies on patients' illness experience using the Narrative Medicine approach: a systematic review. *BMJ Open.* 2016; 6: 1–9.

Fleras A. Theorizing micro-aggressions as Racism 3.0: shifting the discourse. *Canadian Ethnic Studies.* 2016; 48: 1–19.

Garden R. Who speaks for whom? Health humanities and the ethics of representation. *Medical Humanities.* 2015; 41: 77–80.

Gatrell AC, Elliott SJ. 2009. *Geographies of Health. An Introduction.* Chichester: Wiley-Blackwell.

Green C. Being present: the role of narrative medicine in reducing the unequal burden of pain. *Pain.* 2011; 152: 965–66.

Holdsworth C, Robinson J. Parental smoking and children's anxieties: an appropriate strategy for health education? *Children's Geographies.* 2013; 11: 102–16.

Hollin G, Giraud E. Charisma in the clinic. *Social Theory and Health.* 2017; 15: 223–40.

Holt L. Food, feeding, and the material everyday geographies of infants: possibilities and potentials. *Social and Cultural Geography.* 2017; 18: 487–504.

Jewitt S, Ryley H. It's a girl thing: Menstruation, school attendance, spatial mobility and wider gender inequalities in Kenya. *Geoforum.* 2014; 56: 137–47.

Loyd JM. War is not healthy for children and other living things. *Environment and Planning D.* 2009; 27: 403–24.

Makki M, van Vuuren K. Place, identity and stigma: blocks and the 'blockies' of Tara, Queensland, Australia. *Geojournal.* 2017; 82: 1085–99.

Manning L. 1997. The magic wand. In K Fries (ed.) *Staring Back: The Disability Experience from the Inside Out.* New York, NY: Penguin, 165.

McLaughlin J. The medical reshaping of disabled bodies as a response to stigma and a route to normality. *Journal of Medical Humanities.* 2017; 43: 244–50.

Pearce J, Barnett R, Moon G. Sociospatial inequalities in health-related behaviors: pathways linking place and smoking. *Progress in Human Geography.* 2012; 36: 3–24.

Pollack E. 2008. Milk. In: R Nadelhaft, V Bonebakker (eds.) *Imagine What It's Like.* Honolulu, HA: University of Hawaii Press, 111–25.

Schwartz J. Classrooms of spatial justice: counter-spaces and young men of color in a GED program. *Adult Education Quarterly.* 2014; 64: 110–27.

Short B. Those magic carbons: a conversation with Eileen Pollack. October 25, 2009. Available at: https://fictionwritersreview.com/interview/those-magic-carbons-a-conversation-with-eileen-pollack. Last accessed: June 28, 2018.

Smith S, Easterlow D. The strange geographies of health inequalities. *Transactions of the Institute of British Geographers.* 2005; 30: 173–90.

Sziarto KM. Whose reproductive futures? Race-biopolitics and resistance in the Black infant mortality reduction campaigns in Milwaukee. *Environment and Planning D.* 2017; 35: 299–319.

Tsai D. Community-oriented curriculum design for medical humanities. *Kaoshiung Journal of Medical Sciences.* 2008; 24: 373–79.

Viney W, Callard F, Woods A. Critical medical humanities: embracing entanglement, taking risks. *Journal of Medical Humanities.* 2015; 41: 2–7.

Wear D, Aultman JM. The limits of narrative: medical student resistance to confronting inequality and oppression in literature and beyond. *Medical Education.* 2005; 39: 1056–65.

Whitehead A, Woods A (eds.) 2016. *The Edinburgh Companion to the Critical Medical Humanities.* Edinburgh: Edinburgh University Press.

8

CHALLENGING HETERONORMATIVITY IN MEDICINE

William J. Robertson

Introduction

A few years ago, I went to an urgent care clinic because I was experiencing sharp pains in my abdomen. Given my family history, I was concerned it might be gallstones. While palpating my belly, the physician, a middle-aged, straight, white man, casually asked, "Are you married, or do you have a girlfriend?" I can only assume he was trying to make the silence less awkward.

"No," I replied, "but I have a boyfriend."

"Oh," he said, in a sort of disappointed tone.

He removed his hands from my body, removed his gloves, and swivelled on his stool to look at the computer screen. He quickly typed on the keyboard, then turned back to me and said, "I'm going to order an STD panel. It includes an HIV test. Just sit tight and someone will come in to draw some blood." Then he got up and left the room while I lay uncomfortably on the examining table, my face red with a mixture of embarrassment and rage. Why would he suddenly assume that my symptoms were caused by an STI, much less HIV? And even if they somehow were caused by an STI, why wouldn't he ask about my actual sexual practices before ordering a blood panel, which I would have to pay for out of pocket since I did not have health insurance? Why did his question about my relationship status effectively end my encounter with him? Why would he leap to such a conclusion? Was it experiences with previous patients or a case of making assumptions based on ignorance and/or homophobia? What would he tell the nurse, and what would they now be assuming about me when they came to take my blood?

Experiences like mine are not uncommon. Many people I've spoken with—family members, friends, colleagues, research participants, medical students, and even practising physicians—have told me stories about homophobic or heteronormative encounters in the clinic. Medicine absorbs, reflects, and institutionalises all kinds of sociocultural norms and prejudices, including those concerning gender and sexuality. Given the prevalence of heteronormativity in society, it is unsurprising that heteronormativity is pervasive in medical environments. Experiences—or even the knowledge that such experiences occur—with homophobia, transphobia, and heteronormativity in medical settings can lead lesbian, gay, bisexual, transgender, and queer (LGBTQ) people to delay seeking treatment in an effort to avoid feeling embarrassed as well as having to come out to health care providers (Eliason and Schope 2001; Harbin, Beagan, and Goldberg 2012; Baker and Beagan 2014; Whitehead,

Shaver, and Stephenson 2016). If medicine's primary purpose is to *care* for patients, the ongoing and pervasive presence of heteronormative beliefs and practices in medicine should be cause for concern among practitioners.

This chapter highlights and challenges the presence of heteronormativity in medicine. I begin by defining 'heteronormativity' and some important related concepts. I then discuss how medicine is structured to distinguish 'normal' and 'abnormal' and explore how this structure easily lends itself to the enactment of broader sociocultural norms concerning gender and sexuality. Next, I give several reasons why heteronormativity is a problem that medical practitioners should pay close attention to. I conclude with some thoughts about how medical education and practice might push back against the enactment of heteronormativity.

Defining heteronormativity

Literature dating to the mid-1970s and early 1980s has described heterosexuality as an institutionalised and compulsory social system (Rubin 1975; Rich 1980), but Michael Warner coined the term *heteronormativity* in 1991. It refers to the pervasive cultural logic (and its associated discourses and practices) that privileges binary oppositional, complementary, and reproductive heterosexuality as the natural and normal default subject position (see also Katz 1995; Sullivan 2003; Robinson 2016). In this chapter, I expand the term *heteronormative* to also include cisnormativity, which is the implicit view of all people as naturally cisgender (i.e., non-transgender, meaning that a person's gendered sense of self aligns with the gender category to which they were assigned at or before birth). I draw cisnormativity together with heteronormativity primarily for the pragmatic purpose of clarity and brevity. This move is not meant to obscure or ignore the critiques of queer theory concerning the privileging of same-sex sexualities at the expense of gender variance (Stryker 2004, 2006). Indeed, my usage of *heteronormativity* and its derivatives should be considered to include both gender and sexuality, as the two are inextricably linked, and do not refer solely to sexuality.

It is useful to distinguish *heteronormativity* from *heterosexism* and *homo/transphobia*. Whereas *heteronormativity* refers to implicit cultural logics that order a hegemonic sex/gender system and result in the unintentional and non-conscious privileging of cisgendered heterosexuality, *heterosexism* refers to explicit beliefs, discourses, and practices that not only privilege cisgendered heterosexuality as natural and normal but also as culturally/morally/naturally superior. *Homophobia* refers to disgust, hatred, and prejudice towards LGBQ people, while *transphobia* refers to disgust, hatred, and prejudice towards trans people. Heteronormativity and heterosexism can be, but are not necessarily, homo/transphobic since one can believe heterosexuality and/or being cisgender is natural or more moral than being LGBTQ without being disgusted by, hating, or acting in prejudiced ways towards LGBTQ people (see Boellstorff 2004). However, the difference between believing in the naturalness and moral superiority of cisgendered heterosexuality and being disgusted or prejudiced is often blurred or indistinguishable since implicit assumptions and beliefs tend to be made explicit in various ways and can lead to harm (as discussed later in this chapter).

A final term that must be discussed is *homonormativity*. Coined by Lisa Duggan (2002), *homonormativity* refers to discourses and practices that seem to make queer people 'the same' as heterosexual people regarding their desires for relationships, consumption, and social structures. This is most obvious in the ways LGBTQ rights discourses have been overwhelmingly framed around marriage equality over issues such as labour and housing rights or equal access to and better treatment within medical environments. Homonormativity within LGBTQ communities has led to the centring of the experiences, needs, and desires of white middle- and upper-class gay men and lesbians, and thus both heteronormativity and homonormativity should "be understood as part of racialised social formations and white supremacy" (Robinson 2016: 2).

I use *homonormativity* in a similar though slightly different way than outlined above. I think of *homonormativity* as the discourses and beliefs that produce or assume normative ways of being LGBTQ, even where they do not mirror heteronormative social ordering. In simpler terms, *homonormativity* refers to the expectations for how LGBTQ people *should behave as LGBTQ people*. For example, in my ethnographic work in a clinic that specialises in the diagnosis and treatment of anal dysplasia, I have noticed that the clinicians ask male patients who have sex with men if they are a 'top' (only penetrates during sex), 'bottom' (only is penetrated), 'vers' (meaning versatile, prefers both/either), 'vers-top' (prefers to penetrate, but will be penetrated), or 'vers-bottom' (prefers to be penetrated, but will penetrate). These lay categories are charted, becoming medicalised, and inform the clinician's understanding of the patient's risk profile. They also effectuate homonormative ideas about same-sex sexual activity—that it always includes penetration of an anus by a penis, since these categories do not refer to oral or non-penetrative sexual practices such as mutual masturbation. The medicalisation of these lay categories blurs the line between sexual practices and identities (see Young and Meyer 2005; Boellstorff 2011), since many gay men use the categories as identities for determining sexual compatibility.

Heteronormativity and homonormativity rely on social (in)visibility. For example, some LGBQ people can 'pass' as heterosexual because they don't behave in overtly or stereotypically queer ways (heteronormativity makes this possible—indeed, the entire practice of 'coming out of the closet' relies on heteronormativity). Clothing or other bodily adornments may permit trans or non-binary people to hide or alter the appearance of their bodies to be socially recognised as a particular gender. Over the last several decades, LGBTQ rights movements have increased visibility by making LGBTQ lives more perceptible to non-LGBTQ people (e.g., through media). Despite the increasing visibility of LGBTQ people around the world, medical education, training, practice, and knowledge remains largely heteronormative, homophobic, and transphobic (Sanchez et al. 2006; Eliason, Dibble, and Robertson 2011; Schuster 2012).

Ab/normality and the production of heteronormativity in medicine

A key organising principle at the root of contemporary medicine is the normal/pathological dichotomy (Canguilhem 1978; Foucault 1999). 'Normal,' as an enacted category of health or illness, is not a comparison between two individuals but rather of an individual to some established group norm; and 'abnormal' is a deviation from that norm. Physicians see bodies using the medical gaze (Foucault 1994a; Good 1994; Davenport 2000; Prentice 2013), an ability learned through the socialisation process of medical education and training that makes the body a medical object (rather than a whole person) made up of working/dysfunctional parts that can be 'fixed' through technical therapeutic interventions. These processes and their effects are observable, for example, in the practice of diagnosis, which is a complex sociocultural process whereby any number of norms, values, and beliefs are invoked and (re)produced in an effort to make the body into a medical object that can be 'read' by different practitioners in different contexts to achieve certain ends such as curing disease (Mol 2002; Gardner et al. 2011). In this sense, medicine does not simply document categories (e.g., 'male' or 'female') but rather is one part of the broader sociocultural processes that performatively constitutes the categories themselves (Butler 1990, 1993; Hacking 2006; Plemons 2017).

The work of Michel Foucault offers useful insights for the study of heteronormativity in the development of norms and values in medicine. In Foucault's formulation, bodies are contingent upon historically situated sets of discourses, which have a kind of autonomy from individual human subjects in that they have organising effects that lead to different ways of stylising the self. However, there is not a one-way relationship from individual subject to discourse or vice versa, but discourses shape subjects just as subjects shape discourses. Discourses are governed by the rules of the time (Foucault 1994b), which are necessarily driven by power/knowledge. Foucault theorises power as diffuse and capillary, occurring in everyday discourses and practices, and it is through processes of power that normalisation occurs (Foucault 1990, 1995, 1999). If we consider medicine as a discourse, we can see how it both produces 'the truth' about bodies and simultaneously controls their behaviour by directing them to particular actions that align with 'the truth' in an effort to maintain health (and, by extension, a stable population). This authoritative truth is driven by medical claims of expertise over the body. In a Foucauldian frame, medical expertise is not simply the result of implementing scientific research processes in clinical practices, but a modern biopolitical system of power/knowledge that (re)produces discourses about the body and enables the disciplining of bodies through processes of standardi- sation and normalisation.

Importantly, this is not a strictly top-down model because where there is power there is the possibility of resistance (Foucault 1990, 1995). This allows room for individual agency when individual subjects actively stylise themselves in accordance with the expert discourses in order 'to count,' as it were, or to resist the "codes of normalisation" (Foucault 1997: 38) that emerge from clinical knowledge and that permit state recognition. Thus, patients are not merely pas- sive objects upon which such discourses are enacted, but instead are active participants in these productions (for a cogent and compelling example of these forces in action see Plemons 2017). Everyday medical practices and discourses enable expert knowledge to give rise to new distinc- tions and forms—ontologies—of bodies, which do not precede but are produced along with knowledge about them. Bodies-as-medical-objects do not pre-exist medical practices and dis- courses but come into existence—are enacted—through such practices and discourses.

Historically, medical expertise was claimed through jurisdictional boundary conflicts as dif- ferent factions vied for claims to authority over disease, health, and knowledge about bodies (Starr 1984; Ludmerer 1985, 1999; Bonner 1995; Wailoo 1997, 2001, 2011). Arguably, the key factor in establishing this authority was the development of medicine as *a profession* (Abbott 1988; Freidson 1998), which was further solidified by the successes of positivist science in the late 19th and early 20th centuries. This led to a great deal of autonomy within American medicine, which resulted in professional organisations claiming jurisdiction over the educa- tion and credentialing of new physicians. Thus, medical schools (rather than apprenticeships) became a targeted site for the standardised socialisation of medical students into physicians. As medical students develop a physician's habitus, they develop identities as 'experts' of the body (Good 1995; Davenport 2000; Jaye et al. 2006; Prentice 2013; Emmerich 2014). When broader sociocultural ideas about sex/gender and sexuality categories become conflated with medicalised claims about 'normal' and 'abnormal' bodies (i.e., men are males who have penises and testes who are attracted to women who are females who have vaginas and ovaries and are attracted to men), they become naturalised and are assumed to be the default for all people. This is heter- onormativity *par excellence*.

Thus, medical knowledge, grounded in making things normal or abnormal, is enacted through expert discourses and practices, which are bestowed with social authority due to medi- cine's status as a profession with the self-regulatory autonomy. Yet, making things normal or abnormal is always already informed by broader sociocultural mores, so any expert medical knowledge about sex/gender and sexuality will always shape and be shaped by heteronormative cultural beliefs and values (and patients bring these ideas with them into the clinic as well). This blending of heteronormativity into the subject positioning of 'the expert' results in authoritative heteronormative enactments of sex/gender and sexuality in medical practice and discourse, which of course in turn produce more knowledge about 'normal' or 'abnormal' bodies.

The problem of heteronormativity in medicine

Medical providers regularly make heteronormative assumptions about patients in clinical environments (Baker and Beagan 2014; Murphy 2014, 2017; Robertson 2017), but these assumptions often go unnoticed because physicians are trained to think of their practices as scientifically derived and thus objective rather than deeply influenced by their culture and society. There are several reasons why heteronormativity in medicine is a problem that needs to be addressed.

First, heteronormativity can obscure (and arguably reproduce) the health disparities that are unique to LGBTQ people. The medical gaze and its ability to construct the body as a decontextualised medical object can have the effect of ignoring the social determinants of health and illness for LGBTQ patients. Lacking an understanding of the contexts within which patients live can lead to medical environments that reproduce LGBTQ health disparities through contributing to minority stress (Meyer 1995, 2003, 2007), a type of chronic stress that arises from the hostile social environment caused by the incongruence of one's minority status and the dominant heteronormative/heterosexist values that stigmatise minority group members. The chronic minority stress of living in such environments, even when one is not directly subjected to its effects but simply knows that they exist, can produce detrimental health outcomes (Meyer 2007). Thus, when medical environments are heteronormative (and/or heterosexist and/or homophobic), they can reproduce minority stress in LGBTQ people, leading to increased LGBTQ health disparities.

Second, heteronormative/homonormative discourses can have the effect of reducing all LGBTQ health problems to sexual health. LGBTQ health disparities include many more areas of concern than just sexual health such as: disparities in access to treatment, being less likely to have health insurance, experiencing higher incidences of poor mental health, having increased rates of substance abuse (especially tobacco and alcohol), being at higher risk for violence, being more likely to be homeless, having higher rates of some kinds of cancer, and having higher rates of suicide attempts (which is especially high for trans people) (Krehely 2009; Conron, Mimiaga, and Landers 2010; Institute of Medicine 2011; Baptiste-Roberts et al. 2017; HealthyPeople 2018). If providers only think of LGBTQ health as unique sexual health needs when compared to straight and cisgender people, there is a higher likelihood of providers ignoring many of the other unique problems and disparities faced by their LGBTQ patients.

Third, as demonstrated in my opening vignette, heteronormativity can lead to treating LGBTQ people as *inherently* more 'at risk' than straight or cisgender people. This can lead to unnecessary increases in tests or screening procedures, which can increase medical costs as well as burden medical labs and technicians with diagnostic work that is often based on stereotypes rather than sound scientific reasoning. 'Risky' sexual behaviours are a ubiquitous topic of consideration in the health disparities literature, and this focus has been criticised by several scholars (Waldby 1996; Adam 2005; Young and Meyer 2005; Boellstorff 2011). Focusing on behaviour, especially 'risky sexual behaviour,' and developing behavioural and educational interventions often elides the role of identity and subjectivity by collapsing identity into behaviour (for example, asking a patient if they have sex with men, women, or both, and then identifying them as gay, lesbian, or bisexual based on their response). Further, a failure to theorise heterosexuality along similar lines leaves the interplay of heterosexual identity and behaviour unexamined. LGBTQ sexual activity is more easily categorised as risky not necessarily because certain kinds of sexual behaviours among LGBTQ people are inherently more or less risky (after all, heterosexuals engage in oral and anal sexual activities as well), but because certain behaviours are more socioculturally associated with particular groups who are considered abnormal, they are viewed as more 'at risk.' There is no apparent need for labels like 'MSW' (men who have sex with women) or 'WSM' (women who have sex with men) because those behaviours are not considered abnormal in a heteronormative society, and the risks faced by those kinds of sexual activities are considered normal. In fact, issues of heterosexual identity are often simply attributed to gender differences between (cisgender—though this is implicitly assumed in the literature) men and women in studies of different-sex sexual behaviours.

Finally, medical and scientific research regularly treats LGBTQ subjectivities as *aetiological* by seeking to determine 'the cause' of queerness or transness. This is an inherently heteronormative position, since it assumes that queerness and transness are naturally derived deviations that must have some kind of underlying biological cause. Indeed, research into the aetiology of heterosexuality is entirely absent, since it is assumed to be the default 'natural' subject position. This type of thinking and research can potentially result in providers who treat queerness or transness as caused by some inborn biological process, which could then be assumed to be the cause of health disparities rather than that LGBTQ health disparities are the result of sociocultural processes and environments.

These are only a handful of reasons why heteronormativity is a problem for medical practitioners and knowledge producers. One could undoubtedly come up with many more. But the point is that when the medical system that is supposed to help patients contributes to the very problems it is supposedly attempting to solve, it is incumbent upon those within medicine to push back and change the system in ways that are more in line with the ideal of what medicine should be.

Challenging heteronormativity in medicine

The main arena where medicine has attempted to correct for heteronormativity is medical education and training. The prevailing paradigm in challenging heteronormativity and drawing attention to LGBTQ health disparities is *cultural competency*, the purpose of which is to humanise patients and make clinicians more sensitive to patients' sociocultural backgrounds. There are several issues with the cultural competency paradigm, most arguably that it misunderstands or misuses the culture concept such that 'culture' is often used as a synonym for race (Jenks 2011). Such conceptualisations treat culture as a static list of traits associated with particular racial/ethnic (and more recently, sexual and gender minority) groups and make it the job of the physician to be aware of these traits.

While scholars have offered solutions to these problems (e.g., Kleinman and Benson 2006; Jenks 2011), cultural competency continues to ignore the cultural background of providers as well as the cultural environment of the clinic itself (Taylor 2003; Baker and Beagan 2014), which results in a failure to address the heteronormative structuring of medicine. To really challenge heteronormativity in medicine, attention must be paid to the clinical environment as well as to patient–provider interactions. It is simply not enough to recognise that a patient is queer or trans and act more sensitively towards them. Entire clinical environments and institutionalised heteronormative medical structures shape the experiences and practices of all patients and providers in these environments, though this potentially most negatively impacts LGBTQ patients and providers. Both clinical environments and providers, as practising members of heteronormative institutions, are embedded within larger discriminatory and marginalising structures that cultural competency fails to address. Thus, they can inadvertently contribute to the ongoing minority stress of LGBTQ patients rather than alleviating health inequities. In this way, cultural competency might be a stopgap measure, but it should not be considered a final solution to challenging heteronormativity in medicine because changes must also be made at the societal level to interrupt the feedback loop between heteronormative/homophobic social mores and medical knowledge and practice.

Scholarship on racial/ethnic health disparities demonstrates the importance of challenging normativising discourses within biomedical and public health practices, for example by clearly delimiting the kinds of harms that arise out of uncritical normativised ideas about race in medicine (Wailoo 1997, 2001, 2011; Braun et al. 2007; Pollock 2012; Braun 2014). One way to push back against the extant heteronormativity of medical environments is for providers to talk to LGBTQ people about their experiences and work to make changes in their own working environments to make LGBTQ people feel more accepted and less stressed. This could involve clearing out medical environments of heteronormative assumptions in paperwork and health literature. Examples of such actions could be changing intake forms that only provide two boxes for sex/gender to provide more options or a write-in option, providing space for patients to include the gender(s) of their sexual partners on intake forms, including medical literature pamphlets that have pictures of non-heterosexual relationships, and training clinic staff to be more aware of their assumptions about people's gender and sexuality.

Ultimately, medical providers need to be better about recognising the patient's social and cultural contexts, as well as being reflexive about their own sociocultural baggage that fuels heteronormativity, heterosexism, and homophobia both within and outside of the clinic. It is up to all of us—patient and provider alike—to seek out and challenge heteronormativity in our societies. Only then will we have a fighting chance to improve medicine's treatment of queer and trans patients.

References

Abbott A. 1988. *The System of Professions*. Chicago, IL: University of Chicago Press.

Adam BD. Constructing the neoliberal sexual actor: responsibility and care of the self in the discourse of barebackers. *Culture, Health & Sexuality*. 2005; 7: 333–46.

Baker K, Beagan B. Making assumptions, making space: an anthropological critique of cultural competency and its relevance to queer patients. *Medical Anthropology Quarterly*. 2014; 28: 578–98.

Baptiste-Roberts K, Oranuba E, Wets N, Edwards LV. Addressing healthcare disparities among sexual minorities. *Obstetrics and Gynecology Clinics of North America*. 2017; 44: 71–80.

Boellstorff T. But do not identify as gay: a proleptic genealogy of the MSM category. *Cultural Anthropology*. 2011; 26: 287–312.

Boellstorff T. The emergence of political homophobia in Indonesia: masculinity and national belonging. *Ethnos*. 2004; 69: 465–86.

Bonner T. 1995. *Becoming a Physician: Medical Education in Britain, France, Germany, and the United States, 1750–1945*. New York, NY: Oxford University Press.

Braun L. 2014. *Breathing Race into the Machine: The Surprising Career of the Spirometer from Plantation to Genetics*. Minneapolis, MN: University of Minnesota Press.

Braun L, Fausto-Sterling A, Fullwiley D, et al. Racial categories in medical practice: how useful are they? *PLoS Medicine*, 2007; 4: e271.

Butler J. 1990. *Gender Trouble*. New York, NY: Routledge.

Butler J. 1993. *Bodies That Matter*. New York, NY: Routledge.

Canguilhem G. 1978. *On the Normal and the Pathological*. C.N. Fawcett, trans. Boston, MA: D. Reidel Publishing.

Conron KJ, Mimiaga MJ, Landers SJ. A population-based study of sexual orientation identity and gender differences in adult health. *American Journal of Public Health*. 2010; 100: 1953–60.

Davenport BA. Witnessing and the medical gaze: how medical students learn to see at a free clinic for the homeless. *Medical Anthropology Quarterly*. 2000; 14: 310–27.

Duggan L. 2002. The new homonormativity: the sexual politics of neoliberalism. In: R Castronovo and D Nelson (eds.) *Materialising Democracy: Toward a Revitalised Cultural Politics*, 1st ed. Durham, NC: Duke University Press, 175–94.

Eliason MJ, Schope R. Does 'Don't ask don't tell' apply to health care? Lesbian, gay, and bisexual people's disclosure to health care providers. *Journal of the Gay and Lesbian Medical Association*. 2001; 5: 125–34.

Eliason MJ, Dibble SL, Robertson PA. Lesbian, gay, bisexual, and transgender (LGBT) physicians' experiences in the workplace. *Journal of Homosexuality*. 2011; 58: 1355–71.

Emmerich N. Bourdieu's collective enterprise of inculcation: the moral socialisation of and ethical enculturation of medical students. *British Journal of Sociology of Education*. 2014; 36: 1054–72.

Foucault M. 1990. *The History of Sexuality: An Introduction: Volume I*. New York, NY: Vintage Books.

Foucault M. 1994a. *The Birth of the Clinic: An Archaeology of Medical Perception*. New York, NY: Vintage Books.

Foucault M. 1994b. *The Order of Things: An Archaeology of the Human Sciences*. New York, NY: Vintage Books.

Foucault M. 1995. *Discipline and Punish: The Birth of the Prison*. New York, NY: Vintage Books.

Foucault M. 1997. *Society Must Be Defended*. New York, NY: Picador.

Foucault M. 1999. *Abnormal: Lectures at the College de France, 1974–1975*. New York, NY: Picador.

Freidson E. 1998 [1970]. *The Profession of Medicine: A Study in the Sociology of Applied Knowledge*. Chicago, IL: University of Chicago Press.

Gardner J, Dew K, Stubbe M, Dowell T, Macdonald L. Patchwork diagnoses: the production of coherence, uncertainty, and manageable bodies. *Social Science & Medicine* 2011; 7: 843–50.

Good B. 1994. *Medicine, Rationality, and Experience: An Anthropological Perspective*. Cambridge: Cambridge University Press.

Good MD. 1995. *American Medicine: The Quest for Competence*. Los Angeles, CA: University of California Press.

Hacking I. Making up people. *London Review of Books*. 2006; 28: 23–26.

Harbin A, Beagan B, Goldberg L. Discomfort, judgment, and health care for queers. *Journal of Bioethical Inquiry*. 2012; 9: 149–60.

HealthyPeople. 2018. Lesbian, gay, bisexual and transgender health. HealthyPeople 2020. Available at: www.healthypeople.gov/2020/topics-objectives/topic/lesbian-gay-bisexual-and-transgender-health. Last accessed: 27 March 2018.

Institute of Medicine. 2011. *The Health of Lesbian, Gay, Bisexual, and Transgender People: Building a Foundation for Better Understanding*. Washington D.C.: The National Academies Press.

Jaye C, Egan T, Parker S. 'Do as I say, not as I do': medical education and Foucault's normalising technologies of the self. *Anthropology and Medicine*. 2006; 13: 141–55.

Jenks, AC. From 'lists of traits' to 'open-mindedness': emerging issues in cultural competence education. *Culture, Medicine and Psychiatry*. 2011; 35: 209–35.

Karkazis K. 2007. *Fixing Sex: Intersex, Medical Authority, and Lived Experience*. Durham, NC: Duke University Press.

Katz JN. 1995. *The Invention of Heterosexuality*. Chicago, IL: University of Chicago Press.

Kleinman A, Benson P. Anthropology in the clinic: the problem of cultural competency and how to fix it. *PLoS Medicine*. 2006; 3: e294.

Krehely J. 2009. How to close the LGBT health disparities gap. Center for American Progress. Available at: www.americanprogress.org/issues/lgbt/report/2009/12/21/7048/howto-close-the-lgbt-health-disparities-gap. Last accessed: 2 February 2013.

Ludmerer K. 1985. *Learning to Heal: The Development of American Medical Education*. Baltimore, MD: Johns Hopkins University Press.

Ludmerer K. 1999. *Time to Heal: American Medical Education from the Turn of the Century to the Era of Managed Care*. New York, NY: Oxford University Press.

Meyer IH. Minority stress and mental health of gay men. *Journal of Health and Social Behavior*. 1995; 36: 38–56.

Meyer IH. Prejudice, social stress, and mental health in lesbian, gay, and bisexual populations: conceptual issues and research evidence. *Psychological Bulletin*. 2003; 129: 674–97.

Meyer IH. 2007. Prejudice and discrimination as social stressors. In: IH Meyer, ME Northridge (eds.) *The Health of Sexual Minorities*. New York, NY: Springer, 242–67.

Mol A. 2002. *The Body Multiple: Ontology in Medical Practice*. Durham, NC: Duke University Press.

Murphy M. Hiding in plain sight: the production of heteronormativity in medical education. *Journal of Contemporary Ethnography*. 2014; 45: 256–89.

Murphy M. 2017. Everywhere and nowhere simultaneously: the 'absent presence' of sexuality in medical education. *Sexualities*. First published online 26 June 2017.

Plemons E. 2017. *The Look of a Woman: Facial Feminisation Surgery and the Aims of Trans-Medicine*. Durham, NC: Duke University Press.

Pollock A. 2012. *Medicating Race: Heart Disease and Durable Preoccupations with Difference*. Durham, NC: Duke University Press.

Prentice R. 2013. *Bodies in Formation: An Ethnography of Anatomy and Surgery Education*. Durham, NC: Duke University Press.

Rich A. Compulsory heterosexuality and lesbian existence. *Signs* 1980; 5: 631–60.

Robertson W. The irrelevance narrative: queer (in)visibility in medical education and practice. *Medical Anthropology Quarterly*. 2017; 31: 159–76.

Robinson BA. 2016. Heteronormativity and homonormativity. In: NA Naples (ed.) *The Wiley Blackwell Encyclopedia of Gender and Sexuality Studies*. New York, NY: Wiley.

Rubin G. 1975. The traffic in women: notes on the 'political economy' of sex. In: RA Reiter (ed.) *Toward an Anthropology of Women*. New York, NY: Monthly Review Press, 157–210.

Sanchez NF, Rabatin J, Sanchez JP, Hubbard S, Kalet A. Medical students' ability to care for lesbian, gay, bisexual, and transgendered patients. *Family Medicine*. 2006; 38: 21–27.

Schuster MA. On being gay in medicine. *Academic Pediatrics*. 2012; 12: 75–78.

Starr P. 1984. *The Social Transformation of American Medicine*. New York, NY: Basic Books.

Stryker S. Transgender studies: queer theory's evil twin. *GLQ: A Journal of Lesbian and Gay Studies*. 2004; 10: 212–15.

Stryker S. 2006. (De)Subjugated knowledges: an introduction to transgender studies. In: S Stryker, S Whittle (eds.) *The Transgender Studies Reader*. Vol. 1. New York, NY: Routledge, 1–17.

Sullivan N. 2003. *A Critical Introduction to Queer Theory*. New York, NY: New York University Press.

Taylor J. Confronting 'culture' in medicine's 'culture of no culture.' *Academic Medicine*. 2003; 78: 555–59.

Wailoo K. 1997. *Drawing Blood: Technology and Disease Identity in Twentieth-Century America*. Baltimore, MD: Johns Hopkins University Press.

Wailoo K. 2001. *Dying in the City of the Blues: Sickle Cell Anemia and the Politics of Race and Health*. Chapel Hill, NC: University of North Carolina Press.

Wailoo K. 2011. *How Cancer Crossed the Color Line*. New York, NY: Oxford University Press.

Waldby C. 1996. *AIDS and the Body Politic: Biomedicine and Sexual Difference*. New York, NY: Routledge.

Warner M. Introduction: fear of a queer planet. *Social Text*. 1991; 29: 3–17.

Whitehead J, Shaver J, Stephenson R. Outness, stigma, and primary health care utilisation among rural LGBT populations. *PLoS ONE*. 2016; 11: e0146139.

Young RM, Meyer IH. The trouble with 'MSM' and 'WSW': erasure of the sexual-minority person in public health discourse. *American Journal of Public Health*. 2005; 95: 1144–49.

9

MEDICAL NEMESIS 40 YEARS ON

The enduring legacy of Ivan Illich

Seamus O'Mahony

Introduction

Ivan Illich's attack on modern medicine, *Medical Nemesis*, appeared in 1974, famously opening with the statement: "The medical establishment has become a major threat to health." This chapter examines the major themes of the book, and asks whether events since its publication have added weight to Illich's thesis or diminished the book's importance. Illich was born in Vienna in 1926 to a Roman Catholic Croatian aristocrat father and a German mother of Sephardi Jewish origin (Hartch 2015). His parents included among their friends the poet Rainer Maria Rilke, the theologian Jacques Maritain, and the philosopher Rudolf Steiner. Illich was classified 'half-Aryan' as long as his father was alive but, after his death in 1943, the family fled to Italy. Illich initially studied histology and crystallography at the University of Florence, mainly to obtain an identity card under a false name. After the Second World War, he returned to Austria, and enrolled at the University of Salzburg to study history, gaining a PhD. While working on his doctoral research he returned to Italy and began studies for the priesthood at the Gregorian University in Rome. He was ordained in 1951.

Illich's intellectual gifts were quickly recognised by the church. Cardinal Giovanni Montini (later Pope Paul VI) encouraged him to train as a church diplomat at the *Accademia dei Nobili Ecclesiastici*. Illich declined, deciding instead on an academic career. In 1951 he moved to the USA with the intention of post-doctoral study at Princeton, but in New York he came into contact with the Puerto Rican community and decided to work as a pastor with this group instead. In 1956 he was appointed Vice-Rector at the Catholic University in Ponce, Puerto Rico, but was recalled to New York in 1960 after a series of clashes with the local Catholic hierarchy. He subsequently travelled throughout South America, setting up the Centre for Intercultural Formation in Cuernavaca, Mexico in 1961. This was established with the support of the US Catholic hierarchy to prepare North American missionaries for work in South America, providing intensive courses in Spanish and Latin American culture and history. Illich came to question the entire missionary enterprise in South America, effectively sabotaging the programme by openly discouraging would-be missionaries and writing incendiary articles attacking the American Catholic mission in South America.

In 1968, Illich was called to the Vatican to answer charges of heresy. Although no formal conviction was made, Catholic priests were banned from enrolling for courses at the Centre for Intercultural Formation. Later the same year, Illich resigned from the public duties of the priesthood, but, for the rest of his life, continued to regard himself as a priest, and retained a commitment to celibacy. The Centre for Intercultural Formation evolved into *Centro Intercultural de Documentación* (CIDOC), an informal university and language school. CIDOC attracted students from all over the world, its focus shifting from language to social and philosophical issues, and was the intellectual crucible in which Illich developed his ideas on the corruption of Western institutions. During the 1970s he gained a wider audience following the publication of a series of polemical books beginning with *Deschooling Society* in 1971, which argued that educational institutions stifled true learning. His subsequent books had a common theme: that industrialisation and institutionalisation had robbed people of their freedom and handed over fundamental aspects of human life to professions and their institutions, a process of 'de-skilling.' He expanded these ideas in *Tools for Conviviality* (1973) and *Energy and Equity* (1974), in which he argued against mass entertainment and mass transport, respectively. He brought the same thinking to *Medical Nemesis* in 1974.

Illich's intellectual influence peaked in the mid-1970s. CIDOC closed down in 1976 and he subsequently held visiting professorships at various European and American universities. He divided the last decade of his life between Mexico and Bremen, "aristocratically aloof, austere, absorbed but happy" (Obituary 2003). He died of a facial tumour, for which, characteristically, he did not seek medical treatment: "I am not ill, it's not an illness. It is something completely different—a very complicated relationship." Illich collapsed suddenly while at work in his study and died immediately.

Illich was a singular, paradoxical, and slightly absurd figure. Initially regarded as a quasi-Marxist critic of modern consumer capitalism, he grew to be distrusted by the Left and called Marxism 'inhumane.' The Right dismissed him as a communist crank. The church disowned him, although typically, Illich remarked that it was the church that had left *him*. He had immense intellectual gifts; he was fluent in so many languages that he claimed to have no mother tongue. His scholastic hinterland was vast, drawing from theology, philosophy, history, and sociology. He boasted of simple tastes in food and drink, yet a friend wrote after his death that he enjoyed expensive foods and fine wines (Levin 2003). He railed against modern mass transportation and the damage it caused to the environment, yet crossed the Atlantic by jet on countless occasions. He refused to wear a watch, which he referred to as a 'gauge,' yet constantly asked 'gauge bearers' what time it was (ibid.). He preached that educational institutions were a barrier to true learning, yet held visiting professorships at various universities. A charismatic man with a huge circle of friends and disciples, he could be cutting and dismissive to those less gifted, and to those who did not share his views.

After his death in 2002, the psychiatrist and writer Anthony Daniels (2003) wrote:

> Illich was deeply conservative, or at least he would have been had he been born in the Middle Ages. The word reactionary fitted him quite well, insofar as he regarded pre-modern forms of existence as being in many ways superior to our own. He was an anti-Enlightenment figure while he believed in the value of rational argument and of empirical evidence . . . he certainly did not believe in a heaven on earth brought about by rational action on the part of benevolent governments and bureaucracies. He was completely unimpressed by supposed evidence of progress such as declining infant mortality rates, rising life expectancies, or increased levels of consumption. Indeed, he thought modern man was living in a hell of his own creation: the revolution of rising expectations was really the institutionalization of permanent disappointment and therefore of existential bitterness.

Themes of *Medical Nemesis*

There is a degree of confusion around the title of Illich's (1974) medical polemic, *Medical Nemesis*. A further version, *Limits to Medicine: Medical Nemesis—The Expropriation of Health*, was published in January 1975 in Ideas in Progress: "a series of working papers dealing with alternatives to industrial society." A further version of *Limits to Medicine* ("written as a result of the world-wide response which the author received upon publication of the original draft") was published in 1976 (Illich 1976), and is the version I refer to throughout.

Medical Nemesis was a natural development of Illich's ideas on institutions and professions. He argued that modern medicine had hubristically taken on a mission to eradicate pain, sickness, even death. These were, he argued, eternal human realities, which we must learn to cope with: in fact, coping with these verities is what it means to be 'healthy.' Although Illich did not coin the word 'iatrogenesis'—meaning the harm done by doctors—he certainly popularised it. He described three types of iatrogenesis: clinical, or the direct harm done by various medical treatments; social, or the medicalisation of ordinary life; and cultural, meaning the loss of traditional ways of dealing with suffering.

Medicine and the health of populations

Illich argued that scientific medicine had little effect on the overall health of populations. Others had made this argument, most notably the epidemiologist Thomas McKeown (Bynum 2008). Like McKeown, Illich (1976: 1) believed that sanitation, nutrition, and housing were more important determinants of health:

> The study of the evolution of disease patterns provides evidence that during the last century doctors have affected epidemics no more profoundly than did priests in earlier times . . . the combined death rate from scarlet fever, diphtheria, whooping cough, and measles among children up to fifteen shows that nearly 90 per cent of the total decline in mortality between 1860 and 1965 had occurred before the introduction of antibiotics and widespread immunization.

Illich (ibid.) controversially went on to argue that not only did doctors contribute little to the health of populations, they probably did more harm than good: "only modern malnutrition injures more people than iatrogenic disease in its various manifestations." He had a low opinion of doctors ("the medical guild"), who he regarded, cynically, as more concerned with their income and status than the health of their patients: "doctors deploy themselves as they like, more so than other professionals, and they tend to gather where the climate is healthy, where the water is clean, and where people are employed and can pay for their services" (ibid.).

Social iatrogenesis

Illich (ibid.) observed how the founders of the UK National Health Service (NHS) naïvely believed that a free healthcare system would result in a healthier society, and thus less demand for its services. He coined the term 'Sisyphus syndrome,' meaning the more healthcare given to a population, the greater its demand for care. He used the term 'social iatrogenesis' to describe what he saw as the medicalisation of Western society: "medical practice sponsors sickness by reinforcing a morbid society that encourages people to become consumers of curative, preventive, industrial, and environmental medicine." He described how the pharmaceutical industry, enthusiastically supported by the medical profession, benefitted from this medicalisation: "To promote Valium, Hoff-LaRoche spent $200 million in ten years and commissioned some two hundred doctors a year to produce scientific articles about its properties."

Cultural iatrogenesis

Illich (ibid.) went on to argue that 'cultural' iatrogenesis was the most insidious form of iatrogenesis, as it sought to corrupt the essence of what it is to be human. He attacked especially the medicalisation of death:

> The patient's unwillingness to die on his own makes him pathetically dependent. He has now lost his faith in his ability to die, the terminal shape that health can take, and has made the right to be professionally killed into a major issue.

He believed that there is a profound difference between *pain* and *suffering*. Pain, he argued, is a sensation, but suffering is a *practice*. Pain, in the absence of a cultural and spiritual context, is unendurable. Such cultural iatrogenesis had robbed people in modern industrialised societies of the ability to *suffer*, thus rendering pain meaningless:

> Culture makes pain tolerable by integrating it into a meaningful setting; cosmopolitan civilization detaches pain from any subjective or inter-subjective context in order to annihilate it. Culture makes pain tolerable by interpreting its necessity; only pain perceived as curable is intolerable . . . Duty, love, fascination, routines, prayer, and compassion were some of the means that enabled pain to be borne with dignity.
>
> *(ibid.)*

The greatest human pain is death. Through the medicalisation of death, "healthcare has become a monolithic world religion" bringing "the epoch of natural death to an end" so that "Western man has lost the right to preside at his act of dying" (ibid.).

Illich's remedies

Illich's diagnosis of medicine's woes was astute, but his prescriptions were risible. He argued, for example, for "more public support for alpha waves, encounter groups and chiropractic." He advanced rather vague proposals for handing back to lay people responsibility for their health ("the will to self-care among the laity"), limiting the power of doctors ("the professional monopoly of physicians"), insurance companies, and pharmaceutical firms (ibid.). Perhaps it is unreasonable to expect Illich to have provided practical solutions to what he viewed as a spiritual, rather than an organisational, or societal, malaise.

Prose style

Medical Nemesis is not an easy read. The prose is dense, and at times impenetrable. Illich drew not only from the medical literature, but also history, philosophy, sociology, and anthropology. His use of footnotes is even greater than the late writer David Foster Wallace and employed without Wallace's irony: one 39-word sentence has eight footnotes. He defended this use of footnotes: "The footnotes reflect the nature of this text. I assert the right to break the monopoly that academia has exercised over all small print at the bottom of the page" (ibid.). Illich employed this particular style deliberately: he wanted lay people (who, he argued, should take responsibility for their own health) to have access to an extensive bibliography and he wanted to impress medical readers with as much evidence as possible. I suspect that Illich also simply wished to show off: he did not wear his learning lightly. If *Medical Nemesis* had been stripped of repetition, footnotes, and irrelevancies, it might have been a readable long essay. Unreadability, however, is not an insuperable obstacle to success for a book—*Medical Nemesis* was a bestseller and established Illich as a star public intellectual. Illich was a charismatic and accomplished public speaker; I suspect that many bought the book after hearing him speak, and gave up after the first few pages.

Medical Nemesis and Illich's 'apophasis'

A reader unfamiliar with Illich would not guess that the author of *Medical Nemesis* was a Catholic priest. Apophasis may be defined as a kind of theological or philosophical thinking that reveals its true subject by not mentioning this subject (Hartch 2015). The original Greek word means 'denial' or 'negation.' There is a long tradition of Christian apophatic theology, including Meister Eckhart and St John of the Cross. In later life, Illich told his friends that his personal theology was 'apophatic.' His biographer, Todd Hartch (2015), argues that Illich's books, including *Medical Nemesis*, were really about the corruption of Christianity:

> To Illich, the history of the West was thus the tragedy of the institutionalization of Christianity, as the Church, truly the Body of Christ, adopted the false and dangerous guise of an institution . . . If the Church had not succumbed to institutionalization, those other institutions would not even have come into existence. Illich's apophasis, therefore, had two levels. He denied that mandatory schooling was true learning or teaching, that modern medicine was true healing, and that economic development was true compassion; at the deeper level he denied that the Church was a bureaucracy, that the human body was a machine, and that death and suffering could be avoided.

Many years after the publication of *Medical Nemesis*, Illich told his friend, the historian Barbara Duden, that the subject of the book "could as easily have been the postal service because the underlying corruption of the West, not medicine itself, was the true object of his study" (ibid.).

Contemporary reaction to *Medical Nemesis*

The publication of *Medical Nemesis* prompted the *British Medical Journal* to take the unprecedented decision to publish, in December 1974, three individual reviews of the book, along with an editorial comment. Philip Rhodes (1974), Dean of the Faculty of Medicine at the University of Adelaide, like many readers, found Illich's prose style less than engaging: "Such, however, is the obscurity of the language, the imagery, the recourse to mythology, iconography, and selective history that one's interpretation of what the author means could very easily be wrong." Rhodes (ibid.) accused Illich of a lack of originality: "nothing said by Illich has not already been said by some doctor . . . there is nothing really new to be found here." George Discombe (1974), Professor of Chemical Pathology at the Abmadu Bello University, Zaria, Nigeria, was also unimpressed: "Dr Illich betrays a fondness for exotic words, abstract nouns, and emotive phrases—good and proper signs by which to know a mystagogue . . . Illich is revealed as a dealer in Utopias—in the line of Bacon, Rousseau, Karl Marx and G.K. Chesterton." Alex Paton (1974: 573) was the only reviewer of the three who supported Illich: "his argument is closely reasoned, sometimes obscure, often exasperating, but never dull, and fully documented."

The *British Medical Journal* letters page was equally busy. John Bradshaw (1975) wrote:

> The gist of your leading article on Ivan Illich's *Medical Nemesis* is that, while clearly much is wrong with medicine, there is nothing that doctors and other citizens cannot set to rights, that Illich is a somewhat wild man, if interesting, and that one cannot put the clock back . . . I think Illich is not a prophet of industrial (or medical) nemesis: like the rest of us, he is now a witness of its occurrence.

David Horrobin (1977) wrote an entire book—*Medical Hubris: A Reply to Ivan Illich*—refuting Illich's thesis. He mocked Illich as a "classic Old-Testament spellbinder" and, rather patronisingly, "extremely dangerous for people of moderate intelligence." "In almost every situation," wrote Horrobin, "Illich overstates his case and in some he presents a view which to the uninformed must be frankly misleading." He conceded, however, that Illich was "brilliantly eloquent" and "seductively convincing."

Have Illich's prophecies come true?

After the high-water mark of the 1970s, Illich went out of fashion: the medical establishment dismissed him as a crank and moved on. His argument was weakened by the obscurity of his prose, his dismissal of technology, and the impracticality and vagueness of his suggested solutions. It is tempting to regard him as just another historical footnote to the counter-culture of the 1960s and 1970s; yet, 40 years on, much of what he warned against has come to pass. Indeed, there was more than a touch of the Old Testament prophet in Illich's public persona: critics frequently dismissed him in ad hominem attacks as a 'Jeremiah.' When *Medical Nemesis* was published in 1974, US spending on healthcare was 8% of the GDP; it is now 18%. Healthcare makes up 10% of the entire global economy. Medicine has indeed become, in Illich's phrase, "a vast monolithic world religion." Even meliorists such as Atul Gawande (2002) admit that the growth of healthcare as a percentage of the global economy is threatening other aspects of human life, such as transport, housing, and education. Medicalisation has continued unchecked, and Illich would have been wryly amused by the invention of new diseases, such as social anxiety disorder (shyness), male-pattern alopecia (baldness), testosterone-deficiency syndrome (old age), and erectile dysfunction (impotence).

Illich, like the French historian Philippe Ariès (1981), railed against the medicalisation of death. Since 1975, death has moved from the home to the hospital; and hospitals have become a dustbin for all sorts of societal problems, not just dying. Illich assumed that this medicalisation was something doctors actively sought, to enhance their power, but doctors and hospitals did not ask for these problems—society was quite happy to hand them over, as long as the problems could be given a medical gloss. In 2002, Leibovici and Lièvre (866) corrected the Illichian view in the *British Medical Journal*:

> These aspects of medicalization make doctors miserable. The bad things of life: old age, death, pain and handicap are thrust on doctors to keep families and society from facing them. Some of them are an integral part of medicine, and accepted as such. But there is a boundary beyond which medicine has only a small role. When doctors are forced to go beyond that role they do not gain power or control: they suffer.

Illich's prediction of ever-increasing medicalisation has come true, but doctors are as much victims as their patients.

Modern medicine has been called "a culture of excess." In 2011, the Lancet Oncology Commission produced a lengthy report called *Delivering Affordable Cancer Care in High-Income Countries* (Sullivan et al. 2011: 933). The authors, a gathering of the great and the good of modern oncology, concluded (in a passage that could have been written by Illich) that cancer care is in crisis, driven by overuse and futility:

> In developed countries, cancer treatment is becoming a culture of excess. We over-diagnose, overtreat and overpromise. This extends from use of complex technology, surgery and drugs to events related to the acceptance of treatment side-effects. Second, we are a society that focuses almost exclusively on benefit, and such benefit is often small. For example, a 20% improvement in survival for a patient with a non-resectable metastatic solid tumour translates into a benefit of 4–6 weeks at best. Perspective is almost exclusively absent as we focus solely on what is perceived as benefit.

The medical profession and their patients may not be exercised about social and cultural iatrogenesis, but *clinical* iatrogenesis is now recognised as a major societal issue, one in urgent need of fixing. Atul Gawande (2009: 56), in his book *Complications*, summarised the problem:

> In 1991, the *New England Journal of Medicine* published a series of landmark papers from a project known as the Harvard Medical Practice Study—a review of more than thirty thousand hospital admissions in New York State. The study found that nearly 4 percent of hospital patients suffered complications from treatment which either prolonged their hospital stay or resulted in disability or death, and that two-thirds of such complications were due to errors in care. One in four, or 1 percent of admissions, involved actual negligence. It was estimated that, nationwide, upward of forty-four thousand patients die each year at least partly as a result of errors in care.

Many within medicine view with alarm the direction modern healthcare has taken. Denis McCullough, an American gerontologist, wrote: "Economic interests, as well as cultural and social pressures, encourage both an excessive use of health services and an expansion of people's expectations beyond what is realistic, what the health service is able to deliver" (Zuger 2008). The economist Alan Enthoven has argued that increasing spending on medicine will reach a tipping point, beyond which more spending causes more harm than good (Moynihan and Smith 2002). We have seen the rise in the concept of disease 'awareness,' promoted, not infrequently, by pharmaceutical companies. Genetics has the potential to turn us all into 'patients' by identifying our predisposition to various diseases. Guidelines from the European Society of Cardiology on treatment of hypertension and hypercholesterolaemia identified 76% of the adult population of Norway as being at "increased risk" (Getz et al. 2004). This 'disease mongering' (driven mainly by the pharmaceutical industry) has, wrote Iona Heath (2006: e146), "meant a shift of attention from the sick to the well and from the poor to the rich." Illich (1976: 62) himself wrote: "a culture can become prey of a pharmaceutical invasion. Each culture has its poisons, its remedies, its placebos, and its ritual settings for their administration. Most of these are destined for the healthy rather than the sick."

Influence of Illich

Anthony Daniels (2003) spoke for many when he wrote: "My attitude to Illich was composed half of admiration, half of irritation." Illich was a hugely influential intellectual figure in the

1970s and had many disciples, including John Bradshaw, who wrote *Doctors on Trial* in 1978, which reached the Illichian conclusion that: "western doctors today are certainly more productive, directly or indirectly, of ill-health, in every sense, than of health." Illich, naturally, wrote the foreword for Bradshaw's polemic. Richard Smith (2003: 927), then editor of the *British Medical Journal*, wrote this:

> The closest I ever came to a religious experience was listening to Ivan Illich. A charismatic and passionate man, surrounded by the fossils of the academic hierarchy in Edinburgh. He argued that 'the major threat to health in the world is modern medicine.' This was 1974. He convinced me, not least because I felt that what I saw on the wards of the Royal Infirmary of Edinburgh was more for the benefit of doctors than patients.

Illich's marginalisation may have been a defensive response on the part of doctors. Since the 1970s, the dominant ethos in the medical profession has been anti-Illichian. Doctors, patients, politicians, and the pharmaceutical industry formed a broad consensus that more medicine, more healthcare, could only be a good thing. Academic medicine, so powerful in shaping opinion, has developed a relationship with 'industrial partners' that is unhealthily close and uncritical. But a new generation has been influenced by Illich's ideas. A growing resistance is developing within medicine: this movement has various strands, such as the Slow Medicine Movement, founded in Italy in 1989, inspired by the Slow Food Movement. At a meeting of the Slow Medicine Movement in Bologna in 2013, Gianfranco Domenighetti listed the characteristics of health systems as follows: "complexity, uncertainty, opacity, poor measurement, variability in decision-making, asymmetry of information, conflict of interest, and corruption" (Smith 2012). The British Medical Association has backed a 'Too Much Medicine' campaign that shares some of the aims of the Slow Medicine Movement (Godlee 2015).

Medical Nemesis is a paradox: it is bombastic, barely readable, and over-stated, but at its core is a powerful argument. Forty years after its publication, Illich's thesis has only grown in strength.

Acknowledgement

The author and editor would like to acknowledge the editor of *The Journal of the Royal College of Physicians Edinburgh*, Martyn Bracewell, for kindly giving permission to draw on the original article that has subsequently been edited and adapted for this book.

References

Ariès P. 1981. *The Hour of Our Death*. New York, NY: Alfred A. Knopf.

Bradshaw JS. Medical nemesis. *BMJ*. 1975; 1: 94.

Bradshaw JS. 1978. *Doctors on Trial*. London: Wildwood House.

Bynum B. The McKeown thesis. *Lancet*. 2008; 371: 644–5.

Daniels A. Ivan Illich, 1926–2002. *The New Criterion*. January 2003, 21: 78–81.

Discombe GA. Romantic enthusiast. *BMJ*. 1974; 4: 574–6.

Gawande A. 2002. *Complications*. London: Profile Books.

Gawande A. The cost conundrum. *The New Yorker*, 1 June 2009. Available at: www.newyorker.com/magazine/2009/06/01/the-cost-conundrum. Last accessed: 20 January 2018.

Getz L, Kirkengen AL, Hetlevik I et al. Ethical dilemmas arising from implementation of the European guidelines on cardiovascular disease prevention in clinical practice. *Scandinavian Journal of Primary Health Care*. 2004; 22: 202–8.

Godlee F. Too much medicine. *BMJ*. 2015; 350: h1217. Available at: http://dx.doi.org/10.1136/bmj.h1217. Last accessed: 20 January 2018.

Hartch T. 2015. *The Prophet of Cuernavaca: Ivan Illich and the Crisis of the West*. Oxford: Oxford University Press.

Heath I. Combating disease mongering: daunting but nonetheless essential. *PLoS Medicine* 2006; 3: e146. Available at: http://dx.doi.org/10.1371/journal.pmed.0030146. Last accessed: 20 January 2018.

Horrobin D. 1977. *Medical Hubris. A Reply to Ivan Illich*. Montreal: Eden Press.

Illich I. 1974. *Medical Nemesis*. London: Calder & Boyars.

Illich I. 1976. *Limits to Medicine. Medical Nemesis: The Expropriation of Health*. London: Marion Boyars.

Leibovici L, Lièvre M. Medicalisation: peering from inside medicine. *BMJ*. 2002; 324: 866.

Levin L. Ivan Illich. *Journal of Epidemiology and Community Health*. 2003; 57: 925.

Moynihan R, Smith R. Too much medicine? Almost certainly. *BMJ*. 2002; 324: 859.

Obituary. Ivan Illich. *Journal of Epidemiology and Community Health*. 2003; 57: 923–4.

Paton A. 'Medicalization' of health. *BMJ*. 1974; 4: 573–4.

Rhodes P. Indictment of medical care. *BMJ*. 1974; 4: 576–7.

Smith R. Limits to medicine. Medical nemesis: the expropriation of health. *Journal of Epidemiology and Community Health*. 2003; 57: 928.

Smith R. 2012. The case for slow medicine. *BMJ Blogs*. Available at: http://blogs.bmj.com/bmj/2012/12/17/richard-smith-the-case-for-slow-medicine. Last accessed: 20 January 2018.

Sullivan R, Peppercorn J, Sikora K, et al. Delivering affordable cancer care in high-income countries. *Lancet Oncology*. 2011; 12: 933–80.

Zuger A. For the very old, a dose of 'slow medicine.' *The New York Times*, 26 February 2008. Available at: www.nytimes.com/2008/02/26/health/views/26books.html?_r=0. Last accessed: 20 January 2018.

10
HOSPITALAND

Jefferson Wong

Tour of Hospitaland

Welcome, welcome! Welcome to the carnival of horrors! We've recently changed our name to 'Hospitaland' to be able to continue our services, abiding by the newest medical guidelines. Don't worry, though! Upon entering, there's an overwhelming sense of familiarity. To the left is the Patient Centre, where all out-patients and in-patients can enter. Each of them will be given an identification number, and should they desire, they can give up their birth name as well. To the right is a space reserved for the elite medical students, where they will be warmly welcomed to view the spectacle of the ill patient!

The first park is Psyfari, where medical students can observe patients in their primal state, stripped of their identities! Medical students are asked not to feed the patients, though, as bland hospital food must be brought in from the cafeteria and placed just out of arm's reach of the patients. Continuing on to ITU Playground, medical students can practise all of their favourite clinical skills! Every success comes with a prize, and if one cannot succeed, there are many more patients to practise on!

Imagine yourself in Discovery Land, the land of imaging, microscopy and autopsies. Medical students are encouraged to turn their patients into tiny puzzle pieces and forget the entire picture. Patient details and analyses are easier to read on paper anyway. In the Ground Round Maze, try to not get lost in looking for a 'good patient.' Explore all of the patients on the ward round and return to the centre to discuss your best, in other words prognostically worst, findings! Medical students can battle their chosen patients against each other in the 'Sign Colosseum.' Which patient is really the perfect patient? Only time and duration of illness will tell!

For medical students wanting a break, they can take a swim in the Journal Sand Dune or play with the Data Crane. Play with all the patient data that one desires! Afterwards, medical students can find a nice corner in the Theatre, ensuring that they're out of the way while the consultant surgeons perform the operations. At the end of the day, medical students can play their hand in the Pharmacino and place their bets on various drugs and treatments. What's one patient's health worth when you have so many options? Medical students can always go to the Out-Patient Market to see if they can recruit the patient as a new in-patient.

Entry is free for both medical students and patients. Although patients may have a lot to lose, medical students will have a lot to gain!

Themes in Hospitaland

Reprogramming one's mindset

A 'good patient'

Upon entering medical school, medical students are changing the definition of the term 'good patient.' 'Good' no longer refers to the character of the person but now refers to the severity of their illness or how obvious their clinical signs are. The attitudes of medical students are being redirected to always look for the weaker aspects of the patient rather than the positive aspects. For example, medical students would be looking for which limb has colder peripheries rather than asking the patient about their life achievements. Thus, looking at the weaker physical aspects and ignoring the positive characteristics further dehumanises patients. This process of ignoring is the essence of dehumanisation.

Distrust the foolish

When medical students take a medical history from patients, they are taught to distrust the patient's sexual, smoking and drinking history. Medical students are taught to not believe patients when they say that they have not had sex recently. Medical students are also taught to cross-question patients when addressing whether the patients have ever smoked. Most of all, medical students cannot rely on the accuracy of the amount of alcohol that patients reportedly drink. This sense of distrust is like a seed that has been planted that continues to grow and expand into other areas of history taking. More experienced medical students no longer believe that the patients know and understand their diagnoses if they were self-diagnosed. There is a judgement that patients are fickle with their reporting and change their history each time when presenting. Moreover, that broadens to encompass the fact that patients are not to be trusted with medical knowledge. Medical students have become the experts not only in medical knowledge but also in patients' own lives, displacing their self-awareness and autonomy.

Remember 'me'

Furthermore, with patients repeatedly going to get medical treatment at medical centres, they are subconsciously being trained to change the way they speak. People attending medical clinics as patients are encouraged to lose their natural tendency to strike up conversations, to speak freely and to learn about another person's life. They have now been trained to speak a certain way, to use certain words and terms. Specifically, patients have been forced to change the words that they use to present their symptoms, worries and thoughts. For example, a patient will focus on how the symptoms have made them feel poorly and interrupted their ability to carry out their daily activities. They no longer will talk about anything beyond their symptoms and basic daily activities. They will not address their hopes and dreams. They will not talk about the love in their heart. The conversation has become void of deep, meaning-ful talk.

Now patients are only remembered by their medical status, either by a concise history, an interesting presentation, a novel investigation or a rare diagnosis. The patient's name is not remembered and is not supposed to be remembered, as the hospital number is the preferred form of identity to be used in a discussion.

Animalistic dehumanisation

Stripping off clothing: the separation between man and beast

Beginning with the very first interactions with patients, patients are asked to remove their clothes and to re-dress in hospital gowns. This very act resembles the removal of civility for a 'bare life' (Agamben 1995). People are told to remove their clothes and to wear a sheer cloth which exposes their private areas. In public, people are very concerned with their appearance and would never tolerate such requests. But they are giving up this aspect of being civilised to be able to receive treatment. Furthermore, by removing their clothes, they are stripped of their individuality and culture. The clothes they are asked to wear have no flair or personality. The hospital gowns are void of any reference to who the patient is and where they come from.

Private body parts, now public!

In the western world, genitalia are considered private, intimate body parts to be hidden from public view. Medicine changes the term 'private parts' to no longer mean private, sacred and valued, but to now be open for discussion, judgement, criticisms and fault finding. For example, urinary catheterisation and digital rectal exams involve looking at and touching areas on a person that are otherwise considered very private parts of the body. Medical students no longer encounter these body parts as unseen, hidden areas, but regularly perform these procedures on genitals and anuses, where the most private part of a person becomes an open topic to talk about during a coffee break, and even the subject of black humour (Piemonte 2015).

'Maintain' the dignity

Also, the concepts of dignity and respect have changed in the clinical context. In order to listen to difficult-to-hear heart sounds, medical students have to place their stethoscopes directly onto the patient's chest, under their gown. It is implied that the student will not look down the patient's chest unnecessarily, but will instead respect the patient's dignity. The idea, though, is to 'maintain' a patient's dignity, which hints at the notion that their dignity is completely in the hands of the medical student. This takes the term 'dignity' to apply only to the physical aspect of someone's life and removes the meaning of dignity that is normally based on one's character. If dignity is 'stripped' from a patient, what is there to separate the patient from a downtrodden member of society or even a lost animal?

Mechanistic dehumanisation

Nothing but an object

The other major part of dehumanisation is the objectification of a patient. From the first day that they enter medical school, medical students receive constant training in clinical skills and medical investigations on plastic models. Many of the clinical skills and investigations can be embarrassing for both the medic and the patient; however, medical students are taught to be void of those feelings to be able to effectively carry out the procedure. When students perform these procedures on real patients in the wards, the repetitive practice on models can kick in, and inadvertently the students observe and treat the patients like the plastic model, like an object.

Standardise individuality

The constraint of time is the omnipresent watchdog, preventing the patients from talking about other aspects of life which may mean more to them than their current illness. More than that, the constraint of time has forced medical students to stereotype patients based on their presenting histories. This makes efficient pattern recognition possible, but it also groups patients into identifiable labels, which becomes a tick-box exercise to see if a patient fits a certain diagnosis. Time limitations have automated the understandings of patients' lives and re-focused the exploration of a patient's life into more likely and less likely diagnoses rather than emotional journeys and struggles people have gone through in life.

By my command

In the hospital waiting room patients are told to sit and wait with other patients. They have to obey the rules of the hospital and wait for commands from hospital staff. Patients are being ordered to have patience and not to leave the waiting room, in case they miss being called in. They have to conform to the 'inertness' of the waiting room. They must not move around too much in their chair as they might disturb the person sitting next to them. They will have to remain quiet or speak in a low voice so as to be able to hear announcements. They have to sit so that they don't block the walkways or entrances. On top of that, they may be told not to drink any liquids, not to eat foods for over twelve to twenty-four hours and not to empty their bladders until asked to, This concept of following orders by the hospital and hospital staff extends to the rest of the time in the hospital, in particular their interactions with doctors, nurses and specialists. Patients have conformed to the system and lost their ability to take their own initiative. It's as though patients have become a product on an assembly line belt, like a passive player in the medical system.

Welcome to Hospitaland!

References

Agamben G. 1995. *Homo Sacer: Sovereign Power and Bare Life*. Stanford, CA: Stanford University Press.
Piemonte N. 2015. Last Laugh: Gallows Humour and Medical Education. *Journal of Medical Humanities* 36: 379–90.

PART III

Medicine's metaphors and rhetoric

11

DON'T BREATHE A WORD

A psychoanalysis of medicine's inflations

Alan Bleakley

Just as our soul, being air, holds us together, so do breath and air encompass the whole world.

(Anaximenes (585–528 BCE))

My father's death

My father died from pancreatic cancer in 1970—he was just 54 and I was 21, raw and confused. When the cancer found purchase—it started in the pancreas and rapidly spread—he plummeted from feeling out of sorts to a heart-rending fragility. After a short period in hospital he was transferred home—thin, bed bound, often in extreme pain, and eventually drifting in and out of long periods of deep, opiate-induced sleep. From diagnosis to death was less than six months.

When he was diagnosed with terminal cancer, both his family doctor and the consultant oncologist did not reveal the diagnosis to him. They took my mother, my brother and myself aside, told us the diagnosis and prognosis, and asked us to not divulge anything to him. They told my father that he had complications from an operation on his gall bladder (that is how the cancer was first discovered) that would clear up in time. I remember recoiling at the moral dilemma the doctors had set us—to not share the fatal diagnosis with my father but to spin a web of disguise through white lies—yet I joined the charade until the end. My dad, of course, knew that he was seriously ill, but the word 'cancer' was never brought to the table. I was at the bedside when he drew his last breath. Laura Marks (2014) says: "Associated with the soul, animating the lungs, breath is that invisible and usually intangible entity that makes its passage known sonically": the hollow gurgling of the death rattle, then the sigh of resignation, and finally the wholesale withdrawal of noise—the void filled by the family's collective sobs.

Three things in particular struck me about his death: first, the obscene pact of secrecy that we set up with the doctors based around subscription to the stigma that cancer carried; second, the irrational tenacity that we, as a family, showed in sticking religiously to that pact; and third, the oncologist's disturbing language register, describing the 'invasion' of the cancer and how my dad had already 'lost the war.' I found the use of war metaphors particularly confusing because my father had no desire—or energy—to 'fight' his illness. He was a combat veteran, serving in Egypt during WWII; he'd had his fill of war.

Medicine's inflation

In the years after my father's death, I increasingly questioned what I saw as the deception of the doctors and our collusion with this deception, and felt palpable guilt about this. Later, I became aware of the seminal field study of Barney Glaser and Anselm Strauss (1967) that founded 'grounded theory'—in which theory is built up from systematic analysis of data, rather than data being collected to test a prior theory (Nathaniel and Andrews 2010). This study looked at how doctors and nurses in the 1960s interacted with people dying in hospitals from terminal illnesses, particularly cancers. Glaser and Strauss observed that it was common for doctors to enter into a pact with families in which patients were not told of their imminent demise, but were led to believe that they would recover. Cancer carried stigma. Further, nurses were expected to talk with patients about their impending deaths only with the consent of physicians.

This knot of deception—familiar from my father's death—was termed a pact of "closed awareness." Nathaniel and Andrews (2010) described this as an "atmosphere of organized secrecy," where "family members purposely maintain the fiction that the dying patient might recover." Sadly, "This context does not allow patients to close their lives with proper rituals. Because of the organized deception, relatives' grief cannot be expressed openly." In short, this particular posture of medical culture showed an extraordinary level of inflation—where doctors extend their legitimate specialist technical roles into questionable forms of imperialism and authoritarianism as they adopt particular communication strategies, in turn manipulating family members' actions in diverting their natural concern and grief. In other words, the capital of emotional response and grief held within the family comes to be owned and distributed by the medical profession according to its whims, rather than an open and transparent ethical framework. Medicine colonises the voices of patient and family. This was the mid- to late 1960s, and times have changed. It is now standard practice for those dying from cancer to be given their diagnosis and prognosis. However, while the specific culture that Glaser and Strauss explored may be seen as an historical anomaly, medicine's inflations persist.

Cultures take on pomp and egos inflate (as hubris or excessive self-confidence). In physics, inflation means swollen by air or gas; in economics, increase beyond proper limits; in psychology, puffed up with vanity, pride or false notions—a state of mind characterised by an exaggerated sense of self-importance and need for admiration, compensated by feelings of inferiority. Read psychoanalytically, inflation or hubris is then a symptom of basic insecurity (fear of failure; intolerance of ambiguity). Medicine's historical legacy of paternalistic, hierarchical masculine heroism—preferring individualism to collaboration; opaque to the scrutiny of outsiders; refusing to admit to or own its multiple errors; and, at worst, arrogant and self-serving—advertises what psychoanalysts term inflation of the ego, the basis to a Narcissistic Personality Disorder (NPD).

The popular medical website 'Medscape' (www.medscape.com) hosted a discussion about the extent of medical error in which a rash of doctors refused to accept that relatively high rates of medical (particularly surgical) error exist (Stokowski 2016). In a second wave of comments on this theme under the heading 'Doctors in denial?' a nurse said: "Instead of asking what we can do about this problem, most are variations on exclamations of denial." A paediatrician then commented that although medical errors are "hard to accurately quantify, they are hugely underreported . . . people are practicing at the edge of their scope and not appropriately asking for guidance. *Be careful of the ego* and try to be aware of what you don't know" (my emphasis).

The late American neurosurgeon Paul Kalanithi (2016) writes of how he was driven to succeed in medicine to such an extent that it brought his marriage to the edge of ruin. He describes the punishing work schedules and harsh apprenticeship in learning brain surgery, the forming of a tough-minded arrogance as standard identity construction and the impossibly high expectations of success, again driven by fear of failure and intolerance of ambiguity. Tragically, as Kalanithi confesses, his ego was tempered only by the rapidly encroaching shadow of his fatal lung cancer—a humbling by impending death at the beginning of what promised to be a glittering career. The British neurosurgeon Henry Marsh (in Wakefield 2016) writes of a growing awareness only late in his career of his narcissism: "I often think I became a brain-surgeon to justify my own sense of self-importance." He warns that seeking out team members who will challenge and restrain you is essential to check medical hubris and egomania. Doctors shouldn't work in isolation: "People working on their own get out of touch and it corrupts you . . . it's hubris isn't it? The funny thing about medical hubris is that nemesis is visited on the patients rather than the surgeon." That's not a "funny thing," but sad and reprehensible.

Marsh seems to relish the reprehensible. In a recent interview in the UK's *Observer* (Adams 2017), Marsh says that doctors and surgeons "have a very complicated relationship with patients . . . as soon as we have any interaction with patients, we start lying. We have to. There is nothing more frightening for a patient than an anxious or doubtful doctor." This is a good example of 'old school' medical morality, one of double standards grounded in inflation.

Putting medicine on the couch

Overall, medicine does an exceptional job under extreme pressure, but it also shoots itself in the foot unnecessarily. *That* medicine inflicts avoidable physical and psychological wounds on patients, colleagues and doctors is clear, despite the Hippocratic injunction to 'first, do no harm.' *Why* this should be the case is unclear. Here, I suggest that inflation is a major root cause for such slippage, grounded in the culture's refusal of democracy and authentic social justice, including gender equality within its own ranks.

This resistance to democratisation and feminising is itself grounded in an historical-cultural effect—the influence of two guiding metaphors that have shaped medical practice and values since the Enlightenment: the body as a machine and medicine as war, discussed below (Bleakley 2017). These didactic metaphors may be grounded in a wider historical-cultural effect—the "imagination of air" (Hillman 2014), characteristic of early Enlightenment values and practices, discussed later. I will then move through three levels to explain medicine's inflation: first, the refusal of democratisation; second, that such refusal is grounded in the pervasive influence of two key metaphors; and third, that these metaphors in turn are grounded in the discourse of the Enlightenment's scientific 'aerial imagination,' the legacy of which remains potent.

Metaphor 1: the body as machine

Too often the consultant oncologist who diagnosed my father's illness referred to him in terms of the cancer and the afflicted organ, rather than the person, his suffering and sudden shrinking circle of life. Medicine's inflation depends in part upon a parallel and compensatory deflation of patients, while reduction of the complexity of the body to a linear machine suggests intolerance of ambiguity.

Unfettered by the religious observation that prevented Galen (130–210) from dissecting humans, the Flemish doctor Andreas Vesalius (1514–1564) dissected bodies of executed criminals provided by a sympathetic Paduan judge. Vesalius corrected fundamental errors in Galen's work, stemming from extrapolating to the human from animal dissections. Vesalius reduced the body to a shell housing organs, described as the *Fabrica*—Latin for 'something that is made,' or a 'machine.' Vesalius then promoted a mechanical imagination of the body that has shaped medical culture to this day. Patients are reduced to their symptoms, where the body is a set of engineered components: for example, the brain has 'wiring,' the liver is the body's 'factory,' and the kidneys are a 'wastewater filter.' Almost a century after Vesalius, the philosopher René Descartes (1596–1650), on the eve of the Enlightenment, said that "the body is to be regarded as a machine," an automaton. In the wake of Descartes, the celebrated Italian physician Giorgio Baglivi (1668–1706) extended the mechanical imagination of the body through finer grain analogies, where, for example, the stomach was compared to a flask, the teeth to scissors, blood vessels to pipes, and viscera and glands to sieves.

Metaphor 2: medicine as war

I talked earlier of how I was puzzled when the oncologist who was treating my father described cancer as an 'invading' force, a territorialising enemy. I agree with Susan Sontag's (1978) analysis that the use of martial metaphors merely adds to the stigma already suffered by those with cancer—but Sontag goes too far where she demands that metaphors be eradicated from medical discourse altogether. Rather, we need to know why such metaphors are used—where they appeared historically and how they may already be 'dead,' or can—and should—be replaced by other, more helpful, metaphors (Bleakley 2017).

In the Medieval to Early Modern period, my father's cancer would have been ascribed to an imbalance of humours or an excess of vital forces. Illnesses 'lay' on people (passive language) rather than 'attacking' them (active language). Hippocrates (c.460–370 BCE) first named observable tumours 'cancer'—Greek *karkinos*, Latin *carcinos*—after the crab and crayfish, analogous with the sideways creep of tumours ('metastasis' means 'change of position'). The disease was imagined as 'shifty,' scuttling sideways, but not as 'aggressive.'

The martial language of 'aggressive' tumours, and aggressive treatments to combat them, can be traced to the English poet and cleric John Donne's (1573–1631) 1627 sermon: 'Devotions Upon Emergent Occasions.' Donne describes his illness in 1627 as resembling a "siege" and "cannon shot." He thought he was dying from a fever "that blows up the heart," also describing an "illness that invades." But it was the celebrated English physician Thomas Sydenham (1624–1689) who fully embraced militaristic metaphors and created the metaphorical climate that has shaped modern medicine, still in full flow today with personalised drug regimes 'targeting' genetic faults and the ongoing 'war on cancer.'

Sydenham's language is Homeric: "I attack the enemy within," where:

> A murderous array of disease has to be fought against, and the battle is not a battle for the sluggard . . . I steadily investigate the disease, I comprehend its character, and I proceed straight ahead, and in full confidence, towards its annihilation.

Medicine is not for the faint-hearted, but a full-blooded battle reinforcing the dominance of the heroic male. No room for dithering here, but "proceed straight ahead" in full certainty. The scientific imagination of the Enlightenment period embraced a kind of invincibility, becoming psychologically inflated, where now the natural world could be understood and mastered to benefit humankind through technologies. Medicine embraced this same spirit where doctors became heroes. Indeed, the period of medical practice between the 18th and 19th centuries was called 'heroic medicine.' In the absence of knowledge of cures, doctors would treat the ailing body with shock techniques to jolt it back into efficient functioning—bloodletting, purging and sweating. The theory was to re-balance the humours.

By the 19th century, Louis Pasteur (1822–1895) was using the same heroic militaristic language, describing invading armies laying siege to the body that becomes a battlefield.

A "war against cancer" was first described in a lead article in the *British Medical Journal* in 1904. The "fight against cancer" was likened to imperialist domination, the disease described as "darkest Africa" waiting to be discovered and conquered. Later, cancer cells were identified with Bolsheviks, as "anarchic," threatening the stability of the body. Richard Nixon declared a full-scale "war on cancer" in signing the National Cancer Act of 1971, launching a $1.6 billion "federal crusade" to "conquer" cancer, using the most "aggressive" treatments to beat the "invading, killer cells."

In 2011, the 1989 Nobel Prize-winning Director of the National Cancer Institute (NCI), Dr Harold Varmus, was asked at a conference: "Can you give us an overall sense of what we may have accomplished over the last four decades?" Varmus replies: "It's inaccurate, in my view, to think of a war on cancer as though cancer were a single, individual enemy, nor is the metaphor of war exactly right." Corpus linguistic analysis (Semino et al. 2017) shows that in cancer discourse, patients commonly resort to violence and war metaphors. Yet research shows that cancer patients who view their disease as an 'enemy' show higher levels of anxiety and depression, a poorer quality of life, higher levels of pain and less ability to cope overall than those who represent their illness with a different meaning (Bleakley 2017). It is likely that patients use war metaphors unthinkingly. Many do not subscribe to this metaphor complex, but use other, non-martial, metaphors such as cancer as a 'journey.'

Following the poet Wallace Stevens, who said: "The world is presence, not force," we might replace martial medicine with a more feminine, collaborative and tender approach. For example, 'hospital' has the same root as 'hospitality.' Such a lyrical medicine offers an alternative to the standard epic, tragic and dark comic genres of practice (medicine has developed an unsavoury black humour at patients' expense (Piemonte 2015)).

The aerial imagination

The checks and balances that control potential inflation in a democracy, whether in persons or economies, arise from tolerant, collaborative engagement. Where the heroic imagination, and a certain level of intolerance, continues to feed medicine there is no check on inflation. Machine and martial metaphors, however, offer necessary but not sufficient explanations for medicine's inflation. We must also explore what gives these didactic metaphors such impetus and stamina. My suggestion is the legacy of the Enlightenment's 'aerial imagination.' This imagination inflates science beyond its boundaries of an explanatory and exploratory framework to one of imperialism, including domination and control of nature. And in medicine (often in good faith), domination and control of patients' experiences.

Of the realms of nature that might be controlled, the very air we breathe is the most obvious (Kean 2017). This intangible air must first be made tangible through close examination—dissected, measured, weighed—subsequently conquered (human flight), finally controlled (for example, through mass production of soda waters) and made subject to ownership (capitalism's influence upon air quality and access to clean air). James Hillman (2014) describes the rise of a scientific "imagination of air" in terms of the collapse of a Medieval/Renaissance worldview—that of alchemy. When a metal is burned to an ash (calcination) and the residue is weighed, it weighs more than the original metal. The alchemists ascribed this to calcination driving off a substance—phlogiston—that animated the material (think Ariel in Shakespeare's *The Tempest*). Where phlogiston is released, the loss of enervating spirit (the Greek *pneuma*: breath or inspiration) results in heaviness. It took a group of experimental chemists in the 1770s to reject this speculative alchemy, showing that roasted metals gain weight because oxygen is added. One of these chemists, Joseph Priestley, recorded that pumping oxygen into a container with a candle made the flame brighter, and into an enclosed area with mice made the mice livelier, while inhaling pure oxygen led to an exhilarating effect that Priestley suggested might become a popular indulgence. Oxygen inflates.

Priestley, however, would never see 'airs' as capital subject to ownership and unfair re-distribution, a later phenomenon accelerated by the Industrial Revolution and the spread of air pollution. His house in England was burned down because of his dissent from the ortho-doxy of the Church and associated authoritarian politics of the time, and he fled to America, where he sought a more democratic climate. Ironically, Priestley discovered how to carbon-ate water (the basis of sodas) in 1767, thus paving the way for the production of Coca Cola just over a century later. Now, two billion bottles a day are drunk worldwide and Coke has become a symbol of the unacceptable face of commercialism, capitalism and imperialism, the very forces that Priestley despised.

The aerial imagination also materialised through conquering not only the air—the Montgolfier Brothers launched the first hot air balloon flight in 1783—but also the dark. Gas lighting was perfected in 1800, and by 1820 Birmingham, London, Preston, Paris, Vienna, Baltimore and Philadelphia had extensive street lighting, advertising the democratic potential of the new 'airs.'

Combat breathing and the survival of the sickest

The Afro-Caribbean psychiatrist and revolutionary Frantz Fanon described the 'combat breath-ing' of Algerian prisoners of war as a form of resistance in the presence of their French colonist oppressors. This is a literal in-spiration, a collective deep breath to restore energy for acts of resistance: 'breathe in, hold, count to four; breathe in, hold, count to four,' and so on. 'Combat' is used here ironically, for combat breathing is an act of passive resistance as occupation changes the atmosphere of a culture ("you can observe my breathing, but you cannot occupy my breath"). Under occupation, Fanon (1970: 50) suggested that "the individual's breathing is an observed, an occupied breathing. It is a combat breathing."

Sharing an atmosphere involving medical intervention means that the patient can be deprived of breathing space as his or her territory becomes occupied. In my father's case, the whole family was occupied as we colluded with the doctors, thus letting slip the opportunity to adopt combat breathing, or what Homi Bhabha (2004) calls "sly civility"—tactics of resistance that appear to offer conformity with, but subtly undermine, the coloniser's presence: a version of Thoreau's and Gandhi's 'civil disobedience.'

I have described three cures for medicine's inflation: (i) democratising and feminising medicine; (ii) shifting the didactic metaphors that shape medicine and medical practice; and (iii) deflating the imperialistic aerial imagination. In this section, I describe a fourth cure: to undermine medicine's tacit subscription to Utilitarianism, defined as: "the doctrine that an action is right in so far as it promotes happiness, and that the greatest happiness of the greatest number should be the guiding principle of conduct" (*OED*). But one person's "happiness" (and 'health') is another's misery; and the birth lottery leaves many with disabilities and disadvantages where 'health' becomes a relative notion. Further, even the very 'healthy' may risk their lives through challenging sports or lifestyles. One key aspect of medicine's inflation, also a tactic for both legiti-mate and illegitimate occupation of the patient's atmosphere, is to make distinctions between the 'normal' and the 'pathological' that are in fact cultural and can be arbitrary (Canguilhem 1991).

Medicine can democratise (and deflate) under its own steam by challenging long-held sub-scription to ideals of health, embracing the paradoxical value of sickness and suffering. The performance artist and academic Martin O'Brien (2016) describes a "survival of the sick-est," challenging pieties based on holding untenable distinctions between health and sickness.

O'Brien—in an act of sly civility—reverses Darwin's 'survival of the fittest' by imagining a "Zombie Apocalypse" where: "I'd eat you to stay alive. I wouldn't even think twice . . . It's survival of the sickest! If it were the zombie apocalypse, only the infected could survive."

Martin O'Brien has cystic fibrosis (CF), so his breathing works against the grain, as his lungs fill with fluid. This leads to an early death—the average life expectancy for CF is currently 37 years. He needs regular physiotherapy for airway clearance, to free up mucus that would otherwise drown him. But O'Brien has turned his illness and impending death into a paradoxical gift by developing a radical durational performance art around his symptoms and consequent lifestyle (see: martinobrienperformance.com). Here, 'combat breathing' is everyday and therapeutic—an act of resistance against colonising by straight cultural values and standard medical approaches. O'Brien's work advertises Nietzsche's claim that artists can be diagnosticians of culture, challenging cultural norms. He takes the theme of the zombie—the living dead—as an image for the "survival of the sickest" that directly challenges the traditions of the aerial imagination and its inflations, within which conventional modern medicine has been cocooned for three centuries. O'Brien's performance interventions bring medicine down to earth with a bump, puncturing its pieties.

References

Adams T. 2017. 'People talk about the mind–matter problem. It's not a problem for me—mind is matter.' Interview with Henry Marsh. *The Observer, The New Review*, 16.07.17.

Bhabha H. 2004. 2nd ed. *The Location of Culture*. London: Routledge.

Bleakley A. 2017. *Thinking With Metaphors in Medicine: The State of the Art*. London: Routledge.

Canguilhem G. 1991. *The Normal and the Pathological*. New York, NY: Zone Books.

Fanon F 1970. *A Dying Colonialism*. Ringwood: Pelican.

Glaser B, Strauss A. 1967. *Awareness of Dying*. New York, NY: Aldine Publishing Company.

Hillman J. 2014. The imagination of air and the collapse of alchemy, in: J Hillman. *The Uniform Edition of the Writings of James Hillman Volume 5*. Dallas, TX: Dallas Institute Publications, 263–315.

Kalanithi P. 2016. *When Breath Becomes Air*. London: Bodley Head.

Kean S. 2017. *Caesar's Last Breath: The Epic Story of the Air Around Us*. New York, NY: Doubleday.

Marks LU. 2014. Book cover commentary for D. Quinlivan, *The Place of Breath in Cinema*. Edinburgh: Edinburgh University Press.

Marsh H. 2016. *Do No Harm: Stories of Life, Death and Brain Surgery*. London: W&N.

Nathaniel AK, Andrews T. The modifiability of grounded theory. *Grounded Theory Review*. 2010; 9. Available at: http://groundedtheoryreview.com/2010/04/06/751. Last accessed: 9 July 2017.

O'Brien M. 2016. 'If it were the apocalypse, I'd eat you to stay alive.' Available at: www.inbetweentime.co.uk/wp-content/uploads/2016/10/MC_IBT_ProgNotes_MartinOBrien_070217_v01_Web.pdf. Last accessed: 9 July 2017.

Peterkin A, Bleakley, A. 2017. *Staying Human During the Foundation Programme and Beyond*. Boca Raton, FL: CRC Press.

Piemonte N. Last laugh: gallows humor and medical education. *Journal of Medical Humanities*. 2015; 36: 375–90.

Semino E, Demjén Z, Demmen J, et al. The online use of Violence and Journey metaphors by patients with cancer, as compared with health professionals: a mixed methods study. *BMJ Supportive & Palliative Care*. 2017; 7: 60–6.

Sontag S. 1978. *Illness as Metaphor*. New York, NY: Farrar, Straus & Giroux.

Stokowski LA. Who believes that medical error is the third leading cause of hospital deaths? *Medscape*. 26 May 2016. Available at: www.medscape.com/viewarticle/863788. Last accessed: 18 May 2019.

Wakefield M. Henry Marsh: How doctors can become monsters. *The Spectator*. 6 May 2017. Available at: www.spectator.co.uk/2017/05/henry-marsh-how-doctors-can-become-monsters. Last accessed: 18 May 2019.

12

METAPHOR AS ART

A thought experiment

Anita Wohlmann

Research on metaphor has primarily (and for good reasons) foregrounded the problematic sides of metaphors. Metaphors shape experience, they can foreclose options, they suggest norms and cultural values and, in doing so, they may even be lethal, as physician-writer Abraham Verghese (2004) argues in relation to HIV/AIDS metaphors. In psychotherapy and palliative care, metaphors have enjoyed a better reputation. In these disciplines, metaphors are considered helpful tools for patients and doctors to understand problematic thought patterns and change patients' behaviour by rethinking confining metaphors (Kirmayer 1993; Ogden 1997). In end-of-life contexts, metaphors offer a protective "veil" for patients who need to avoid or postpone, for a moment, the "glare of reality" (Hutchings 1998). When patients use metaphors, they often do so to explain what an illness experience is like. In lack of a language of illness (Woolf 1926), figurative speech makes the inexplicable expressible (Conway 2013).

Metaphors are prevalent in the language of health care professionals. When doctors use metaphors in conversation with patients, metaphors help explain complicated, abstract issues (Casarett et al. 2010). However, metaphors as epistemological or pedagogical tools can be somewhat arbitrary because they are subject to a doctor's personal tastes and whims (Trogen 2017). For this reason, researchers have subjected metaphors to evidence-based methods so that the effectiveness of a metaphor in communicating an intended meaning can be better determined (Kendall-Taylor and Haydon 2016). Others have suggested that—given the side-effects of metaphors—we should refrain from using them (Sontag 1978) or increase "metaphoric literacy" (Holmes 2011: 272). These approaches reflect valid concerns and fit with evidence-based medicine and its preference for quantitative study designs, which psycholinguists, cognitive scientists and neurobiologists can offer. From the perspective of literary criticism, such approaches are seen more critically. Marjorie Garber (2011: 235) argues, for example, that the use of metaphors for distinct, predefined purposes is a form of instrumentalisation that problematically seeks to "read *through* metaphor." Such pursuits kill the magic of metaphor by taming its strangeness, incongruity and absurdity.

In an era in which evidence-based logics and quantitative methodologies prevail yet have been found insufficient, more holistic and interdisciplinary approaches to health and healing have pointed to other rationales and methodologies to understand and respond to the paradoxes and ambiguities of health and illness. Literature and art, so one of the arguments goes, can offer a different way of seeing illness and understanding its experience. Similarly, figurative language, such as metaphor, invites us to see something in a different way, to consider the literal and material object as well as a potential meaning beyond what is immediately there. In what follows, I ask what it would imply if we understood metaphors not only as handy tools but also as small works of art. In *The Transfiguration of the Commonplace* (1981), the philosopher and art critic Arthur C. Danto suggests that metaphors and artworks share a similar structure:[1] They invite us to see a common object, such as a consumer product, as something else (e.g., Andy Warhol's *Brillo Box* or Marcel Duchamp's 'ready-mades'). Artworks and metaphors transfigure a common object that we thought we knew and, in doing so, they change our ways of seeing it. Art and metaphor suggest a meaning beyond the literal and, therefore, they can (and need to) be interpreted. In fact, it is the act of interpretation, "the complexity of responsive understanding," that constitutes a work of art (Danto 1981: 175; Bahlmann 2015: 42–43).

To see metaphor as art—a meta-metaphor so to speak—may add important nuances to the use and understanding of metaphors in medicine. What follows is a thought experiment[2] that is founded, like all metaphors, on a mistake: a metaphor is *not* an artwork, just as much as a warrior who is compared to a lion is *not* a lion (Bode 2017: 146). But there is something about the notion of metaphor as artwork that illuminates what metaphors can also be, and it is this process, this mapping of features from artwork (source) to metaphor (target), that I am interested in. To explore this connection, I will draw on art philosophy, phenomenology and literary criticism, particularly the work of Arthur C. Danto, John Dewey, Siri Hustvedt, Mark Doty and Walker Percy, who have explored concepts of relationality and aesthetic experience to describe the imaginative space in which art and metaphor happen. In comparing metaphor to art, I will try to identify some of the properties of art that might be productively transferred to metaphors and, by illustrating these features with specific examples, I hope to show how this thought experiment might illuminate properties of metaphors that are potentially useful in medical/health humanities.

Metaphors are paradoxical because they are both true and false. The American novelist and essayist Walker Percy, a graduate from Columbia University College of Physicians and Surgeons, argues that metaphors are "mistakes: misnamings, misunderstandings, or misrememberings" (1958: 80). Despite their inherent falseness, metaphors may light up something that feels true. Metaphors can startle and astonish us and entail an "authentic poetic experience"— what [Richard Palmer] Blackmur calls 'that heightened, that excited sense of being'" (ibid.). Metaphors thus stimulate the imagination; they surprise, make strange and open up new ways of perceiving. In *Art as Experience* (1934: 55), John Dewey argues that the encounter with a work of art implies that we "undergo an experience," which he defines as a form of surrender and "yielding of the self." The beholder is not asked to identify, to attach "a proper tag or label" (ibid.), but to perceive: he sees something "for the sake of seeing what is there" (ibid.: 54), and this "act of perception proceeds by waves that extend serially throughout the entire organism . . . The perceived object or scene is emotionally pervaded throughout" (ibid.: 55). Dewey emphasises that perceiving is not a passive act. Instead, "to perceive, a beholder must *create* his own experience" (ibid.: 56). One might say that in encountering a work of art, something starts to resonate within us, but this is not a passive form of waiting until (or if at all) something will happen. Instead, "There is work done on the part of the percipient as there is on the part of the artist" (ibid.: 56). Similar to how Percy and Blackmur understand an encounter with a metaphor, an encounter with art in Dewey's sense relies on aesthetic perception as much as it depends on creation and recreation. According to Dewey, "Perception is an act of the going-out of energy in order to receive . . . We must summon energy and pitch it at a responsive key in order to *take* in" (ibid.: 55). Similarly, in Danto's concept, simply perceiving an object as a work of art is not enough: Rather, as Katharina Bahlmann (2015: 43) suggests, it is a decision or attitude to see something as a work of art, to interpret and read it as art. As a consequence, interpretation—and thus the collaborative, dialogic interaction that artworks invite—is fundamental to their structure. To illustrate how these properties of artworks might be transferred to metaphors, I will examine a number of metaphors used by poets, doctors and patients.

In Norman Dubie's (1986) poem 'The Funeral,' the lyrical 'I' remembers his childhood and his youngest aunt. In the last stanza, the aunt's burial is described, and we learn about her illness by means of a striking simile:[3] "The cancer ate her like horse piss eats deep snow." When I read the comparison for the first time, it triggered a number of sensory impressions from my childhood: I could hear the sound that melting snow makes once a warm fluid meets the icy surface, and I could see the steam that forms in the crystal-clear air. Even today, I can imagine the hole in the snow's otherwise perfect and pure whiteness, and the yellow edges that have ripped open the even surface. And I remember the moment of surprise, when horses urinate; the sudden gush of fluid and the inevitability of the process. Letting myself get carried away with this simile implies a double temporality: The experience happens here and now when I surrender, as Dewey calls it, to the simile and its sensuous evocations. But it is also an image that has a haunting quality, one that I experienced before and that "resonates years after reading it" (Addonizio and Laux 1997: 95).

A more analytic approach to Dubie's simile adds further nuances to the aesthetic experience that metaphors trigger. We can identify the source domains (urine and snow) and the target domains (cancer and aunt). In the process of understanding the metaphor, we map the properties of the source domain onto the respective target: cancer is compared to the horse's urine, and the aunt is likened to the snow. Establishing a link between cancer and urine is a novel and fresh way of seeing cancer, whereas the comparison of a young woman to the purity of snow feels more familiar (think of Snow White). The association with urine gives cancer and the way it ravages the snow-like young woman an air of mundanity and triviality. There is also a beastly and animalistic quality because the urine in Dubie's metaphor comes from an animal. Cancer-as-urine appears as dirty, ignominious, disgraceful. Moreover, urine implies consumption and waste, which is echoed in "the offal's pail" that the lyric 'I' and his aunt carried to the fox, when she was still well. The urine soils what used to be pure; it destroys in a rush and thus seems inevitable and inescapable.

This more analytic reading, as I want to argue in line with Siri Hustvedt (2010), does not replace my initial response; nor does the subjective reaction invalidate the latter reading. Instead, the analytic reading adds to the earlier, more impulsive reading. Similarly, Hustvedt (ibid.: 36) describes a notion of accruing insight and understanding to the interpretative process. In her essay 'Embodied Vision,' Hustvedt discusses the role of subjective, embodied responses and the role of imagination and relationality when she renders her first reaction to a painting by Francisco de Zurbarán, *Still Life With Lemons, Oranges, and a Rose* (1633):

> I cannot track the initial unconscious milliseconds of my response to the picture, but I knew the image hit me instantly and bodily . . . [an] observer would have pronounced me to be in a state of heightened emotion and attention.
>
> *(ibid.: 33)*

In her essay, Hustvedt tries to understand "the visual experience" of that moment and comes to realise that when she looked at the painting, "an imaginary elsewhere . . . has opened up," a sudden recognition that is paired with a more reflexive consciousness (ibid.: 31), which Hustvedt ascribes to "*the way* they [the objects] are painted" (ibid.: 35; original emphasis). She describes how she falls into a kind of reverie . . . an active, ongoing, shifting, physical, mental response to what I was seeing, one that included emotion—but which one? A form of awe . . . a strong lifting sensation inside me, as I am rising up and out of myself . . . a form of *transference* of my memories and my lived past onto the painting.

(ibid.: 35–36; original emphasis)

According to Hustvedt, looking at a work of art is an intersubjective dialogue and a leap from the given, factual and real into a world of imaginative play, where we can pretend to be someone else or detach the original meaning of a thing and replace it with something else (ibid.: 37). This capacity is one that children develop early in their lives: When children play, Hustvedt argues, they pretend that a stick is a horse, and this transference is similar to the space where art happens, "the fictional space of human life, the world of play and its transformations" (ibid.: 37–38). Similarly, as I want to suggest in line with Danto, metaphors are a playground of the imagination where the transfer or mapping of features results in imaginative mistakes and playful pretence that can entail new ways of seeing. Moreover, such playful, imaginative interaction can trigger a shock or a moment of surprise; it can cause a defamiliarisation of something we thought we knew well.

In medical education, it is often the reverse movement—namely the familiarising quality of metaphor—that is used for pedagogical or mnemonic purposes. Typically, as Alan Bleakley (2017) argues in *Thinking with Metaphors in Medicine*, metaphors serve as tools for explanation, quick identification and labelling. In this sense, they are not meant to invite sustained perception and the recreation of an aesthetic experience. Can metaphors in medicine still be a space where art or aesthetic experience happens? Bleakley (ibid.: 93) seems sceptical of this notion when he describes how pedagogical metaphors are instrumentalised for rote learning in order to speed up memorisation, help students to quickly identify patterns or symptoms and reduce uncertainty. While culinary metaphors in medicine abound, as Bleakley observes, they are used as mnemonic metaphors and are stripped of any prolonged aesthetic perception, even though culinary metaphors link 'hard facts' to embodied experiences of taste and smell. To illustrate his point, Bleakley refers to a blog by a study group, in which a student offers a description of her learning experience that is guided by metaphors. She gives an extensive list of metaphors (or "food analogies," as she calls them), such as coffee bean sign, strawberry cervix, oat cell carcinoma or café au lait spots.[4] Interestingly, the student starts her blog by elaborating on one particular metaphor, the Oreo cookie sign:

Who likes oreo [sic] cookies? I came to know about the Oreo Cookie sign today! It's seen on a chest x ray (lateral view) when there is a pericardial effusion! The anterior most layer (the chocolate part!) is the epicardial fat. The mid layer (the cream part . . . yumm!) Is the fluid. And the posterior layer (again, the chocolate part) is the pericardial fat!

(ibid.: 88)

In this description of how the Oreo cookie metaphor works as a means to diagnose pericardial effusion, I see a pleasure of (re)creating an imaginative space that the comparison has opened up for the student. The text suggests the student's sensory delight and pleasure in thinking with the metaphor. As readers, we become witness to the student's joy in exploring an absurd and surprising comparison, which is a new way of seeing pericardial effusion. The Oreo cookie metaphor has activated the student's perception, and she is intrigued both as a future medical professional interested in facts and knowledge and as an embodied individual who is imaginatively tasting the Oreo ("yumm!") and sharing her culinary preferences. The number of exclamation marks (five in six sentences) suggests a vividness and excitement, which might be an echo of the first encounter with the metaphor, which the student may have had earlier the same day and which is still accessible when she writes down her thoughts. The initial question "Who likes Oreo cookies?" appears to me as a reaching out to fellow students; it is a desire to share this moment of pleasure with others and an invitation to enter the imaginative space of the metaphor with her. Reading the student's interpretation of the Oreo cookie metaphor, we are invited to access with her this imaginative space of the culinary metaphor, this moment of pretence, in which a very real, literal symptom is, for a while, something entirely different. In this sense, metaphors in medicine—similar to artworks—are about creation, recreation, experience and perception; they suggest a particular way of seeing the world, and they are an invitation to explore.

Dubie's cancer metaphor and the student's cookie comparison are invitations to explore an object or experience with imagination and creativity. Physicians use similar techniques when they invent new metaphors to explain unfamiliar terms, difficult diagnoses and diseases to their patients. A study by David Casarett et al. (2010) examines the communication of doctors with their patients and found that doctors are quite resourceful in suggesting metaphors and analogies to their patients. Following the poet Mark Doty (2010: 79–80), creating a new metaphor is a continuing inquiry "into experience in search of meaning" and, since a new metaphor suggests "an individual way of seeing," it is also a form of self-portraiture.

Patients, too, invent new and striking comparisons to convey the idiosyncratic experience of their condition. In his autobiography *Jolly Lad*, recovering alcoholic John Doran (2015: 176),[5] for example, explores a metaphor that expresses to him what happens when an alcoholic decides to stop drinking:

> Picture a reservoir surrounded by mountains. You have been tasked with draining the massive body of water away to repopulate the area. But once the water has gone you are faced with the former town that was initially flooded and the now wrecked buildings which need to be pulled down. Call several construction firms. People have been fly tipping here for years. There is tons of rubbish here. You will need help to clean the area up. There are corpses wrapped in carpet and chains. It was the ideal place to dump bodies. You'll need to call the police and the coroner's office. The press are on their way. There are rotten and half eaten animal carcasses that need to be cleared up and disposed of. Environmental health needs to be involved. You have never seen so many mangled shopping trollies, broken children's bikes and unwanted cars. The clearance job will be massive. There are burst canisters of toxic waste that have long since leached into the ground. It will be years before you can do anything with this land. The water was merely the stuff that was making this area look picturesque. What you have left in its place is an area of outstanding natural horror. It probably feels like you should have left well enough alone.

Doran offers here an imaginative exploration of what might be considered a detailed painting of a wasteland or horrific crime scene. Doran invites us to enter this image with him; he gives orders via imperatives and addresses an imaginary reader, "you," to participate in the description that is focalised through the narrator. He unfolds, before the eyes of his readers, a visual scenario that has narrative qualities. The narrator's gesture of reaching out to his readers and inviting them to envision the wasteland with him is similar to what the writer and literary critic Anatole Broyard (1992) hopes his doctor will do: In *Intoxicated by My Illness*, Broyard imagines a doctor who offers metaphors to his patients that are imaginative, daring and original. Broyard hopes that his doctor will enter his patient's condition and look "around at it from the inside," as if it were a house (ibid.: 42–43). Similar to Doran's wasteland, Broyard uses a specific space as a source domain, which allows him to roam about and explore different areas. In Broyard's illness-as-house metaphor, the doctor is a "kind landlord," the patient is the tenant, and together, they try to find out how they can make the premises more "liveable" (ibid.: 43).

Doran's elaborate metaphor, which one might also label an allegory, "a systematised metaphor" with a series of similarities (Bode 2017: 149), strikes me as a particularly detailed description. It seems as if Doran's narrator is describing a film scene or a painting that he has in his mind. In the act of meticulously describing what he sees or imagines, he unfolds this particular landscape, its objects and inhabitants before his own and his readers' eyes. Similar to an ekphrastic exercise, one might say, Doran's elaborate passage translates a painting into words and, in doing so, he brings his character's singular experience "vividly before our eyes" (Karastathi 2015: 96). In the ancient world, ekphrasis was a rhetorical exercise for students to train their rhetorical skills (ibid.: 93). When ekphrastic passages appear in a narrative, as Sylvia Karastathi (ibid.: 95, 109) explains, they produce a "freeze-time effect," because they refocus our attention and decelerate the reading process. In doing so, the elaborate description of a mental image makes space for a moment of heightened perception, in which the sequence of events, the question "what happens next?", is momentarily suspended. This potential for deceleration and refocus of attention towards the present moment is an intriguing effect that also seems to apply to Doran's careful description of the wasteland or the student's delight in the Oreo cookie metaphor. With this shift of focus, the use of metaphors can be likened to miniature art works: When metaphors suggest a new way of seeing a common, familiar thing, they invite us to suspend for a moment what we know and to welcome the playful pretence and the patent mistake. In this sense, metaphors can be refreshing and may (re)connect us to our sensory perceptions and singular experiences.

Metaphors, like artworks, are, without a doubt, far from being innocent pleasures. Works of art can (and are supposed to) be troubling, controversial and charged. And yet, there are good reasons why art and literature are increasingly used in medical/health humanities to counter what researchers in the field of health care have identified as reductionism and estrangement, burnout and lack of empathy. Neither art nor metaphor are solutions to these problems per se, but they offer, as I have tried to show, a mode to reinvigorate language and perception, shift one's perspective and use imagination. Contrary to much of the existing research on metaphors in medicine, metaphors are not static or frozen. They are alive and entail a creative, collaborative and dialogic exchange. In this sense, when we hear or read a metaphor, "we are not only witness to the results of another person's intentional play in his or her fictive space, we are free to play ourselves, to muse and dream and question and theorize," Hustvedt (2010: 38) argues in relation to works of art. Moreover, we come to understand something about ourselves when we engage with the vision of another. Hustvedt suggests that an artwork (or metaphor, as I would add)

> reflects the vision of the other, the artist, that we have made our own because it answers something within us that we understand is true. This truth may be only a feeling, only a humming resonance we cannot put into words, or it may become a vast discursive statement, but it must be there for the enchantment to happen—that excursion into you that is also I.
>
> *(ibid.)*

Looking at artworks has become a pedagogical intervention in medical education. Medical student Eliza Miller (2010: 17), for example, compares caring for pictures with caring for patients. Of course, as she points out, "a patient is not a painting," yet looking at art involves "'slow looking' and creative discussion," which Miller finds reinvigorating and important for her work. However, as with many interventions from medical/health humanities to clinical practice, the question is how such elements "could be brought to the wards" (ibid.: 17). Making space and finding time for deceleration, for the freeze-time that imagination and play entails, is certainly a challenge, and it can lead astray. And yet, there may be more to be found in the process than to be lost. Ultimately, and contrary to a museum visit, an approach to metaphors as artworks can easily be integrated into everyday routines. It might be worth a try to follow, for a moment, a metaphor's invitation to imagine, to pretend, to play and roam in the figurative domain, and to be mindful of what is suggested and how our sensory system and imaginative mind respond.

Notes

1 I am grateful to Dr Katharina Bahlmann, who introduced Danto's work to me. Her ideas and suggestions have been a great inspiration for this essay.
2 In my research project on metaphors, this idea is still at an early stage. Therefore, some of the suggestions here are still undeveloped and will be elaborated more fully elsewhere.
3 Similes, like metaphors, are based on comparisons and thus on seeing-something-as-something-else. Contrary to metaphors, similes make the comparative gesture transparent through 'like' or 'as.'
4 Source: www.medicowesome.com/2015/02/study-group-discussion-food-analogies.html, accessed February 18, 2018.
5 I am very grateful to my colleague Dr Emily J. Hogg, who shared this metaphor with me.

Acknowledgements

This paper was conceived as part of the research programme 'The Uses of Literature' at the University of Southern Denmark (SDU), funded by the Danish National Research Foundation (grant no. DNRF127), and as part of the research project 'Body and Metaphor: Narrative-Based Metaphor Analysis in Medical Humanities' at Johannes Gutenberg University Mainz, funded by the German Research Foundation (grant no. WO 2139/2–1).

References

Addonizio K, Laux D. 1997. *The poet's companion: A guide to the pleasures of writing poetry.* London: Norton.
Bahlmann K. 2015. *Arthur C. Danto und das Phantasma vom 'Ende der Kunst.'* Paderborn: Wilhelm Fink.
Bleakley A. 2017. *Thinking with metaphors in medicine: The state of the art.* London: Routledge.
Bode C. 2017. Tropes. In: M Rosendahl Thomsen, L Horne Kjældgaard, L Møller, et al (eds.) *Literature: An Introduction to Theory and Analysis.* London: Bloomsbury.
Broyard A. 1992. *Intoxicated by my illness and other writings on life and death.* New York, NY: Fawcett Columbine.
Casarett D, Pickard A, Fishman J, et al. Can metaphors and analogies improve communication with seriously ill patients? *Journal of Palliative Medicine.* 2010; 13: 255–260.
Conway K. 2013. *Beyond words: Illness and the limits of expression.* Albuquerque, NM: University of New Mexico Press.
Danto A. 1981. *The transfiguration of the commonplace: A philosophy of art.* Cambridge, MA: Harvard University Press.
Dewey J. 1934, 2005. *Art as experience.* New York, NY: Penguin.
Doran J. 2015. *Jolly lad.* London: Strange Attractor.
Doty M. 2010. *The art of description: World into word.* Minneapolis, MN: Graywolf.
Dubie N. 1986. The funeral. In: *The springhouse.* New York, NY: Norton.
Garber M. 2011. *The use and abuse of literature.* New York, NY: Anchor Books.
Holmes M. After Sontag: Reclaiming metaphor. In: M. Hanne (ed.) *Binocular vision: Narrative and metaphor in medicine.* Special issue of *Genre.* 2011; 44: 239–261.

Hustvedt S. Embodied visions: What does it mean to look at a work of art? *The Yale Review*. 2010; 98: 22–38.

Hutchings D. Communicating with metaphor: A dance with many veils. *The American Journal of Hospice and Palliative Care*. 1998; September/October: 282–284.

Karastathi S. 2015. Ekphrasis and the novel/narrative fiction. In: G. Rippl (ed.) *Handbook of intermediality: Literature—Image—Sound—Music*. Berlin: De Gruyter, 92–112.

Kendall-Taylor N, Haydon A. Using metaphor to translate the science of resilience and developmental outcomes. *Public Understanding of Science*. 2016; 25: 576–587.

Kirmayer L. Healing and the invention of metaphor: The effectiveness of symbols revisited. *Culture, Medicine, and Psychiatry*. 1993; 17: 161–195.

Miller E. Caring for pictures, caring for patients: Medical students at the Frick. *The Frick Collection: Members' Magazine*. Fall 2010: 16–17.

Ogden T. Reverie and metaphor: Some thoughts on how I work as a psychoanalyst. *International Journal of Psychoanalysis*. 1997; 78: 719–732.

Percy W. Metaphor as mistake. *The Sewanee Review*. 1958; 66: 79–99.

Sontag S. 1978, 2002. *Illness as metaphor and AIDS and its metaphors*. London: Penguin.

Trogen B. The evidence-based metaphor. *JAMA*. 2017; 317: 1411–1412.

Verghese A. Hope and clarity. *New York Times Magazine*, 2004; February 22.

Woolf V. 1926, 2012. *On being ill*. Ashfield, MA: Paris Press.

13

THE PRACTICE OF METAPHOR

Shane Neilson

The doctors I admire

The doctors I admire most have not been titans of knowledge, preternaturally dextrous surgical wizards, or empathic wells into which a patient's pain can be poured to the cleansing, cathartic benefit of all. Nor have my favourites been tireless and error-free machines that provide consummate, efficacious care from sunup to sundown. Have these offered perfect models of health using their own vigorous, fit, and radiant selves as proof? No. The doctors I admire are, instead, creative practitioners able to communicate with patients using metaphor. Such doctors routinely encounter a problem or a means of seeing a problem that a patient cannot comprehend, reach into an improvisational bag of metaphor, and, in the midst of a moment of clinical difficulty with patient and doctor at an impasse, rhetorically construct a bridge to understanding. These doctors appreciate the power inherent to metaphor, a power that effects the sudden revelation of a previously unknown truth, that allows a thing to be seen both for what it is and is not. This chimera can, in my witnessed experience, make all the difference. Being able to think metaphorically, however, takes a good deal of practice.

Paraphrasing Kathryn Montgomery, Alan Bleakley (2017: 3) describes medicine as "*phronesis*—theory put to practical use in activity, or, better, as performance . . . and—most importantly—in working with patients to develop meanings for their illnesses, largely through appropriate metaphorical framing." With the ubiquity and use of metaphor in medical practice established by Bleakley in his foundational *Thinking With Metaphors in Medicine: The State of the Art*, this chapter is intended to demonstrate the utility of a specific framework for metaphor use in medical practice that originates not from speciality clinic—the usual purview of analysis in the small subfield of medical metaphor studies—but from the family practice milieu. This difference is important, for the majority of physicians currently practising in the Western world are generalists, and general practice has a distinct philosophy. As Bleakley (ibid.) maintains when it comes to the study of metaphor in medicine, "context matters." It is important that, in the medical humanities, the research conducted by humanists not reproduce the errors of biomedical research and largely ignore general practice altogether.

After demonstrating a resonant historical metaphoric intervention by Galen with one of his own patients, I explain what 'metaphoric intervention' is using examples from my own training, illness experience, and practice career. The purpose of presenting this assemblage or narrative record is threefold: first, to suggest what clinical conditions are required for metaphoric intervention by a family doctor in a family practice clinic; second, to offer a praxis that has, in my experience, been valuable in allowing patients to perceive both benefits and harms with a given proposition; and third, to describe an enactment of metaphoric intervention in the discipline of medicine itself, a purpose that requires a small preface. In *Words With Power*, Northrop Frye (2007: 22) defined the "descriptive mode" of language—one of five levels of language, the others being conceptual, rhetorical, imaginative, and kerygmatic—as "the one in which we are reading to get information about something in the world outside the book . . . [w]ords or signifiers are, in theory, being subordinated to what they signify, servomechanisms to the information they convey." Frye shrewdly points out that scientific discourse with its "servo-mechanistic" level of language tries to exchange rhetoric for description as much as possible, and yet the descriptive mode of prose is the easiest to bend to the purpose of disseminating lies via its obscuring of the ideology behind description. Thus my third objective can be re-stated as suggesting that clinical medicine is as much a relational and scientific practice as it is a creative one, and it is this creativity function that requires emphasis in contemporary pedagogy. This chapter can be taken to offer 'proof' to minds in thrall to the evidence-based regime, but a proof that can never be expressed as statistics and only as itself, according to a metaphorical process.

The why of metaphoric intervention

There are many ways to communicate with patients, and many relational styles. Doctors might prefer a professional tone that does not reach deeply into the language's richer resources of expression; they might speak more colloquially, preferring a friendly approach that does dig into idiom, metonymy, and metaphor. Whatever the style, metaphor-based interventions can be undertaken on a contingent basis to move an encounter forward, if only to reveal the stakes of a particular choice.

To define my terms: two key building blocks for my concept of metaphor are (a) the common understanding of metaphor in which a comparison is made between two things and (b) the Greek etymological basis of the word that involves the prefix *meta*, meaning 'after, with, across,' and *pherein*, meaning 'to carry.' The composite of these creates a literal 'carrying across.' Two more building blocks come from Jeffery Donaldson's (2015: 8) Frygian-inflected definition of metaphor in *Missing Link: The Evolution of Metaphor and the Metaphor of Evolution*: (i) "the active relation of elements in space"; and (ii) metaphor as both "an *is* and an *is not*." As can be determined from my definition, which cunningly places components in relation with one another, I consider metaphor to be a relational process that brings into view likeness and unlikeness. Likeness is the more easily apparent part of the relational process, but unlikeness is, as yet, an untapped field in medical metaphor studies and I will show the important role it has to play in clinical care a little later in this paper when discussing Jane, a recent patient of mine, and Mrs X, a patient from my training.

Using metaphor when communicating to patients can be placed under the baggy monster of 'Narrative Medicine,' defined by Rita Charon (2006: 4) as "medicine practised with [the] narrative skills of recognizing, absorbing, interpreting, and being moved by the stories of illness,"[1] but in truth both the use of medical metaphor and the broader medical project Charon defines are ancient. For example, *The Hippocratic Corpus* contains some case histories, especially *Of the Epidemics*, which employ judicious metaphoric language to great effect. Therein, a Silenus is described as having "heaviness of the head" and "muddy urine" (*Internet Classics Archive*: np), suggesting powers of observation that seem more acute than if the symptoms and signs were related in purely descriptive language. Yet that group of physicians tended not to write in the first person, resulting in a less self-conscious relational style that is required to illustrate occasions of metaphoric intervention. As Nissen and Wynn (2014: 4) write in 'The History of the Case Report,' Galen was among the first to employ a "more conversational tone" in which he "places himself in the text in the first person, being an active agent in the case description." Although Galen was not the kind of doctor to engage in what I will term 'decentred sharing' later in this paper, for his ego is usually front and centre in his writings, I nevertheless transcribe a metaphorical intervention he conducted on a friend who struck two of his slaves with a scabbarded sword, injuring them severely. Full of remorse for having acted in anger, the friend approached Galen, and

> handed over his whip, stripped off his clothes, and bade me to flog him for what he had done while in the violent grip of his cursed anger—for that is what he called it. When I laughed (and this was a reasonable reaction), he fell on his knees and begged me to do what he asked. It was very clear that the more he kept importuning me and asking to be flogged, the more he was making me laugh. When we had wasted enough time in begging and laughing, I promised him that I would flog him if he would himself grant me the one very small thing which I was going to ask. When he did promise, I urged him to pay attention to me while I had a few words to say to him, since this was my request. When he had promised that he would do so, I spoke to him at some length and admonished him that it was necessary to train the irascible element within us. This is the way, obviously, that I flogged him and not in the way he asked.
>
> *(Harkins 1963: 40–1)*

Galen's metaphoric intervention is to surprise with performative truth, putting the link between violence to others and spiritual violence to the self within spatial relation. Also placed in relation here is the literal relationship between friends and the witty reclaiming of the 'flogging' metaphor from violence to, instead, that of spiritual instruction. It is perhaps significant that the anecdote appears within an English translation of *On the Passions and Errors of the Soul*, a volume designed to instruct a reader in the proper manner to lead a good life and achieve wisdom so as to not succumb to disease that results from both bodily disorders and disorders of the soul.

As you might intuit from Galen's example, an adequate metaphoric praxis is not the application of easy, so-called 'dead metaphors' that merely apply human predicaments to material, inanimate referents. Though Galen does deploy the basic maxim 'know thyself' as an overarching imperative to avoid disease, one could think of this maxim as his single identification of governing cultural meta-metaphor; he then goes to great lengths to unpack that meta-metaphor in his text, rendering it instead as a process rather than as a thing. He provides many instructive, relational examples of just how to achieve its end result.

An obvious dead metaphor of the modern era is the 'heart as pump.' In the twentieth century, a million cardiologists and cardiac surgeons have explained to hundreds of millions of patients what congestive heart failure is, or valvular disease is, in mechanical terms. Such metaphors are part of a medical script that is contained, expected, and which has no creative power, for there is no longer new material being transformed into something else and back, nor are there minds previously unaware of the coming transformation, nor is there a practitioner aware of the necessity of a new transformation to occur. Worse still, the script destroys the possibility for alternative formulations.

Before new metaphors come in clinical situations, there is just the difficulty, the situation waiting for the carrying across. As will be demonstrated in my narrative record of metaphoric interventions, parts of the powers inherent to my practice of metaphoric intervention are the personal stakes involved—before the instance in which the metaphoric intervention is necessitated, there is the doctor and the patient as separate category, as juxtaposed 'source' and 'target.' When the metaphoric intervention suddenly is required, and that requirement is subsequently perceived by the practitioner, then what was once a dyadic encounter becomes increasingly intersubjective in both the aforementioned 'like and unlike' senses, destabilising the pathophysiological focus of medical diagnostics/therapeutics on the one hand and also potentially exorcising the stuckness of dysfunction on the other. Metaphor can become both spur and bond, both tool of identification and juxtaposition of difference. For the clinicians reading this, the following metaphor interventions can act, as they did in a paediatric pain study Bleakley (2017: 2) comments upon, as "an heuristic, perhaps even as a comfort blanket." The fact does not entail diminishment, for as Donaldson (2015: 328) knows, all "[m]etaphor is heuristic in principle."

The how of metaphoric intervention

I begin this section by relating constructive examples of metaphoric interventions from my own training period and from my illness experience to highlight the relationship between practice, experience, and metaphor that demonstrates the utility of metaphor in everyday doctoring. I start with the frame of *decentred sharing*, a helpful theoretical model that is itself metaphorical; I move to a metaphorical intervention involving *family* by a skilled clinician that I witnessed as a medical student; and I present a metaphoric intervention involving *choice* that made me reckon with a previously unacknowledged truth. From here I provide a further two examples from my professional practice that loosely adhere to the model of 'decentred sharing.'

Decentred sharing

A metaphor that constitutively informs my overall practice is *decentred sharing*. I picked this up from a psychologist attached to the Family Practice Unit at Memorial University of Newfoundland. Back then (and probably still), first-year family medicine residents were expected to attend a series of half-day sessions devoted to improving interviewing skills. During one of those sessions, the psychologist explained how she occasionally shared information and experience from her own life with patients, but only according to the ethic of what she casually called 'decentred sharing.' Although the session was almost over, I delayed the group's departure by asking "Just exactly what does 'decentred sharing' *mean*?" Having, I expect, found us rather uncommunicative as a group to that point in the morning, the psychologist seemed delighted at the question. She explained:

> I share data and affect from my own life only if such sharing passes a test I apply in my mind. I ask myself, "Is sharing X meant to help the person who is dealing with X, or am I sharing it because I want to burden them with *my* X? Am I seeking relief for myself?" If I share my experience for the benefit of others, then I generally won't be trying to meet my own needs. I won't share to impose my own greater authority on them. I won't share to shame them and show that I chose better despite similar circumstances. I'll be sharing for a constructive, rather than a destructive, purpose. That's decentred sharing.

As she spoke, I began to create a visual metaphor that concretised 'decentred sharing.' I envisioned the word *share* within a circle, but somehow skewed to the left, as close to the circle's margin as possible. Next to the circle I envisioned another circle without a word inside, an empty circle.

Having reached the age of forty-two, I've buried my parents; have three children, two of whom have chronic illnesses; and possess a chronic illness myself. There is a range of life experience here that can be of use for working with patients, but I repeatedly check my motivation for metaphor by recalling the overarching metaphor of 'decentred sharing.' I deliberately ask myself whether I'm seeking care by revealing personal experience, or if I'm making my metaphors from off-centre. One has to apply the intervention at the right time, and if the objective is to force someone into choosing the path I myself took in any given situation, then the didacticism inherent to such sharing will inevitably be resisted. Instead, my motivation is often to suggest a homology of experience, a recognition of the inherent difficulty of the predicament, and to place next to the patient an alternative, a way of proceeding or enduring that is useful insofar as it exists as an option, not as a judgement or prescription.

The family metaphor

During my clinical training, an internist routinely relied on a metaphor of 'family' when she talked to difficult patients. (By using the word 'difficult' I recognise I am relying upon another metaphor, but any clinician reading this text will understand the shorthand.) The metaphor she used was actually part of a metaphor system in which caregivers could be likened to family, or the fact of her own family could be introduced as a means to identify with patients who were having problems with their family. To be concrete, her metaphor was *Your Family = Me* or *My Family*. One example from my rich exposure to her well-developed metaphor use comes immediately to mind: a delirious old woman who had metastatic small cell lung cancer was dying on the ward. She routinely caused problems for the nurses, intentionally throwing food around the room, refusing to take medication, and cursing at will. After receiving a plea from nursing staff to 'Talk to Mrs X!', a dying patient who was never once visited in the hospital by a next of kin, the internist went to the bedside and started to chat.

"I know who you are!" said the cachectic old lady.

"But I want to know more about you, I don't know you well enough!" said the internist with a slight smile.

"Why do you want to know about me? All you need to know about me is that I'm dying. Soon I'll be dead, dead, dead!"

The internist sat down by the bedside, putting her head level with the old woman's, and waited for more, which certainly came.[2]

"Why can't you make it easier for me to breathe? And the nurses are stupid. Why can't they bring me my pills on time? They're always late, and you know that don't you? Well of course you do. You see them. And you don't do anything about it." The old lady's left hand flew about like a conductor's. Her right arm was splinted from a pathologic fracture.

"It is certainly hard to be here," said the internist. "Many of my family members died in a hospital. Some of them felt like you do."

"Oh, so you *understand* now, do you? You *get me*! You *finally* get me!" Enraged, she shook her balled left fist. (Her anger reflects a great truth about metaphor: at the cusp of realisation, when we are about to or have just deployed our metaphoric interventions, practitioners must reckon with unlikeness. The presence of unlikeness means, thankfully, that the metaphor isn't just rejectable, although that is what might happen. The metaphor is, instead, applicable because of its possible shadow side of likeness, which is yet to come.)

"Oh, I don't know what it's like to die, no, though I have watched a lot of people die. Including my mother and father. And I was very angry and scared. Also sad."

I looked around this ward room. The three other patients, previously terrorised by the dying old lady, were now peeking around their curtains.

"And did you have anything to say to them that made dying all right, doctor?" the old lady asked.

"No. But when I have a patient who reminds me of my parents, it means I've thought of them again. And the old fear I faced so badly, I find, has faded and what's left is what was always there—love."

"So you *love* me, then, is that it! Ha ha ha. *Love*."

"I love enough to listen, maybe. Where is your family?"

As it turned out, the old lady had five days left to live, and of those, she was conscious for four. Each of those days, she repeatedly asked for her 'daughter'—the doctor, though it was never clear if this was done purely in sarcasm, or out of satire, or if the old woman sometimes did feel warmly disposed to the attending doctor. We never could be sure, likeness and unlikeness informing that relationship to the core—including the original source. The old woman had no family, of course, or none willing to visit her after decades-long estrangement.

Yet the intervention largely worked: the nurses were able to do their work without scolding, and the old woman was able to die—however cloying you might find this instance—amongst metaphorical family, all because the attending physician subtly deployed a metaphor of family, juxtaposing her own experience with that of the old lady, confessing that things are not the same and yet, in another sense, they are. This juxtaposition was accomplished with patience but also a technique of rhetorically insisting on the metaphor's likeness and provisionality in every line of speech. With this intervention, the internist changed meaning for the patient by putting one thing in relation to another, effecting "imaginative transformations that occur when non-literal relations are expressed" (Bleakley 2017: 6).

The choice metaphor

During an acute worsening of my own illness, when I was involuntarily admitted to the Nova Scotia Hospital, I spent a few hours staring at the wall in my own room. Eventually summoning the resolve to die, I left my room and stared down the old hospital's long corridor to a large window I was certain I could pitch myself through. A few stories up, the fall would have killed me. I stood in the darkness for about ten minutes until a nurse's aide found me and insisted upon the metaphor of choice. Slight, small, and moustached, that old Bluenoser listened to me ramble about death. I must have seemed unsure. When my speech trailed off into a long ellipse, he said,

> Shane, we can keep you inside, safe from the troubles of outside. But you can always find a way to die. You've always got your own self wherever you are. We keep you in here so that we can help you to choose to live. You could run down the hall and smash through the glass; or you could choose to stay and come play cards with me. Either way, what you choose now will help set your choices going forward. Because you see, if I call someone and we assign a 24-hour watcher, then you'll be stuck in these same choices, the unhealthy ones. And if you run through the glass, then you'll be dead and unable to make any more choices. But if you decide to make the healthy choice and do the work to settle and be a bit social, then I bet your next set of healthy choices won't be as hard, or as strange to you.

I looked down the hallway, wondering if running down it was something chosen. At that moment, I was operating according to a morbid destiny framework, feeling vaguely compelled to act. I did not think then that I had a choice; I knew only metaphors involving 'death as relief and silence.' But now a metaphor of choice challenged the hegemony of certain self-inflicted doom and hypothetical solace. By suggesting that I could choose and embedding my possible choice in a broad chronology that took me out of present distress, the nurse's aide showed me a different path to take—a dramatic and concrete example of Bleakley's (ibid.) observation that "medical metaphors . . . provid[e] a framework for theorizing and shaping practice interventions in clinical settings."

Personification

A common problem my patients face when accepting their illnesses and coming to terms with them is determining what their illnesses means for them, or what Bleakley (ibid.) calls "identity constructions" that are in particular guided by cultural meta-metaphors of 'medicine as war' and 'the body as a machine.' Denial is partially instigated by stigma, and what a disease might mean for individuals is influenced by prevailing cultural norms. The stigma internalised by so many of my patients with mental health concerns tends to be expressed along lines pre-set by the aforementioned metaphors. Take Jane, who resists a diagnosis of major depressive disorder and panic disorder because, for her (and many others like her), they constitute a form of weakness. I, too, once thought this way about myself, and thus I make my way through this encounter with an awareness of what that same self-assessment felt like, what it meant:

> "I've always tried to take care of things on my own and I've never asked for help before," she said in my office, her eyes downcast, snow spattering her coat. "But this is just too hard and I can't get through the day without crying. I'm a weak person. I'm falling apart."

The 'weak' and 'falling apart' ventures are body-as-machine metaphors, in which the selfhood of the suffering individual is instead conceptualised as an automaton that is breaking down or already broken and which can no longer do work. According to the meta-metaphor's entailment, if a machine cannot do work, it is useless.

I mention the possibility of treatment.

"I don't want a crutch!" she exclaims.

This statement is also a legacy of the 'body as a machine' meta-metaphor—Jane is refusing repair for her broken-down body.

"If I can't do my work, then I can't pass at school and then I can't graduate. I won't be able to have a life and do what everyone else seems able to do."

Following Jane's rendition of catastrophisation, I ready the metaphoric intervention of *personification*. I try to separate out selfhood and value judgement of the self from illness, not by insisting on the fundamentally metaphoric explanation of 'chemical imbalance in the brain' that many of my colleagues use, which is (at best) neutral in its implications, but rather by isolating dysfunction as authored by illness from Jane's larger, richer life. When Jane mentions that she is suffering panic attacks several times a day, but is also avoiding making any meaningful inroads to doing work because it "makes me anxious," I make my move, using a sublimated rhetoric of decentred sharing as represented in the following 'we' pronoun use.

At this point, I pretend I am looking at the person known as Anxiety. Whenever I mention 'it' or its name, 'anxiety,' I look away from Jane and towards 'it'—inaugurating what Bleakley (ibid.) insists is an important valence of metaphor in medicine, that of "performance" in which "non-verbal as well as verbal metaphors such as gesture, proximity, expression and habitual style" are considered. I continue,

> I tend to think of anxiety as a person. That person, Anxiety, wants to control us. For example, when you think of school, you quickly become overcome with anxiety. You try to force thoughts of school from your mind in a process called avoidance, but the more you do this—the more you avoid school—the stronger anxiety gets. Soon it returns with the force of panic attacks. Anxiety makes you think about what *it* wants. The more you try to avoid it, the more you have to pointedly ignore what is clearly happening: Anxiety has turned you against yourself. It has left you with no option. You can't work because it makes you anxious; but you're not working, which is making you anxious.

I then switch and refer to Anxiety as an "elephant in the room" that is being avoided through a tragicomically ineffective routine.

> Anxiety is pretty strong now, as strong and as big as an elephant. It's in this room. And what is its message? Probably for us to do our work, to live up to our responsibilities, which is also the cause of the anxiety in some way, in that if we don't do our work, there will be consequences we would rather not face. But to defer dealing with this message, a message we're calling Anxiety, we have to not look at it even more.

I now slowly push myself against my examining room wall, moving back in my chair and extending my body away from the patient, miming that the elephant is getting bigger—the metaphor now performative. My pronoun use switches to the personal:

> I've tried to forget about what I need to do, but forgetting works only serves to make the elephant bigger and stronger. Now I have to ignore Anxiety even more, despite the accumulating evidence of the necessity of dealing with it, in order to make Anxiety go away. So I do.

I am now pressed against the wall, with my head turned to the side, miming being squished by an invisible elephant. I return to personification:

> This is what Anxiety wants—it wants you to feel it, it wants to control you, it wants you to avoid doing things so that it can get more powerful. Anxiety wants you to think of yourself as weak because then you are agreeing that you can be controlled. It wants you to reject treatment on the premise of weakness. It is afraid that you might get better and it will have to go away.

I've used a script like this at least once a month, and the message seems to get through, possibly because of the inherent unfairness baked into this metaphoric construction of control. Who wants to be controlled in such a sadistic (but actually masochistic) manner? People tend to move past their stuckness when their plight is presented in this way. The script can also be a spur to shifting their construction of illness meaning away from 'body as machine' and stigmatised experience. An elegant feature to this script is its inversion of paradox. Rather than allowing anxiety to be, simultaneously, cause and consequence of suffering as outlined above in a self-justifying and perpetuating system, I separate it from the self through personification. If she follows me that far, Jane can see Anxiety as something that is not her but that also is within her power to recover from. In other words, it *is* and *is not* her—personification separates it from her self, but yet is nevertheless clearly within her subjective experience, albeit removed from its throne. In this way, I've pushed back against the destructive meta-metaphor of 'the body as machine' by precipitating out Jane's self *and* by mobilising a resistance within the entailments governed by the meta-metaphor. Think of the 'body-as-machine' meta-metaphor as a Trojan Horse containing the intervention above in which agency is granted to the suffering person who is newly encouraged to recognise a control dynamic and to assume her own determination or the right to operate the machine. This dual resistance—stepping out and staying within the meta-metaphor—does work prescribed by Anita Wohlmann, who investigates how "the plurisignifying potential of metaphors [can] be activated and conceptualized so that limiting and harmful metaphors become liberating and productive" (in Bleakley ibid.: 20). Put another way, the unlikeness of the metaphor's relationality can be mined from within and productively re-deployed.

Balance and wholes

Because the previous examples have involved a very high affective quality, a less extreme example from this past January is apropos. In that month, I met a patient for the first time who required a particular accommodation in the university setting because of his chronic psychiatric illness (see Appendix to this chapter). With that functional matter quickly dispatched, I began to talk to him a little more about his current state of health. In just a few minutes, we reached an impasse around the subject of medication. His issue was that he had been on many medication trials before, always experienced side effects, and had encountered many stigmatising medical professionals on his journey. And yet it was apparent to me, for several strong reasons, that medication was very much indicated as a protective measure.

"I don't want to go on drugs," he concluded, "because I'm doing a lot of other things now that are good for my health."

Engaging in decentred sharing along the lines of my own mental health experience would be perilous in this situation, not because I don't have similar experiences or have had similar views in the past, but rather because self-disclosure always has an element of risk and such disclosures can't be taken back once they occur. Instead, I offered him metaphors of *balance*[3] and *wholes*. I derived both of these metaphors on the spot. According to the metaphor of balance, we can influence our current level of well-being by performing a series of acts that work to put our health in equilibrium. Sometimes these acts are inherently unbalanced, however; the acts are done to compensate for something missing that is meant to be present for our selves to be in balance. By relying too much on a compensation tactic to achieve balance, we exist in a paradox of unbalance to achieve balance. I concluded the explanation to say,

> Sometimes what didn't work before will work better now because we have become slightly different people with the passage of time. Like you say, I agree that there is currently no pressing need for medication. But that can change and part of balance is employing an approach to our health that accepts the range of possibilities to keep it in balance.

I proceeded to the metaphor of wholes:

> There are parts of us that keep us well, parts of us that are neutral, and then other parts that work to make us unwell. Sometimes, though, the parts that keep us unwell are the parts that we don't want to see or that we see as being something else—in the

most dangerous situations, as good things. A possibility here is that you're making medication a part that becomes the whole of your diagnosis. What can happen with a lot of people is that they associate their medication with their illness and by a process of magical thinking, they figure that by not taking medication, they are no longer unwell. Sometimes stigma can be as sneaky as being the thing that we reject in the form of little pills.

Although he didn't leave the room with a prescription, nor did he promise to think about things, the key is that the doctor (me) perceived a real health risk in the future while respecting the patient's reluctance to take medication that, at least based on the natural history of the condition, is indicated. Metaphor constituted a way to bring up the topic of pharmacotherapy in a hypothetical way that was non-impositional and even uncertain. I presented a couple of metaphors that were meant to sit next to the patient's aversion to pharmacotherapy, as a prelude to possible adoption. Metaphors were used in a persuasive manner to avoid what had obviously brought confrontation with other doctors in the past. There was no 'A-ha!' moment to be had here, only—to use a metaphor—a small chip to be made in the edifice of his reluctance.

Notes

1 Sometimes when I read of narrative medicine as a thing I recall Frye's (2007: 18) witticism about narrative as a sacred, weighty *thing* after he describes some salient features of narrative: "I recall these exceedingly obvious points to emphasize the primary role of narrative or sequence in holding together every mode of verbal expression from the Bible to the telephone directory."
2 In this way the internist performatively enacts metaphor, which Donaldson (2015: 35) calls "an expression of spatial relation—or seeing relation as an expression of space," space being "the radical environment of metaphor, its allowing condition."
3 The Hippocratic corpus uses metaphors of balance all the time, the famous humoral system being one grand metaphor of balance. Here's a more subtle balance metaphor from *Aphorisms* that doesn't involve the humours: "A slender restricted diet is always dangerous in chronic diseases, and also in acute diseases, where it is not requisite. And again, a diet brought to the extreme point of attenuation is dangerous; and repletion, when in the extreme, is also dangerous" (*Internet Classics Archive*: np).

References

Bleakley A. 2017. *Thinking With Metaphors in Medicine: The State of the Art*. London: Routledge.
Charon R. 2006. *Narrative Medicine: Honoring the Stories of Illness*. Oxford: Oxford University Press.
Donaldson J. 2015. *Missing Link: The Evolution of Metaphor and the Metaphor of Evolution*. Montreal: McGill-Queens.
Frye N. 2007. *Words With Power*. Toronto: Penguin.
Harkins PW. 1963. *Galen on the Passions and Errors of the Soul*. Columbus, OH: Ohio State University Press.
Hippocrates. *Of the Epidemics*. Available at: http://classics.mit.edu/Hippocrates/epidemics.html. Last accessed: 30 October 2018.
Nissen T, Wynn R. The history of the case report: a selective review. *JRSM Open*. 2014; 5: 4.

Appendix

(Permission has been obtained from the patient to publish the excerpt below.)

Excerpt from actual chart note

I explained that if he doesn't have a goal, he's likely not to make progress, and simply subsist in the therapeutic process. He might make slow movement with gradual chipping away and perspective framing etc. but it won't be as useful a process if **X** doesn't want something from it.

I then offered a few goals of my own just in the current moment in order to show him that I have goals operating all the time:

- to see my patients and do a competent job
- to return home to Oakville in one piece on the 401
- to contribute to the functioning of my home upon return

After hearing this, **X** nominated the **(redacted)** goal that I know he already has operative.

I tried to engage in a metaphorical process in which my left hand was **X**, my right hand was a goal, and in between was an avoidance process that became bigger and bigger. My right hand began to drift from my left. I used an example I came up with on the spot, the 'caveman' example who wants to be warm and dreams of fire but never puts the sticks together to make fire because he convinced himself it was too difficult and unpleasant to rub sticks together and survive.

X seemed to understand. But whether he will make any movement is hard to tell. At any rate, **(redacted)** is not really a goal, it's an outcome and the goal is diminishing the duration of his avoidance process by having him change behaviour.

14

MEDICAL SLANG

Symptom or solution?

Nicole M. Piemonte

Introduction

Metaphorical language, especially the use of culinary metaphors, is ubiquitous in medical education and practice. Rarely, however, is this language seen for what it is—creative, imaginative, and even psychologically protective—and is instead considered succinct and accurately descriptive. This chapter explores the complexity of metaphorical language and medical slang and how they point to the underlying culture of medicine that distances clinicians and learners from the existential weight of serious illness, suffering, and death. It argues that practitioners' and trainees' inabilities to recognise the dissonance created by using aesthetically appealing metaphors to describe sources of pain and suffering is a symptom of a much larger problem in medicine—namely, the tendency to overlook the all-too-human elements of medical care. While using metaphors or slang to describe potentially devastating illnesses is not inherently problematic, failing to see the tension between what seriously ill patients go through and how clinicians talk about and 'manage' sickness can be. As such, this chapter concludes by calling on educators to help their students see patient encounters as more than routine moments of one's day and to bring these future clinicians back to a kind of care defined by compassion, vulnerability, and connection.

A blueberry muffin baby

I first started thinking about metaphors in medicine when I was in graduate school. At the time my partner was a medical student at the same university, so I often found myself futilely tuning out the group study sessions he hosted for his friends while I agonised over my dissertation in the bedroom of our tiny apartment. I can recall rather clearly the time I overheard them talking about the differential diagnosis for a 'blueberry muffin baby.' I remember thinking to myself—wow, that sounds adorable; what a cute way to describe a newborn. I was, in fact, so delighted by the image I'd conjured in my mind that I went over to where they were studying and asked them about it. You might imagine my horror when they told me that the bluish marks on the skin that define the blueberry muffin baby signify underlying causes that range from blood disorders or infections like herpes and syphilis to congenital leukaemia and even metastatic neuroblastoma. They told me that other symptoms can be an enlarged liver or spleen, congenital blindness and deafness, micro or macrocephaly, and seizures.

Comingled with a sense of how tragic it would be to give birth to such a sick baby was an unshakeable feeling that referring to a devastating constellation of symptoms as a 'blueberry muffin baby' was somehow *wrong*. Isn't it strange, I asked the medical students in my apartment that night, to use such an endearing term for a baby who might die? Not really, they said—it's a pretty accurate description of how the condition physically manifests. Conceptually, of course, I understood how the term functioned. The metaphor or resemblance was descriptive; it succinctly captured the tangible signs of underlying pathology— and did so in a way that medical novices would remember. As Matthew Wynia (1995) points out, comparing medical conditions to familiar, concrete objects, such as food, makes them easier to remember and recall.[1] But emotionally, I couldn't quite close the gap that such a strange juxtaposition created.

That night I learned that while my unease with such terms was uncommon, the use of culinary metaphors like the blueberry muffin baby is, indeed, anything but. There are strawberry tongues and cherry haemangiomas, pear-shaped hearts, olive-sized masses, port-wine stains, and, of course, Adam's apples. Add to this a variety of medical slang—some made famous by Samuel Shem's *The House of God*, like 'turf' and 'GOMER'[2]—and any patient might be surprised to hear his or her potentially serious situation discussed in such terms. Even more surprising, to me at least, is that my friends in medical school didn't seem to recognise this dissonance.

Why culinary metaphors?

Wynia (1995: 437) suggests that culinary metaphors are prolific in medicine because they serve as a comforting diversion—they keep one tethered to 'humanity,' to the 'the 'real' world of nonmedical, benign, and even pleasant things.' I think Wynia is right that this language serves as a 'comforting diversion,' but it seems to me the diversion has a different, albeit unintentional, motivation. Rather than keeping the clinician or clinician-learner connected to the world—a messy, rather capricious world filled with suffering, illness, and mortality— these metaphors might be doing just the opposite. In other words, using such language may be a way to unconsciously distance oneself from the existential precariousness that signs and symptoms of disease point to. A blueberry muffin baby, for instance, is emotionally and psychologically easier to hold than a newborn child arbitrarily fated to die.

Pena and Andrade-Filho (2010) claim that analogies in medicine are paradoxical in that they celebrate aesthetically uplifting images that so often refer to suffering and death. This paradox, however, is rarely seen as such. Most often, semantic manoeuvres like these are seen as accurate, objective descriptions of clinical presentations, rather than a strange marriage of levity and tragedy. And even at a more basic level, medical metaphors are rarely viewed as imaginative and creative, but rather for their utility— useful descriptors that facilitate memorisation or succinct, effective communication. As Alan Bleakley (2017: 46) puts it, "Medicine is laced with metaphor, yet its public face refuses this, claiming plain language, concrete thinking . . . This suggests that medicine suffers from a split between its conscious public persona and its unconscious structure."

Language, epistemology, and practice

So what is this "public persona" of medicine to which Bleakley alludes? The culture in which clinicians practise and trainees learn is predominantly shaped by the epistemology of medicine— what doctors know and how they come to know it (Montgomery 2005). Within medicine, the 'knowable' is believed to be the observable and measurable—usually empirical, scientific facts—and how one comes to know those facts is through observations or via measurements, lab tests, microscopy, imaging, and so on. This is, in part, a result of the fact that traditional accounts of medicine are dominated by a discursive system grounded in an epistemological theory of the body as an anatomical/physiological/biochemical structure that is best known and understood through the methods of science and through the impartial observations of the physician (Komesaroff 2001).

On its face, the assumption that medicine is a scientific endeavour is reasonable, considering that clinicians often rely on technology and scientific modalities to 'reveal' the workings of the biological body. But, because epistemologies carry with them a certain kind of ethos, they can shape ideas of the specific dispositions and values that will allow one to properly secure knowledge. The contemporary epistemic virtues of scientific medicine, for example, include notions of objectivity, rigour, and detachment. These virtues are rooted in a cultivation of a particular 'scientific self' who attempts to suppress aspects of his or her subjective self—a kind of 'willed willessness' in the quest for 'Truth' (Daston and Galison 2010). In becoming this particular scientific self, knowing and knower become one; the knower is one who must resist the temptations of imagination and subjectivity. Thus, when medicine is conceived of as an applied science, and when one of the epistemic virtues of this science is objectivity, students and doctors may come to see the adoption of an objective stance towards a patient and her illness as good, noble, or right—despite the fact that scientific objectivity can occlude the very human elements of illness and medicine, resulting in narrow and insufficient care of the suffering other.

While objectivity—and even the distance and detachment required to remain objective—is viewed as essential to sound, 'scientific' medicine, Montgomery (2005: 36) points out that doctors have the "good sense not to practise that way." Good doctors, of course, know there is much more to clinical practice than objective observations and measurements. And yet, a medical culture that presents itself as objective and claims plain language and concrete thinking is the same culture that fails to account for the tension created by metaphors that render serious conditions innocuous.

It should be said, however, that conceiving of medicine this way is understandable, for several reasons. First, while seeing the body as a biological entity in need of physical intervention can result in a thin view of what it means to be a doctor, doing so makes sense because *it so often works*. The fact that many doctors can discern our physical maladies and effectively ameliorate them through scientific thinking is a very good thing and something to be celebrated. Second, maintaining objectivity and clinical distance when patients suffer intensely or unjustly is understandable, and perhaps nearly inevitable, since it is difficult to witness such suffering, especially when it reminds us of our own mortality. As the German philosopher Martin Heidegger (1962: 295, emphasis in original) would put it, "for the most part," we cover up our trajectory towards death by "fleeing *in the face* of it." Avoiding the existential reality of death—and its harbingers like pain and suffering—may simply be part of our nature as mortal beings.

Arthur Frank, a sociologist who suffered a heart attack at age thirty-nine and a serious cancer diagnosis the following year, reminds us of this very point, but within the context of medicine. He says that voices of patients can be hard for clinicians to hear, as they "bespeak conditions of embodiment that most of us would rather forget our own vulnerability to" (Frank 1997: 84). Sickness and death can be terrifying, painful, and ugly, and viewing these events as biological breakdowns is easier to emotionally manage. A tangible, pathological object that requires medical intervention is much less anxiety-provoking than a person whose existence has become conspicuously tenuous. In an earlier work, Frank (1991) explains how his illness experience revealed to him that patients and doctors usually discuss medical issues very differently. Frank points out that typically, when patients talk about what is happening to them, they engage in "illness talk"—that is, language that describes their lived experience of being ill; what is happening to not only their bodies but also their identities and sense of self. In contrast, most clinicians, according to Frank, engage in "disease talk"—language about the biological happenings of the body as object that tends to drown out the voice of 'illness talk' during the clinical encounter:

> Because the disease terms refer to measurements, they are 'objective.' Thus, in disease talk *my* body, my ongoing experience of being alive, becomes *the* body, an object to be measured and thus objectified. 'Objective' talk about disease is always medical talk. Patients quickly learn to express themselves in these terms, but in using medical expressions ill persons lose themselves: the body I experience cannot be reduced to the body someone else measures.
>
> *(Frank 1991: 12, emphasis in original)*

The particular discourse of the culture of medicine facilitates knowledge production, and the way in which things are discussed, or left unaddressed, creates and informs both physicians' and patients' realities and how they interpret their experiences. For Frank, the dominant discourse of medicine—that is, medicine's public persona—significantly limits the responses of both patients and doctors when they are confronted with the kind of suffering that cannot be distilled into the language of disease. Frank writes:

> Medical treatment, whether in an office or hospital or on the phone, is designed to make everyone believe that only the disease—what is measurable and mechanical—can be discussed . . . I know I am supposed to ask only about the disease, but what I feel is the illness. The questions I want to ask about my life are not allowed, not speakable, not even thinkable. The gap between what I feel and what I feel allowed to say widens and deepens and swallows my voice.
>
> *(Frank 1991: 13)*

Conflicting messages

While Frank rightly points out the constrictive language used in the clinical space that so narrowly prescribes the patient's role, it still leaves us to wonder about the metaphorical language clinicians use out of earshot of patients—language that, as we've seen above, can be creative, illustrative, and even poetic. How is it that patients can feel that the most 'appropriate' way to discuss their illness with their doctors is through objective language about their biological bodies, while their doctors—once they leave the room—talk to their colleagues, their students, their staff about patients in subjective terms laden with metaphors, anecdotes, and even jokes? What exactly happens when physicians cross the threshold between a patient's room and the halls of the hospital?

I've written elsewhere about gallows humour in medicine—jokes made 'behind the scenes' in order to defuse traumatic, serious, or emotionally painful experiences like death—arguing that we should be less concerned about when and whether using gallows humour is appropriate in medicine and more concerned about how its mere existence is a symptom of a much deeper problem: namely, the medical world's failure to appropriately address the complexity of illness, suffering, and death (Piemonte 2015). We haven't given our clinicians and students the language or the space to reflect on the emotional rigours of confronting human vulnerability and mortality, and yet we expect them to be 'professional' or build 'resilience' or pay attention to their own 'wellness' in the midst of it all. It's no wonder that some physicians defy their oaths of professionalism and altruism—making jokes at the expense of their patients or focusing myopically on objective, narrow, biological dysfunction—when we've trained them to become experts and specialists in a field suffuse with uncertainty, human emotion, and unanswerable questions about the meaning of life and death.

So, while rhetorical manoeuvres like gallows humour and medical slang are more expansive and creative than the limiting language of biological disease that Frank finds so alienating, it seems they serve the same function in medicine: to render distressing experiences banal and manageable. Said otherwise, when the clinician sees the body as object or attempts to laugh at the absurdity of death and suffering, he or she doesn't have to experience the vulnerability that comes with being all too human. Physician Danielle Ofri (2013) speaks to this point as she looks back on her training:

> As much as we empathise with our patients, part of protecting our inner core may require drawing an unconscious demarcation between 'us' and 'them.' I can recall, as a resident, the palpable relief of leaving the hospital at the end of a long night, something I generally thought about in physical terms—getting out of grubby scrubs, the promise of a hot shower and edible food. But it was more than that: There was also the awkward relief of leaving behind the graphic reminder of what could befall my own body. Somewhere, deep down, I needed to convince myself that we doctors were a different species from our patients.

The more time I spend in medical education, the more I see this unconscious demarcation everywhere I turn. When I was in my early twenties, I cared for my mother for a little over two years while she was dying of ovarian cancer. At the time, I had no theory to make sense of the practice of medicine, nor did I really see medicine as very problematic. Yet, even then, I felt a palpable boundary between my mother (and myself) and those who cared for her. And nowhere was this boundary more noticeable than at the threshold of her hospital room. Outside her door on the oncology floor, nurses laughed and chatted about their weekends; doctors, technicians, and students flitted about, hustling to finish their daily work. While the laughter always stopped at her room's entrance, and while each of her caregivers remembered to walk in grim-faced and serious, they knew they always got to walk back out—out into a universe that still made sense to them. Outside my mother's door, the busyness of everyday continued on, while our whole world was collapsing on the other side.

Heidegger (1962: 83) reminds us that physical space is always more than just space; it is not simply the measurable area containing material objects, but the "*wherein* [that] I live," the space where we dwell. My mother and I were dwelling in a space of sickness, fear, and inevitable death. We counted the minutes that passed differently than did her caregivers, knowing our time together was tragically finite. We hung on to doctors' words, scrutinised every gesture and look and pause, and were crushed under the weight of statements that were considered 'bad news' to her doctors and completely life shattering to us. A few years later, I would read the words of Simone de Beauvoir (1985: 73) as she described caring for her mother who was dying of stomach cancer, and they would capture it all for me: "The world had shrunk to the size of her room . . . My real life took place at her side."

The greatest struggle I've faced in my time teaching medical students and residents is helping them recognise the thresholds they cross every day. Rarely can they see the strange tension between their daily routine and the experience of their patients in the hospital bed before them. The great American writer Anatole Broyard (1990) once said after receiving his cancer diagnosis, "To most physicians my illness is a routine incident in their rounds, while for me it's the crisis of my life. I would feel better if I had a doctor who, at least, perceived this incongruity."

The words 'at least' are important here. Those of us in medical education get so caught up in things like trying to define empathy and debating about whether it is teachable, in hammering down the minutiae of ethical principles, in developing mnemonics to help our students learn how to appropriately break bad news, that we fail to see that it is all so much simpler. We need only to get our students to see that medicine is full of people who may be having the crisis of their lives, and who are, simultaneously and absurdly, also just items on a to-do list. Our job is simply to help them recognise this incongruity, to recognise that they participate in a medical system that unconsciously encourages them *not* to see patients as whole people with rich and sometimes tragic lives, but as 'things to do' and—at least in the United States—as 'relative value units' needed for reimbursement and compensation.[3]

Medical education as socialisation

Clinicians and learners rarely acknowledge the tension that results from seeing patients as items on a list, but this is not to say any of them intentionally reduce their encounters with patients to contractual exchanges devoid of human connection. Few, if any, future clinicians choose medicine because they want to practise it this way. Rather, at least from my vantage point, I watch the slow creep of disillusionment grab hold of students and residents in ways they can't even see. The wheels of modern medicine are fast and fierce, and yet the process of getting caught up in them is gradual and imperceptible. Like my friends who couldn't feel the dissonance when referring to a dying newborn as a blueberry muffin baby—seeing it only as an accurate description of physical pathology, as a phrase that could help them memorise information for a standardised exam—medical trainees rarely see the incoherence of the systems in which they participate. And this is, in large part, a result of the fact that very few of their mentors point out the painful moments when their deepest values collide with the everyday work they are required to do.

For years, scholars in medical education have discussed the 'hidden curriculum,' which is the implicit value system communicated to students on the wards through their interactions with peers and mentors conflicting with the espoused values of the formal curriculum. Unfortunately, the hidden curriculum's emphasis on efficiency, compliance, and the acquisition of knowledge, coupled with its tendency to focus on biological disease processes and technical intervention, undermines the explicit values of professionalism and leaves little room to focus on what kind of person the doctor should be (Olthuis and Dekkers 2003). This is a serious problem, given that medical education does, in fact, significantly shape the kind of doctors (and people) students are becoming.

It is interesting to think about how much of this hidden curriculum is determined by language and the 'appropriate' ways to talk within medicine. Bleakley (2017: 91) makes this connection when discussing the function of metaphors:

> Metaphors are part of the historical fabric of medical culture into which students are integrated (inclusion), while interested non-medics . . . are refused or vetted (exclusion) as 'medicine watchers.' This is a process of socialisation leading to an identity construction, associated particularly with gaining legitimate entry into a community of practice as expertise develops.

The way doctors, nurses, and other professionals talk about patients is a result of (and also perpetuates) the cultural scripts that define who is 'in' medicine and who is 'out.' At the same time, these scripts implicitly communicate what is okay to talk about, to think about, and to feel something about. I see the downstream effects of this when residents come to my office to express some of the pain they're in and end up spending most of their time apologising for their emotions and saying there 'must be something wrong with them' for feeling the way they do about suffering patients. 'I feel like my brain is broken or something,' one resident told me. 'My attending was in the room with me when it happened, but he's fine. Why can't I just get over it?'

While residents and medical students often tell me how strange it is that no one talks to them or 'debriefs' them about deaths in the hospital, those who acknowledge the moral distress of *everyday* medicine are certainly in the minority. More often than not, our young doctors start to see themselves as cogs in a massive machine, and some have forgotten why they chose a life in medicine in the first place. During a workshop I led with residents at my hospital a few months ago, which was intended to help them reconnect to the reasons they chose medicine, one senior resident said to the group: "I haven't felt connected to those reasons in two and a half years, which, I guess, is exactly how long I've been in residency."

Saying what we really mean

When I hear these things, I can't help but feel deep compassion for our doctors, our nurses, and our students. Medicine is hard and messy, and it requires an amount of emotional labour that few people recognise when they sign on for the job. We ask our caregivers to be on the frontlines of human suffering and stare it straight in the eye; yet, we poorly equip them to do so. So, instead, they spend most of their time trying to avert their gaze.

What we need, then, at least as a starting place, is an educational system acknowledging that medicine is not an exact science and that it demands more of a person than acquiring and applying knowledge. Throughout medical training, the idea of attending to patients as whole people who suffer in complex ways should hold as much weight as learning the biology and pathophysiology of disease. Students should be told that the education they are undertaking has as much to do with their character as it does with their intellect (Montgomery 2005). Students need to be introduced to new, expansive ways of thinking and talking about medical care, which I believe (like many of the contributors to this book) are afforded by real engagement with the arts and humanities—particularly narrative, poetry, and film that speak to the lived experience of illness. And this kind of learning must be incorporated thoughtfully throughout training and not simply tacked on as an afterthought.

We must also accept the fact that caring for sick people requires a place for reflection and expression of human emotion. We need to encourage our current and future caregivers to see that the metaphors they use, the non-biological terms they avoid—the rhetorical gymnastics they unconsciously engage in to evade vulnerability—matter. Emphasis should be placed on discussing the lived experience of illness, suffering, and death, rather than just their biological realities, and our caregivers should be encouraged to see the tensions between the ways they talk about illness and how patients actually experience it.

It should be said that asking our clinicians and trainees to acknowledge these things requires them to also see their own vulnerability, their own potential for suffering and death. And we can't ask them to do so if we are unwilling to attend to their pain, frustration, or disappointment. At a very basic level, those who are called to care for us need our care, too. They need broader, more flexible scripts that account for suffering—their patients and their own—and we all need to be willing to listen.

Notes

1 Wynia's paper also offers an extensive list of culinary metaphors used in medicine.
2 Turf means to 'get rid' of a difficult patient by handing them off to another team. GOMER stands for Get Out of My Emergency Room, usually referring to an elderly patient who is unable to communicate

his or her symptoms and often turfed from one department to another. For an extensive list of medical slang and acronyms, see http://messybeast.com/dragonqueen/medical-acronyms.htm.

3 According to the National Health Policy Forum, "Medicare uses a physician fee schedule to determine payments for over 7,500 physician services. The fee for each service depends on its relative value units (RVUs), which rank on a common scale the resources used to provide each service. These resources include the physician's work, the expenses of the physician's practise, and professional liability insurance." See 'The Basics: Relative Value Units': www.nhpf.org/library/the-basics/Basics_RVUs_01-12-15.pdf.

References

Bleakley A. 2017. *Thinking with Metaphors in Medicine: The State of the Art*. New York, NY: Routledge.

Broyard A. Doctor talk to me. *New York Times*. August 26, 1990. Available at: www.nytimes.com/1990/08/26/magazine/doctor-talk-to-me.html. Last accessed: February 13, 2018.

Daston LJ, Galison P. 2010. *Objectivity*. New York, NY: Zone Books.

de Beauvoir S. 1985. *A Very Easy Death*. New York, NY: Pantheon.

Doctors' Slang, Medical Slang and Medical Acronyms and Veterinary Acronyms & Vet Slang. Available at: http://messybeast.com/dragonqueen/medical-acronyms.htm. Last accessed: November 26, 2017.

Frank AW. 1991. *At the Will of the Body*. Boston, MA: Houghton Mifflin.

Frank AW. 1997. *The Wounded Storyteller: Body, Illness, and Ethics*. Chicago, IL: University of Chicago Press.

Heidegger M. 1962. *Being and Time*. Translated by John Macquarrie and Edward Robinson. New York, NY: Harper and Row.

Komesaroff P. 2001. The many faces of the clinic: a Levinasian view. In: SK Toombs (ed.) *Handbook of Phenomenology and Medicine*. Dordrecht, NL: Kluwer Academic Publishers, 317–30.

Montgomery K. 2005. *How Doctors Think: Clinical Judgment and the Practice of Medicine*. New York, NY: Oxford University Press.

Ofri, D. Why doctors don't take sick days. *The New York Times*. November 15, 2013. Available at: www.nytimes.com/2013/11/16/opinion/sunday/why-doctors-dont-take-sick-days.html. Last accessed: March 30, 2018.

Olthuis G, Dekkers W. Medical education, palliative care and moral attitude: some objectives and future perspectives. *Medical Education*. 2003; 37: 928–33.

Pena GP, de Souza Andrade-Filho J. Analogies in Medicine: Valuable for learning, reasoning, remembering and naming. *Advances in Health Science Education*. 2010; 15: 609–19.

Piemonte N. Last laughs: gallows humor and medical education. *Journal of Medical Humanities*. 2015; 36: 375–90.

Shem S. 1978. *The House of God*. New York, NY: Richard Marek Publishers.

Wynia MK. Culinary metaphors in medicine. *Infectious Diseases in Clinical Practice*. 1995; 4: 437–40.

15

AGEISM AND RHETORIC

Judy Z. Segal

If we do not know what we are going to be, we cannot know what we are: let us recognise ourselves in this old man or in that old woman.

(Simone de Beauvoir 1970: 5)

Preface

At the centre of debates on North American campuses about freedom of expression is the question of how much words matter, of what speech actually *does*. Recently, Paul Russell, Professor of Philosophy at my university (British Columbia), wrote the following, as he argued publicly for the primacy of free speech:

> When I was a child the old adage was "sticks and stones may break my bones . . .," which was meant to emphasize that there was a real and significant difference between physical violence and threats and words and language that was merely abusive and offensive. This allowed for a real measure of tolerance and freedom of expression.[1]

To be fair, I should note that Russell conceded that the adage "may well be too simple," but he went on to say that he abhors the adoption of its opposite: that "words can be used as weapons." But, of course, words *can* be used as weapons. We know that; children know it. When I linger at my granddaughter's daycare at pick-up time, I sometimes have occasion to witness the casual, rhetorical, cruelty of four-year-olds.

My chapter makes two arguments, the first subsumed in the second. First, medical humanities ought centrally to include rhetorical studies, a discipline concerned with what words *do*. Rhetoricians study persuasion, broadly defined, and not only in formal contexts of political or forensic speech-making, but also in contexts of everyday life—including, importantly, life lived in an idiom of health and illness. A rhetorical perspective considers persuasions that sometimes go unnoticed; included among these persuasions are acts of speech that we may identify as *microaggressions*: small acts of symbolic violence. My second argument is about ageism—and the way it is perpetuated, in part, rhetorically. I can begin by asking you, reader, what came to mind when, moments ago, I used the word, "granddaughter"? Did my authorial skin wrinkle unattractively? Did I become a little frail? Did my memory become unreliable? Anyway, would you prefer not to identify with me? David Archard (2009: 568) begins his review of Helen Small's *The Long Life* by saying that the first reason not to like old age is its proximity to death. He is, I believe, not entirely right. What he calls the second reason is more salient, I think: he says that age brings "a failing of powers, debility and senility at worst" (ibid.).[2] The dislike of old age is a dislike of the perceived condition of oldness itself. This account, from Martha Nussbaum, is chilling, but not, I think, completely wrong:

> [D]isgust is always at some level self-disgust, as one perceives animality in others and shuns it in oneself. But with aging the truth is front and centre: it really is for oneself that one fears. Stigma learned early and toward others gradually becomes self-stigma and self-exclusion, as one's own aging body is seen as a site of decay and future death— by oneself, as well as by others.
>
> *(Nussbaum and Levmore 2017: 114)*

And, still, disdain for people who are old (including, at some point, oneself) is, importantly, an effect of ageist rhetoric. Margaret Morganroth Gullette (2017a: abstract; original emphasis) writes, forcefully, "*Language* shapes thought, and *ageist* language invisibly spreads *ageist* thinking."

Ageism: an introduction

Healthy ageing and *successful ageing* are current narrative options for becoming old, ostensibly supplying a counter-rhetoric to the more entrenched narrative of decline in ageing. The new, consumerist, take on ageing is problematic, as many critics have noted (see, for example, Gullette 2004; Sinding and Gray 2005; Katz 2009; Lamb 2014): for one thing, it is an option available only to some people—those who are both well resourced and lucky. It creates an ideal, largely commercially sponsored, of an existence often unattainable, and it is represented, typically, in the figure of the young-old, rather than the old-old, person. Furthermore, "successful ageing" attributes responsibility for quality of life in late life to individuals, personalising risk and distributing moral blame.

Narrative replacement could not, in any case, ever really *be* replacement—because a narrative of decline is always already present in a narrative of successful ageing: we age successfully against, and within the terms of, a narrative of decline. Indeed, decline as a feature of ageing is what rhetorician Kenneth Burke (1954/1984: 74, italics in original) might call a "piety," where "piety," disconnected from its religious sense, signifies instead "*the sense of what properly goes with what.*" Ageing goes with decline, as piety speaks to "a desire to round things out, to fit experiences together in a unified whole" (ibid.: 1954/1984: 74).[3] So, even in the presence of any (putatively) resistant discourse, the messages about ageing we encounter day to day refer to "the grey tsunami,"[4] the prevalence of dementia, the high cost of health care for an ageing population, and the general sense that, as age theorist Margaret Cruikshank (2013: 36) notes, critically, "the business of being old is to be sick." Ageing is not one of the topics addressed in Jonathan Metzl and Anna Kirkland's (2010: 2) *Against Health*, but the book's central critique fits:

> Health is a desired state, but it is also a prescribed state and an ideological position . . . [T]he term is used to make moral judgments, convey prejudice, sell products, or even to exclude whole groups of persons from health care.

The expectation of decline in health and ability is a prominent feature in a rhetoric of ageism—although the primacy of health and ability in discourse about ageing is itself problematic, as I will argue—but we can recognise other features of age stereotyping as well. In the North American context in which I write, to be old is, in some cases, to be rich, and wealth may spawn social resentment about generational inequity.[5] Bridie Jabour (2016) writes in the *Guardian* that "intergenerational warfare" is not about age but rather class. In some cases, to be old is to be poor, and poverty may spawn social resentment about a looming financial burden. Sentiment against old people, that is, has some of the features of sentiment against immigrants: they suck up resources that should belong to others; if they support themselves by working, they suck up jobs not rightfully theirs.

Anti-ageing medicine and post-human research further affirm that old age is despicable and in need of annihilation. Still, while it seems possible that scientific advances will make 80 the new 50—at least for some—such advances probably won't solve the problem of a dreaded old age, only bump it into another decade of life. In her graphic memoir, *Can't We Talk about Something More Pleasant?*, Roz Chast (2014: 20) says wryly,

> I could see that [my parents] were slowly leaving the sphere of TV commercial old age (Spry! Totally independent!! Just like a normal adult, but with silver hair!!!)—and moving into the part of old age that was scarier, harder to talk about, and not a part of this culture.

Deep old age, whenever it may occur, is "not a part of this culture."

Meanwhile, a young and attractive old age wedges its way into acceptability. In 2014, *People* Magazine raised the age of possibility for "beauty at any age" from 59 to 69, feeling the need, it seemed, to give a nod to Meryl Streep, Susan Sarandon, and other celebrated women in their 60s—including, at the time, Helen Mirren, who has become a kind of poster elder. (Mirren is now over 70, which poses an interesting challenge to the magazine.) In 2017, *Allure* Magazine, in one of its glossy, appearance-obsessed issues, proclaimed an editorial commitment to "the end of anti-aging." Editor, Michelle Lee (2017: 30), in fact, wrote, "Changing the way we think about aging starts with changing the way we talk about aging." But how utterly disingenuous: what is the ageing that Lee is no longer "anti"? It's Helen-Mirren ageing. Helen Mirren is the issue's "cover girl" and is the subject of a photographic feature in which she appears pleasantly glamorous. Mirren also appears in an ad for a *L'Oréal* moisturiser that promises to "get your rosy tone back." Writing about this issue of *Allure*, Amanda Hess (2017: 15) notes, "As the business of fighting aging has consumed the culture, it has produced a secondary aversion—not just to the signs of aging but to the signs that we're trying to stop the signs of aging." Aversions all around.

Oldness, that is, is not simply a quality of persons; it is a social category loaded in a particular way. This is not to say old age is a social construction; it is as material as a state of being can be. But there is a social and discursive element to it. Like sexism, racism, homophobia, transphobia, and other frames of discrimination, ageism is a "system of inflicted sufferings." It is ageism, not ageing itself, that, as Margaret Morganroth Gullette (2017b: xiv) argues, constitutes the "alleged problem" of greying nations: "aging [is] the trigger of ageism," and ageism is the process by which old people become "minor defective characters in someone else's story" (ibid.: xv). Old age is anticipated and viewed negatively from an ever-diminishing distance; then we arrive there. But, as we are, the luckiest of us, old or pre-old (and as we are all pre-dead), we need some way of understanding old age outside of both decline and the neoliberal moralism of age defiance. What are the rhetorical contours of ageism and what might a less harmful rhetoric of age look like?

My subject position

I have revealed that I am part of the population I am writing about. I am old, although by some typologies, young-old; I am, at this writing, almost 70. While I don't believe one has to be old to write about oldness, I am certain that being old has given me access to rhetorical activity that was less apparent to me not simply in my youth and middle-age, but even up to about five years ago, when I began having repeatedly to answer the question, "Are you still working?" As Elaine Showalter (2014: xi) writes in her introduction to Lynne Segal's *Out of Time*, being old, like being fat, is a stigmatised identity that is always already *out*. This being the case, I believe that, as aphorisms go, "you're only as old as you look"—which clocks how other people see, and therefore treat, you—makes at least as much sense as "you're only as old as you feel." The designation "retired" is itself a classifying premise that erases individuality, history, and diversity. People who were once differently employed are often now gathered under a single head, and described simply as "retired." The word, currently, to me, means "being made tired again": simply trying to maintain adult status as an old person can be exhausting. In routine ticket purchases, I find it re-tiring to have to say whether I am a Senior OR an Adult, since, apparently, it is impossible, when buying a ticket, to be both. I protest each time. Last year, I wrote to the Vancouver Aquarium, which I had recently visited with my granddaughter, to ask why, if they have two ticket-price categories for Children—under and over four—they might not have two categories for Adults: under and over 65. They found the suggestion worth ignoring.

This essay is not my first requiring me to think carefully about my subject position—beyond acknowledging that I am a white (well, sort of: Jewish), heterosexual, cis woman, living in Canada, middle class, from a working-class family of origin. In 2006, I began to write about breast-cancer narratives. I was interested, primarily, in what seemed to me the coercive function of the publicly circulating, dominant, story of breast cancer:

> I found a lump; I was diagnosed; I was terrified; I fought; things were hard (but I made the best of them); I beat cancer (at least temporarily); now I'm a better person; in many ways, cancer is the best thing that ever happened to me.[6]

My interest in breast-cancer narratives was that of a rhetorical scholar: how does this discourse act in the world, I wanted to know; what does it do for, and to, people who have/had breast cancer; what questions does it answer?; what regulatory function does it serve? In 2009, I was diagnosed with breast cancer—and I came to see, from my new "standpoint" (Harding 1993), some of the rhetorical habits that perpetuate a particular version of breast-cancer experience. I wrote another essay, this one on the discursive formation of the breast-cancer patient (as myself).[7] That second essay also engaged, explicitly, with the shift in my investigator position, from objective-enough researcher, to someone with what Harding (ibid.) would call "a stronger objectivity." As an observer-participant (slightly different from a participant-observer), I was perched at the margin of a medico-social scene—and from there, I could see things I couldn't see before. How does the standard story assert itself? Well, for one thing, it turns out that, sometimes, even your closest friends can't stop telling you how brave you are (despite there being little evidence of that virtue), how you'll beat your disease—and, as a corollary, how disappointing you'll be if you fail (in other words, if you die). Before I had breast cancer, I knew *that* people conducted a kind of narrative pedagogy of how to be ill; when I was undergoing treatment, I learned *how*: they sometimes did it, across a table, at dinner, sitting back in their chairs, folding their arms, and looking at you like they wished you'd stop talking, when you began to voice your fear and anxiety, when you abandoned, and so, obviated for them, the positive *persona* of the cancer patient as "survivor."

Lately, I have been doing that sort of unbidden and relentlessly embodied research again—but now on old age. I have, for some time, been interested in ageism as a topic in the rhetoric of health and medicine (and as a topic *beyond* health and medicine). But now that I am old, my rhetorical sensors are irretrievably trained on what we talk about when we talk about ageing, and on rhetorical aggressions, many of them microaggressions, directed at people who are old—and, worryingly, *by* people who are old, at each other, and themselves. I am observing the discursive construction of, once again, me.

I have absorbed the ageism I have observed. Although I have never lied about my age (I have thought about lying *up*; I look okay for 70, but amazing for 80)—I do exactly the things Gullette (2017b: 168) says people like her, and me, do: we make some effort, usually unconsciously, to "pass for younger": "We enter a room of potential ageists with *the same* presence, speak with *the same* rapidity." "Passing might cover anything," Gullette says, ". . . clothing, athleticism, tech purchases, vocabulary, ways of walking—by means of which we 'mime the dominant' we have long been."

Methodology and theory

Along with being a member of an aggregate of old people, I am a member of an aggregate of rhetoricians of health and medicine. There are now many of us. We have a long list of publications, including increasingly many monographs (see, for example, Condit 1999; Scott 2003; Segal 2005; Berkenkotter 2008; Keränen 2010; Johnson 2014; Graham 2015; Derkatch 2016; Jensen 2016; Teston 2017; Koerber 2018). We have our own academic conferences and participate in more general rhetoric conferences and in thematic, inquiry-based, interdisciplinary conferences. We have a new journal, *Rhetoric of Health and Medicine*, its inaugural issue published in May 2018.

As we have grown as a (sub)discipline, we have become more and more attentive to methodology. In giving methodological accounts of our work, we are ourselves rhetorically motivated: we wish to persuade our audiences of the empirical value of our work. In 2018, Routledge published an essay collection: *Methodologies for the Rhetoric of Health and Medicine*, edited by Lisa Meloncon and J. Blake Scott (also editors of the aforementioned journal). *Methodologies* promises a "thorough and nuanced explanation of the exigencies, values, epistemological assumptions, limitations, affordances, and adaptations of methodology [in rhetoric of health and medicine]" (Meloncon and Scott 2018: 11). Meloncon and Scott aim, they say, by representing plural and sometimes "messy" research methods, to advance the recognition of Rhetoric of Health and Medicine "as a pragmatically multifarious and discernible area of study that can inform Rhetorical Studies and other areas, such as the medical humanities, medical education, health communication, health policy-making, medical research, and the practice of medicine" (ibid.: 19).

Meloncon and Scott expand my own (Segal 2005, 2009) account of rhetorical methodology—but avoid, they say, my argument that rhetoricians of health and medicine necessarily use what has been traditionally identified as "rhetorical theory" (Meloncon and Scott 2018: 7). That is, they distance themselves from the following, which I did write: "Rhetorical criticism is criticism performed by a rhetorical critic. The statement is more than tautological. A rhetorical critic is a person trained within a scholarly tradition into a rhetorical subjectivity suggesting lines of inquiry and a procedure for thinking" (Segal 2005: 7); that procedure, I have also said, is "intentionally underspecified" (ibid.: 9), so that rhetorical criticism, like rhetoric itself, can respond to local conditions. But Meloncon and Scott (2018: 5) and I agree that rhetorical analysis is procedurally capacious; it exhibits what they themselves call "methodological mutability"—"a willingness and even obligation to pragmatically and ethically adjust aspects of methodology to changing existences, conditions, and relationships." Moreover, rhetorical criticism is both interdisciplinary (rhetorical criticism is a part of disabilities studies, gender studies, science and technology studies, and so on) and *poly*disciplinary: it can form many alliances, and co-sponsor inquiry with anthropology or history or philosophy, for example.

Central to my rhetorical project on ageing is Burke's (1969: 73) assertion that human agents use words "to form attitudes or to induce actions in other human agents"—and that they do this, in general, simply by deploying language, as they must, "dramatistically," as a form of symbolic action (Burke 1966: 44). Pertinent to my project also is Ian Hacking's "dynamic nominalism": his nuancing of *static nominalism* (things are what we name them) and *realism* (things are; then we name them). Hacking (2002: 113) writes, "[N]umerous kinds of human beings and human acts come into being hand in hand with our invention of the ways to name them." This process, he says, of "making up people" "changes the spaces of possibilities for personhood" (ibid.: 107). *Old people*, I would argue, works just this way, naming both a class and a classification. Hacking (1999: 105) explains too what he calls "indifferent" and "interactive" kinds: "[C]alling a quark a quark makes no difference to the quark," he says—and this indifference is not true of people: "self-aware people . . . may understand how they are classified and rethink themselves accordingly" (ibid.: 108).[8] This is not to say there is nothing quark-like about old age: a person who loses their sight in old age, for example, will not regain sight because of what is said about it: old age is an interactive kind with elements of indifference. Kristen Ellison (2014: 23), mobilising terms offered by Lévi-Strauss, writes about being old as a "raw" state, and about the significations of oldness—what culture has done to being old—as a "cooked" one. Finally, my project, like many others in rhetorical criticism, is ameliorative in motive,[9] although it would be hubristic to suggest that rhetorical description is itself more than a small symbolic action.

Rhetorical observations

As others who write about age have noted, one of the peculiar things about ageism is that it is discrimination that takes as its object ourselves[10]—our future selves in the case of much ageism, but also, as has been noted, our present ones: old people may be, and frequently are, ageist, wanting to dissociate from others of their age; embarrassed, really, to be old. Age theorist Ashton Applewhite (2016: 1) writes tellingly about her misguided wish not to be identified with a colleague her own age, while a kind of false-consciousness emerges in Martha Nussbaum's (2016: 149) account of the anger she feels when someone assumes they are stronger and more capable than she is, and offers her help in (her example) hoisting her luggage into an overhead bin. Margaret Morganroth Gullette (2017b: 174) writes about shame and shaming in old age: "Shame at 'aging' is . . . a painful, wordless sensation of being wrong, foisted on members of the minority age-classes by hostile exterior forces." The shame experienced by virtue of being old is an affect we have been training for all our lives, having internalised an ageism we could not help but learn. Gullette quotes a study by Isaacs and Bearison on the preference of children as young as six not to sit with older adults (cited in Gullette 2011: 6)—and Martha Nussbaum reports that "preverbal [!] children already show avoidance behavior when given a choice between an older and a younger person" (Nussbaum and Levmore 2017: 112). I have attached this observation to myself in a benign, but sad, really, sort of way: I sometimes find myself trying to demonstrate to my granddaughter, now almost five, that I am absolutely the most fun adult she has ever met. It never occurred to me, when I was a parent of young children, to perform fun as a kind of labour.

How have we become persuaded to dread and to despise old age as we do? A birthday card says, "Don't worry, you don't look your age."[11] A storefront salon, advertising "non-invasive skin therapy," posts a sign that screams "STOP AGING." A friend introduces her older brother as her "older brother," and he makes a joke that everyone seems to get: "Are you saying I'm *old*?" (that is, have you insulted me?). A Facebook friend, who has had an unpleasant encounter with an older stranger, shares her experience in a post cleverly written as an open letter to "Grannies"—because what she has selected for attention, among all possible features, is the offender's age (and gender). A lighthearted newspaper article provides tips on "how to survive a family vacation with the grandparents." The author empathises with young family members who may have to tolerate the unreasonable, and laughable, demands of grandparents: "Will you feel obliged to give in to a nightly request to eat at 5 p.m.?" (Davis 2017). That complaint is only slightly less disturbing than this one, as the article continues: "[A]s baby boomers—who've apparently been stashing their wealth away for just this kind of moment—age, they're opting to open the coffers for time with their offspring's offspring" (ibid.). That is, wealth, even when it is shared, is material for resentment and ridicule. The article is written in jocular fashion, but jocular is the worst kind of ageism—in part because it gets a kind of rhetorical pass. The following is from a "Shouts and Murmurs" article in a recent *New Yorker*—and I quote it at length, because it was published in the *New Yorker*!:

> How can we make sure our loved ones are prepared for life's joys and challenges? . . . You have to let *go*. You have to allow your parents to make mistakes—that's the only way he or she will learn. You have to let your parent get her heart broken by a man in her assisted-living facility who she thinks is Warren Beatty. You have to let your parent slip and fall on the playground when he is wandering there, lost, after setting out on an errand he can't recall. You have to let your parent give the wrong answer, because otherwise how will he or she ever really learn who Ariana Grande is? . . . If you rush to your parent's side every time he breaks his hip, how will he learn that there are consequences to breaking a hip?
>
> *(Frazer 2017)*

A salesperson in a travel store advises an older customer against buying the luggage whose high price comes from its lifetime guarantee, because, he says, she won't need it—"How many years do you have left to travel? Ten?"—placing her (actually, it was me) on an actuarial table of consumption. Ageist metaphors travel unnoticed in the discourse of everyday life: sympathy goes to the "sandwich generation," without consideration for the person(s) thereby consigned to be the suffocating piece of bread at the top. Ashton Applewhite maintains a blog, "Yo, is this ageist?", where contributors describe various scenarios and pose that question. Usually, the answer is "Yes."

Ageist rhetoric includes not only these discursive acts of disregard and disrespect, but also microaggressions in the form of public representations of old people, ubiquitously. Other commentators have written about representations of age in multiple locations—theatre, film, television, popular culture, advertising, the popular press (see, for example, Blakesborough 2008, on television; Rosanova 2010, on the popular press; Chivers 2011, on film; Ellison 2014, on advertising; Lipscomb 2016, on theatre; and Marshall and Rahmn 2016, on popular culture)—and I would be able to offer no more than a drive-by look at these sources, primary and secondary. I wish only to acknowledge that, currently, not all representations of old people row in the same direction: that is, they are not all terrible. Looking, for a moment, at the medium formerly known as television, we may observe, for example, that "Grace and Frankie"

(Kauffman and Morris 2015–present), starring Jane Fonda and Lily Tomlin (aged 80 and 78, respectively, as I write), is less ageist than was "Hot in Cleveland" (Martin), starring Betty White (aged 93 when the series ended in 2015). Fonda and Tomlin play characters in their 70s, with complex lives; episode themes are often age related, involving health and illness, work and retirement, sex, romance, memory, parenthood, grandparenthood . . . but to be old is not the characters' *raison d'être*. The themes of "Hot in Cleveland," on the other hand, were less variable and less complex—and White's purpose in the ensemble cast was, almost invariably, to be, comically, old.[12]

Rhetorical theory offers a construct helpful in considering what are still the most common—that is, negative—views of old people: it offers the idea itself of a speaker's perceived bad character. Unfolding "bad character" in relation to mental illness, Jenell Johnson writes about the removal, in 1972, of Thomas Eagleton from the Democratic presidential ticket. Eagleton was the vice-presidential candidate running with George McGovern, and he was dropped following the revelation that he had previously been admitted to hospital with a diagnosis of depression. Johnson (2010: 461) writes about the public association, especially at the time, of mental illness with *stigma*: "a constitutive rhetorical act that also produces a disabling rhetorical effect": *kakoethos* or "bad character." A Disabilities Studies understanding of rhetorical disability, Johnson argues, "directs attention to the variety of barriers that prevent certain rhetors from achieving rhetoricity with certain audiences" (ibid.). I would argue that old people occupy such a position of bad character—drawn into a stigmatising perception that they are intellectually unreliable or emotionally labile and so not to be trusted as speakers: rhetorically disabled.

The idea of the *kakoethos* of old people in general—and political figures in particular, if we take up Johnson's own focus—invites us to examine the intersection of age and gender. An example is the 2016 US primaries and presidential election, where the three most prominent figures in the contest were about the same age: they were all around, or over, 70. But only Hillary Clinton was both old and a woman. In the spring of 2016, I Googled "Bernie Sanders 'too old,'" "Donald Trump 'too old,'" and "Hillary Clinton 'too old.'" One of my discoveries, interesting in itself, was that Sanders' age was a less salient feature of his identity than was his socialism (perhaps the way out of being on the receiving end of ageism is to be known as embodying something more shocking than oldness). My Google findings: for "Bernie Sanders 'too old,'" there were 256,000 results, including many articles on why Sanders' age didn't matter to his candidacy. For "Hillary Clinton 'too old,'" there were nearly 2 million results. Clinton's grandmotherhood was a favourite topic of comment, although Clinton had seven times fewer grandchildren than Sanders, and was six years younger.[13] There were comments on her "wrinkles" and her glasses, and a report that a Republican primary candidate "accused" Clinton of using a walker to arrive at a photoshoot. "Accused" her of it. When Clinton did not immediately disclose the pneumonia that caused her to stumble at a campaign stop, commentators and other commenters spoke of her *secret* life as opposed to simply her *private* life. For "Donald Trump 'too old,'" I found 505,000 results: about twice as many as for Sanders and four times fewer than for Clinton. Being old while a woman is a sufficient condition for rhetorical disability.

Conclusion

I said earlier that rhetoricians often have ambitions of amelioration, and so I conclude by offering some thoughts on revising the rhetoric of old age. Simply, people, when they are young, must come to understand themselves as continuous with the people they will be when they are old: everyone is damaged by ageism. The goal is identification, explained by Kenneth Burke (1969: 1–23) as the condition, the means, and the goal of rhetoric.[14] I invoke the epithet at the head of my essay, from Simone de Beauvoir (1970: 5): "If we do not know what we are going to be, we cannot know what we are: let us recognise ourselves in this old man or in that old woman."

This is an excerpt from an essay by Susan Sontag (1972: 29, 33), written when she was 39:

> [There is no] abnormality in the anguish and anger that people who are really old, in their seventies and eighties, feel about the implacable waning of their powers, physical and mental. It is a shipwreck, no matter with what courage elderly people insist on continuing the voyage . . . Aging is a movable doom.

And this is an excerpt from an essay by Sontag's son, David Reiff (2008: np), written shortly after her death:

> [N]o amount of familiarity could lessen the degree to which the idea of death was unbearable to [my mother]. In her eyes, mortality seemed as unjust as murder . . . In her mind, even at 71, my mother was always starting fresh, figuratively as well as literally turning a new page.

In the first excerpt, there is nothing more to be feared than old age; in the second, nothing more to be wished for. The value of a life lived old is one that Sontag could see most clearly from her deathbed. Her original failure was a failure of identification and continuity.

So, I offer for consideration a small move under a heading that might read, "amelioration through complex, temporal, narrative representations of humans." "Orange Is the New Black" (Kohan), based on Piper Kerman's (2010) memoir of the same name, is set in now two US federal prisons for women. Episodes move attention back and forth between younger and older characters, not only because the main characters are age-diverse, but also because the show's signature structure includes revealing the backstories of inmates and other characters—answering the question, "How did [this person] get here?" We are, in each episode, reminded that the old characters used to be young—and young characters used to be younger—and we witness their identities as continuous, or, at least, integrated, as they have aged. (So often, on other programmes, the flashbacks of older characters to younger selves are only sentimental reflections on happier times; the assumption is always that young is the better state.) A telling sequence on OINB occurs in the final moments of the last episode of Season 2 (2013). The character of Miss Rosa, played by Barbara Rosenblat, had been introduced to viewers as an older inmate with cancer: bald, acerbic, and dying. That is how the audience knows her—until we are introduced to "young Rosa," a mischievous and energetic compulsive thief, played by Stephanie Andujar. The final moments of the episode find (old) Rosa escaping from prison, her fellow inmates having plotted successfully for her to die free; she drives away in a stolen prison van. As Rosa is seen behind the wheel, her face softens back in time; the effect is of reverse time-lapse photography, as, digitally, Rosenblat is transformed into Andujar. Rosa is reclassified in this transformation: lifted out of her age cohort and returned to the context of her own life. Representations of characters with complex, integrated identities, it seems to me, are a mass media corrective to ageism.

One takeaway message that emerges from observations of rhetoric and ageism is that ageism will not be solved within a discourse of health alone—including "successful" or "healthy" ageing (interesting how the two have become interchangeable). Becoming old is not simply a matter of waning health or waxing decline; becoming old is growing into a person as complex as, arguably more complex than, that person when they were young. Here is something that's hard to miss in a hospital: typically, in the West at least, old people are low on the hierarchy of humans; we see old people, and we don't aspire to be them. And who could blame us? We may have just received a social-media post with an image of a smiling old man eating sushi—he's someone's dad—and we have read appreciative comments that are mostly versions of "So cute," as if he were a cat. In the culture of the hospital, however, being old is not the lowest thing you can be; being young is. The hierarchy is flipped. If you're 90, and reclining on a gurney as you wait for imaging, you are an unmarked kind. If you're 30, waiting in that horizontal line for your tumour-hunting scan, you are the most pathetic person in the room, the one from whom others avert their eyes. We face challenges, including health challenges, at every age.[15] Health is a part of any conversation about old age; of course it is. But "healthy ageing" will not end ageism. Only inclusion will, and that will come, in part, through a shift from a rhetoric of classification (that is how we "make up people") to a rhetoric of identification.[16]

Notes

1 The quotation appeared at Russell's academic.edu page, available at: www.academia.edu/35143248/UBC_free_speech_for_Wente_excerpts_2017.docx.
    If the page becomes inaccessible, Russell can be found quoted in Wente (2017).

2 The well-worn retort, in response to those who complain about their old age, is "consider the alternative." Currently, however, confronted with those alternatives, one could be forgiven for thinking, "Give me a minute." See, for example, Ehrenreich (2018). On the idea of death as preferable to deep old age, see, for example, Ezekiel Emanuel's essay (2014) in which he explains his wish to die at 75.

3 "Piety" for Burke is a "scheme of orientation." "The orientation may be right or wrong; it can guide or misguide." It is pious for the bird to fly with the flock—even if the flock is following a bird mistaken in its rise to flight (1984: 76).

4 Andrea Charise writes of a rhetoric of "imminent catastrophe": an "ominous rhetoric of rising, swamping, tides, and disease—amplified by the authoritative tones of medical and health policy expertise" (2012: 3).

5 I live in a city where many of the people who live in multimillion-dollar (although often *very ordinary*) houses bought them for tens of thousands of dollars 40 years earlier; many people, shut out from the notoriously hideous Vancouver housing market, resent politicians, developers, offshore investors, and . . . old people.

6 See Segal (2007). Diane Price Herndl, also writing about breast-cancer narratives as genre, notes this often implicit coda: "Be like me" (2006: 232).

7 See Segal (2015).

8 Hacking continues, "I do not necessarily mean that . . . individuals, on their own, become aware of how they are classified, and thus react to the classification. Of course they may, but the interaction occurs in the larger matrix of institutions and practices surrounding this classification" (1999: 103).

9 Rhetorical criticism has a history of ameliorative intention. See, for example, Roderick Hart (1994).

10 Cruikshank writes, for example, "A white person who 'others' a black will not herself become black, but a thirty-year-old who 'others' someone over seventy-five may well live to join the minority that now seems so distant" (2013: 6).

11 Birthday cards are well-known locations for ageism (and other offenses). See, for example, Martincin (2016).

12 Turner (2015: 212) writes an encomium to Betty White, praising her both for the longevity of her career and for her "consistent use of blue humor and her multiple portrayals of ageism and sexism." I respectfully both agree and disagree. On "Hot in Cleveland," White's sexuality is not portrayed *qua* sexuality but *qua* comedy; evidence is that it plays with a laugh track.

13 Defining "cultural age," Woodward (2006: 183) writes, "[O]lder women who are the same chronological age as men are considered to be 'older' than men."

14 Burke (1966: 5) describes the principle of continuity and discontinuity.

15 S. Lochlann Jain, who was diagnosed with cancer at the age of 36, writes, "If you're going to die at forty, shouldn't you be able to get the senior discount at the movies when you're thirty-five? Does the senior's discount reward a long life, or proximity to death?" (2013: 29).

16 Narratives, as we know, can sponsor identification. See, for example, Loe (2011) and Woodward (2003).

References

Applewhite A. In: Yo, is this ageist? Available at: http://yoisthisageist.com. Last accessed: 10 February 2018.

Applewhite A. 2016. *This Chair Rocks: A Manifesto Against Ageism.* New York, NY: Networked Books.

Archard D. Review of Helen Small, "The Long Life." *Philosophical Quarterly.* 2009; 59: 568–70.

Berkenkotter C. 2008. *Patient Tales: Case Histories and Uses of Narrative in Psychiatry.* Columbia, SC: University of South Carolina Press.

Blakeborough D. "Old people are useless": Representations of aging on *The Simpsons. Canadian Journal on Aging.* 2008; 27: 57–67.

Burke K. 1966. *Language as Symbolic Action: Essays on Life, Literature, and Method.* Berkeley, CA: University of California Press.

Burke K. 1969. *A Rhetoric of Motives.* Berkeley, CA: University of California Press.

Burke K. 1984/1954. *Permanence and Change,* 3rd ed. Berkeley, CA: University of California Press.

Charise A. "Let the reader think of the burden": Old age and the crisis of capacity. *Occasion: Interdisciplinary Studies in the Humanities.* 2012; 4: 1–16.

Chast R. 2014. *Can't We Talk about Something More Pleasant?* New York, NY: Bloomsbury.

Chivers S. 2011. *The Silvering Screen: Old Age and Disability in Cinema.* Toronto: University of Toronto Press.

Condit CM. 1999. *The Meanings of the Gene: Public Debates about Human Heredity.* Madison, WI: University of Wisconsin Press.

Cruikshank M. 2013/2003 (3rd ed.). *Learning to Be Old: Gender, Culture, and Aging.* Lanham, MD: Rowman and Littlefield.

Davis HG. 2017. How to survive a family vacation with the grandparents. *The Globe and Mail,* 13 December. Available at: www.theglobeandmail.com/life/travel/how-to-survive-a-family-vacation-with-the-grandparents/article37315085/#c-image-0. Last accessed: 28 May 2018.

de Beauvoir S. 1996/1970. *The Coming of Age.* New York, NY: Norton.

Derkatch C. 2016. *Bounding Biomedicine: Evidence and Rhetoric in the New Science of Alternative Medicine.* Chicago, IL: University of Chicago Press.

Ehrenreich B. 2018. *Natural Causes: An Epidemic of Wellness, the Certainty of Dying, and Killing Ourselves to Live Longer.* New York, NY: Twelve Books.

Ellison KL. Age transcended: A semiotic and rhetorical analysis of the discourse of agelessness in North American anti-aging skin care advertisements. *Journal of Aging Studies.* 2014; 29: 20–31.

Emanuel EJ. 2014. Why I hope to die at 75, *The Atlantic* (October). Available at: www.theatlantic.com/magazine/archive/2014/10/why-i-hope-to-die-at-75/379329. Last accessed: 6 June 2018.

Frazer C. 2017. Our parents are our future. *The New Yorker,* 25 September. Available at: www.newyorker.com/magazine/2017/09/25/our-parents-are-our-future. Last accessed: 28 May 2018.

Graham SS. 2015. *The Politics of Pain Medicine: A Rhetorical-Ontological Inquiry.* Chicago, IL: University of Chicago Press.

Gullette MM. 2004. *Aged by Culture.* Chicago, IL: University of Chicago Press.

Gullette MM. 2011. *Agewise: Fighting the New Ageism in America.* Chicago, IL: University of Chicago Press.

Gullette MM. 2017a. Margaret Morganroth Gullette: Against "aging"—How to talk about growing older. *Theory Culture & Society,* 21 December. Available at: www.theoryculturesociety.org/margaret-morganroth-gullette-aging-talk-growing-older. Last accessed: 24 May 2018.

Gullette MM. 2017b. *Ending Ageism, or How Not to Shoot Old People.* New Brunswick, NJ: Rutgers University Press.

Hacking I. 1999. *The Social Construction of What?* Cambridge, MA: Harvard University Press.

Hacking I. 2002. *Historical Ontology.* Cambridge, MA: Harvard University Press.

Harding S. 1993. Rethinking standpoint epistemology: What is "strong objectivity"? In: L Alcott, E Porter (eds.) *Feminist Epistemologies.* New York, NY: Routledge, 49–82.

Hart R. 1994. Wandering with rhetorical criticism. In: W Nothstine, C Blair C, G Copeland (eds.) *Critical Questions: Invention, Creativity, and the Criticism of Discourse and Media.* New York, NY: St. Martin's Press, 71–81.

Herndl DP. Our breasts, our selves: Identity, community, and ethics in cancer autobiographies. *Signs: Journal of Women in Culture and Society.* 2006; 32: 221–45.

Hess A. 2017. Old money. *New York Times Magazine,* 17 September, 13–15.

Jabour B. 2016. Boomers and millennials: This is not intergenerational warfare, it's class warfare. *The Guardian*, 6 April. Available at: www.theguardian.com/commentisfree/2016/apr/06/boomers-and-millennials-this-is-not-intergenerational-warfare-its-class-warfare. Last accessed: 4 June 2018.

Jain, SL. 2013. *Malignant: How Cancer Becomes Us*. Berkeley and Los Angeles, CA: University of California Press.

Jensen RE. 2016. *Infertility: Tracing the History of a Transformative Term*. Pennsylvania, PA: Pennsylvania State University Press.

Johnson J. The skeleton on the couch: The Eagleton affair, rhetorical disability, and the stigma of mental illness. *Rhetoric Society Quarterly* 2010; 40: 459–78.

Johnson J. 2014. *American Lobotomy: A Rhetorical History*. Ann Arbor, MI: University of Michigan Press.

Katz S. 2009. *Cultural Aging: Life Course, Lifestyle, and Senior Worlds*. Toronto: University of Toronto Press.

Kauffman M, Morris HJ (creators). *Grace and Frankie*, 2015–present [Netflix]. Okay Goodnight and Skydance Television, United States.

Keränen L. 2010. *Scientific Characters: Rhetoric, Politics, and Trust in Breast Cancer Research*. Tuscaloosa, AL: University of Alabama Press.

Keränen L. 2014. "This weird, incurable disease": Competing diagnoses in the rhetoric of Morgellons. In: T Jones, D Wear, LD Friedman (eds.) *Health Humanities Reader*. New Brunswick, NJ: Rutgers University Press, 36–49.

Kerman P. 2010. *Orange Is the New Black: My Year in a Women's Prison*. New York, NY: Spiegel & Grau.

Koerber A. 2018. *From Hysteria to Hormones: A Rhetorical History*. University Park, PA: Pennsylvania State University Press.

Kohan J (creator). *Orange Is the New Black*, 2013–present [Netflix]. Lionsgate Television and Tilted Productions, United States.

Lamb S. Permanent personhood or meaningful decline? Toward a critical anthropology of successful aging. *Journal of Aging Studies*. 2014; 29: 41–52.

Lee M. The end of "anti-aging." *Allure* 2017: 30.

Lipscomb VB. 2016. *Performing Age in Modern Drama*. London: Palgrave Macmillan.

Loe M. 2011. *Aging Our Way: Independent Elders, Interdependent Lives*. Oxford: Oxford University Press.

Martin S (creator). *Hot in Cleveland*, 2010–2015 [TV Land]. Hazy Mills Productions, SamJen Productions, and TV Land Original Productions, United States.

Martincin K. 2016. Is your birthday card a microaggression? APA Counselling Psychology Division: Older Adult Special Interest Group (nd). Available at: https://div17oasig.wordpress.com/2015/03/09/is-your-birthday-card-a-microaggression. Last accessed: 16 May 2018.

Meloncon L, Scott JB. 2018. Introduction: Manifesting methodologies for the rhetoric of health and medicine. In: L Meloncon, JB Scott (eds.) *Methodologies for the Rhetoric of Health and Medicine*. New York, NY: Routledge, 1–23.

Metzl JM, Kirkland A (eds.) 2010. *Against Health: How Health Became the New Morality*. New York, NY: New York University Press.

Nussbaum MC. 2016. *Anger and Forgiveness: Resentment, Generosity, Justice*. New York, NY: Oxford.

Nussbaum MC, Levmore S. 2017. *Aging Thoughtfully: Conversations about Retirement, Romance, Wrinkles, and Regret*. Oxford: Oxford University Press.

Reiff D. 2008. Why I had to lie to my dying mother. *The Observer*, 18 May. Available at: www.theguardian.com/books/2008/may/18/society. Last accessed: 6 June 2018.

Rozanova J. Discourse of successful aging in the *Globe and Mail*. *Canadian Journal of Age Studies*. 2010; 213–22.

Scott JB. 2003. *Risky Rhetoric: AIDS and the Cultural Practices of HIV Testing*. Carbondale, IL: Southern Illinois University Press.

Segal JZ. 2005. *Health and the Rhetoric of Medicine*. Carbondale, IL: Southern Illinois University Press.

Segal JZ. Breast cancer narratives as public rhetoric: Genre itself and the maintenance of ignorance. *Linguistics and the Human Sciences*. 2007; 3: 3–24.

Segal JZ. 2009. Rhetoric of health and medicine. In: A Lunsford (ed.) *Sage Handbook of Rhetorical Studies*. Thousand Oaks, CA: Sage Publications, 227–45.

Segal JZ. 2015. The view from here and there: Objectivity and the rhetoric of breast cancer. In: F Padovani, A Richardson, JY Tsou (eds.) *Objectivity in Science: New Perspectives from Science and Technology Studies*. Dordrecht: Springer.

Segal L. 2014. *Out of Time: The Pleasures and Perils of Ageing*. New York, NY: Verso.

Showalter E. 2014. Introduction to *Out of Time: The Pleasures and Perils of Ageing* by Segal L. New York, NY: Verso.

Sinding C, Gray R. Active aging—spunky survivorship? Discourses and experiences of the years beyond breast cancer. *Journal of Aging Studies.* 2005; 19: 147–61.

Sontag S. 1972. The double standard of aging. *The Saturday Review,* 23 September, 29–38.

Teston C. 2017. *Bodies in Flux: Scientific Methods for Negotiating Medical Uncertainty.* Chicago, IL: University of Chicago Press.

Turner KM. 2015. The Betty White moment: The rhetoric of constructing aging and sexuality. In: N Jones, B Batchelor (eds.) *Aging Heroes: Growing Old in Popular Culture.* Lanham, MD: Rowman and Littlefield, 211–22.

Wente M. 2017. What's so scary about free speech on campus? *The Globe and Mail,* 14 November. Available at: www.theglobeandmail.com/opinion/whats-so-scary-about-free-speech-on-campus/article36948480. Last accessed: 14 November 2017.

Woodward K. 2003. Against wisdom: The social politics of anger and aging. *Journal of Aging Studies.* 17: 55–67.

Woodward K. Performing age, performing gender. *NWSA [National Women's Studies Association] Journal.* 2006; 18: 162–89.

16

THE RHETORICAL POSSIBILITIES OF A MULTI-METAPHORICAL VIEW OF CLINICAL SUPERVISION

Lorelei Lingard and Mark Goldszmidt

Every way of seeing is a way of not seeing.

(K. Burke)

Metaphor matters because it creates expectations.

(James Geary)

We've been systematically exploring clinical supervision for almost 20 years in medical education, resulting in careful definitions, guides, recommendations and practical tips (Kilminster and Jolly 2000; Kilminster et al. 2007; Martin, Copley and Tyack 2014). Notwithstanding this knowledge, fundamental gaps in our understanding persist. Supervisory practice has been described as "the least investigated, discussed and developed aspect of clinical teaching" (Kilminster and Jolly 2000: 827). While the supervisory relationship has been identified as the single most important factor in supervision, it has been acknowledged that much remains unknown about it, including the influence of context, the variability of relationships, the implications of teams and the role of judgement (Kilminster et al. 2007). And a discomfiting sense persists that "despite the importance of clinical supervision to professional development and practice, there is a lack of research regarding how it is best conducted . . . [and] a lack of awareness among practitioners regarding effective supervisory strategies" (Martin, Copley and Tyack 2014: 202). How can we know so much about clinical supervision, and yet understand so little? This chapter argues that the answer lies at least in part in the metaphors we have used to describe and understand it.

Conceptual framework: what's in a metaphor?

As "wordlings" (Burke 1966), human beings are hopelessly entangled with metaphor. Metaphor is a way of thinking in new ways, releasing persuasive and imaginative power. Far from being merely a stylistic or literary device, metaphor structures everyday life in ways we hardly notice because they are mostly unconscious (Lakoff and Johnson 1980). Thus, metaphor constitutes a powerful, everyday rhetoric through which we reflect and reproduce our beliefs about our world. It also offers a way to *reimagine* that world, to realise what Kenneth Burke espoused as the curative power of language. Championing the imaginative possibilities of metaphor in medicine and medical education, Bleakley (2017: 33) argued that medicine "needs better metaphors" and better attunement to them in physicians and trainees. By "better" metaphors, he meant those that open up new possibilities by embracing uncertainty, confronting complexity and affirming collectivism. His book on metaphors in medicine is a call to "realize the power of metaphor in medicine—for both good and bad—[and] to recognize the central place of the imagination in medicine" (ibid.: 214).

This chapter takes up that call, with a specific focus on the discourse of clinical supervision. First, we excavate some conventional metaphors of clinical supervision, with particular attention to the literature on definitions, guides and frameworks. Then we imagine new metaphors for clinical supervision, drawing on naturalistic research conducted over the past decade. Our analytical strategy is to attend to how each metaphor persuades by selecting, directing and deflecting our attention (Burke 1966).

Conventional metaphors: how do we currently know clinical supervision?

In the literature on clinical supervision, conventional metaphors abound. We will organise them in terms of Lakoff and Johnson's (1980) typology of orientational, ontological and structural metaphors. Orientational metaphors, in which concepts are spatially related to each other (e.g., up or down, in or out, deep or shallow), are evident in key terms such as *under supervision, oversee* and even *observe* (which comes from the Latin *observare*, to watch over). Etymologically, the verb 'to supervise' is itself an orientational metaphor, 'to look over' from Medieval Latin *supervisus* (McDonald 1964: 643), which has been absorbed into normal usage such that its status *as* metaphor is concealed.

Ontological metaphors, representing the abstract as concrete, also abound. Supervision is a *container* inside of which we find other things (e.g., clinical supervision should include practices such as observation and feedback); supervision is an *entity* that can be structured or built (e.g., *models* of supervision, supervisory *arrangements*); and supervision is a *substance* of which we increase or decrease the *levels, amounts, quantity* or *intensity*. The last of these underpins the common metaphor of clinical supervision as a 'balancing act' between trainee learning and patient safety. Too little supervision and patients might be hurt; too much and trainees might not develop their expertise.

Structural metaphors, in which one concept is understood and expressed in terms of another, also recur. These include the metaphor of supervision-as-relationship, which engenders notions of relationship *building, quality, commitment* and *roles*. The metaphor of supervision-as-transaction manifests in such concepts as *providing* supervision, and supervision *contracts, partnerships* and *products*. And the metaphor of supervision-as-machine is evident in efforts to enumerate its various *parts*, characterise its *inputs* or *elements* and assess its *outcomes* and *effects*.

Such conventional metaphors perpetuate into common sense a set of assumptions. We would draw attention to four of these. The first is the binary assumption: clinical supervision is a balance between two competing forces or values. Most often, the binary is represented as patient safety and trainee learning. The second is the realism assumption: clinical supervision exists independent of perception—thus the focus on concrete dimensions in frameworks and limited attention to context and nuance. The third is the linearity assumption: clinical supervision is a relationship in which power is hierarchically structured. For the most part, supervisors are considered to exert their power over trainees. And the fourth is the neutrality assumption:

clinical supervision is a cognitive, dispassionate practice, not an affective one. Aside from some attention to conflict and trust, the influence of emotion on supervision is ignored in our conventional metaphors.

These assumptions have consequences. They simplify rather than complexify our understanding of clinical supervision, concretising the abstract, sanitising the messy. They translate the question of *how* supervision is realised into *how much* supervision is provided. They homogenise into idealised norms an array of nuanced, variable relationships emerging at the intersection of multiple, competing exigencies. Is it any wonder, then, that we understand little about how supervision actually unfolds?

Emerging metaphors: how can we otherwise understand clinical supervision?

This section of the chapter imagines 13 metaphors to expand our conventional conceptualisations of clinical supervision. They are organised, loosely, according to the assumption(s) they trouble. The organisation is not developmental: we do not intend to suggest a trajectory towards the 'perfect' metaphor. There is no perfect metaphor. Rather, we hope to illustrate how different metaphors draw our attention to different aspects of clinical supervision, and to reflect on how they may help us to productively trouble deep-seated assumptions about what clinical supervision is, and should be.

Metaphors that trouble the binary assumption

The ontological metaphor of 'balancing' patient safety and trainee learning—picture a set of weighing scales—helps us to acknowledge that these two values are in relationship and that their relationship is often one of tension. However, the metaphor is limiting in its assumption that, as one side goes up, the other must, according to the laws of physics, go down: more supervision increases patient safety but decreases learner independence, less supervision decreases patient safety but increases learner independence. Following this ontological metaphor, we draw conclusions and create policies (RCPSC 2013). But the metaphor is overly simplistic.

To trouble the ontology of 'balancing,' let's consider a metaphor like *the supervisory juggling act*. This metaphor is inspired by Goldszmidt et al.'s (2015) study of clinical supervision in internal medicine, in which attending physicians combined a triad of supervisory practices—teaching, supervision and patient care—into four recurring supervisory 'styles': direct care, empowerment, mixed practice and minimalist. Importantly, Goldszmidt et al. realised that the combinations of the three practices into a particular supervisory style (what we would conceptualise as 'juggling') was neither random nor idiosyncratic: it constituted a response to broader organisational forces in the clinical training environment such as wait lists and bed census tracking. For example, direct care supervision (in which teaching and supervision receded, and the supervisor took over patient care from the trainees) was a common response to the pressure to discharge patients. An advantage of the juggling metaphor is that the number of objects in the air is not dictated: Goldszmidt et al. conceptualised a triad, but one could justifiably imagine expanding the triad (e.g., adding assessment) or subdividing it (e.g., breaking teaching into multiple dimensions). The focus of the juggling metaphor is not a number; the focus is rather on what emerging research (e.g., Steinert, Basi and Nugus 2017) recognises as a multiplicity of practices combined according to context.

Another metaphor that troubles the binary comes from Kennedy et al. (2007), who described how clinical supervisors created the illusion of independence for trainees through backstage oversight. The illusion was achieved by enacting supervisory strategies outside the view and awareness of the trainee, such as viewing test results in the electronic health record. Through **supervision by illusion**, supervisors can transcend the binary trade-off between 'increase' and 'decrease,' and find ways to achieve both.

Conventional metaphors foreground another binary: the supervisory dyad of faculty and trainee. Focusing on the dyad deflects our attention from understanding **supervision as diffusion**. Supervision takes place in workplace settings where activity is collective, and trainees access that collective strategically. Junior trainees seek guidance from more senior trainees before taking questions to their faculty supervisor. Trainees access the expertise of other health professionals such as nurses (Tamuz et al. 2011), while organisational structures (such as rotation schedules), genre systems and policies (such as pharmacy checks on medication orders) also participate in the diffused system of supervision (Cadieux and Goldszmidt 2017).

Metaphors that trouble the realism assumption

As the illusion and diffusion metaphors begin to suggest, supervision is not always what it seems. We can further trouble the realism assumption by imagining **supervision as performance**. Following Goffman's (1959) representation of life as a theatre (and embodied in Kennedy's notion of 'backstage oversight'), the metaphor of 'performance' highlights that both supervisors and trainees are acting a part *for* particular audiences, embodying motivations, following norms and having effects. For example, in a programme of research exploring oral case presentations delivered by trainees to supervisors during morning rounds, Lingard et al. (2003) argued that these are 'presentations' of not only the patient but also the trainee. The supervisor has not witnessed much of what the trainee has done (history interview, physical examination, ordering of labs): the case presentation represents a performance of those actions for the supervisory audience. In this regard, the performance has two motivations: it transfers information about the patient, and it stands in as a 'proxy' for the trainee's competence in unobserved tasks (Kennedy et al. 2008: S91).

This proxy function—*fluency as competency*—participates in the extended metaphors of both illusion and performance. It does rhetorical work, persuading the supervisor that the trainee is either competent due to a fluent narrative, or incompetent due to a dysfluent one (Kennedy and Lingard 2007). The representation is not always straightforward: trainees who *sound* competent but are not can fool faculty. Beyond the supervisory exchange, fluency as competency does rhetorical work to enable a human resource system in which trainees *do* much of the clinical work in the teaching hospital and supervisors *hear* about that work but participate only partially in it. Our tacit acceptance of the illusion of supervision—made possible when we use fluent telling as a proxy for competent doing and thinking—is necessary to maintain this clinical training system. Without it, clinical supervision is untenable: we do not have the supervisory resources to physically oversee all the trainee labour in a teaching hospital.

The realism assumption sets us up to understand supervision as a product that supervisors *provide* and trainees *receive*. But supervision is not merely transmission. **Supervision is co-construction.** By the co-construction metaphor, we intend to represent both how supervisor and trainee work together and how they *know together*. In a study of laparoscopic surgery training, Cope et al. (2015) found that much of the supervisory interaction centred on "visual cue interpretation" through two dialogic sequences. In "guided co-construction," the supervisor focused the trainee's eye to see what the supervisor was seeing. In "authentic co-construction," neither supervisor nor trainee appeared certain of what they were seeing, so they created knowledge collaboratively. "Authentic co-construction" is not limited to the operating theatre; research in general practice has also described how supervisors "manage with" senior trainees to collaboratively understand clinical problems (Brown et al. 2018). Authentic co-construction draws our attention to a feature of clinical supervision rarely visible in conventional metaphors: sometimes supervisors are uncertain, and the 'supervision' is a mutual process of coming to know.

Metaphors that trouble the linearity assumption

Taking this line of thinking a bit further, we can acknowledge that supervisors may not have as much control as we have conventionally thought, or as they'd like. Notwithstanding the etymology of the word—'over seeing from on high'—supervision is not simply a case of linear power relations.

It has been our experience that clinical supervisors who appear at research meetings during a stint on the wards often look like they're ***weathering a storm***. This metaphor troubles the linearity assumption by zooming us out from our usual focus on supervisor and trainee to see them from a distance, sharing a tiny boat on a dark sea, buffeted from all sides by wind and wave, steering a course dictated at least as much by the elements as by any preplanned destination. We can play with the storm metaphor to reimagine the problem of 'supervisor control.' We might picture both trainee and supervisor in the same boat and realise that the supervisor does not control the elements and cannot protect the trainee from them. We might picture them in two different boats carelessly lashed together, reflecting their differing motivations and perceptions of the supervisory encounter. Or we might picture them in the same boat, pulling the rudder in different directions. Baranova and Goldszmidt (2018) have recently found that supervisors and trainees on inpatient teaching teams may disagree about fundamental aspects of the 'storm,' such as the purpose of a hospital admission. These disagreements can have them pulling in opposite directions with their definition of patient problems and their perceived solutions, with one narrowly defining the presenting problem and targeting timely discharge and the other broadly defining a constellation of problems and advocating more holistic care. More senior-level trainees may be particularly likely to resist their supervisor, using strategies such as 'doing without reviewing,' or waiting for the supervisor to rotate off the team and then re-negotiating plans with another supervisor.

Such research represents supervision as entanglement, rather than as linear power relations. And entanglements are multiple and unpredictable, as Apramian et al.'s (2015) metaphor of ***thresholding*** suggests. Exploring how faculty's individual procedural variations shaped supervision in surgery, they found that each supervisor had a distinct threshold between principles (how things must be done, such as appropriate tissue handling) and preferences (how things might be done, such as the selection of suture types). Trainees engaged in 'thresholding,' trying to recognise and respond appropriately to these thresholds as they worked with different surgical supervisors. The metaphor of 'thresholding' expands our thinking in three important ways. First, in spotlighting the subjectivity of supervision, it challenges the assumption that individual supervisors represent a community standard and can be interchanged without undermining the integrity of that standard (Apramian et al. 2019). Second, the thresholding metaphor orients us to the complex ways in which trainees engage in supervision: they quickly recognise that thresholds are multiple and moving; they readily accommodate the irony that reproducing one supervisor's preference may mean violating another's principle; they periodically resist a threshold but rarely do so explicitly; and they gradually form their own thresholds out of the experience of negotiating those of others. Third, thresholding begs the question: 'is "competence" in the eye of the beholder, just a supervisor's recognition of their own thresholds mirrored back to them?'

Another metaphor of entanglement is Sebok-Syer et al.'s (2018) theory of **coupling**. In interviews with faculty and senior postgraduate trainees, they heard repeatedly about the difficulty of identifying independent trainee performances on which to base competency assessments. Most trainee performances were perceived not to be independent at all, but to be profoundly interdependent—with supervisors, other trainees, healthcare professionals and system factors. Sebok-Syer et al. (ibid.) used the metaphor of 'coupling' to conceptualise clinical performances as joint performances, and trainees and supervisors as implicated in and by one another's actions. The metaphor of coupling begs some critical questions for assessment, including: how do we judge individual competence if performance is fundamentally interdependent? And how can we persist in translating interdependent performances into assessment tools that assume independence?

The metaphor's theoretical roots in organisational science direct our attention to supervision as a complex system, and provide a vocabulary for exploring the nature and degree of interdependence of system components (Orton and Weick 1990; Lingard et al. 2014). The coupling metaphor also carries another meaning, one with overtones of personal and physical intimacy. This metaphorical meaning creates an uncomfortable clash by bringing together sexual entanglement and supervisory entanglement. Our code of medical professionalism makes such a metaphor taboo, and so we are conditioned to ignore it. But, following Burke's (1961) theory of "perspective by incongruity," an uncomfortable metaphor holds the most potential to help us see in new ways. This includes spotlighting dark corners we have carefully kept in the shadows. One dark corner is the emotionality of supervision.

Metaphors that trouble the neutrality assumption

Our conventional metaphors of clinical supervision are void of emotion. This void is not specific to clinical supervision: emotions are largely ignored across the field of medical education, in both its scientific endeavours and its professional socialisation processes (McNaughton and LeBlanc 2012). The void is also not specific to medical education; a theoretical review from behavioural psychotherapy criticised its "heartless accounts" of clinical supervision (Lombardo, Milne and Proctor 2009: 207). The absence of emotion in our conceptualisations of clinical supervision has profound rhetorical effects; in eliding emotion, we make it not just invisible, but unspeakable. This is particularly problematic with regards to darker emotions such as fear, despair, hurt and anger.

Many physicians experience a crippling combination of responsibility and powerlessness in today's healthcare environment. Just as fatigue, burnout, stress and loss of empathy plague clinical practice, so too do they influence clinical supervision. The metaphor of **Atlas's burden**—for the Titan condemned to hold up the sky for eternity—might capture the despair that descends when a faculty supervisor finds herself with 25 patients (plus eight more admitted overnight), one senior resident (going home post call), two junior residents and an off-service resident, three medical students, demanding pages from central administration (regarding bed census), an expectation to teach (something, anything!) during morning rounds, and requests from residents for (now overdue) Entrustable-Professional-Activity assessments. Faced with this situation, supervisors may try to hold up the sky single-handedly, enacting medicine's values of strength, endurance and heroism. But the Atlas's burden metaphor challenges the hero narrative, foregrounding a sense of vulnerability, futility and despair. The solution to 'hold up the sky' will often produce in supervisors the sensation of staggering under the weight of their obligations as teachers, supervisors and care providers, failing to make visible progress in any of these, and realising that tomorrow will bring more of the same.

What about trainees' experience of the emotionality of clinical supervision? According to a study of comics drawn by medical students, they wish they could wake from their *supervision nightmare* (George and Green 2015). Almost half of trainee drawings used horror-genre images to represent the emotionally harrowing aspects of supervision. Among the powerful metaphors in trainees' drawings, clinical workplaces were dank dungeons and post-apocalyptic landscapes, supervisors were demons, devils and monsters, and trainees were sleep-deprived zombies and victims of violent castigation.

Published guidelines, definitions and tips on clinical supervision ignore these darker emotional dimensions. Interestingly, more positive emotions are largely absent as well. One exception is the notion of trust, which is prominently featured in both published frameworks and research. In fact, *supervision as entrustment* is coming into common parlance with the implementation of competency-based medical education (ten Cate et al. 2016). However, trust in this conceptuali-sation is portrayed as a cognitive more than an affective dimension; it is depicted as a judgement that supervisors make, rather than an emotion that supervisors and trainees experience.

Finally, we should note the emergence of *supervision by surveillance*. Martin et al. (2017) reported that 97% of supervisors in their study conducted backstage oversight of trainees' deci-sion and actions by accessing the electronic medical record remotely. As medical education becomes increasingly enamoured with the prospects of "big data" (Arora 2018), "learning analytics" (Cirigliano et al. 2017) and "dashboards" (Boscardin et al. 2017), supervision by surveillance is moving towards automation and institutionalisation. Current discussions of big data envision its integration with observation, feedback and coaching for meaningful track-ing of trainee performance. But given concerns about faculty capacity to supply the increased assessment information required for Competency-Based Medical Education (CBME), supervi-sion by surveillance could quickly outstrip faculty-generated insights. In naming this metaphor into being, we hope to encourage debate about the assumption of neutrality inherent in it: are data neutral?

Conclusion: what are the rhetorical possibilities of a multi-metaphorical view?

In excavating, analysing and extending our metaphors of clinical supervision, we hope to open up new rhetorical possibilities. By 'rhetorical' here, we echo Burke's argument for the curative potential of language. All language is 'symbolic action,' not only describing but also constructing our attitudes and actions. Metaphors have particular constructive power, being both pervasive and possessed of the ability to help us to see in new ways.

Conventional metaphors of clinical supervision reproduce a particular conceptualisation of clinical supervision as binary, realist, linear and neutral. This has consequences. Ontologically, it orients us to understand supervision as a matter of trade-offs, objective behaviours, hierarchical power structures and dispassionate interactions. Epistemologically, it predisposes us to assemble instrumental knowledge about clinical supervision such as tips, guidelines and definitions, and it orients us to ask 'how much?' rather than 'how?' questions. Rhetorically, our conventional metaphors limit what we can say, see, know, understand and do about clinical supervision. Most problematically, they deflect our attention away from understanding what is an unpredictable practice at the intersection of multiple, competing and powerful forces, both human and mate-rial, in the clinical training environment.

We have offered 13 metaphors to help us see clinical supervision in new ways: juggling, illusion, diffusion, performance, fluency, co-construction, weathering a storm, thresholding, coupling, Atlas's burden, nightmare, entrustment and surveillance. Some of these metaphors, like *thresholding* and *coupling*, we've drawn from recent naturalistic research into how supervision works. Others, like *diffusion* and *surveillance*, we've named into being to prompt reflection and debate. Our intent is that this set of new metaphors will serve as 'better' metaphors in Bleakley's (2017) sense that they open up possibilities by troubling assumptions about what supervision is, or what it should become. However, the real possibility lies not in any individual metaphor. The rhetorical possibilities for 'seeing differently' are maximised from a multi-metaphorical approach.

A multi-metaphorical approach can attune us to the endless manifestations, the inherent complexities and the glaring contradictions that make up clinical supervision. By reflecting our experience through multiple metaphors, we can see that clinical supervision is both real and relative, both practice and performance. It is made up of both binaries and multiples. It manifests as both linear hierarchy and nonlinear entanglement. It engages both cognition and affect. We offer this kaleidoscopic view of clinical supervision as a way to cultivate critical awareness. Most of us have a limited store of conventional conceptualisations of clinical supervision. A multi-metaphorical approach can help us to identify our default conceptualisations and question the assumptions that underpin them. It can help us to ask what different conceptualisations might mean for our attitudes and actions as supervisors or trainees. It can prompt us to explore the dominant conceptualisations in our particular clinical training contexts, and to ask what purposes they serve there. It can alert us to the implications of new conceptualisations that are fast becoming common sense in our field. And it can mobilise us to imagine an increasingly elaborate suite of metaphors that, together, better represent the nuanced, relational, situational phenomenon that is clinical supervision.

References

Apramian T, Cristancho S, Watling C, et al. Thresholds of principle and preference: exploring procedural variation in postgraduate surgical education. *Academic Medicine.* 2015; 90: S70–6.

Apramian T, Cristancho S, Sener A, Lingard L. How do thresholds of principle and preference influence Surgeon assessments of learner performance? *Annals of Surgery.* 2019; 268: 385–90.

Arora VM. Harnessing the power of big data to improve graduate medical education: big idea or bust? *Academic Medicine.* 2018; 93: 833–4.

Baranova K, Goldszmidt M. 2018. Roles in tension: it's time to start talking about the purpose of a hospital admission. Canadian Conference on Medical Education, Halifax, NS.

Bleakley A. 2017. *Thinking with Metaphors in Medicine: The State of the Art.* New York, NY: Routledge.

Boscardin C, Fergus KB, Hellevig B, Hauer KE. Twelve tips to promote successful development of a learner performance dashboard within a medical education program. *Medical Teacher.* 2017; 9: 1–7.

Brown J, Nestel D, Clement T, Goldszmidt M. The supervisory encounter and the senior GP trainee: managing for, through and with. *Medical Education.* 2018; 52: 192–205.

Burke K. 1961. *The Philosophy of Literary Form: Studies in Symbolic Action.* New York, NY: Vintage Books.

Burke K. 1966. *Language as Symbolic Action: Essays on Life, Literature, and Method.* Berkeley, CA: University of California Press.

Cadieux DC, Goldszmidt M. It's not just what you know: junior trainees' approach to follow-up and documentation *Medical Education.* 2017: 51: 812–25.

Cirigliano MM, Guthrie C, Pusic MV, et al. "Yes, and . . .": Exploring the future of learning analytics in medical education. *Teaching and Learning in Medicine.* 2017; 29: 368–72.

Cope A, Bezemer J, Kneebone R, Lingard L. "You see?": teaching and learning how to interpret visual cues during surgery. *Medical Education.* 2015; 49: 1103–16.

George DR, Green MJ. Lessons learned from comics produced by medical students: art of darkness. *JAMA.* 2015; 314: 2345–6.

Goffman E. 1959. *The Presentation of Self in Everyday Life.* Garden City, NY: Doubleday.

Goldszmidt M, Dornan T, van Merriënboer J, et al. Attending physician variability: a model of four supervisory styles. *Academic Medicine.* 2015; 90: 1541–6.

Kennedy TJ, Lingard L, Baker GR, et al. Clinical oversight: conceptualizing the relationship between supervision and safety. *Journal of General Internal Medicine.* 2007; 22: 1080–5.

Kennedy TJ, Lingard L. Questioning competence: a discourse analysis of attending physicians' use of questions to assess trainee competence. *Academic Medicine.* 2007; 82: S12–S15.

Kennedy TJT, Regehr G, Baker GR, Lingard L. Point-of-care assessment of medical trainee competence for independent clinical work. *Academic Medicine.* 2008; 83: S89–S92.

Kilminster S, Jolly B. Effective supervision in clinical practice settings: a literature review. *Medical Education.* 2000; 34: 827–40.

Kilminster S, Cottrell D, Grant J, Jolly B. AMEE Guide No. 27: effective educational and clinical supervision. *Medical Teacher.* 2007; 29: 2–19.

Lakoff G, Johnson M. 1980. *Metaphors We Live By.* Chicago, IL: University of Chicago Press.

Lingard L, Garwood, K, Schryer, C, Spafford, M. (2003). A certain art of uncertainty: case presentation and the development of professional identity. *Social Science and Medicine.* 56: 603–17.

Lingard L, McDougall A, Levstik M, et al. Using loose coupling theory to understand interprofessional collaborative practice on a transplantation team. *Journal of Research in Interprofessional Practice and Education.* 2014; 3: 1–17.

Lombardo C, Milne D, Proctor R. Getting to the heart of clinical supervision: a theoretical review of the role of emotions in professional development. *Behavioural and Cognitive Psychotherapy.* 2009; 37: 207–19.

Martin P, Copley J, Tyack Z. Twelve tips for effective clinical supervision based on a narrative literature review and expert opinion. *Medical Teacher.* 2014; 36: 201–7.

Martin SK, Tulla K, Meltzer DO, et al. Attending physician remote access of the electronic health record and implications for resident supervision: a mixed methods study. *Journal of Graduate Medical Education.* 2017; 9: 706–13.

McDonald AM. 1964. *Chamber's Etymological English Dictionary.* London: WR Chambers, Ltd.

McNaughton N, LeBlanc V. 2012. Perturbations: the central role of emotional competence in medical training. In: B Hodges, L Lingard (eds.) *The Question of Competence: Reconsidering Medical Education in the Twenty-First Century.* Ithaca, NY: Cornell University Press, 70–96.

Orton JD, Weick KE. Loosely coupled systems: a reconceptualization. *Academy of Management Review.* 1990; 15: 203–23.

Royal College of Physicians and Surgeons of Canada. (2013). *General Standards of Accreditation: The Descriptors Document.* Available at: www.royalcollege.ca/portal/page/portal/rc/common/documents/accreditation/accreditation_blue_book_b_descriptors_e.pdf. Last accessed: April 22, 2018.

Sebok-Syer, Chahine S, Watling C, et al. Considering the interdependence of trainee clinical performance: implications for assessment and entrustment. *Med Educ.* 2018. April 19. doi: 10.1111/medu.13588.

Steinert Y, Basi M, Nugus P. How physicians teach in the clinical setting: the embedded roles of teaching and clinical care. *Medical Teacher.* 2017; 39: 1238–44.

Tamuz M, Giardina TD, Thomas EJ, et al. Rethinking resident supervision to improve safety: from hierarchical to interprofessional models. *British Journal of Hospital Medicine.* 2011; 68: 448–56.

Ten Cate O, Hart D, Ankel F, et al. international competency-based medical education collaborators: entrustment decision making in clinical training. *Academic Medicine.* 2016; 91: 191–8.

17

THE CHAOTIC NARRATIVES OF ANTI-VACCINATION

Katherine Shwetz

Narratives of anti-vaccination

Let us briefly compare two stories: in one, a sinister governmental force conspires with powerful corporations to inject a mysterious toxin into the bloodstreams of the unsuspecting public, who must rally together in order to stop the conspiracy.

In another story, parents immunise their children, protecting them from vaccine-preventable diseases. The children do not fall ill, nor do they endanger the health of others. In short, as a blogger using the pseudonym 'Humble Mom' on *Moms Who Vax* put it in their own consideration of these two different narratives, "nothing happen[s]." "The anti-vaccine movement, to be honest," the blogger wrote, "is a lot more interesting than reality. Their rants and theories are the stuff of trashy novels and Michael Bay movies." From a public health point of view, 'nothing happens' is a fantastic result, but from a narrative perspective it is considerably less exciting.[1] The first story has all the makings of a good thriller: a conspiracy plot, a clear antagonist (Big Pharma and the government, in cahoots), and a group of plucky and morally righteous protagonists working to reveal the truth.

The attractive, dynamic quality of the anti-vax story, compared to the static and unchanging narrative of the public health pro-vaccine narrative, is a key factor in the ongoing problem of scepticism about vaccines. Mistrust or suspicion of vaccine science—despite the extensive evidence suggesting that vaccines are not only safe, but one of biomedicine's greatest triumphs—is an ongoing and growing problem faced by contemporary healthcare workers (Dubé et al. 2015). Healthcare providers have tried a wide range of strategies to combat this mistrust. These strategies range from aggressive education campaigns, social media, text message reminders, open conversation, and authoritative action on the part of doctors, to interpersonal interventions by everyone from nurses to local religious leaders (Dempsey and Zimet 2015; Dubé et al. 2015). While many of these strategies may prove to be helpful, there has yet to be any conclusive evidence to suggest that any one approach is substantially more effective than another (ibid.).

One of the major weak spots of many of pro-vaccine activities is that they are overwhelmingly tailored to a person who does not understand vaccine science, and are thus largely education-based. However, starting from what Dubé et al. (ibid.: 4191) call an assumption of a "knowledge-deficit" on the parent of vaccine-suspicious groups "assum[es] that vaccine hesitant individuals would change their mind if given the proper information." This is not the case.

Counter-intuitive though it may seem, anti-vaccine movements are generally not born out of misinformation or ignorance. In fact, many of the people who belong to vaccine-sceptical communities have a higher than average "health literacy" (Kitta 2012: 507). As Andrea Kitta (ibid.) argues, the emphasis on education in efforts to reduce vaccine mistrust is a "deficient" model: she observes that focusing on educating people about vaccines "fundamentally misconstrues how different publics mobilize and interpret 'scientific' perspectives," when—as Mark Navin (2013: 244) points out—vaccine-sceptical communities are "insufficiently committed to truth-oriented inquiry," and are drawn to these mistrustful beliefs for reasons other than ignorance.

Vaccine hesitancy and anti-vax movements are thus not a problem of education, or facts (or at least, they are not *only* a problem of education). Mistrust of vaccines is the result of complex factors, many of which are unrelated to the medical realities of vaccination. Some potential sources of vaccine scepticism are a "struggl[e] with state control over individual choice" (Kitta and Goldberg 2017: 510), the influence of peer groups (ibid.), a neoliberal veneration of individual choice (Reich 2014: 680), or a mistrust of the Western medical system in general (Navin 2013: 249), to name only a few of the manifold potential reasons. As is evident in some of the aforementioned potential sources of vaccine mistrust, the relationship between the root cause of vaccine mistrust and the actual experience of vaccination is loose at best. On a surface level, vaccines have very little to do with a neoliberal attitude that fetishises individual choice, but these two factors may be related on an unconscious or emotional plane. The relationship between many of the factors that lead to vaccine mistrust is thus not literal, but figurative. Vaccines are transformed into powerful symbols that stand in for bigger, more abstract ideas of governmental control, scepticism of modern science, or fear of the vulnerability of human bodies.[2] If we accept that vaccines play a symbolic role in vaccine-sceptical communities, it follows that resistance to vaccines is—at least in part—a narrative problem, and it will therefore require a narrative solution.

The stories told by vaccine-suspicious groups are rarely *only* about vaccination; instead, as Eula Biss (2015) writes, these narratives are fuelled by a "labyrinthine network of interlocking anxieties" that exceed the limits of vaccines themselves. Considered purely as a narrative, the stories told by anti-vaccination movements are more engaging than the stories told by healthcare professionals and vaccine advocates, in part because anti-vaccination stories are flexible, free of the adherence to evidence and facts that scientific and medical narratives must have. Indeed, as Shelby and Ernst (2013) have argued, effective storytelling has become one of the most powerful tools in the arsenal of those seeking to sway vaccine-hesitant parents into outright vaccine refusal. Shelby and Ernst (2013: 1796) point out that:

> with little or no science or evidence-based information to back up claims of vaccine danger, anti-vaccine activists have relied on the profound power of storytelling to infect an entire generation of parents with fear and doubt. And so some may argue that the success of the anti-vaccine movement is due to the fact that they have told a better story.

In order to respond better to vaccine mistrust, then, healthcare professionals on the frontlines of immunisation must learn to be just as dexterous in their narrative abilities as are the vaccine-sceptical groups. Healthcare professionals need to recognise the narrative conventions of anti-vaccination stories, so that they can be alert to the figurative fears that may be informing the vaccine-hesitant opinions.

Responding to vaccine hesitancy as a narrative problem will require "narrative competency," to use Rita Charon's (2008) phrase, or 'close reading skills,' to use a common term from my home discipline of English. Close reading—a qualitative methodology that involves "the detailed analysis of the complex interrelations and ambiguities (multiple meanings) of the verbal and figurative components within a work" (Abrams 1999: 181)—can help unpack the often confusing anecdotes offered by anti-vaccination groups by revealing the symbolic and other non-literal forces that power these narratives. Anecdotes can seem impossible to respond to; as Shelby and Ernst (2013: 1796) astutely observe, "personal accounts, particularly as utilized by the anti-vaccine movement, are seemingly immune to facts," but all forms of narrative—personal or otherwise—are ripe for narrative analysis that can be used to direct a more effective response to the underlying issues in vaccine scepticism.

So what kinds of narratives are being told in anti-vax and vaccine-hesitant communities? The narratives that emerge from the vaccine-sceptical communities are as complex and heterogeneous as the issue as a whole, but there are recognisable patterns in many of the personal anecdotes from the anti-vax community. If healthcare professionals can develop both a richer understanding of the generic conventions of chaos narratives and an ability to 'close read' the nuances of each individual narrative, it will be possible for them to better understand the deeper, more amorphous anxieties that underwrite resistance to vaccine science.

Many of these anxieties are harnessed into the form of a "chaos narrative," a genre of medical anecdote first theorised by Arthur Frank (1995) in *The Wounded Storyteller*. In *The Wounded Storyteller*, Frank (ibid.: 75) suggests that illness narratives can be subdivided into three general categories: restitution narratives, which detail a return from illness to total health (what Frank calls the "[y]esterday I was healthy, today I'm sick, but tomorrow I'll be healthy again" plot [ibid.: 77]); quest narratives, which figure illness as a constructive, educational quest that "is defined by the ill person's belief that something is to be gained through the experience" (ibid.: 115); and chaos narratives, where the "plot imagines life never getting better" (ibid.: 97). Of these three general categories, chaos narratives are the most frightening. In a chaos narrative, the experience of illness is imagined as a descent into a disordered, unhappy life from which the ill person can never return. Both quest and restitution narratives presume some kind of 'return' from the debilitating experience of being ill, but there is no cure for chaos.

The narrative structure—the different features that make up a story's unique form—of chaos narratives features chaos in both form (how the story is told) and content (what happens in the story). The way that the story is told often reflects in form—sentence structure, vocabulary, and figurative language such as metaphor or symbolism—the content of the story. A traditional chaos narrative, for example, can often be identified by sentences that are themselves disordered and chaotic instead of clearly written and grammatically succinct. Classic chaos illness narratives are frequently characterised as "an anti-narrative of time without sequence, telling without mediation, and speaking about oneself without being fully able to reflect on oneself" (ibid.: 99). Many of the features commonly found in chaos narratives lend themselves well to the different factors that feed into mistrust of vaccines. For example, chaos narrative "feeds on the sense that no one is in control. People living these stories regularly accuse medicine of seeking to maintain its pretense of control—its restitution narrative—at the expense of denying the suffering of what it cannot treat" (ibid.: 100). The tellers of these personal anecdotes do not always set out to tell a story that deliberately fits into the chaos narrative format; rather, all of Frank's three forms of illness narrative speak to shared cultural understandings of the relationship between illness and the human experience, and these understandings are reflected in the narrative patterns in anecdotes. The mistrust of the medical establishment in chaos narratives is well suited to the narrative goals of vaccine-resistant communities, who also frequently accuse doctors of "seeking to maintain [a] pretense of control" over vaccine-preventable diseases and attempt to reveal this controlling impulse in story. The ill person who is the subject of a chaos narrative is what Frank (ibid.: 104) calls a "chaotic body," which is

Contingent, monadic, lacking desire, and dissociated . . . It is often victim to dominating bodies, which make it the object of their force. It is scandal to mirroring bodies, since it shows how easily the images they use to construct themselves can be stripped away. To the disciplined body, the chaotic body represents weakness and inability to resist. The dominating, mirroring, and disciplined bodies each suppress the possibility that they could become chaotic; the chaotic body is the other against which these bodies define themselves. But they claim no empathic relation to this body; it represents only what they fear for themselves.

Many of the above features of chaos narratives—the sense that the ill person is "victim to dominating bodies," for example—are an excellent fit for the sense of "struggling with state control over individual choice" (Kitta and Goldberg 2017: 510) found in many vaccine-resistant narratives. Narratives of vaccine scepticism make one significant change to the chaos narrative genre: in the vaccine-resistant chaos narrative, chaos is not a precondition of existence or the result of the inevitable, unavoidable experience of illness. The chaos has a clear cause and is deliberately inflicted upon innocent victims by a powerful force.

As an example, consider the following three personal anecdotes from the vaccine-sceptical website *Parent Voices Following Vaccination*:

Sophia was perfect up till 13 months—met all milestones and was perfect in every way. At 13 months she developed a small cellulitis rash on her forehead and was given a week of intravenous antibiotics, then had the MMR jab a month later. Straight away she lost eye contact lost her words and became like a zombie—would not engage with anyone, had chronic diarrhoea for 8 months, stimming, spinning, toe walking, screaming, not sleeping, terrified of going anywhere. The whole thing is disgusting and akin to murdering our child and I will do anything to get justice for this.

The above anecdote has all the features of a classic chaos narrative. The language used describes the descent from a perfect state of health to an endless, catastrophic state of illness. Sophia's childhood is described using words that evoke a sense of utopia: the word "perfect" is used twice to describe her experience, and she is detailed as having "met all milestones." The turn in the narrative comes with the "MMR jab"—and here, even the word "jab" (as opposed to a more neutral word like "injection") suggests a violent act that is out of proportion to the "small cellulitis rash on her forehead." After the "jab," Sophia's "self" is lost, which suggests that the doctors have taken her away. The narrative communicates this loss by using language that dehumanises the child: she changes from the "perfect" kid to "a zombie." The symptoms that are described as emerging after the vaccine are listed in a long, continuous sentence that suggests an unending sensation of suffering for the family. It is worth noting that this catalogue of misery blends medical and emotional symptoms: Sophia suffers from "chronic diarrhoea" but is also "terrified of going anywhere." The mix of emotional and physical symptoms is characteristic of chaos narratives, which frequently feature bodies "being swept along, without control" (Frank 1995: 102). The final phrase picks up the "zombie" metaphor used in the third sentence: the vaccination is "akin to murdering our child," suggesting that the chaos is so complete that Sophia's newly chaotic body is no longer human, and something monstrous has taken her place. Setting aside the deeply ableist connotations of comparing a child with autism to a zombie, close reading the anecdote reveals how a fear of chaos, and a sense of profound loss, undergirds this particular narrative about vaccines.

Similar references to chaos and loss can be found in many personal anecdotes on the website. In another one, a parent writes that:

After the MMR atop the many other vaccinations, we watched as our son left us from the inside out. His last sentence was "that is a red car" as he pointed to it over my shoulder. It has been very hard. His Dad, sisters and brothers know what we witnessed and have been battling to bring him back ever since. I know that my son is a victim of vaccinations, in my gut! He just began leaving us all of a sudden after his MMR. I believe, in hindsight, it is a combination of all of the many vaccinations. I did report and even entered a contract with Waddell-LaBlanc in New Orleans, LA. Their firm split off and once I checked to see if Baker's name or mine was on the national list, it was not. Something has to be done. We are losing our children to greed by big pharma!

The phrasing here echoes many of the same features found in the anecdote about Sophia, particularly in the repeated emphasis on "losing" a child: this parent claims that their "son left us from the inside out," their family has been trying to "bring him back," the child "began leaving us all of a sudden," and the final call to a collective "we" when the parent writes that "we are losing our children to greed." A feeling of erasure compounds the narrative of loss: neither the son nor the parent finds their name on the "national list." This chaotic anecdote focuses on two kinds of loss: that of the child, who "left us from the inside out," and of the family's visibility, as seen in the language that repeatedly suggests testimony ("we watched," the family "know[s] what we witnessed," "I know," "I believe," etc.). The anecdote explicitly attributes this chaos to "greed by big pharma," although it does not provide any specifics about how or why "greed" played into their experience.

The final example I offer (although there are countless similar examples available on this website and on many other online collections of anti-vax anecdotes) again echoes the sense of loss:

My son was a perfect wonderfully funny 15 month old before the MMR on that fateful day in January 2006. I realize now that each vaccine in turn did have a detrimental effect on his little immune system but, all in all he lasted it out until the MMR tipped him directly over the edge. He slipped away little by little over about a month after the shot, he had the worst bright yellow watery diahrea (sic) for approx 3 months constantly. All his words disappeared, it was so much of a regression, the poor little man didn't even recognize his own name and he stopped eating (which lasted 2 years) until I had healed his gut again from the damage that had been done. The eye contact was gone, the smiles gone, the laughter gone, the colour in his cheeks gone, everything was replaced with a shadow of my little boy. Our world fell apart my son was trapped inside a very painful and scary world. I have no doubt that his peanut and egg allergy are from the vaccine injury and ingredients but we could have lived with that. The MMR was just one shot too many. My sons (sic) tests reveal a high level of Aluminum, there is mercury and lead there too, amongst others. What do you do when you look back and know in your heart that your intuition was trying to tell you something? trying to tell you that this felt wrong, every shot!, every vaccine appointment ! a really bad feeling. The only way you live with that is to try and recover that baby back every day, every minute for the next however many years it takes. Some people cannot do that, some people have lost their child forever. I hope parents wake up to the lies soon, & start listening to the parents who have nothing to gain from anything but telling the truth.

As in the first two anecdotes, a major part of the chaos narrative is the construction of lost identity. The child goes from being "perfect wonderfully funny" to "a shadow" of their former self. The moments of reflection posed in this anecdote are classic examples of a chaos narrative, in that they follow an experience of illness that is a descent into an impossibly disordered state. The child's illness in this narrative is profoundly destructive: the family's "world fell apart," and the child is "trapped inside a very painful and scary world." This anecdote also picks up again on the suggestion that vaccines turn a full person into a shell that has been emptied of all identity or sense of self: "Some people have lost their child forever," states the parent in this anecdote, claiming that they "try and recover that baby back every day, every minute" (despite the fact that their child is still living).

Each of these three examples suggests that vaccines can lead to the loss of a high-functioning, presumably idealised child. It is telling that while these three examples are all part of the "overnight autism" cliché (Shelby and Ernst 2013) frequently found in such vaccine-mistrustful narratives, the phrasing of this onset of symptoms as total loss of the child is telling. Part of the repeated insistence on blame in the narrative may be due to the desire to identify a clear cause for the inexplicable and difficult experience of having a child with autism. If, as Eula Biss (2015) argues in her book *On Immunity*, part of what fuels vaccine scepticism is the desire to keep children safe, to protect them, then it is essential to understand the undercurrent of fear that vaccines could lead to not just injury but a kind of death of the self. For healthcare providers fighting the dangerous scepticism of vaccine-resistant communities, understanding how a fear of chaos and loss may be fuelling or motivating parents can help shape more targeted responses to these narratives.

Notes

1 There have been some inspiring efforts on the part of scientists and activists such as Dr Natasha Crowcroft to tell more exciting and narratively dynamic stories about vaccination. For an example, see Crowcroft's talk, 'The Invisible Heroes of Vaccination.' See also the blog post 'The Greatest (Non) Story Ever Told' on the blog *Moms Who Vax*, cited in Shelby and Ernst (2013) and referenced here.
2 For an excellent exploration of this last cause, see Eula Biss's (2015) *On Immunity*.

References

Abrams M. 1999. *A Glossary of Literary Terms*. 7th ed. Stamford, CT: Thomson Learning.
Biss E. 2015. *On Immunity*. Minneapolis, MN: Graywolf.
Charon R. 2008. *Narrative Medicine: Honoring the Stories of Illness*. Oxford: Oxford University Press.
Dempsey AF, Zimet GD. Interventions to improve adolescent vaccination: what may work and what still needs to be tested. *Vaccine* 2015; 33 Suppl 4: D106–113.
Dubé E, Gagnon D, MacDonald NE and the SAGE Working Group on Vaccine Hesitancy. Strategies intended to address vaccine hesitancy: review of published reviews. *Vaccine* 2015; 33: 4191–203.
Frank A. 1995. *The Wounded Storyteller: Body, Illness, and Ethics*. Chicago, IL: University of Chicago Press.
Fu LY, et al. Educational interventions to increase HPV vaccination acceptance: a systematic review. *Vaccine* 2014; 32: 1901–20.
'Humble Mom.' The Greatest (Non) Story Ever Told." *Moms Who Vax Blog*, 17 September 2012. Available at: momswhovax.blogspot.com/2012/09/moms-who-vax-greatest-non-story-never.html. Last accessed: 3 July 2018.
Jarrett C, et al. Strategies for addressing vaccine hesitancy: a systematic review. *Vaccine* 2015; 33: 4180–90.
Kata A. Anti-vaccine activists, Web 2.0, and the postmodern paradigm: an overview of tactics and tropes used online by the anti-vaccination movement. *Vaccine* 2012; 30: 3778–89.
Kitta A. 2012. *Vaccine and Public Concern in History: Legend, Rumor, and Risk Perception*. New York, NY: Routledge.
Kitta A, Goldberg DS. The significance of folklore for vaccine policy: discarding the deficit model. *Critical Public Health* 2017; 27: 506–14.

Navin M. Competing epistemic spaces: how social epistemology helps explain and evaluate vaccine denialism. *Social Theory and Practice* 2013; 39: 241–64.

Parent Voices Following Vaccination. Available at: www.followingvaccinations.com. Last accessed: 29 May 2018.

PHO Talks: the invisible heroes of immunisation. 2017. Directed by N. Crowcroft. Available at: www. youtube.com/watch?v=uvWrKCwk6AI. Last accessed: 29 May 2018.

Reich J. Neoliberal mothering and vaccine refusal: imagined gated communities and the privilege of choice. *Gender & Society* 2014; 28: 679–704.

Shelby A, Ernst K. Story and Science: How providers and parents can utilize storytelling to combat anti-vaccine misinformation. *Human Vaccines and Immunotherapeutics* 2013; 9: 1795–801.

18
THOUGHT CURFEW
Empathy's endgame?

David Cotterrell

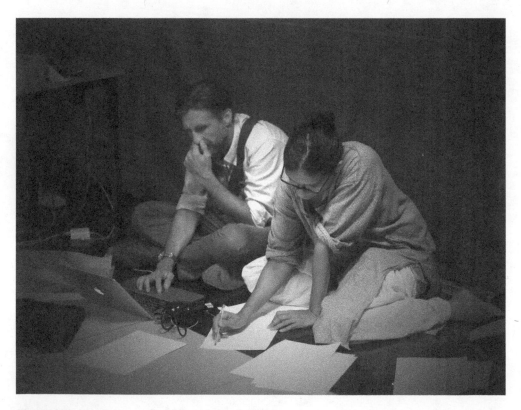

Figure 18.1   David Cotterrell and Ruwanthie de Chickera

This chapter is written from the subjective first-person view of the artist. It may appear idiosyncratic and tangential. But if the subject of the chapter is 'empathy,' and empathy is defined as "The ability to understand and share the feelings of another" (OED), perhaps it seems reasonable to request both the reader and the writer to attempt to meet through a confessional moment of solidarity. The narrative may appear to be framed within the development of a play, but it is actually focused on a question and therefore offers a philosophical inquiry. The question offers a choice: is empathy an advantage in all forms of contemporary society; or is this most cherished of human skills actually a hindrance to the effective delivery of progress within a technologically enhanced environment?

The conceit

I recently collaborated with the playwright and theatre director Ruwanthie de Chickera on the writing and development of a play. My collaborator had already defined its title—'Thought Curfew'—before I was invited to share an intellectual journey with her. Within the context of current events in Rwanda, and within the contexts of our independent practices in London and Colombo, my role (and our challenge) was to embrace and explore the concept of 'thought curfew.' This was to be addressed through developing a short story into a play embracing both theatre and visual art; and relating to our respective moral perspectives on our contemporary worlds. In Sri Lanka, London and Rwanda, the co-director and I wrestled with our misgivings and the challenges of mixing methodologies, languages and references. We progressed the production through earnest conversations, frustrating debates and theatrical-devising workshops. In the summer of 2018 it premiered in Kigali. It may tour globally, or it may never be seen again. It is captured here through the word and the lens.

To write the script and to understand the decision-making that would inform the tone, narrative, characterisation and context of the production, we had to test the logic of the conceit, itself as resonant and ambiguous as the title. To understand whether there could be any coherent development of something that we could both defend, we had to ask ourselves: 'in which world, however nihilistic, stylised or allegorical, could such a term appear credible?' The question we posed is: 'How could a "thought curfew" come about?' Could we extrapolate from the present or should this exist only as a dark fairy tale, an unimaginable otherness?

Perhaps there had been an appalling event—such a catastrophic attack that a population felt a collective existential threat. A government with a tendency to prefer authoritarianism might use this moment—a 'state of emergency'—to implement protective measures. Perhaps widespread monitoring could be justified. There might be reason to mandate comprehensive access to civilian correspondence. Perhaps CCTV and other forms of location-based data collection could extend from high-value sites to common sites of congregation. The human cost of monitoring the comprehensive feeds would be onerous. Potentially, 3D facial recognition software could be deployed, and algorithms could at least begin to filter the daunting mass of data. Location-aware phones would be hacked; TVs become listening devices; home automation would double as home monitoring; and debit cards would directly feed the location of their users into a correlated database of medical records, tax status and debt liabilities. Before long, the system would either grind to a halt or become so complex that it would consume the sum of all spare human labour, with vast farms of supercomputers and countless gigawatts of energy at play. The system would become comprehensive beyond belief, even surveying its own surveillance. It would become a form of artistry, with the original cause seeming almost trivial compared to the internal logic and beauty of the evolved systems design. With all the futuristic efficiency of a fibreoptic backbone or a maglev network, the conveyancing of data and the fault-tolerant complexity would become a point of national pride. As with the national pride of overcoming the enormous obstacles and technical challenges needed to become a nuclear power, the purpose of the system is overlooked in its self-sustaining demand for upgrades, refinement

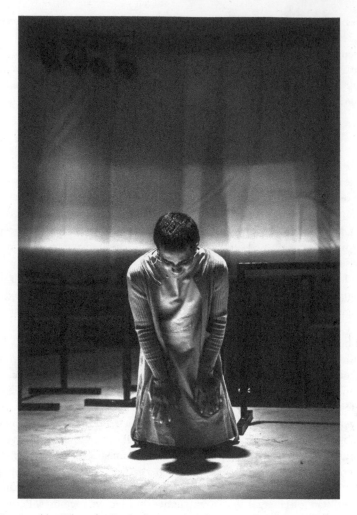

Figure 18.2   How could a 'Thought Curfew' come about?

and perpetuation. The gloss on the system replaces the system itself. It becomes clear that the algorithms are strong and the prediction of deviance is with merit, but the faith in the system is not total. The system may have unforced errors leading to false positives. Even worse, there is a suspicion that without human backup the system may not be ready to adapt to new counter-measures by enemies of the state. Reluctantly, the state increases its network of informers. But the mass employment of special constables, reserve military and other trusted irregular forces is costly. The state has already invested heavily in the automated infrastructure, and potentially the deployment of the population to the task is beyond its economic capacity. The narrative of fear is resurrected and accelerated. Patriotism and paranoia of infiltrators is promoted. Volunteers are requested. Rewards are offered. Volunteers discreetly and in large numbers come forward. It is hard to know the scale of the volunteer monitoring force. What does become evident is that few words are spoken in a way that might suggest lack of loyalty without a quiet and timely removal of the offender from society, workplace, school or family. The system is complete. Assurances are made that the failsafe algorithmic and human societal safety net is now robust, oversight is in place; the double check removes potential abuses, and with perpetual vigilance, prevention of risk can be sustained. A massive public health 'net' has been established.

There is a noticeable change in behaviour—not sudden, but more evident as the net developed and behavioural shifts that might be perceived locally as incremental were viewed as dramatic from abroad. Initially, words relating to 'terrorism' seemed to lead to a response, but later a suspicion that phrases related to quality of 'economic engagement,' 'work ethic' and even 'personal values' might lead to being flagged, followed and cautioned.

Behavioural change followed. Email caution, key word avoidance, teenagers' playful evasion of CCTV, leaving phones at home, testing response times—all gradually revealed that the penalties and lack of humour, public shaming and community disapproval had led to a broad compliance. Total compliance appeared to be effective through the instigation of the volunteer monitoring force and the sustaining of majority consent. Office workers took care to avoid certain subjects, while conversations between friends became a little anodyne, and partners found themselves speaking less to each other than they might have done before. A population, united by an external sense of purpose, undertook an internal process of careful suppression of vocalised thought. However, in the heat of an argument, at a moment of exhaustion, in the delirium of sleep, in the crying of pain, people would realise with horror that they had failed to edit their expression. Through misadventure or mistake, individuals could fall foul of the system instigated to protect them. Reports of examples made, of conspirators identified, of subversives and terrorists confessing, continued to surface. Despite the care with which citizens tried to live their lives, the risk of disgrace and denouncement remained present. Slippage led to outrage—public humiliation and shame, private grief.

These reports caused massive anxiety to those who were not sure whether they trusted their inner demons to remain hidden from their peers. The state observed that some of these well-publicised occurrences appeared to cause a disturbing level of sympathy for the subject that appeared to transgress from the societal compact for mutual defence.

In parallel, research scientists—led by the team that had once been credited with the development of Ritalin—had been working hard to understand the inability of the mind to focus within constraints. An experimental psychostimulant pharmaceutical treatment was developed which appeared to suppress some of the less task-oriented thought patterns. It was first available as an oral prescription-based drug. It had minimal short-term side effects and appeared to perform well over longer-term trials. In fact, it offered certain benefits: a reduction in anxiety, perhaps credited to reduced fear of retribution, but potentially caused by a diminished tendency to prevaricate, was reported by many participants. It was licensed and released to the market. Within two years, the drug was widely available and commonly adopted. While the self-regulating initiative of individual users was reaping significant societal benefits—as evidenced by a marked reduction in accusations and arrests—the reliance on a single pharmaceutical supplier and the need for patients to conscientiously manage their own dosage presented risks. Moreover, the original research group controversially proposed the development of the drug as a mandatory vaccine. It was a step too far for Parliament.

Even in a climate of existential threat to the population, the enforced and irreversible censorship of the population seemed to be beyond the scope of a benign state. A voluntary trial was proposed. This should only be implemented if the subjects of the treatment willingly adopted it. In spite of an extraordinary level of (highly repressed) disquiet, trials were approved. Early tests suggested that the vaccine rendered the subject fully capable of satisfactory social interaction, complex engagement with tasks, affection and happiness (the chief components of 'wellbeing'). Depression, anxiety, doubt and dissatisfaction were reduced to be almost undetectable. The end result appeared to be the creation of a model member of society: contented, accepting and without conflict, incapable of posing a threat to the system, to themselves or to others. The question of whether anyone might choose to have his or her ability to resist suppressed was a fascinating social experiment, and as the first few volunteers came forward they were initially treated with a level of macabre curiosity before later claiming their status as minor celebrities. The vaccine was so successful that the initial subjects were soon allowed out of isolation, returning to their families and workplaces. Family members remarked that their returning spouses, children and parents appeared to be simply kinder, more content versions of their previous selves. The trial was completed and the programme continued voluntarily, more discreetly, but with increased capacity. Those choosing to inoculate themselves were not required to announce the decision to employers, partners or children. For distant observers and local dissenters, the vaccine became known as the 'Thought Curfew.' More potent varieties appeared and could be obtained on the dark web, at a price—for many, a price worth paying.

OK, so it's a bit far fetched and more than a little derivative. It sounds like *1984, Brave New World, The Stepford Wives* and a range of other haunting and lauded dystopian classics. Despite this, something resonated, not necessarily with literature but perhaps more with a

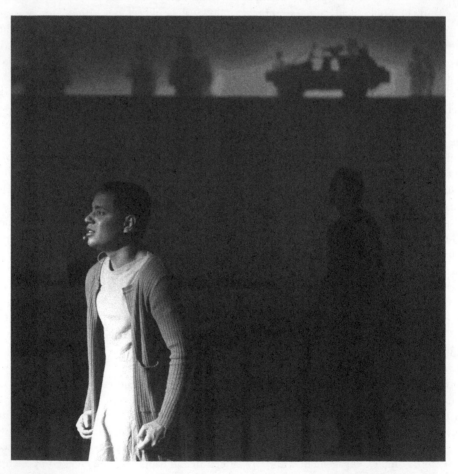

Figure 18.3   Perhaps there had been an appalling event. We are mentally designed with the capacity to deliberate, but our body appears more responsive to certainty

quiet question that is running through a range of arenas in contemporary society. I stepped away from my residual trauma of watching *One Flew Over the Cuckoo's Nest* a bit too early in my childhood and tried to understand how it could be that someone might voluntarily choose to prohibit part of their mental function.

The context

The prevarication, angst, continual search for alternatives, outcome visualisation, consideration of the repercussions, fear and visceral imagining of failure are all natural safeguards within our mental apparatuses. They protect us from misadventure, and allow us to balance probabilities, moral alternatives and risks. Without them, we might foolishly confront unknown circumstances and unknowingly jeopardise our lives or too flippantly leap to judgement over others. However, there are times when the alternatives are not helpful or even when awareness of them can cause us harm.

I think I have always been scared of heights. I think that potentially all of us are, or at least should be. The fear of heights (or at least the fear of falling) is a natural respect for the fragility of our bodies under the influence of gravity-induced impact. A surprisingly short fall can break the spine and cause catastrophic damage. The irony is that the fear is not always linked to the risk of falling. We may fear the idea of falling even more as a far-fetched fantasy than as a practical likelihood. We imagine falling forward when standing near a cliff, yet we are unlikely to fear sudden inabilities to stand when pausing in the street. The chance of losing our footing may not be massively different, but the imagined outcome is of a different order of severity. When climbing a rock face, or even a ladder, there may be a moment when the imagination overtakes practical functioning, and instead of saving us from our naivety, begins to manifest the danger that will place us in jeopardy. The wonderfully named phenomenon 'Elvis-leg,' or 'Sewing-Machine leg,' describes the awful experience of a limb appearing to vibrate when resting on the rung of a ladder, a rope or even the ball of the foot. I have experienced this many times and found it interesting as an apparently involuntary physical response to situations. There are a range of ways of stopping this debilitating physical experience. Perhaps lowering the heel to contact with a surface, or simply shifting the weight from the ball of the foot, can cause the spasm to pass. However, because the condition is a combination of physical tension and mental anxiety, I discovered that the most effective is to try to not think about the circumstance, the risk or the fear.

I realised that the best tactic to overcome this experience is to try not to think at all. By all means assess and prepare in advance, but once committed, the time may have passed to consider alternative outcomes. I found that building a rhythm, breaking down the task into rudimentary simple actions, emptying your mind and, most importantly, trying not to let the mind wander seemed to work.

I wondered whether this decisiveness—innate or learned—might have been what the playground leaders must have had. I mused as to whether this might have enabled me to score a goal rather than spend my childhood running up and down the pitch and desperately trying to find someone to pass the ball to. Is this the mysterious skill that was retained by the kids who fought for dominance physically and verbally amongst their 9-year-old peers? Perhaps this was why I had always been a pacifist, mystified by others' ability to overcome all of the doubt and concern, the compassion and the fear that might lead them to cross a threshold to deliberately harm another person. Part of it may have been a moral position, but part of it might simply have been that I was incapable of delivering within that structure of interaction. I wasn't able to mentally claim to the certainty and finality of the act. I couldn't decouple my anxiety and prevarication enough to fully commit to defending myself or attacking another to the level at which I might have a chance of overcoming a more engaged and focused adversary. Aware of my limitations, I always opted for negotiation, frequently attempted to engender empathy, and occasionally tried to build enough ambiguity to encourage an opponent to experience the same uncertainty, ensuring that I would never be a risk to the world.

The overthinking of a scenario can cause everything from sex to violence to become impossible. We are mentally designed with the capacity to deliberate, but our body appears more responsive to certainty. Popular culture and social media offer credit to the machismo of mountain-bikers, test pilots, athletes, surgeons, soldiers and others who appear to defer anxiety in order to function without hesitation at times when the rest of us might feel it more appropriate to wrestle with the viability, morality or practicality of the daunting challenge that we have imposed, or has been imposed on us. Perhaps we don't want the climber to experience the paralysing fear of uncertainty. I can understand why the possibility of an unexpected moment of doubt within the special forces soldier being remotely monitored breaching a compound might seem undesirable as a character trait within the Pentagon. In this circumstance, it might seem reasonable to think that a soldier's deferral of moral and existential parallel narratives might be safer for the individual and for those within their team. It could be that we might be quite happy to know that the surgeon had taken a pill to ensure that he wouldn't be struggling with emotional and professional stress while leading a team in a high-risk operation. It could be that we might be quite content to feel that the success of the operation was not entirely contingent on the performance of a human at all. Indeed, the performance-enhancing drug Modafinil ('Daffy') has been trialled (in simulated conditions) on sleep-deprived surgeons and found to have some beneficial effects in improving concentration or fighting exhaustion (Sugden et al. 2012).

The consent

There has been an acceptance of the need to moderate risk and to embrace mitigation strategies within our lives. From the driving license to the parking sensor, we are reminded of the need to recognise the difference between domains amenable to personal judgement and contexts of deferred decision-making. We quietly adopt and accept advances in navigation, monitoring and enforcement that reduce our capacity for errors and protect us from our tendency to err, increasingly supported by technologies. There are indications that we may be at a tipping point in our reliance on the role of the human decision-maker within some areas. Driverless cars are trialling across the USA, deliveries by drone are being tentatively licensed and research institutes and technology companies are developing prototype robotic carers.

This maturing of artificial intelligence for domestic, commercial and humanitarian purposes is happening neither in isolation nor without extraordinary governmental and industrial investment. While support reflects a range of utopian and entrepreneurial aspirations, the funding of at least part of this accomplishment cannot be decoupled entirely from the military research programmes of wealthy nations. Perhaps it is not strange that the contexts of greatest perceived personal and institutional risk are the contexts where we may begin to see the most energetic promotion of the benefits of delegation of roles to machines. As we begin to accept the advantages of self-regulating power stations, online diagnoses and self-checkout shopping, the starker issues regarding the essential ethical changes that we are embracing may be tested with much greater consequences, thousands of miles from home.

The death or injury of soldiers, however much reduced through technological advancement, is a risk for any government. In democratic countries, the public view of repatriation of bodies or the enhanced awareness of the long-term implications of battlefield injury have proved to be challenging for any government seeking to engage militarily with global concerns. While other factors may dominate in some circumstances, the public consent for conflict is supported by the level of consensus for the moral defensibility of the intervention, and reduced through the awareness of the human cost. It could be argued that a greater moral justification creates tolerance for a greater level of risk. If this statement is accepted, then there are one or two ways to improve the viability of sustaining public consent for a military action. One is to develop more compelling ways to explain the moral imperative leaving conflict as the only justifiable option. The second is to reduce the risk to a country's combatants of serious injury or death. In the absence of a strong argument for war, potentially a population that doesn't have to witness its cost can tolerate war for longer. While infantry in recent conflicts have still been very visible, as technology progresses certain operations can now be delegated entirely to longer-distance, over-the-horizon, remotely monitored or even autonomous firing systems. The possibility of the same or similar dominance of the ground must prove a compelling notion for any political and military leader. However, when technology has potentially moved faster than the ethical issues it has raised, the future role of human responsibility has not yet been confirmed.

At a time when autonomous weapons are now amongst us, or at least above us, we are still placated by the idea that there is a human operator who will have to retain ownership of the moral fallout from the violence that may be enacted—for example, the PTSD of drone operators is well documented. The fact is that the potential for doubt, for empathy and compassion, however deeply suppressed through the endless training of drills, repetition and rehearsal, remains as a key notional safeguard against the unconstrained unleashing of institutional violence.

It may seem strange to concatenate institutional violence with institutional compassion, but this was potentially the other domain that was elevated within our thought experiment. As an area where the pressure on individuals is extreme, while the institutional and societal tolerance for failure is poorly expressed, surgeons offered a group that we imagined might benefit from periodically electing to reduce their capacity to feel. Comparing the role of surgeons with soldiers is contentious. Soldiers have historically been institutionally instrumentalised, experimented upon and sacrificed. Surgeons are potentially the elite knowledge-and-skills base of an institution, and their individual expertise is prized and rewarded. As a society, our tolerance for human error, crisis of confidence and existential angst for surgeons may not be significantly greater than the Pentagon's acceptance of these human characteristics within the military. Our awareness of risk and accountability has increased through the emergence of greater transparency, more effective statistical analysis and more aggressive litigation and insurance claims. We want our surgeons to advance their techniques and ideas, but we are also not enthusiastic for acceptance of the risks associated with human involvement. Without the level of the US Defence Advanced Research Projects Agency (DARPA) or the UK Defence Science and Technology Laboratory (DSTL) support that the military attracts, but still with extraordinary governmental and private investment, surgery could be argued to be about to follow a parallel path.

In an era of advanced keyhole surgery, credible potential for robot-assisted procedures exists (Adams 2018; Campbell 2018). Robotics is well advanced in prostate surgery for example and wider implementation is only hampered by cost and training. If surgery is being controlled and monitored via cameras and haptic feedback devices in the operating theatre, surgeons can remotely control instruments from thousands of miles away. With the promise of steadier hands and more accurate interventions, there is already engagement of precision technology to mediate human-to-human interaction. If the experience in the operating theatre is mediated through technology, the progression to intelligent, angst-free, computer oversight of the procedure is not a science-fiction fantasy. Patients now expect to be briefed on the percentage risks of procedures prior to consenting to them. This may be a more important metric than our ability to trust or relate to the remote figure of the surgeon or anaesthetist. When offered the risk profile of a routine operation being conducted partially or entirely by autonomous robot as opposed to a consultant surgeon, the question arises: will we still elect to prioritise the human when the robot surpasses the practitioner's success rate?

These two domains are radically different, but both represent an imminent moment where we may be ready individually or societally to accept that the reassurance of believing that a member of our species is engaged in fundamental, critical, actions on our behalf is no longer necessary. The question that we as a society have to address at a rapid pace, before it is rendered moot by our iterative adoption of technology, is: what, if anything, would be lost if we progress to completely remove the empathic potential of the human from situations that present us with risk?

The curfew

Our play became an allegorical journey through a stylised landscape. It was a landscape viewed from a child's eyes as the infant attempted to escape from the insanity of the rapidly pervasive thought curfew. Our backstory was never revealed and, in many ways, remained redundant in the dystopian fairy tale of fear and alienation that evolved to claim the title of the production. On the stage in Kigali, the child travelled from the safely mediated domestic consumption of the world's problems through the landscape's peripheral refugee disenfranchisement. She travelled on to witness development-sector response and finally to confront the military boundary of humanitarian space. As she migrated, running from the Thought Curfew, she found it had continually overtaken her. She observed and was terrified by the pervasiveness of 'the unthinkable' as she saw the varied methodologies of society being sustained without space, mandate or ability for critical awareness or reflection.

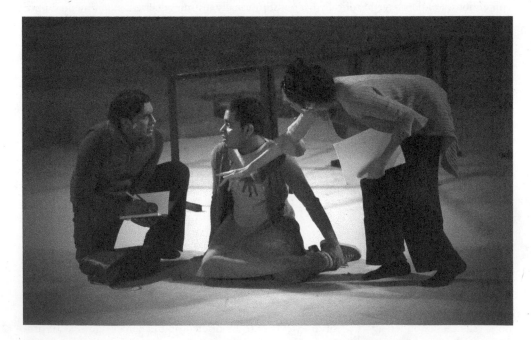

Figure 18.4 Our play became an allegorical journey through a stylised landscape

The script played with the imaginary vocabulary of theatre to stretch time, space and the credibility of her journey. The unthinking behaviour that she was witnessing was playful, absurd, pointless and sinister. The fantasy made no pretence at realism and was as plausible as a mental flight of fancy as a physical odyssey. In reality, the script was derived from observed behaviour, language and dialogue in each of these contradictory landscapes. Her 'Uncanny Valley'[1] experience was due to a subtle shift in her ability to believe and trust in the words spoken to her and the sincerity behind them. There are no direct threats to the main character, yet she finds the world alien and dangerous. Her nightmare was not of a 'Thought Curfew' but of a world that appeared to be capable of suppressing human empathy. The landscape of the Thought Curfew is tragically ineffective, but in her mind the tragedy was not simply a loss of utility. The fear that she acted out for the audience was more poignant. Without empathy, without human doubt, fear and anxiety, she saw a world that continued to function but without the self-criticism needed to understand why.

In the rapid technological progress and human-feeling regress that we are witnessing, we are likely to develop methods of selectively removing our reliance on human discretion through increasingly effective deferred decision-making, and robust institutional (other-directed) methodologies and directives. The question our dystopian exercise raised is: if we institutionalise the delivery of our goals, what may be required to mandate that we continue to sensitively evolve our understanding of the value, purpose and meaning of our actions?

Note

1 A term coined by the robotics professor, Masahiro Mori (first introduced in its current form in the 1978 book *Robots: Fact, Fiction, and Prediction*, written by Jasia Reichardt), to describe the unsettling relationship between human and avatar.

References

Adams T. 2018. The robot will see you now: could computers take over medicine entirely? *The Observer Magazine*. 29 July 2018, 18–21. Available at: www.theguardian.com/technology/2018/jul/29/the-robot-will-see-you-now-could-computers-take-over-medicine-entirely. Last accessed: 2 August 2018.

Campbell D. 2018. The robot will see you now: how AI could revolutionise the NHS. *The Guardian*. 11 June 2018. Available at: www.theguardian.com/society/2018/jun/11/the-robot-will-see-you-now-how-ai-could-revolutionise-nhs. Last accessed: 2 August 2018.

Sugden C, Housden CR, Aggarwal R, et al. Effect of pharmacological enhancement on the cognitive and clinical psychomotor performance of sleep-deprived doctors: a randomized controlled trial. *Annals of Surgery*. 2012; 255: 222–27.

Acknowledgements

Photographs (Figures 18.1–18.4) by Prauda Buwaneka. Images courtesy of the author and artists.

David Cotterrell would like to thank Ruwanthie de Chickera who was the co-creator of the theatrical project that forms the context for this text, and Prauda Buwaneka who documented the development and realisation of the work.

PART IV

Medicine as performance and public engagement

19

THE PERFORMING ARTS IN MEDICINE AND MEDICAL EDUCATION

Claire Hooker and James Dalton

> Imagination is the ally of both lying and truth-telling. It is double-edged; it has its uses and abuses, its privileges and penalties. On the one hand, it is one of our most powerful tools for knowing reality, and on the other it reverts to its original idolatrous form of image-making which is inevitably destructive of truth.
>
> *(Farber 1974)*

> I think that the only acceptable practical consequences of what Sartre has said is to link this theoretical insight to the practice of creativity—and not that of authenticity. From the idea that the self is not given to us, I think there is only one practical consequence: we have to create ourselves as a work of art.
>
> *(Foucault 1984)*

> 'Be slick at this! Be slick at that! We need acting lessons!'
>
> *(Medical student, reported in Sinclair 1997)*

Introduction

It is almost never OK for a medical student to stumble when beginning to build her repertoire of professional performance. Instead, there is a gap between the impression the student must give—of confidence and authority, with just the right amount of eye contact and sympathetic tone—and the student's inner fears and feelings. As a result, medical students (and doctors) often parse 'performing' the role of doctor as akin to 'fake it till you make it.' This gap between the public performance of doctoring and private unspoken views and feelings is one that neither students nor their teachers are very keen to acknowledge (Whorwell and Shanahan 2016).

This chapter is about the gap, this tendency to understand performance in medicine as a form of faking. We argue that the gap springs in part from anxieties that lie at the core of modern medicine, the uneasy awareness of how far short both medical practice and patient lived experience fall from the ideal of physician authority and scientific certainty. Our contention is that contemporary theatre in medicine is powerful because it requires that we-the-audience confront the gap, in one way or another. Performance traditions slip between ideas of real and fake fluidly. They encourage play in the tension. They occupy, as anthropologist Victor Turner would describe it, a subjunctive mode—in language, this is the 'what if' that opens the door to *poiesis* (Turner 1990: 11–12).

We claim that there are methods of accessing this subjunctive mode that can address the anxiety about authenticity in the performative aspect of medicine. While some constrained theatre practices in medical education (notably the mimetic acting encouraged by standardised patients and empathy scores) might only make the gap wider, many contemporary theatre practices in medical education work that gap, even without intending to. Different modes of performance may provide students and doctors with space to enact a state of 'what if' when encountering anxieties of real/fake in their practice of medicine.

This chapter presents ways in which such a merging of performing arts and medical performance can manifest through a series of shifts via the subjunctive mode. We examine mimesis (a first subjunctive shift, 'what if I were a doctor?'); how rehearsing back stage and modelling front stage have shaped performance in medicine; the beginnings of critical mimesis (a second subjunctive shift, 'what if that were me?') in the possibilities in role play in medical education; aesthetic drama (a third subjunctive shift, 'what if I am not the expert?') where being implicated as audience to illness narratives shifts performing empathy from 'showing' to 'being affected'; and contemporary improvisation and other forms of performance play (a fourth subjunctive shift, 'what if we are here together?') where 'authenticity' is a transitory emergence from enactments of professionalism in performances that are co-created and partial.

Scene I: <set in the past>

The notion that doctoring is a performance is as enduring as medical traditions themselves. Most healing traditions from around the world have placed performance at the heart of practice (Porter 1999; Gemi-Iordanou et al. 2014). Indeed, the mythologised originary context for European medicine—Classical Greece, c. 2500 years ago, the era that gave us the Hippocratic corpus—entwined performance and ritual in the practice of Asklepian physicians (Roth 2008; Mitchell-Boyask 2009; Oberhelman 2013). In those temples, and in many other healing traditions across multiple societies and cultures, the religious healers of the day (priests, shamans, medicine men, witch doctors, *sangomas*) would enact rituals of music, dance and drama. In ritualistic healing practices, the performance of the healer was, and still is, inseparable from the process of healing.

Are these performances deceptions? Are they fake? In a myriad of cultures and traditions, performative healing had, and has, both power and integrity. Performances were often deep and risky engagements between the healer and the sick, in many cases including mediations with spirits or a spiritual world. The healer's body becomes an instrument of healing in such performances, and bears real costs in fatigue and pain. For many of those who witness or experience such events, this is the quintessence of a caring and ethical engagement that honours, through engagement, the struggles of suffering.

And yet, deception and confusion have an equally long presence in the history of healing. The slipperiness of what it means to *act a part* has a long history in theorising illness and medical care. Implicitly or explicitly, the fancy that doctoring requires counterfeit—beneficially intended, or otherwise—has been embedded every way we looked in medicine and medical education. Consider this extract from the famed Hippocratic corpus (not the Oath):

> Perform your medical duties calmly and adroitly, concealing most things from the patient while you are attending to him. Give necessary orders with cheerfulness and sincerity, turning his attention away from what is being done to him; sometimes

reprove sharply and sometimes comfort with solicitude and attention, revealing nothing of the patient's future or present condition, for many patients through this course have taken a turn for the worse.

(Palmieri and Stern 2009: 164)

This beneficent deception had its social politics. The status of folk healers was disputed in the ancient world as it is in the contemporary one. Elite rationalist Hippocratic corpus writers scoffed at the supernatural beliefs and remedies of traditional healers, terming them conjurers, purifactors, vagabonds and quacks (McNamara 2004).

The development of scientific medicine from the seventeenth century, and the processes of professionalisation in medicine in the late nineteenth and early twentieth century, similarly joined the epistemic project of science-based medicine to the social project of reinforcing the status, authority and power of its socially elite practitioners. Scientific medicine pursued certainty and truth through reductive methods: the truth of clockwork, anatomised bodies; of what could be seen under the microscopes of the clever, brutal pathologists of the Paris Hospitals (Warner 2003); and of dose-responses observed in the artificial conditions of randomised (later, controlled) trials. This version of medicine formed as a precipitate from the early modern drive to distil the world into conceptual binaries—hard/soft, cognition/emotion, mind/body, precision/care, objective/subjective, masculine/feminine, public/private, rational/empathetic, healthy/diseased—if one half of each opposition exemplified knowledge, discovery and victory over the diminishing mysteries of disease, then it defined the values of medical science and its executors. Doctors were, and mostly still are, supposed to be objective, rational, precise and cognitive in their public, professional role; to display traits from the undesired list of constructed opposites would counter the integrity of the doctor, would mark him (not her) as not medical. Even to suggest that his was a role performed, a surface mask, courted risk in a modern world where authenticity was constructed in opposition to the counterfeit of performance (Latour 1993).

In the early twentieth century, medical education narrowed to training students in scientific methods. The famed Flexner Report (1910), which advocated this, also recommended the closure of five out of seven medical schools dedicated to enrolling black students, and all medical schools for women (Byrd and Clayton 2002). New regulations—much needed—to safeguard patients from unscrupulous quackery, including faith healing, also suppressed Indigenous and other traditional healers, and ridiculed their performance-based practices.

We suggest that the greater their social prestige, the more physicians have claimed power and authority over their patients on the basis of their technical knowledge and expertise, and the more they have been likely to deceive their patients. They perform deliberate deceptions to control their patients ("turn his attention from what is done to him") and conceal the limitations and uncertainty of medical practice such as context effects (Arnold, Finniss and Kerridge 2014). They deceive because they are conscious of the tenuousness of the performance: the anxiety of being seen through tends to haunt social elites.

Scene II: an air of verisimilitude—'front stage' and 'back stage' as a theory of social action in medicine

These are hardly new observations. The 'theatre' has been a foundational metaphor for sociological theories of medical practice. This is because so many twentieth-century sociologists were struck by the artifice and theatricality of quotidian medical practice. They were also interested in the 'applied' question of how student doctors were 'socialised' into their professional role and identity (Collyer 2015).

The pre-eminent theorist remains Erving Goffman, whose studies of self-presentation in a number of fields, including medicine, prompted him to apply images of the theatre as the basis for analysing social action ('dramaturgical analysis') (Goffman 1959). Goffman was an acute observer of the gaps between what medical students and doctors presented to their patients, and what they presented to each other (Goffman 1961); and between either of these, and what they thought and said privately (or to ethnographic researchers). Consequently the artifice of performance was central to his theorisation not only of medicine, but also of everyday life.

Goffman's key insight was how *all* social interaction is inherently performative. He observed how performance was functional: each actor uses his or her performance to attempt to control the action; and seeks agreed-upon definitions of the situation through inter-act-ion with others, adjusting their performance to maintain coherence of role and to respond to the different situations available to them (Jacobsen and Kristiansen 2015). A core tool is 'impression management,' in which actors present performances that are idealised in ways that support preferred definitions of their roles and of the contextual situations. Goffman highlighted the theatricality of medicine—its many props and costumes, its rituals, the operating theatre as a theatrical space. He captured how students and doctors feel that 'medical performance' often equates with 'impression management.'

Goffman theorised the gap as the distance between 'front stage,' where performances are presented to the audience of patient or colleague, and 'back stage,' where performances are rehearsed, props prepared and where contradictory thoughts might be acknowledged. He not only acknowledged, but also theorised, the *weakness* of the 'front stage' performance. This is most vivid in medical education, where medical students learn to assume a 'cloak of competence' (Haas and Shaffir 1977) in order to manage patients' impressions of their authority, and to inveigle them into compliance with their treatment, despite discomfort and indignity. The cloak of competence conceals medical students' uneasy sense of charlatanism; the 'mask' of professionalism that they adopt enables them to claim social status, to define the situation and efficiently manipulate their interactions with patients. It underpins students' and doctors' capacity to objectify patients, so that their inappropriate emotional or even sexual responses can be shut off, and hence leave their role as doctor undisturbed.

Since Goffman gave a sociological language and scholarly validation to the idea that doctors are always acting an inherently counterfeit part, the gap between 'front stage' and 'back stage' in medical practice has continued to fascinate (see e.g. the work of performance artists such as ORLAN (Brodzinski 2014)). Revelations of the 'back stage' have become a core theme in popular culture. The gap is central to popular confessional medical autoethnography and autobiography (Foxton 2012), is frequently explored in more literary writing (Lam 2008; Hitchcock 2009; Shem 2009) and, of course, has been the core structure of the ever-growing quantity of television medical dramas from the first season of 'M.A.S.H' to the present day of 'Scrubs' and 'House.' Funny and brutal, in these texts doctors discuss 'Hollywood' calls (a false performance of resuscitation), GOMERS ('get out of my emergency room'), ways to avoid patients, how to fabricate appointments and how to offer false reassurance.

Scene III: mimesis—simulation and sensibility

In acknowledging that there is a 'front stage' for the performance of a role, and that such a role carries with it a historical 'genre'—the style and normative competencies of how doctors are expected to appear and act—we arrive at the crucial mechanism of mimesis in medical education.

Medical students learn their professional performance through a first subjunctive shift, 'what if I were a doctor?' They watch senior consultants at work, they sculpt their manner to meet examination criteria, and they absorb the 'hidden curriculum' in the nuances of behaviour. Such source material, implicitly and explicitly marked as successful by the upward career trajectories of those who 'play the part,' is bundled up in a role that medical students reinforce through regular opportunities for rehearsal over the course of their education. Students begin to build their own professional performance repertoire through mimesis—a concept that connoted 'impersonation,' 'representation' and 'imitation' in Ancient Greek aesthetics (Halliwell 2009) and that remains a critical and contested tool for understanding the relationship between performer and character in contemporary theatre practice (Diamond 1997; Carlson 2016b).

Depending on where they study, medical students may be given the opportunity for rehearsal in a simulation setting, which can range from virtual learning environments employing artificial mannequins with features that enable the practice of surgery, intubation or other procedures, to high-intensity specialised situation simulations with experienced professional actors (such as an emergency response to a serious road accident or to terrorist attack), to undertaking short role plays either with trained actors or their peers.

High-tech simulation events can be akin to the dress rehearsal, with the focus on technical mastery—for example, of specific surgical skills. As with a dress rehearsal, the advantage of simulation is in embedding specific skills by practising them, but without the real-world consequences of endangering flesh-and-blood patients. Students may even make mistakes and be able to learn from them. 'Performance' here connotes mastery through an embodied dexterity only acquired by practice, and matches the narrow meanings of performance used for management (Morrissey 2015).

The fit between performance, medical practice and the interior experiences of students is more complicated in the small series of staged role plays that most medical students (at least those in the Anglophone 'West') encounter: breaking bad news, responding to an angry, weeping or aggressive patient, and assessment in an 'objective structured clinical examination' (OSCE). In an OSCE, students rotate through a range of 'stations,' at each of which they must examine and assess 'standardised patients' (SPs)—actors who have carefully scripted details about the patient whose part they play, complete with symptoms and physical history, along with social circumstances, beliefs and concerns (Wallace 2006). Candidates achieve marks for each step that they perform correctly. The skills assessed include a range of highly specified communication skills, and may include how students address the SP, how they physically position themselves in relation to the SP, their eye contact and the forms of their display of empathy, or response to the SP's emotions.

It is here that the gap can begin to yawn and widen, because both student and SP are performing according to an artificial ritual script, rather than actually engaging with one another. In this gap the exclusive spotlight on the doctor–patient dyad alienated the contours of reality, with no inclusion of policy and material constraints, or populations of healthcare institutions, as if such complexities did not exist.

The transmutation of empathy—a moment defined by the suspension of judgement and spontaneous, deep connection with another human being—into a scorable behavioural display for a counterfeit patient (Jamison 2014) creates a profound epistemic and ethical gap, to the importance of which we return below. The OSCE can become a scene in which the medical student covers her or his inner feelings with a practised swirl of his or her invisible imaginary cloak of competence, or the equally concealing mask of scored empathy.

The constraints imposed by standardisation, both of the false patients and of the suite of communication skills that the student is required to perform, can erode students' 'sensibilities,' their capacities to feel into the fine grain and unique texture of interaction with an individual patient, or to respond with creativity, imagination or sensitivity (Bleakley 2015). Worse, they can cultivate a medical fantasy that the students' meagre repertoires—both technically, in doses of pharmaceutical medication; and performatively, in pitch, intonation, dynamics and timing—will be sufficient to encounter the all-ages, all-walks-of-life, all-backgrounds radical alterity of their patients and the variations and inherent uncertainties of their illnesses (Bleakley 2018). The OSCE can become a rack of good intentions producing not simulations, but simulacra, copies without originals, fabrications whose unreality are confirmed by the very goals for which they were created (ibid.).

Yet medical students often feel they gain important practice by acting in these small scenes, and educators find that this practice enables a range of performances and constructions of meaning and identity. These rehearsals are often valued, and—in embodied practice—resist standardisation. The imagined future in which the students will play their part but with the consequential suffering of real patients—the subjunctive shift—gives the performance power. In a similar way, the technical prowess that produces entertaining deception at a magic show is a joy shared between magician and audience (Kneebone 2017).

Medical students can be tender, tearful and courageous when attending simulated patients at a simulated car crash or terrorist attack (Brodzinski 2010). Students and SPs, all embodied actors, cannot remain entirely cognitive—they are *affected* in the performance (Marshall and Hooker 2016). Students can accommodate a second subjunctive shift—'what if it were me?' There's nothing inauthentic in this play with repertoire, this construction of a style. We might consider this the beginning of a *critical* mimesis (Irigaray 1985: 76).

Scene IV: so much more real than life—authenticity and expertise

Theatre people are all liars, charlatans, scavengers and fly-by-nights.

(Simon McBurney)

I love acting. It is so much more real than life.

(Oscar Wilde)

Since the 'first wave' of medical humanities (Bleakley 2015; Whitehead and Woods 2016), medical students have been sent to the theatre to watch performances. Instead of being participants in what Victor Turner and Richard Schechner—colleagues of Erving Goffman's—termed the 'social drama,' the conflicts and challenges they might encounter in their everyday of medical practice, they become audience to an 'aesthetic drama'; that is, one that all parties (actors and audience) recognise as not-real, as deliberately staged (Brodzinski 2010).

Typically, such medical students would be exposed to works like Margaret Edson's *W;t, The Elephant Man* or Sarah Kane's *4.48 Psychosis*—works *about* illness, told from the perspective of patients. As with reading literary works about illness experiences, the most common rationale for going to the theatre is to give doctors insight into the lived experience of patienthood and illness and, as a result, to cultivate empathy for their patients. We could recast this in Turner and Schechner's terms: in the aesthetic drama, the medical students see a representation of the social dramas of illness, only with particular features emphasised or slightly shifted; they will then incorporate some of the insights and subtle actions of the aesthetic drama into the social drama of their interactions with patients (Brodzinski 2010). The perceived practical outcome of seeing such theatre might suggest why medical students aren't generally taken to see highly theatrical or abstract absurdist theatre or avant-garde performance art.

Although the artifice of theatre is known and accepted by definition in aesthetic drama, medical students are generally still there to learn something 'real' about patients' experiences—as though 'patient experience' is 'real' and not itself a construction (Scott 1991). Increasingly, there are more opportunities for such experiences to be encountered in the theatre by students, echoing a strong desire for telling illness stories in contemporary culture. Pathography has grown exponentially as a literary genre over the past few decades (Whitehead 2014). This growth is part of a wider turn to 'documentary theatre' (Reinelt 2009), which encompasses a range of forms that include verbatim theatre (actors performing 'word-for-word' accounts collected by interviewing people), testimonial theatre (actors performing transcripts of public inquiries), autobiographical performance (the performer telling their own story) and documentary drama (a theatre company translates the assemblage of factual objects and accounts and generates a performance text from these with added artistic license).

Perhaps ironically, the theatre is considered "a way of re-establishing trust and truth, where these values have been found lacking in institutions" (Schulze 2017: 195), especially the media (Anderson and Wilkinson 2007). Though theatre is also constructed and partial in how it represents reality, its framing as a form of 'make-believe'—where the event of performance only refers to events that happened in another place, at another time—inoculates it from the kind of accusations of inauthenticity other forms of public address may receive. Its potency comes from its not claiming to be completely true. Theatre holds a particular power, however, where the performance features a trace of lived experience, a call to the audience that the spoken words, like the actors' bodies, have been brought in from an outside world (Carlson 2016a); the primary source material used in 'theatre for health' (Brodzinski 2014; Shah and Greer 2018). While medical students worry or joke about how they counterfeit a doctor, verbatim theatre, documentary theatre forms and theatre for health are consumed by audiences and theatre makers hungry for 'authenticity' (Brown and Wake 2010; Bleakley 2018) amid life in hyperreality (Bleakley 2015).

The desire for authenticity is intrinsically connected to the forms of social disempowerment that these theatre works address. Documentary theatre makers work within the traditions of theatre for change, of which Augusto Boal's *Theatre of the Oppressed* is best known. Verbatim and other documentary theatre works are typically oriented to representing the stories and voices of those whose social marginalisation is reflected in their absences or stereotyped representation in public and popular culture. The purpose of documentary theatre is often framed as a form of 'consciousness raising,' allowing audiences to better see and understand their own social circumstances and to make others aware of the existence and qualities of social problems (Wilkinson 2007; Madsen 2018).

This rationale underpins theatre works about illness, the sort that medical students might see. Such works provide a platform for the voices of patients and sufferers of stigmatised, mental and chronic illnesses, groups defined by disenfranchisement within medicine. And as audience, with no need to present their role or reach for their cloak of competence, medical students can allow another subjunctive shift—'what if I'm not the expert?' Documentary theatre forms often deliberately position their informants as the experts. Indeed, some include non-trained performers precisely because they have lived experience of the production's subject—for example, Lara Veitch, whose experiences with cancer featured significantly in Brian Lobel and Bryony Kimming's *A Pacifist's Guide to the War on Cancer* (2016). Rather than being seen as amateurs on an alien stage, such performers become 'experts of the everyday'—a term used by prolific 'reality theatre' company Rimini Protokoll for their collaborators from outside mainstream performing arts (Mumford 2013).

Authenticity here is a matter of communal holding by all gathered in the audience—lived experiences shared in public are potent. Caroline Wake, in her analysis of headphone verbatim theatre piece *Stories of Love and Hate*, employs sociologist Nick Couldry's observation that neoliberalism's push to maximise efficiency for profit smothers the time-consuming task of consultation, be it with a firm's clients, a business's customers, the *polis* of a city or, we might add, patients and staff in a healthcare system (Wake 2014). The result for Couldry is a 'crisis of voice,' and Wake adds that this becomes a "social laryngitis . . . whereby individuals and collectives inflame their throats not by shouting but by strangling their voices even before they emerge" (ibid.: 82).

An audience witnessing documentary theatre becomes part of re-voicing the non-consulted. The power of these works—remarked on time and again by audiences that become tearful, discomfited, uplifted and otherwise affected (Massumi 2015)—has long been recognised to have transformative effects. Audiences, implicated in the performance, do not merely experience emotion or achieve catharsis in the Aristotelian way, but often articulate deeper, ethically inflected shifts in their sense of self and new commitments to values-based social action (Boal 1979; Wilkinson 2007; Anderson and Wilkinson 2007; Madsen 2018). Consciousness raised becomes 'conscientisation,' critical consciousness.

Of course, many medical students are well enough equipped with Goffmanian armour to mock such works, or otherwise enact their own resistance to normative, morally dictatorial pedagogies. And in both medicine and theatre, there are many concerns about how easily a form intended to empower can be recolonised by social elites. Patients' narratives can become simply a resource for a performance of medical virtue (Garden 2007); patients' voices can become compulsory confessions, used for a medical performance of pastoral care (Mayes 2009); and the voices of the voiceless achieve distinction for middle-class theatre makers, not for themselves (Gibson 2011). Similarly, the turn to 'research-based theatre' (Balfour 2009; Belliveau and Lea 2016) might be methodologically sophisticated, but is also constructed by the defensive epistemic norms and anxieties of health research, and the inexorable constraints of neoliberal university outputs, impacts and achievements, subsuming and re-rationalising the labour of the 'experts of the everyday' by a dramaturgical scientific gaze seeking to incorporate only that which is 'evidence-based.'

As this suggests, while staging patients in the role of expert can deliver narratives of healthcare to doctors and medical students from beyond the spectrum of their daily experiences, the audience will still interpret what they watch through their own cultural sensibilities, assumptions and prejudices (Geertz 1983). The question we must turn to then is: 'how might the performing arts challenge the ways in which doctors are trained to see and, in seeing, how they are taught to respond?'

Entr'acte: <smoke machine> seeking 'empathy'

Jealous in honour, sudden and quick in quarrel, seeking the bubble reputation even in the cannon's mouth.

(Jacques, As You Like It, *Act II Scene vii)*

While medical students get sent to the (aesthetic) theatre to gain insight into patients' experiences, the rationale is typically an intention to build students' empathy. It is hard to overstate the frequency or passion with which empathy is desired as professional fabric for medical students and doctors, or the extent of academic literature now devoted to the term (Pedersen 2007; Bleakley 2015; Hooker 2015).

Other than occasional pleas on websites (see for example thedailybeast.com/how-being-a-doctor-became-the-most-miserable-profession), there are no exhortations to cultivate empathy *for doctors,* and no plays or novels recommended to medical students for that purpose. One of our observations has been that, so long as no one offers empathy *to* medical students, enabling embodied insight into how it transforms (Marshall and Hooker 2016), calls for new doctors to show empathy to patients cannot have much effect. Medical students and junior doctors are not only treated as powerless and disenfranchised in the hierarchies of medicine, but, resultingly, often experience abuse and mistreatment at the hands of their senior consultant instructors—close to 90% experience or witness 'teaching by humiliation,' for example, across several English-speaking countries (Scott et al. 2015). Under these conditions, precisely what did we collectively expect to result from mimesis?

Empathy is a 'weasel word' with not only varied, but also contradictory, definitions (Pedersen 2007; Bleakley 2015; Hooker 2015). Notionally a moment in which a doctor feels with or for a patient, it has just as often been the occasion for medical self-congratulation (Garden 2007). Notionally a basis for care, medical schools, health care institutions and governments have been all too eager to offer it as a means of coping with the deficits that patient disempowerment and uncoordinated, under-funded health care education and institutions produce.

If we look directly at what has, until now, been made invisible—namely, the extent of bullying, harassment and mistreatment in healthcare workplaces, the subject of the 2017 verbatim theatre work *Grace Under Pressure* (Williams and Dwyer 2017)—our attention, as audience, is shifted from empathy for the suffering of individual characters to the hierarchical structures that perpetuate abuse, mimetically reproducing it from one generation of arrogant, ethically deformed, mostly male, senior clinicians to the next. This is the shift made by Bertolt Brecht, Augusto Boal and other theatre makers whose practice aimed at using theatre to produce social change. Instead of an Aristotelian concept of theatre, in which the audience achieves catharsis through empathy with the (tragic) protagonist—the model on which medical humanities implicitly relies—Brecht used aesthetic, overtly stylised theatre to *distance* the audience from the protagonist, in order to replace empathy for a character with insight into the social structures that produced his or her suffering (Robinson 2016). Boal dispensed with empathy by handing the power to act to the audience, who he termed 'spect-actors' (Boal 1979).

Theorisations of empathy that actually pay attention to the philosophical origins of the term in phenomenology (see Zahavi and Stein, cited in Hooker 2015)—virtually absent in medical education, and directly at odds with the most common instrument used to measure medical students' 'empathy'—understand it as deeply and intrinsically connected to the body, though in ways more complicated and vested in *interaction* than the concept of 'mirror neurons' can presently accommodate.

But when medical students are exhorted to 'demonstrate' empathy, they are not provided with ways of cultivating it where it occurs—in the body. Medical students are not taught to acknowledge their bodies. Instead, they are taught to *deny* their fatigue, their hunger, their dehydration and their stress. They are not given space to build an embodied, aesthetic sense of transient but profound ethical relations—what Nussbaum calls "fine awareness and rich responsibility" and Bleakley, following Rancière, calls "sensibility" (Nussbaum 1990; Bleakley 2015). Returning medical students to their bodies is something that performance can offer to the medical humanities (Watson 2011; Singh, Khosla and Sridhar 2012; Larsen, Friis and Heape 2018).

Indeed, empathy has been theorised as something *done-in-performance*—as intense, social-emotional labour performed in ways similar to the deep acting performed by stage and screen actors trained in Lee Strasberg's method-acting tradition (Larson and Yao 2005). This idea encapsulates the ways in which empathy is not so much a 'feeling' as it is *process*. Empathy is *what happens*—the transient and powerful capacities that bodies have when they are *affected* (Marshall and Hooker 2016).

For these reasons, several scholars have emphasised that empathy, like consciousness raising, implies moral relations: it is not enough to 'feel with' someone suffering: such a feeling brings with it ethical requirements to act (although what action to take is rarely simple, exact or obvious) (Bolaki 2016). Kate Rossiter makes this argument specifically with reference to the play *W;t*—one of the most canonical theatre works in the medical humanities (Rossiter 2012).

Scene V: that within which passes show—improvising the future

. . . to live truthfully under given imaginary circumstances.

(Sanford Meisner)

'Microethics' (Komesaroff 2008) and care ethics (Noddings 2002)—the ethics of being-in-relation to others—require connection. In the medical humanities, there has long been concern about the alienating effects of replacing forms of touch, such as palpation, percussion and auscultation, with technology and flows of data (Castel 1991; Verghese and Horwitz 2009). Perhaps the SP needs the antidote of the slight awkwardness, the intense, multivalent communication, of touch.

Hence, the current shift in medical education towards the interactive performance approaches drawn from Boal's *Theatre of the Oppressed*—Forum Theatre is particularly popular as a means of making patient experience more visible to the medical spect-actors (Boynton 2009; Hammer et al. 2011; Watson 2011; Berkun 2013; Shochet et al. 2013; Atluru 2016; Arnett 2017; Baker 2017; Boynton 2009; Buck 2017; Dudeck and McClure 2018; Hoffmann-Longtin, Rossing and Weinstein 2018; Larsen, Friis and Heape 2018)—and from specific performance schools such as Meisner and Lecoq and the Chicago tradition of improvisation originating from the work of Viola Spolin (Watson 2011). These approaches recognise and explicitly challenge hegemonic medicine's anxiety to achieve certainty, neutrality and objectivity, to standardise and to measure (Bleakley 2015), which are so at odds with the lived experience of clinical practice, where patients are so much more variable (physiologically and circumstantially) than the blunt instrument of treatments averaged through randomised controlled trials (RCTs).

Improvisation offers a way of addressing the unexpected, how to be open to input in a manner that accepts it and adds to it (the 'yes and . . .' principle) (Watson 2011). Performance practice acknowledges and deepens the embodied skills and intuitive, embodied knowledge of medical specialisations, of which surgery is the pre-eminent example (Kneebone 2018). It speaks to the subjunctive 'what if I was a doctor?' Dreyfus and Dreyfus (1986: 30) emphasise that the central criterion for expertise is that the practitioner does not follow explicit rules, but responds to the affordances presented by the situation (cf. ibid.: 63, n.32). What makes someone an expert is less the quality of their knowledge or technique than their experience *as they act*. This includes the capacity to enter a 'flow state' in which cognitive, emotional and physiological integration result in seamless, quality performances that can include expert improvisation such as those given by jazz musicians, hip-hop dance artists, magicians and plein-air painters (Bergamin 2016; Whorwell and Shanahan 2016). 'Improv practice' helps students respond to the 'pimping' public interrogation method by which they are often taught. It enables increased capacity to handle criticism and feedback, absorbing and reflecting it in the process of being a doctor (conscious leadership). Because students gain responsive tools, it can reduce performance anxiety (Watson 2011; Scott et al. 2017).

But 'improv,' clowning, playback and other forms of interactive performance are not just another instrument for building yet another set of standardised skills. They are self-reportedly 'transformative' (Anderson and Wilkinson 2007; Balfour 2009; Larsen, Friis and Heape 2018). The paradigm of 'enactment' provides a framework for understanding why—because of the profound and unavoidable construction of the self that occurs not as a result, but in the process, of inter-act-ion with others. Because improvising requires confronting uncertainty and hence often unexpectedly profound vulnerability, clinicians may be surprised at the sudden degree of emotion present; for example, particularly of anxiety—it can more significantly *affect* a sense of identity.

In the paradigm of 'enactment,' perception itself is theorised as a social, rather than an individual, phenomenon: perception is enactive, relational and specific to an environment (Zarrilli 2007). This enables a fourth subjunctive shift: 'what if medicine really was ensemble, or collaboration?' Meaning and understanding—for example, the co-constructed knowledge of a particular patient's chronic pain or medically unexplained symptoms—emerges best from co-creation, whereas 'impression management' and struggles between the actors (patient, doctor and others in the health system) to define the scene and their roles is notoriously disastrous (Stone 2012). This theatre is a theatre not of meaning but of "forces, intensities, present affects" (Zarrilli 2007). Meaning emerges from "having intentions, acting, and getting a response" (Larsen, Friis and Heape 2018), a social process that occurs *in the act of doing it* (ibid.: 151).

This approach develops the ethical maturity of professionals (doctors or otherwise). The capacity for this deep *ethical* development has been theorised in divergent ways—for example, as the cultivation of 'sensibility' (Bleakley 2015), as 'care' (Thompson 2015), as 'tenderness' (Cixous, cited in Bleakley 2015), as fine awareness and rich responsibility (Nussbaum 1990) and as the 'microethics' of clinical practice (Komesaroff 2008). We join these others in suggesting that it is this ethical development, rather than 'empathy' (more of a secondary consequence of ethical maturation), that is primarily sought by theatre and performance in the medical humanities (Rossiter 2012). Here we suggest additionally that this ethical maturation is a richer concept than the 'authenticity' or 'presence' that are often held up as the desired opposite to 'performance' (Bleakley et al. 2011; Auton 2018)—indeed, 'presence' can be understood as a verb, not an enigmatic noun, created in the act of performance (Macneill 2014).

Scene VI: finale

Theatre is a space shaped by action in public, where people come together to witness and enact meaning and affect. Performance practice involves what Norbert Elias referred to as "the paradox of involvement and detachment," the capability of being part of the emergent flow of the action, affected and re-acting to it (Larsen, Friis and Heape 2018), and simultaneously an observer of it. Such capacities are a critical component of the *phronesis*—practical wisdom—that several analysts have identified as a core component of being—doing—a good doctor (Little 2003).

Theatre offers the means to inhabit the gap between authentic and pretend *and in this way* strengthens the ethical integrity of medicine. Authenticity is not the question, at least not 'authenticity' imagined as what lies underneath the cloak of competence or as a still presence amid the flux of performance. Rather, authenticity exists transiently, in enactment, in the creating of self—as Foucault might suggest, as a work of art. Performing arts practices entering medical education highlight the capacity for health as a translational, collaborative engagement between all participants (Kristeva et al. 2018), each interpellated as expert, drawing on their own embodiment of illness, dis-ease, biomedicine, healthcare protocols and the like: each listening to, and responding with, one another in direct attendance. Rather than a site for anxiety, the gap becomes a 'what if?', an invitation to shift medicine and healthcare delivery from contained, individualised experiences of illness and the neoliberal systems that manage them towards co-present, polyvocal enactments of healing.

References

Anderson M, Wilkinson L. A resurgence of verbatim theatre: Authenticity, empathy and transformation. *Australasian Drama Studies*. 2007; 50: 153–69.

Arnett B. 2017. *The Complete Improviser*. (Bookbaby: on demand).

Arnold MH, Finniss DG, Kerridge I. Medicine's inconvenient truth: The placebo and nocebo effect. *Internal Medicine Journal*. 2014; 44: 398–405.

Atluru A. 2016. What improv can teach tomorrow's doctors. *The Atlantic*. August 24 2016. Available at: www.theatlantic.com/education/archive/2016/08/what-improv-can-teach-tomorrows-doctors/497177. Last accessed: 11 November 2018.

Auton E. 2018. *Performance or Presence? Examining the Private Parts of Medical Education*. University of NSW.

Baker B. 2017. Improvisation for the doctor–patient connection. In: LinkedIn September 15, 2017. Available at: www.linkedin.com/pulse/improvisation-doctor-patient-connection-bob-baker-md. Last accessed: 11 November 2018.

Balfour M. The politics of intention: Looking for a theatre of little changes. *Research in Drama Education: The Journal of Applied Theatre and Performance*. 2009; 14: 347–59.

Belliveau G, Lea G (eds.) 2016. *Research-Based Theatre as Artistic Methodology*. Chicago, IL: Intellect.

Bergamin JA. Being-in-the-flow: Expert coping as beyond both thought and automaticity. *Phenomenology and the Cognitive Sciences*. 2016; 16: 403–24.

Berkun S. 2013. What I learned from improv class. In *Scott Berkun*, April 16, 2013. Available at: http://scottberkun.com/2013/what-i-learned-from-improv-class. Last accessed: 11 November 2018.

Bleakley A. 2015. *Medical Humanities and Medical Education: How the Medical Humanities Can Shape Better Doctors*. London: Routledge.

Bleakley A. Bad faith, medical education, and post-truth. *Perspectives on Medical Education*. 2018; 7: 3–4.

Bleakley A, Bligh J, Browne J. 2011. *Medical Education for the Future: Identity, Power, Location*. Dordrecht: Springer.

Boal A. 1979. *Theatre of the Oppressed*. Sydney: Pluto Press.

Bolaki S. 2016. *Illness as Many Narratives* London: Edinburgh University Press.

Boynton B. 2009. *Confident Voices: The Nurses' Guide to Improving Communication and Creating Positive Workplaces*. (CreateSpace Independent Publishing Platform).

Brodzinski E. 2010. *Theatre in Health and Care*. Basingstoke: Palgrave Macmillan.

Brodzinski E. 2014. Performance anxiety: The relationship between social and aesthetic drama in medicine and health. In: V Bates, A Bleakley, S Goodman (eds.) *Medicine, Health and the Arts: Approaches to Medical Humanities*. London: Routledge.

Brown P, Wake C. 2010. *Verbatim: Staging Memory and Community*. Strawberry Hills, NSW: Currency Press.

Buck JH. 2017. *Medical Improv: A New Way to Improve Communication!* (CreateSpace Independent Publishing Platform).

Byrd WM, Clayton L. 2002. *An American Health Dilemma: Race, Medicine, and Health Care in the United States 1900–2000*. New York, NY: Routledge.

Carlson M. 2016a. The imitation of what? In: *Shattering Hamlet's Mirror: Theatre and Reality*. Ann Arbor, MI: University of Michigan Press.

Carlson M. 2016b. Verbatim. In: *Shattering Hamlet's Mirror: Theatre and Reality*. Ann Arbor, MI: University of Michigan Press.

Castel R. 1991. From dangerousness to risk. In: G Burchell, C Gordon, P Miller (eds.) *The Foucault Effect: Studies in Governmentality*. Chicago, IL: University of Chicago Press.

Collyer F. 2015. *The Palgrave Handbook of Social Theory in Health, Illness, and Medicine*. Basingstoke: Palgrave Macmillan.

Diamond E. 1997. *Unmaking Mimesis: Essays on Feminism and Theater*. London: Routledge.

Dreyfus HL, Dreyfus SE. 1986. *Mind Over Machine: The Power of Human Intuition and Expertise in the Era of the Computer*. New York, NY: Free Press.

Dudeck TR, McClure C. 2018. *Applied Improvisation: Leading, Collaborating, and Creating Beyond the Theatre*. London: Bloomsbury Publishing.

Farber L. Lying on the couch. *Review of Existential Psychology and Psychiatry*. 1974; 13: 125–35.

Foucault M. 1984. On the genealogy of ethics: Overview of a work in progress. In: P Rabinow (ed.) *The Foucault Reader*. New York, NY: Pantheon.

Foxton M. 2012. *Bedside Stories: Confessions of a Junior Doctor*. London: Atlantic Books Limited.

Garden R. The problem of empathy: Medicine and the humanities. *New Literary History: A Journal of Theory and Interpretation*. 2007; 38: 551–67.

Geertz C. 1983. Art as a cultural system. In: *Local Knowledge: Further Essays in Interpretive Anthropology*. New York, NY: Basic Books.

Gemi-Iordanou E, Gordon S, Matthew R, McInnes E. 2014. *Medicine, Healing and Performance*. Oxford: Oxbow Books.

Gibson J. Saying it right: Creating ethical verbatim theatre. *NEO: Journal for Higher Degree Students in the Social Sciences and Humanities*. 2011; 4: 1–18.

Goffman E. 1959. *The Presentation of Self in Everyday Life*. New York, NY: Anchor Books.

Goffman E. 1961. *Asylums: Essays on the Social Situation of Mental Patients and Other Inmates*. Garden City, NY: Anchor Books.

Haas J, Shaffir W. The professionalization of medical students: Developing competence and a cloak of competence. *Symbolic Interaction*. 1977; 1: 71–88.

Halliwell S. 2009. Mimesis and the history of aesthetics. In: S Halliwell, *The Aesthetics of Mimesis: Ancient Texts and Modern Problems*. Princeton, NJ: Princeton University Press, 1–56.

Hammer RR, Rian JD, Gregory JK, et al. Telling the patient's story: Using theatre training to improve case presentation skills. *Medical Humanities*. 2011; 37: 18–22.

Hitchcock K. 2009. *Little White Slips*. Canberra: Pan Macmillan Australia.

Hoffmann-Longtin K, Rossing JP, Weinstein E. Twelve tips for using applied improvisation in medical education. *Medical Teacher*. 2018; 40: 351–56.

Hooker C. Understanding empathy: Why phenomenology and hermeneutics can help medical education and practice. *Medicine, Health Care and Philosophy*. 2015; 18: 541–52.

Irigaray L. 1985. The power of discourse and the subordination of the feminine. In: *This Sex Which Is Not One*. Ithaca, NY: Cornell University Press, 68–85.

Jacobsen MH, Kristiansen S. 2015. Goffman's sociology of everyday life interaction. In: *The Social Thought of Erving Goffman*. Thousand Oaks, CA: SAGE Publications, 67–84.

Jamison L. 2014. *The Empathy Exams: Essays*. London: Granta Publications.

Kneebone RL. Performing magic, performing medicine. *The Lancet*. 2017; 389: 148–9.

Kneebone RL. Introducing 'In Practice.' *The Lancet*. 2018; 391: 723.

Komesaroff P. 2008. *Experiments in Love and Death: Medicine, Postmodernism, Microethics and the Body*. Melbourne: Melbourne University Press.

Kristeva J, Moro MR, Ødemark J, Engebretsen E. Cultural crossings of care: An appeal to the medical humanities. *Medical Humanities* 2018; 44: 55–58.

Lam V. 2008. *Bloodletting and Miraculous Cures*. New York, NY: HarperCollins Publishers.

Larsen H, Friis P, Heape C. Improvising in the vulnerable encounter: Using improvised participatory theatre in change for healthcare practice. *Arts and Humanities in Higher Education*. 2018; 17: 148–65.

Larson EB, Yao X. Clinical empathy as emotional labor in the patient–physician relationship. *JAMA*. 2005; 293: 1100–6.

Latour B. 1993. *We Have Never Been Modern*. Cambridge, MA: Harvard University Press.

Little M. 2003. *Restoring Humane Values to Medicine: A Miles Little Reader*. Sydney: Desert Pea Press.

Macneill P. 2014. Presence in performance: An enigmatic quality. In: P Macneill (ed.) *Ethics and the Arts* Dordrecht: Springer, 137–49.

Madsen W. Raising social consciousness through verbatim theatre: A realist evaluation. *Arts & Health*. 2018; 10: 181–94.

Marshall GRE, Hooker C. Empathy and affect: What can empathied bodies do? *Medical Humanities*. 2016; 42: 128–34.

Massumi B. 2015. *Politics of Affect*. Hoboken, NJ: Wiley.

Mayes C. Pastoral power and the confessing subject in patient-centred communication. *Journal of Bioethical Inquiry*. 2009; 6: 483–93.

McNamara L. Conjurers, purifiers, vagabonds and quacks: The clinical roles of the folk and Hippocratic healers of Classical Greece. *Iris: Journal of the Classical Association of Victoria*. 2004; 16–17: 2–25.

Mitchell-Boyask R. The art of medicine: Plague and theatre in ancient Athens. *The Lancet*. 2009; 373: 374–5.

Morrissey J. Regimes of performance: Practices of the normalised self in the neoliberal university. *British Journal of Sociology of Education*. 2015; 36: 614–34.

Mumford M. Rimini Protokoll's reality theatre and intercultural encounter: Towards an ethical art of partial proximity. *Contemporary Theatre Review*. 2013; 23: 153–65.

Noddings N. 2002. *Starting at Home: Caring and Social Policy*. San Francisco, CA: University of California Press.

Nussbaum M. 1990. *Love's Knowledge*. Oxford: Oxford University Press.

Oberhelman S. 2013. *Dreams, Healing, and Medicine in Greece: From Antiquity to the Present*. London: Routledge.

Palmieri JJ, Stern TA. Lies in the doctor–patient relationship. *Primary Care Companion to the Journal of Clinical Psychiatry*. 2009; 11: 163–8.

Pedersen R. Empathy: A wolf in sheep's clothing? *Medicine, Health Care and Philosophy*. 2007; 11: 325–35.

Porter R. 1999. *The Greatest Benefit to Mankind: A Medical History of Humanity from Antiquity to the Present*. London: Fontana Press.

Reinelt J. 2009. The promise of documentary. In: A Forsyth, C Megson (eds.) *Get Real: Documentary Theatre Past and Present*. London: Palgrave Macmillan, 6–23.

Robinson A. 2016. An A to Z of theory. Augusto Boal: Theatre of the Oppressed. *Ceasefire*. 29 March 2016. Available at: https://ceasefiremagazine.co.uk/augusto-boal-theatre-oppressed. Last accessed: 18 May 2019.

Rossiter K. Bearing response-ability: Theater, ethics and medical education. *Journal of Medical Humanities*. 2012; 33: 1–14.

Roth D. 2008. Reciprocal influences between rhetoric and medicine in ancient Greece. University of Iowa. PhD Thesis. Available at: https://ir.uiowa.edu/cgi/viewcontent.cgi?article=1188&context=etd. Last accessed: 11 November 2018.

Schulze D. 2017. *Authenticity in Contemporary Theatre and Performance: Make It Real*. London: Bloomsbury Publishing.

Scott J. The evidence of experience. *Critical Inquiry*. 1991; 17: 773–97.

Scott K, Berlec S, Nash L, et al. Grace under pressure: A drama-based approach to tackling mistreatment of medical students. *Medical Humanities*. 2017; 43: 68–70.

Scott K, Caldwell P, Barnes E, Barrett J. 'Teaching by humiliation' and mistreatment of medical students in clinical rotations: A pilot study. *The Medical Journal of Australia*. 2015; 203: 185.

Shah S, Greer S. Polio monologues: Translating ethnographic text into verbatim theatre. *Qualitative Research*. 2018; 18: 53–69.

Shem S. 2009. *House of God*. London: Transworld.

Shochet R, King J, Levine R, et al. 'Thinking on my feet': An improvisation course to enhance students' confidence and responsiveness in the medical interview. *Education for Primary Care*. 2013; 24: 119–24.

Sinclair S. 1997. *Making Doctors: An Institutional Apprenticeship*. Oxford: Berg.

Singh S, Khosla J, Sridhar S. Exploring medical humanities through Theatre of the Oppressed. *Indian Journal of Psychiatry*. 2012; 54: 296–7.

Stone L. On botany and gardening: Diagnosis and uncertainty in the GP consultation. *Australian Family Practice*. 2012; 41: 795–8.

Thompson J. Towards an aesthetics of care. *Research in Drama Education: The Journal of Applied Theatre and Performance*. 2015; 20: 430–41.

Turner V. 1990. Are there universals of performance in myth, ritual, and drama? In: R Schechner, W Appel (eds.) *By Means of Performance: Intercultural Studies of Theatre and Ritual*. Cambridge: Cambridge University Press, 8–18.

Verghese A, Horwitz RI. In praise of the physical examination. *British Medical Journal*. 2009; 339: b5448.

Wake C. The politics and poetics of listening: Attending headphone verbatim theatre in post-Cronulla Australia. *Theatre Research International*. 2014; 39: 82–100.

Wallace P. 2006. *Coaching Standardized Patients: For Use in the Assessment of Clinical Competence*. New York, NY: Springer.

Warner JH. 2003. *Against the Spirit of System: The French Impulse in Nineteenth Century American Medicine*. New York, NY: Johns Hopkins University Press.

Watson K. Perspective: Serious play—Teaching medical skills with improvisational theater techniques. *Academic Medicine*. 2011; 86: 1260–5.

Whitehead A. 2014. The medical humanities: A literary perspective. In: V Bates, A Bleakley, S Goodman (eds.) *Medicine, Health and the Arts: Approaches to the Medical Humanities*. London: Routledge.

Whitehead A, Woods A (eds.). 2016. *The Edinburgh Companion to the Critical Medical Humanities*. Edinburgh: Edinburgh University Press.

Whorwell PJ, Shanahan F. In the performing art of medicine: The doctor as actor. *QJM: An International Journal of Medicine*. 2016; 109: 159–60.

Wilkinson LA. 2007. Creating verbatim theatre: Exploring the gap between public inquiry and private pain. University of Sydney.

Williams D, Dwyer P. 2017. *Grace Under Pressure*. Sydney: Currency Press.

Zarrilli PB. An enactive approach to understanding acting. *Theatre Journal*. 2007; 59: 635–47.

20

A MANIFESTO FOR ARTISTS' BOOKS AND THE MEDICAL HUMANITIES

Stella Bolaki

In the old art the writer writes texts.

In the new art the writer makes books.

(Ulises Carrión)

What is (not) an artist's book?

The artist's book "integrates the formal means of its realization and production with its thematic or aesthetic issues".[1] Rather than a mere container for ideas, it underscores its materiality, its **BOOKNESS**.

The artist's book refuses to relinquish its allegiances to either art or to the book. But it has many more allegiances.

Johanna Drucker has sketched out a "zone" for the artist's book, made by "the intersection" of many "individual fields of activity":

> fine printing, independent publishing, the craft tradition of book arts, conceptual art, painting and other traditional arts, politically motivated art activity and activist production, performance of both traditional and experimental varieties, concrete poetry, experimental music, computer and electronic arts, and last but not least, the tradition of the illustrated book, *the livre d'artiste*.[2]

Artists' books are committed to a permanent process of reinvention. "Anything can be considered a book if that is the artist's intention."[3]

The aesthetic and political characteristics of artists' books

Created for one-on-one *sensual* interaction, artists' books are *intimate*.

Unlike the untouchable painting hanging on a gallery wall, they are "uniquely accessible."[4]

Unlike the dancer and the musician who "produce and consume their aesthetic product" but are themselves "instruments for yet a further audience," the reader of an artist's book is "both performer and audience."[5]

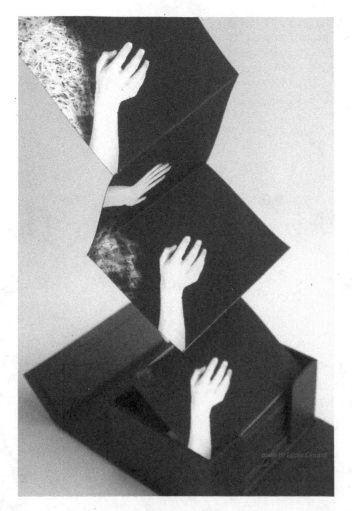

Figure 20.1   David Paton, *Speaking in Tongues: Digitally Speaking/Speaking Digitally* (2015). Digital print on Innova Smooth Cotton High White. Photo by Egidija Čiricaitė

Artists' books are a radical format of bringing art to a wider public. They circulate outside the gallery system. Most art works don't get passed from hand to hand. One doesn't just "happen to 'find' a Jackson Pollock painting . . . among one's things" or on the shelves of a bookshop. Books have the "capacity to be in the world with an independence and mobility unlike that of any other work of art."[6]

Not all books have such a free life, of course, but the **democratic** myth of the book is still alive. The space of the artist's book is THE WORLD. Not just the art world.

The book as matter and metaphor

Books are corporeal. They have a body and skin. Too often a **cracked** spine.

In the language of typography and publishing, we refer to the "body" of the text. And whatever is attached to that body is described with terms such as headers, footers, glossaries and appendices.

Artists' books are "lived bodies." Claudia Kolgen's book *Ein Hauch von Erinnerungen* (*A Hint of Remembrance*) "breathes through a small aperture in the dark grey cover as you open and close it, forcing air in and out of the white rubber bellows, lungs."[7]

The book has rich metaphorical associations. We talk of "turning the page, or of starting a new chapter in our lives. We shelter, disguise or hide ourselves between covers."

As Clare Best affirms, "we are all **BOOK**."[8]

The binding of a book is a *scar*. This is a metaphor but it is also where the pages of the book stitch together and come apart.

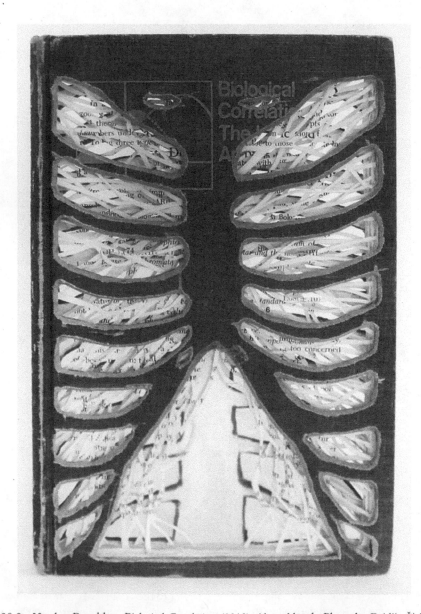

Figure 20.2   Heather Beardsley, *Biological Correlations* (2013). Altered book. Photo by Egidija Čiricaitė

Some books hide their *scars*. Others flaunt them.

If "writing good iambic pentameter feels like putting *stitches* into the eternally gaping wound of being human,"[9] artists' books "literally process" experiences through "*stitches*, glue and tears."[10]

Artists' books and the medical humanities

In the *first wave* of medical humanities, the subjective experience of illness is articulated through narrative.

In the *second wave* of medical humanities, illness experiences are articulated through **embodied**, **performative**, e p i s o d i c and **hy**b*rid* forms of expression.

An artist's book "consists of various elements, one of which might be text.

A text that is part of a book isn't necessarily the most essential or important part of that book."[11]

An artist's book may contain as many words as a narrative but these are embedded in the matter of the book, where they appear in "a **more intentional**, MORE EVIDENT, **deeper way**."[12]

Linearity, coherence and closure have been privileged in illness narratives. But illness experiences "may lack a beginning" (its causes hidden) or an ending, "where resolution is reached."[13]

The basic internal dialogue of any book form is sequence and breaks. Artists' books may follow a linear movement or consist of a collection of "fragments, glimpses and moments," focusing on "the embodied and now."[14]

First-wave medical humanities engage in listening and proxy-experience.

Second-wave medical humanities demand embodied interaction and participation.

In order to read text, "knowing the alphabet is enough."[15]

In order to read artists' books, one must **PLAY** their various elements as if they were a "musical score."[16]

Conventional illness narratives establish an "inter-subjective communication.

Inter-subjective communication occurs in an abstract, ideal, impalpable space."

In the case of artists' books, "communication is still inter-subjective, but it occurs in a concrete, real, physical space—the page."[17]

To make a book is . . .

"Enclosure and intimacy are two familiar features of the book's {spatial embrace}."[18]

But the space of the book is intimate and public at the same time.

Books balance

enclosure

and

EXPOSURE.

A relation between "enclosure" and "exposure"[19] also describes many people's lived experience of illness.

To make a book is "to gain power over objects."[20]

To make a book is "to create physical form for ideas."[21]

To make a book is to claim the aesthetic and imaginative elements of illness communication.

To make a book is "to have a voice in the world."[22] Even when the book contains no words.

While making a book can assert the artist's will or mastery of the material world, it can also be a form of "exciting intimacy with nonbeing." Eve Sedgwick described the making of her textile books as "a meditative practice of emptiness" and added: "It feels wonderful to exist and to be active in that space of suspended agency." She was exploring the very "**material**" issue of her mortality through physical means.[23]

To make a book is to share your experience with other people. The exchange happens in the intimate space between page and reader.

To make a book is to "intervene into the social order."[24] This is especially true in the case of transforming existing books through textual, visual and material manipulations, when parts of a work are cut out or altered to make it NEW.

To make a book is "to effect change in the way medical professionals interact with their patients."[25] Martha Hall brought her artists' books to the consultation room and used them to communicate with her physicians while living with breast cancer.

If illness narratives are both "affective" and "effective,"[26] artists' books show that very clearly through the "*intimate* **authority**" that they offer.[27]

Patient ⌷ doctor relations

Like every patient, each artist's book is unique.

Rather than "constituting a series of preformatted boxes to check," as in the electronic patient record, a book "opens up, often in different directions."[28]

Just like patients, artists' books can be seen from a distance, behind a display glass, or *close at hand*.

Just as turning or unfolding a book's pages reveals more than its cover, so "reading" a patient involves more than looking at a set of body scans.

As multisensory spaces artists' books renew faith in "medicine's old-fashioned tool: *human touch*."[29] But examining artists' books goes beyond a diagnostic touch.

Books expect to be *caressed*, not palpated.

Unlike "palpation," the "caress" does not seek to "disclose"; to arrive at an appropriate course of action or a clinical diagnosis.

Instead, "it *searches*."

It is "a movement unto the invisible."[30] As expansive as the process of reading.

Artists' books do not just "call upon the doctor's narrative competence."

They demand a different set of competences or rituals: "the ability to open, and open up to, the book,

and let its mysteries or provocations generate inquiry."[31]

The book has the power to bridge the gap in patient doctor relations as the patient⌷doctor sit together, "joined where parts of the book touch each of them, the book spread across their laps."[32]

This is no book recipe for cultivating empathy.

It may lead to disbelief, denial, discomfort. Compassionate words or silence.

Unsettling silence or silence attesting to presence and witnessing.

The radical pedagogy of artists' books

How to mobilise the *aesthetic* and **political** characteristics of artists' books to **democratise** the *culture* of **medicine**?

How to challenge the invisibility and "epistemic injustice" that patients experience daily?[33]

How to provide alternatives to militaristic, hierarchical and market values within medical care?

How to resist dehumanising metaphors such as *the body as machine*?

How to work towards a "medical aesthetics"?[34]

In the place of an ~~instrumental~~ and ~~technical~~ medical education we need a

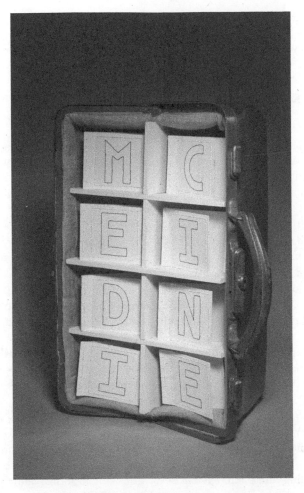

Figure 20.3 Susannah Ronnie, *Books as Medicine* (2014). Paper, transparent paper and card with topstitch thread, leather case. Photo by Colin Davison

radical pedagogy.

We need new metaphors that draw on the imaginative richness, intimacy and complexity of artists' books.

It is important to communicate illness experiences through alternative, more versatile and expressive forms.

But we also need to change habitual ways of perceiving the body so that it is not reduced to the "object of the biomedical gaze."[35] As "objects of wonder,"[36] artists' books can inspire a new sense of mystery and beauty when it comes to the body's materiality.

Artists' books and the medical humanities call for a sensibility attuned to "moments of enchantment," what Jane Bennett calls *"an ethic of enchanted materialism."*[37]

To make books is to resist the "disenchantment story" around medical care.[38]

To make books will not magically make financial pressures and lack of time disappear. But it can create a space to recapture strength and motivation to fight for the improvement of relationships, services and systems.

Sara Ahmed writes:

> We can be shattered by what we come up against.
>
> And then we come up against it **again**.
>
> We can be exhausted by what we come up against.
>
> And then we come up against it **again**.[39]

To make books is to produce new modes of enchantment that don't "guarantee" generosity and ethical responses but make them "more possible."

Artists' books and the medical humanities insist that "repeated acts" of enchantment are required to respond to what we come up against, again and again.[40]

With new "energy and inspiration."[41]

Artists' books and the medical humanities resist the exclusion of "multisensory experience" from "the realm of knowledge."[42]

Artists' books and the medical humanities resist the reduction of experimentation and creativity to the mere provision of technical training.

To make books is to **PLAY BY THE BOOK**, but not by the idiomatic book.

Artists' books "might look and feel different from traditional medical textbooks but they are of equal **HEFT**."[43]

The radical pedagogy of artists' books amounts to a **politics of provocation**.

The radical pedagogy of artists' books amounts to a politics of beauty.

The flip side of the politics of provocation is a politics of **beauty**.[44]

***

Even though manifestos do not require justifications, this text serves as a commentary (an appendix to the main body, if you like) about my choice to write in the form of a manifesto, and to write a manifesto on artists' books and the medical humanities, in particular. Manifestos have a performativity to them, whether it comes from the forceful utterances they consist of—imagining and willing things into existence—or from certain formal and typographic choices their writers make. As my chapter appears in this volume's section on 'performance and public engagement,' writing about an innovative art form that is created to be handled—'played' or 'performed' *through* a performative and playful type of writing—seemed fitting. The artist's book, as an example of "intermedia" (Higgins 1984) that combines text, image and various methods of production, is not the same as performance art, but it is equally embodied and performative, while also being less ephemeral than performance—more tangible, as a result of the book's tactility and materiality.

As my epigraph reveals, the manifesto was largely inspired by Ulises Carrión's *The New Art of Making Books*, originally written in Spanish and published in 1975. As a poet and maker of books, Carrión was influential in conceptualising the artist's book genre (even though he preferred the term *bookwork*). *The New Art of Making Books* consists of 141 statements in six sections about the making of a new and different kind of book—"books that are conceived as an expressive unity . . . where the message is the sum of all the material and formal elements" (Klima 1998: 36)—that fundamentally challenges our reading experience.

In 'A Manifesto for Artists' Books and the Medical Humanities' I draw on Carrión's affirmation of a new bolder aesthetic and on his radical statements that compare the *old* (text) and the *new* (book) in order to approach debates in the medical humanities. Specifically: the privileging of narrative at the expense of alternative forms of representing illness experience; and linked to

that, the emphasis on "narrative competence" (Charon 2006) within the field of medical education. In my manifesto I map the old and the new aesthetic onto the first and second 'wave' of
the medical humanities respectively (Bleakley 2015; Whitehead and Woods 2016). In this way,
I mobilise the provocations of *both* the tradition of artists' books, approached as part of a cultural
revolution that started in the 1960s seeking to democratise art, and of the medical humanities
field in its current, more critical, shape. The manifesto is polyphonic and engages in what, following Audrey Shafer, I have called "critical interloping": as I quote, mix and riff off critics,
artists and educators who have written powerfully not only about illness narratives, the medical
humanities and medical education, but also about books, materiality, activism and pedagogy, I
take delight in welcoming "interlopers from distant disciplines to the cause of medical humanities" (Bolaki 2016: 13).

The critique of the first wave's emphasis on narrative has been met with a turn towards art
forms like performance art, graphic medicine and digital storytelling, and away from a mere focus
on the humanising and instrumental applications of the arts to consider instead their democratising and radical potential. The artist's book, I contend through this manifesto, is a multimodal
and multisensory medium that has affinities with these subversive and less utilitarian art forms.
Despite continuing debate on whether its portability, durability and inexpensive nature necessarily translate into wide accessibility (Lyons 1985), the artist's book is viewed as "fundamentally
democratic as it imagines every reader as a potential contributor to the dialogue it engages" and
"mirrors values to social groups still groping for an identity and a sense of collective purpose"
(Wallis 1998: 101). As such, it can be mobilised to democratise the culture of medicine.

As it does not relinquish its allegiances to either art or to the book (the most common being
the codex form, which is made with pages fixed in a rigid sequence by being clasped on one
side), the artist's book is a productive format for rethinking debates surrounding narrativity in
the medical humanities and the role of affect within illness narrative scholarship (Wasson 2018).
While they don't exclude language or narrative, artists' books can be situated within both the
'performative' and the 'material' turns that resonate with the critical medical humanities; one
must learn to 'perform' books through touch as much as 'read' them. Reading them requires
not only interacting with words and images but also paying attention to their shape, size, format,
colour, texture, typography and even fragrance and sound. Their advantage over literary narratives of illness is that they invite a non-diagnostic participatory touch that not only establishes a
clear association between aesthetic/sensuous experience and verbal or visual communication, but
also makes ethical demands on readers that complicate simplistic models of empathy. This is the
book's radical pedagogy celebrated in the 'Artists' Books and the Medical Humanities' manifesto.

In the remaining part of this commentary, I elaborate on these points and others from the
manifesto, while drawing on examples from a research and public engagement project I led on
artists' books and the medical humanities in 2016. This consisted of an interdisciplinary symposium, an exhibition of contemporary artists' books entitled *Prescriptions* (Beaney Art Museum,
Canterbury, 22 April to 25 September 2016) and a series of bookmaking workshops whose aim
was to allow a wide range of patients, health professionals and members of the public to experience the material and performative power of this medium in practice.[45]

Through their expressive richness and versatility artists' books can enhance the ways in
which we think about, and experience, our bodies. As *material* artefacts, and as a result of the
associations of the book with the body, books mediate *embodied* experiences of illness more
directly than literary narratives. Many of the works included in *Prescriptions* used the book and its
elements as a metaphor for the body or as metaphors for particular kinds of illness. For example,
an open, yet 'frozen' book was used by Ashley Fitzgerald to corporealise a rare condition of the
nervous system in *G. B. S.* (standing for Guillain-Barré Syndrome) (Figure 20.4). Lizanne van

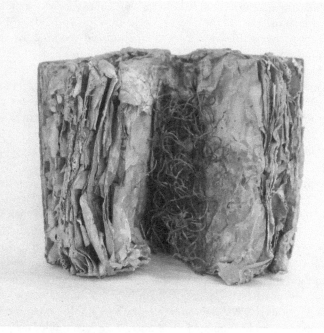

Figure 20.4 Ashley Scott Fitzgerald, *G.B.S.* (2015). Altered book. Photo by Egidija Čiricaitė

Essen's sculptural book *Osteoporosis* exhibited the characteristic holey appearance of osteoporotic bone to display rather than inform about this condition.[46] Artists' books can also bear the body's marks and hold its traces through the inclusion of body scans, pathology lab bags and even fingerprints and hairs in their multi-textured matter. These objects do not merely function as signs, but have a material presence; they return us to their embodied use by the people they belonged to and invite us to attend to our own embodied experience when touching them.

'Illness as a journey' is a dominant way of representing illness experience, but non-linear or open-ended narratives are better suited to some experiences, such as chronic illness. Whether it is telling a story through the concertina form that allows temporal development or offering simultaneity of moments within a single page, artists find voice and meaning in the shaping of their books and stories. Theirs are affective accounts that capture *lived* experiences of illness in a *palpable* way: for example, what waiting for diagnosis and treatment feels like in Anne Parfitt's *Diary of an Illness* (Figure 20.5), which consists of repeated sequential drawings, each drawing "an imitation of the previous, yet never identical . . . mirroring the indistinguishable yet unique nature of each moment" (Parfitt 2017: 74); or how medical events can dominate one's life in Martha A. Hall's *The Rest of My Life II* (Figure 20.6) that consists of an overwhelming amount of medical appointment cards stitched together into a book. As we read in one of its pages, the book becomes a kind of "pulse-taking . . . the present being stitched together—over and over." In retaining sequential regularity, one of the book form's major structural features, but refusing closure, works like these expand awareness of the complexity of illness experiences that resist established forms of narration. The focus on the ever-present or enduring nature of illness experience, which can't be measured in objective time, also reveals that patients rarely constitute the temporality of illness in the same way as their physicians.

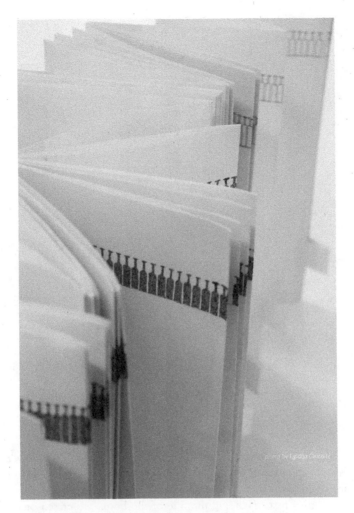

Figure 20.5　Anne Parfitt, *Diary of an Illness* (2000–2001). Ink on paper. Photo by Egidija Čiricaitė

Clinicians, scholars and members of the public have privileged particular types of evidence and ways of presenting or sharing knowledge about health (third-person reports, medical data and illness representations that rely on language or favour triumph stories). This generates "epistemic injustice" (Kidd and Carel 2017) and leads to stigma, silence and, sometimes, poor treatment. Artists' books counter epistemic injustice through the "intimate authority" (Drucker 2011) they offer, even when they treat the invisibility and the often depersonalising experience of being a patient. For example, for her book *Unknown*, also part of a live performance, Carole Cluer considered the number of people diagnosed with breast cancer in the same year as her (45,704 in 2004). Her book consists of pages and pages of identical-looking hand-drawn grids of blue dots (based on the measurements grids and tattoos used when one has radiotherapy), each one representing one person, anonymous like her. While *Unknown* retains affective distance through the system of order it devises and its lack of text, it makes us feel beyond what we can merely see as its content translates into physical sensations that move our bodies. In other cases,

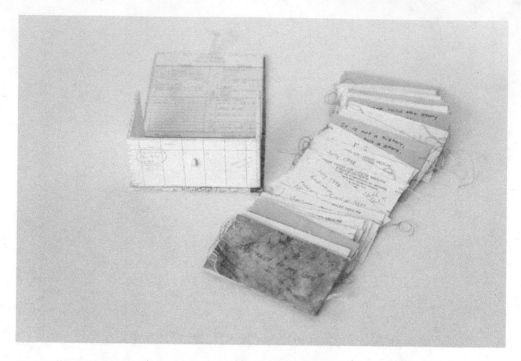

Figure 20.6 Martha Hall, *The Rest of My Life II* (2003). Handmade box covered in colour copies of the artist's planning calendar, accordion with hand stitching and original paste covers. Maine Women Writers Collection, University of New England, Portland, ME. Photo by Laura Taylor

the intervention into medical culture is more forceful as in Hall's *What You Don't Want to Know about Breast Cancer*, an altered version of a publication by the National Cancer Institute. Its pages are stitched, stapled, torn, glued, cut, crumpled, marked and resequenced. Moreover, many of the words in the original text, including the title of the book, are erased or highlighted with black ink. Through this performative, angry book, Hall 'writes back' to the official medical narrative and reclaims some of her agency as a patient.

Dominant metaphors in medical education, such as 'the body as machine,' perpetuate the dehumanising and objectifying aspects of medical care. Artists' books can disperse the medical gaze by opening up the idea of the body as traditionally understood by medicine. They can help reignite a sense of wonder and mystery when it comes to confronting our bodies' materiality (Evans 2016) or their interactions with medical equipment. In the case of the *Prescriptions* exhibition, brain lesions on an MRI scan and arthroscopies of knees were re-contextualised through their visual similarity to stars and a lunar landscape in Egidija Čiricaitė's *Innumerable as the Stars of Night* and Véronique Chance's *In the Absence of Running* respectively. *On Innards* is a collaborative book by Amanda Couch, Andrew Hladky, Mindy Lee and Richard Nash embodied through its multitude of folds: the intestines. It is held together by a mesenteric binding, which, when unwound, allows the book to be fully experienced by the reader. The body experiencing loss of consciousness became associated with stories of enchanted sleep in Julie Brixey-Williams's *Rosebud*, a bookwork created after reading the entire tale of *The Sleeping Beauty* into an anaesthetic machine that drew the breathing patterns as a series of flow loop waveforms. Finally, the body was mapped differently in Lise Melhorn-Boe's meander book

Body Map that consists of square pages, each with a section of the artist's photographed body. Hand-printed text on top of the photos contains personal references (written directly on each part of the body) and researched information about environmental hazards (written around the body). In all these ways, artists' books can "re-enchant" (Willis, Waddington and Marsden 2013: 67) illness narratives as they invest in alternative images that fall outside strictly clinical frameworks. By defamiliarising habitual modes of perception, they can pave the way for new educational metaphors (Bleakley 2017) and promote a more sensately fluent clinical practice at a time of increasing reliance on medical imaging and simulation technologies.

The slow movement through which artists' books have to be handled, given their fragility and vulnerability, can become a metaphor for the kind of gentle care a patient may want. However, this dimension of artists' books also adds "a ritualistic element to the act of reading" and creates "a space for a contemplative experience" (Strand 2017: 90) that engages both body and mind. Whether it is reading or instead making books, as in the case of my project's workshops (Isworth 2017), book arts practices encourage a kind of mindfulness that can redress the emphasis on reflective *writing* models within medical education (Belling 2012) as vehicles for understanding patient experience.

One such vehicle within narrative medicine is Rita Charon's 'parallel chart.' As its name suggests, this chart "parallels the hospital chart but uses ordinary language to render the medical experience palpable, to make it both tangible and sentient" (Langellier 2009: 156). As Kristin Langellier puts it "in performative terms," the parallel chart "repeats the hospital chart but as different, remaking and redoing it as a critical intervention" (ibid.). When we pay attention to its performative aspects, the parallel chart can be seen as "enacting performance as critical pedagogy" (ibid.: 155). Following Langellier, we can bind narrative medicine not only to performance but also to book arts and in this way make even more palpable the aspects of "embodied making (a storytext) and doing (reading it with others)" (ibid.) that are occluded when the focus falls on textuality rather than physicality.

Even as critical medical humanities—specifically one of its streams situated in the humanities—encourages us to widen the frame of enquiry beyond the boundaries of the patient–doctor encounter, with respect to the clinical setting, it importantly asks us to consider: "what else . . . is in the room, and with what forms or modes of agency might it be associated?" For example, "how might we account for non-human-objects and presences"? (Whitehead and Woods 2016: 2). The book as object has agency. In the case of Hall's interactions with the medical community, her books allowed her to bridge the distance, literally, as her doctor and she had to draw their chairs closer to read one of her books together in the consultation room (Bolaki 2016: 77).[47] The book placed between doctor and patient becomes an intimate space of connection in the 'here' and of complete immersion in the 'now.' Provided, of course, that the patient is willing to share her story in this way and the doctor is willing to open, and open up to, the book's performative joys and ethical demands.

Notes

1 Drucker 2004: ?
2 Ibid.
3 Bodman and Sowden 2010: 7.
4 Klima 1998: 16.
5 Mitchell 1996: 166.
6 Drucker 2004: 358.
7 JM Walton qtd. in Bolaki 2016: 87, n.29.
8 Best 2016.
9 Campo 1997: 116.

10 Wellbery 2017: 19.
11 Carrión 1985: 40.
12 Carrión 1985: 34.
13 Wasson 2017.
14 Wasson 2017; Wasson 2018: 6.
15 Carrión 1985: 42.
16 Mitchell 1996: 162.
17 Carrión 1985: 35–36.
18 Drucker 2004: 360.
19 Drucker 2011: 14.
20 Niffeneger 2011: 12.
21 Niffeneger 2011: 13.
22 Hall 2003: 15.
23 Sedgwick 2011: 69–70; 83.
24 Drucker 2004: 109.
25 Hall 2003: 15.
26 Diedrich 2007: xvii.
27 Drucker 2011: 14.
28 Wellbery 2017: 20
29 Verghese 2011.
30 E. Levinas qtd. in Bolaki 2016: 60.
31 Wellbery 2017: 20
32 Ibid.
33 Kidd and Carel 2017.
34 Bleakley 2015: 105.
35 Evans 2016: 345.
36 Drucker 2004: viii.
37 Bennett 2001: 156–57.
38 Ibid.: 174.
39 Ahmed 2017: 163.
40 Bennett 2001: 156–57.
41 Ibid.: 174.
42 Tanner 2006: 209.
43 Miller and Tuttle 2017: 12.
44 M. Klawiter qtd. in Bolaki 2016: 49.
45 To see more about the project's activities, visit https://research.kent.ac.uk/artistsbooks.
46 All examples of artists' books mentioned in the essay refer to the exhibition *Prescriptions*. (Also see Bolaki and Čiricaitė 2017).
47 Also see Martha Hall's documentary *I Make Books* (2004), Maine Women Writers Collection, www.une.edu/mwwc.

References

Ahmed S. 2017. *Living a Feminist Life*. Durham, NC: Duke University Press.
Belling C. A Happy Doctor's Escape from Narrative: Reflection in *Saturday*. *Medical Humanities*. 2012; 38: 2–6.
Bennett J. 2001. *The Enchantment of Modern Life: Attachments, Crossings, and Ethics*. Princeton, NJ: Princeton University Press.
Best C. 2016. I Am Book, *BMJ*, Medical Humanities Blog. Available at: http://blogs.bmj.com/medical-humanities/2016/07/01/i-am-book-clare-best. Last accessed: 20 April 2018.
Bleakley A. 2015. *Medical Humanities and Medical Education: How the Medical Humanities Can Shape Better Doctors*. London: Routledge.
Bleakley A. 2017. *Thinking with Metaphors in Medicine: The State of the Art*. London: Routledge.
Bodman S, Sowden T. 2010. A Manifesto for the Book. [online]. What Will Be the Canon for the Artist's Book in the 21st Century? Available at: www.bookarts.uwe.ac.uk/canon. Last accessed: 20 April 2018.
Bolaki S. 2016. *Illness as Many Narratives: Arts, Medicine and Culture*. Edinburgh: Edinburgh University Press.

Bolaki S, Čiricaitė E (eds.) 2017. *Prescriptions: Artists' Books on Wellbeing and Medicine*. London: Natrix Natrix Press.

Campo R. 1997. *The Desire to Heal: A Doctor's Education in Empathy, Identity, and Poetry*. New York, NY: Norton.

Carrión U. 1985. The New Art of Making Books. In: J Lyons (ed.) *Artists' Books: A Critical Anthology and Sourcebook*. Rochester, NY: Visual Studies Workshop Press Layton, 31–43.

Charon R. 2006. *Narrative Medicine: Honoring the Stories of Illness*. New York, NY: Oxford University Press.

Diedrich L. 2007. *Treatments: Language, Politics, and the Culture of Illness*. Minneapolis, MN: University of Minnesota Press.

Drucker J. 2004. *The Century of Artists' Books*. New York, NY: Granary Books.

Drucker J. 2011. Intimate Authority: Women, Books, and the Public–Private Paradox. In: K Wasserman (ed.) *The Book as Art: Artists' Books from the National Museum of Women in the Arts*. New York, NY: Princeton Architectural Press, 14–17.

Evans M. 2016. Medical Humanities and the Place of Wonder. In: A Whitehead, A Woods (eds.) *The Edinburgh Companion to the Critical Medical Humanities*. Edinburgh: Edinburgh University Press, 339–55.

Hall MA. 2003. Artist's Statement. In: *Holding In, Holding On: Artist's Books by Martha Hall*. Exhibition catalogue. Mortimer Rare Book Room, Smith College, 10–15.

Higgins D. 1984. *Horizons: The Poetics and Theory of the Intermedia*. Carbondale, IL: Southern Illinois University Press.

Isworth E. 2017. "We Make Books": Reflections on Artists' Books and the Medical Humanities Workshops. In: S Bolaki, E Čiricaitė (eds.) *Prescriptions: Artists' Books on Wellbeing and Medicine*. London: Natrix Natrix Press, 23–31.

Kidd IJ, Carel H. Epistemic Injustice and Illness. *Journal of Applied Philosophy*. 2017; 34: 172–90.

Klima S. 1998. *Artists' Books: A Critical Survey of the Literature*. New York, NY: Granary Books.

Langellier KM. Performing Narrative Medicine. *Journal of Applied Communication Research*. 2009; 37: 151–58.

Lyons J. (Ed.) 1985. *Artists' Books: A Critical Anthology and Sourcebook*. New York, NY: Visual Studies Workshop Press.

Miller C, Tuttle JS. 2017. "I make books so I won't die": Artists' Books in the Archives and Classroom. In: S Bolaki, E. Čiricaitė (eds.) *Prescriptions: Artists' Books on Wellbeing and Medicine*. London: Natrix Natrix Press, 11–17.

Mitchell B. 1996. The Secret Life of the Book: The Livre d'Artiste and the Act of Reading. In: L Edson (ed.) *Conjunctions: Verbal–Visual Relations*. San Diego, CA: San Diego University Press, 161–67.

Niffeneger A. 2011. What Does It Mean to Make a Book? In: K Wasserman (ed.) *The Book as Art: Artists' Books from the National Museum of Women in the Arts*. New York, NY: Princeton Architectural Press, 12–13.

Parfitt A. 2017. Diary of an Illness: Artist's Statement. In: S Bolaki, E Čiricaitė (eds.) *Prescriptions: Artists' Books on Wellbeing and Medicine*. London: Natrix Natrix Press, 74.

Sedgwick EK. 2011. Making Things, Practicing Emptiness. In: J Goldberg (ed.) *The Weather in Proust*. Durham, NC: Duke University Press, 69–122.

Strand RA. 2017. Arabesque 3: Artist's Statement. In: S. Bolaki, E. Čiricaitė (eds.) *Prescriptions: Artists' Books on Wellbeing and Medicine*. London: Natrix Natrix Press, 90.

Tanner LE. 2006. *Lost Bodies: Inhabiting the Borders of Life and Death*. Ithaca, NY: Cornell University Press.

Verghese A. 2011. A Doctor's Touch. [online]. TEDGlobal. Available at: www.ted.com/talks/abraham_verghese_a_doctor_s_touch. Last accessed: 20 April 2018.

Wallis B. 1998. The Artist's Book and Postmodernism. In: C Lauf, C Phillpot (eds.) *Artist/Author: Contemporary Artists' Books*. New York, NY: The American Federation of Arts, 93–101.

Wasson S. 2017. *Translating Chronic Pain: Creative Manifesto*. [online]. Available at: www.lancaster.ac.uk/translating-pain. Last accessed: 20 April 2018.

Wasson S. 2018. Before Narrative: Episodic Reading and Representations of Chronic Pain. *Medical Humanities*, Published Online First, 1–7. Available at: http://mh.bmj.com/content/early/2018/01/11/medhum-2017-011223. Last accessed: 20 April 2018.

Wellbery C. 2017. Inter-face: Artists' Books as Mutual Inquiry. In: S Bolaki, E Čiricaitė (eds.) *Prescriptions: Artists' Books on Wellbeing and Medicine*. London: Natrix Natrix Press, 18–22.

Whitehead A, Woods A. (eds.) 2016. *The Edinburgh Companion to the Critical Medical Humanities*. Edinburgh: Edinburgh University Press.

Willis M, Waddington K, Marsden R. Imaginary Investments: Illness Narratives Beyond the Gaze. *Journal of Literature and Science*. 2013; 6: 55–73.

21

GRASPING EMERGENCY CARE THROUGH POP CULTURE

The truths and lies of film, television and other video-based media

Henry A. Curtis

Pop culture consumers

What influences are pop culture, video-based media exerting on the world of emergency medicine? Do they reflect, forecast, interpret or influence the culture of emergency care?

Sarah is a pop culture consumer. She chooses which of her display devices will transport her to fabricated and documented medical realities today. Viewing a dramatic film, she weeps during scenes of quiet death due to terminal illness, the surrounding family and friends all elegantly attended to by the attentive physician. Next, she stands witness to the televised heroic resuscitation of an assuredly unsurvivable injury. Wow! Physicians can cure anything! She switches to the news. Now she must judge the physician whose incompetence was failing. A young child could have lived if only this physician had done something different. Anything! The remote switches again, now to suffering due to news of an incurable virus. Nausea sets into the pit of her stomach. A constellation of symptoms erupts. The emergency department will sort it out. 9–1–1.

Dr Muse is also a pop culture consumer. She endures the news berating the emergency physicians responsible for contributing to the unsustainable cost of healthcare. Spending on advanced imaging during emergency department stays is an easy target. She switches to an episode of 'House' (2009), in which a child suffers Gadolinium-contrast toxicity due to inappropriately ordered magnetic resonance imaging and requires haemodialysis. Time for work. She dons her scrubs.

For Sarah, this is a disjointed journey. Paramedic gives her a medication under the tongue. Registration clerk takes her license. Triage nurse checks her vital signs. Transporter shuttles her to a hard, uncomfortable bed in the emergency department. Bedside nurse draws her blood into four vials. Radiology tech takes an X-ray, shielding her pelvis with lead. The doctor arrives. Surely, she will understand the gravity of the situation, perform a head-to-toe exam, listen to her story and order an MRI. Then Sarah is jolted, as if being woken from a dream. The nurse encourages her to sign the discharge papers. What did the doctor say? Did she even examine me? What about my MRI? Why did I feel bad? I can eat a cracker now. Does this mean I am healthy again?

Pop culture, in stark contrast to high culture, embodies cultural products manufactured for mass consumption (Crossman 2018). Video-based media, a highly accessible and appealing product line, includes media resources found ubiquitously in narrative film and documentary works, televised fictional and reality shows, televised and internet-based news, 3D 360 virtual reality experiences, social media posts and attachments, and video hosting communities such as YouTube and Vimeo. These products populate a reservoir of media representations and images, which are transported via personal vehicle, ambulance or aircraft to the gritty ground where emergency healthcare reality meets the truths and lies of video-based mass entertainment. In this venue, physicians will emulate the heroes and loathe the villains while patients seek to reconcile their expectations. Amidst the suffering and joy of people of all races, ages, gender and beliefs a shared truth emerges in the raw, energetic and unpredictable emergency department.

Five images portrayed by media representations of emergency medicine and medicine in emergencies will be examined: doctor–patient relationship, replacing the bedside assessment with technology, bias and diversity, journey of a doctor over a lifetime and future thinking in emergency pop culture.

Doctor–patient relationship

'Patients always lie' is the golden rule of Gregory House, M.D. Above all, never trust the patient if you want to uncover the mystery and solve the case. Elaine can be trusted to be a 'difficult patient,' according to her chart that followed her from doctor to doctor while seeking treatment for a rash during a 'Seinfeld' episode (1996). Pop culture warns doctors to not trust patients and to covertly label the difficult patients in order to propagate immutable impressions. Physicians are shown depictions of placing blame and judgement on drug-seeking patients for their behaviours. They also learn the effectiveness of dehumanising and objectifying patients by referring to them as their symptomatologies rather than their names.

Doctors have strengths, weaknesses, insecurities, bad personality traits, desires, goals and dreams. They are humanised. They commit adultery, act arrogantly, insult others and aspire to greedy ambitions. They are people who make mistakes, misdiagnosing and giving lethal doses of medications. Many have fallen victim to the crisis of our time, addiction to pain medication. Dr Carter confesses his drug addiction to Dr Benton ('ER,' 2000) while House, M.D. justifies his to the team.

Doctors can dispense vigilante justice. Sometimes doctors wish to punish patients for bad behaviour. A foolish soldier got a pool ball stuck in his mouth and was threatened with a rectal temperature and unnecessary major surgery during a 'M*A*S*H*' episode (1982). Other times doctors tread beyond threats and serve as judge, jury and executioner. Dr Greene finds himself alone in an elevator on the way to the operating room with a man alleged to be a child molester who has just tried to kill his wife and baby ('ER,' 2001). Ventricular tachycardia ensues. Dr Greene charges the defibrillator but discharges the energy into the air, watching the man die.

Patients' impressions have also been formed in various contexts in which doctors have been portrayed as dutiful to family ('ER,' 1997), home wreckers who steal girlfriends ('House,' 2007) and medical mavericks responding to crises with limited resources, attempting feats for which they are not qualified ('ER,' 1994). Additionally, the moral ambiguity of physicians has often been questioned.

There is an expectation that emergency physicians function as detectives who infallibly solve medical and nonmedical emergencies and urgencies, delivering miracle cures for all ailments. This reputation holds regardless of how many other specialists have been unable to 'fix' this problem. A fine way to shock a patient is to explain to him or her that the diagnostic duty of an emergency physician is to rule out emergencies and urgencies rather than ruling in any cause of symptoms. On TV, most patients present with acute disease that can be cured rather than chronic disease that festers (Ye and Ward 2010). Television doctors have access to unlimited resources without concern for cost. They are able to generate a new result every three minutes (Lapostolle et al. 2013). Most emergency physicians have limited use of high-value equipment, must consider the cost of testing and are deprived of the precious resource of time. Many are mandated to see, diagnose, treat and disposition patients whom they have never met before within three hours.

The realities of the outcomes surrounding many emergencies are incorrectly represented by video-based mass media. For instance, cardiac arrest, the gravest medical emergency, is shown by pop culture to have exorbitant rates of neurologically intact survival. This Dutch angle from reality engenders false beliefs from patients and family members, who are influenced by unrealistic hopes when considering advanced directives and end-of-life decision-making. When a patient does not survive a cardiac arrest, families are dissatisfied with the abilities of the doctor and may go on to file a complaint or outright litigation.

Besides curing biomedical disease, patients want doctors to address their social, economic and psychological concerns. Physicians often find themselves in clinical situations that cannot be solved with a biomedical science algorithm, but instead require attention to the patient's experience of suffering, hope, dying or death. There are many instances in which TV doctors inspire patients with a will to live, reunite estranged family members and mend broken social connections. It is crushing to patients whose 'other needs' are surprisingly not met in the emergency department. A man who lays carpet for a living visits Highland Hospital and asks an emergency physician for an immediate audience with a specialist, pain medication, disability enrolment and access to a primary care physician—all things that the physician is unwilling or unable to attend to ('The Waiting Room,' 2014).

Many times, it is not so easy to say 'no' to importunate patients with unrealistic expectations. In worship of patient satisfaction scores such as Press Ganey, external pressures force doctors to give patients 'it all' by delivering care which is flawless, fast, friendly and free. Waters can be muddied when entitled customers of the hospital demand a spa experience (Barton et al. 2010) rather than genuine human connection and compassionate care. One of the largest deterrents of patient experience is long perceived waiting times during the course of emergency department visits—if only there were an editor who could make quick cuts to speed up the action in the hospital. Patients also pursue the notion of one-stop shopping so that during their visit for a runny nose they can also have next week's blood work collected and diagnostic imaging performed.

Aside from the aforementioned challenges, there are other barriers to overcome for a successful consultation between emergency physician and patient. Doctors in emergency departments are interrupted up to once every six minutes (Chisholm et al. 2000) and interrupt patients every 18 seconds (Beckman and Frankel 1984). While there are times when it is imperative to reprioritise and multi-task, the majority of these infractions reduce the value of the patient consultation, minimising the amount and content of time, with no gain. One 'Scrubs' (2003) episode offers an interesting perspective, marking time to interruption at the bedside with a digital stopwatch. Communication can also be dampened when intermediaries such as translators, caregivers, family members and parents speaking for children juxtapose their translation of the senders' and receivers' intended exchange.

Ideally, once there is a provisional diagnosis, a therapeutic goal is agreed upon through shared decision-making so that the patient is compliant with the treatment plan that includes medications, procedures and other interventions. Unfortunately, in life things do not always go according to plan. The film *Knocked Up* (2007) lends a good example of how the best-laid plans sometimes go to waste. A gravid patient about to give birth according to her birth plan is initially unwilling to heed the advice of a physician with poor bedside manner to change the course based upon an evolving threat to the foetus. Other barriers to treatment plan compliance include uninformed consent, socioeconomic disadvantage and focus on chief complaint rather than chief concern.

Replacing the bedside assessment with technology

Chief complaint. Electronic medical record review. Genetic testing. Cardiac monitoring. EKG. Labs. Imaging. Phone call. Review of data complete. Meeting the patient—that is an after-thought. 'Your tests are fine,' albeit not at all related to your chief concern. 'You don't have an emergency right now'—follow up with someone who cares. The oversaturation of data in the healthcare workplace has created a state in which choices must be made. How much of our limited time should be spent analysing the data vs. speaking with the patient?

We are approaching an age in which genetic testing may predetermine patient health, medical clearance and career opportunities. *Gattaca* (1997) glimpses an alarming future real-ity in which the best person for a space mission is nearly excluded from his dream because of his genetic makeup. What other dreams will be shattered by the science of genetics in the near future?

Our society is becoming more subject to its technology master who collects, stores, interprets and visualises data. Such data are best collected from our machines rather than direct interface with people themselves. In House, M.D.'s world there is little incentive to consult with a patient because biomedical science data collection presides over patient story. Even during codes, the cues for signs of life come from the machine rather than the patient. 'House' (2009) demonstrates our reliance while holding down a medical alert test button which convinces a resuscitation team to attempt an airway on a presumed dying patient who had in actuality just fallen asleep.

Technology takes clinician presence away from the bedside. ZDoggMD, a Free Open Access Meducation enthusiast, documents physician compulsion for electronic health record docu-mentation (Damania 2015). Physicians feel compelled to rush away from patients and towards computers, spending more time documenting care than providing it. While some have rushed towards the bedside toting their computers on wheels in an effort to combine charting with patient interaction, their swayed attention towards records and testing yet away from the patient can at best be considered offensive. Sacrificing time at the bedside often means denying patients the social ritual of the physical exam so espoused by Abraham Verghese (Costanzo and Verghese 2018). When physicians and patients do not build mutual trust, can meaningful and effective care be delivered?

Bias and diversity

We live in a world of limited resources dispensed according to preference. At the emergency department, preference is given to the wealthy, famous, friends, family members, board members and donors. This can take many forms such as being pampered at triage, being communicated to with clearer explanations of medical decision-making, receiving unlimited specialist physi-cians scrambling to the bedside, obtaining the results of investigations near immediately, being infused with sufficient medication to ensure that there is never a discomforting moment, having a private room and, of course, achieving it all super expedited. In some freestanding emer-gency rooms, services such as dog walking and child pick-up are even offered (Sullivan 2018).

Preference can furthermore mean the difference between life and death. In *Contagion* (2011), Alan Krumwiede alleges that a high-ranking member of the CDC warned his friend of a health crisis in Chicago before warning the public, so that she could escape.

It is written into the physician code of ethics to treat all people with equality, yet are all immune to the consequences of implicit bias? This wretch lurks under our consciousness but may surface under stressful conditions, influencing how physicians communicate with, and make decisions for, patients (Burgess 2017). In the emergency department, it is imperative to strive for a culture of inclusion and to be aware of groups vulnerable to potential bias—consider race, ethnic group, age, religion, gender orientation, socioeconomic class, stigmatised disease, obesity, intoxication, drug use, frequent emergency department use and homelessness. Additional 'at-risk' populations include the incarcerated, impoverished and disabled and those with poor language skills, mental illness and low health literacy. Entry into the emergency department is indiscriminate. Anyone can walk through the doors any time with any condition. Vigilance against discrimination is paramount. Additionally, care must be taken to avoid bias against members of the healthcare team. Jeanie Boulet goes to the hospital's HIV clinic and is warned by a clinic patient to seek treatment elsewhere so that she doesn't get reassigned to a job without patient contact ('ER,' 1996).

Pop culture has a privileged position of influence, in that it has the eyes and the ears of the world beholden to the representations and images it produces. Shows such as 'ER' have flaunted diversity, representing doctors as LGBTQ, immigrants, young, old, disabled and sufferers of chronic disease, yet they have fallen short, under-representing the diversity of patient mix found in today's emergency departments (Primack et al. 2012). Why are the reflections of video-based mass entertainment in such a state of distortion?

Journey of a doctor over a lifetime

Physicians-to-be may heed the call to the journey when aspiring to find a means of helping others, desiring a means of gainful employment, needing to give back, wishing to save others and undergoing transformative medical experiences (McHarg, Mattick and Knight 2007). Many are affected by pop culture's window to this world, depicting scenes with alluring images of heroism, comradery and connection to humanity.

Moreover, pop culture parades the inherent challenges of this career choice. Brutal realities of medical education are highlighted on TV shows such as 'ER,' 'Scrubs,' and 'Grey's Anatomy.' Graduating physicians have high debt loads, with median educational debt for medical education at $180,000 and undergraduate education at $20,000 along with non-education debt of around $8000 (Paul and Skiba 2016). Despite this cost of education, salaries for residents remain low while they continue to work long hours. An episode of 'Scrubs' (2002) makes light of their plight as J.D. resorts to stealing hospital pudding and toilet paper. Medical students and residents are encouraged by the heroes and tormented by the villains of medical education along the path (Foster and Roberts 2016). There is a high risk of falling victim to exhausting episodes of pimping or brief episodes of belittling from higher-level residents or staff physicians. Medical students must learn how to deal with 'not knowing' and to 'tolerate ambiguities' (Bleakley 2015), while wrestling with feelings of insecurity and competition with their peers. Students experience an emotional rollercoaster during rites of passage conveying moments of celebration when donning the white coat, tragedy when experiencing the death of a young person for the first time and honour when making the first incision on a cadaver. Chief Weber's recital of the Hippocratic Oath reminds physicians that being a doctor is a higher calling with great responsibility to society, often characterised by self-sacrifice ('Grey's Anatomy,' 2010). Personal identity is under threat, to be exchanged for professional identity. One day the disconnected physician may wake, look into the mirror at a new image of his or her self and see that he or she has morphed into a hero like George Clooney, or antihero like Gregory House.

After graduating undergraduate and graduate medical education, the real lessons of being an emergency physician begin. New physicians must accustom themselves to taking full responsibility for everything that happens in the department and to be highly functional in a myriad of highly complex and unpredictable situations. Healthcare metrics, measuring profit and volume, replace grading systems based on mastery of meaningful concepts and knowledge (Branch et al. 2017). House, M.D (2004) comments that: "treating illnesses is why we became doctors. Treating patients is what makes most doctors miserable." Thinking of patients in terms of profit and volume can contribute to a shift towards a hostile viewpoint of patients. Physicians have become de-centred in healthcare, losing control of their practice. Formularies determine which drugs can be prescribed. Insurance executives dictate who gets seen, what tests can be ordered and what procedures can be performed. Politicians make laws that direct care options. Administrators track the metrics with consequence and prescribe management pathways and protocols that can influence physician decision-making (Derlet et al. 2016). Physicians are even forced to shuffle patients to waiting areas of the hospital, pending dispositions dependent on insurance approval of necessary operations and therapy (*Article 99*, 1992).

Another highly significant contributor that impacts the patient–physician encounter is physician wellness. Given all of the pressures of balancing a demanding life in medicine with other social, family and spiritual priorities, there is a high risk of succumbing to depression, poor self-care and burnout, yet many live happy, balanced lives. On 'Scrubs' (2009), Elliot points out to Turk how he focuses on the good parts of medicine while she focuses on the bad, which is why she believes she would stop being a doctor if given the opportunity. Turk's resilience is fortified by his belief that his actions can have positive impacts, that he does have some control, tenacity is worthwhile and that setbacks are inevitable and surmountable (Howe, Smajdor and Stockl 2012). It is equally important to have a support network and to be able to discuss mistakes and vulnerabilities with a peer rather than dwelling on them. Humour is another valuable tool of wellness. Many medical school classes humorously depict the challenges of medical school life through music videos (Harvard Medical School 2014). One 'M*A*S*H*' (1980) episode makes light of pretending that someone has died to fluster the responding physician. Perhaps most importantly, physicians should continuously rejuvenate themselves by pursuing a search for meaning in their day-to-day practice.

Future thinking in emergency pop culture

Medical encounters are likely to continue to migrate from physical to virtual spaces. These virtual spaces allow online consultation through email, synchronous video, asynchronous video, instant messaging and virtual reality environments. The case for telemedicine is persuasive for patients who want to receive empathetic healthcare in an accessible and immediate manner at a reduced cost (Yellowlees, Richard Chan and Burke Parish 2015) in a quiet space that is mutually convenient. Prehospital applications are being developed by emergency services personnel and can be expanded to connect community first responders to physicians while they are providing medical assistance during the waiting period before professional first responders arrive on the scene. 'Grey's Anatomy' (2015) highlights utilisation of this technology where Ruby is coached over the phone to perform cardiopulmonary resuscitation to the beat of 'Staying Alive.'

Patients are wearing devices such as contact lenses, jewellery, watches and embedded in their clothing that collect large streams of continuous remote biosensor data. Data are also collected from devices such as asthma inhalers and there is much work towards the development of Nano sensor technology circulating through the bloodstream, which could usher in an era of pre-diagnosis of inevitable or highly probable future medical emergencies. Patients receive tracking, updates and warnings through the connected apps that display this data. Information is often collected in online clouds where there is a concerning risk that our privacy may be invaded by distributing such sensitive information to unauthorised personnel. In a scene from *The Circle* (2017), set in a shielded underground locale, Mae and Ty discuss the ramifications of this unauthorised access to our private health information.

Artificial intelligence is replacing human skills. AI can already identify pulmonary tuberculosis better than radiologists. Virtual assistants are poised to collect and record elements of history of present illness and review of systems. Future forecasts suggest that AI may generate differential diagnoses with big data, suggest high-value testing based on patient presentation, encourage low-cost care pathways and monitor, interpret and respond to streaming physiologic data. How far will machine learning advance? In *Elysium* (2013), a dystopian future is depicted in which the doctor is now an uncaring machine. It dispenses pills to keep a victim of a radiological accident functional for five days while he awaits certain death with no social or psychological support.

It is certain that pop culture's mass entertainment media will continue to reflect movements and shape reality within healthcare in the future. As virtual, mixed and augmented reality gain popularity, viewers may experience these future forecasts in more immersive ways than ever before.

Controlling the narrative

Pop culture, video-based media portray intimate and memorable stories forming public impressions of physicians and how they respond to emergencies. These images exert substantial influence on the patient–physician consultation, the social contract and physicians' roles within the healthcare industry. Physicians should heed the visceral response to take control of their lives and tell it their way before others create the narrative.

Consider producing content yourself or collaborate with those in the film, television and virtual reality industries. Capture attention with compelling stories. Make it personal. Be bold and creative. Chant mantras. Focus on the interests and needs of the viewers. Distribute far and wide using video-friendly social media tools. Above all, tell your stories your way.

Control the narrative!

References

Article 99. Dir. Howard Deutch. Perf. Ray Liotta, Kiefer Sutherland, Forest Whitaker. March 13, 1992.

Barton M, et al. My best Press Ganey scores yet. *Emergency Physicians Monthly*; 2010. Available from: http://epmonthly.com/article/my-best-press-ganey-scores-yet-video. Last accessed: July 31, 2018.

Beckman HB, Frankel RM. The effect of physician behavior on the collection of data. *Annals of Internal Medicine*. 1984; 101: 692–6.

Bleakley A. 2015. *Medical Humanities and Medical Education: How the Medical Humanities Can Shape Better Doctors*. London: Taylor and Francis. Kindle Edition.

Branch WT, Jr., Weil AB, Gilligan MC, et al. How physicians draw satisfaction and overcome barriers in their practices: 'It sustains me.' *Patient Education and Counseling*. 2017; 100: 2320–30.

Burgess DJ, Beach MC, Saha S. Mindfulness practice: A promising approach to reducing the effects of clinician implicit bias on patients. *Patient Education and Counseling*. 2017; 100: 372–6.

Chisholm CD, Collison EK, Nelson DR, Cordell WH. Emergency department workplace interruptions: Are emergency physicians 'interrupt-driven' and 'multitasking'? *Academic Emergency Medicine*. 2000; 7: 1239–43.

Contagion. Dir. Steven Soderbergh. Perf. Matt Damon, Kate Winslet, Jude Law. September 9, 2011.

Costanzo C, Verghese A. The physical examination as ritual: Social sciences and embodiment in the context of the physical examination. *Medical Clinics of North America*. 2018; 102: 425–31.

Crossman A. Sociological definition of popular culture: The history and genesis of pop culture. ThoughtCo, April 22, 2018. Available at: www.thoughtco.com/popular-culture-definition-3026453. Last accessed July 31, 2018.

Damania Z. 2015. EHR state of mind. Available from: http://zdoggmd.com/ehr-state-of-mind. Last accessed: August 2, 2018.

Derlet RW, McNamara RM, Plantz SH, et al. Corporate and hospital profiteering in emergency medicine: Problems of the past, present, and future. *Journal of Emergency Medicine*. 2016; 50: 902–9.

Elysium. Dir. Neil Blomkamp. Perf. Matt Damon, Jodie Foster, Sharlto Copley. August 9, 2013.

ER, '24 hours' Season 1, Episode 1, September 19, 1994.

ER, 'Doctor Carter, I Presume' Season 3, Episode 1, September 26, 1996.

ER, 'Fathers and Sons' Season 4, Episode 7, November 13, 1997.

ER, 'May Day' Season 6, Episode 22, May 18, 2000.

ER, 'Rampage' Season 7, Episode 22, May 17, 2001.

Foster K, Roberts C. The heroic and the villainous: A qualitative study characterising the role models that shaped senior doctors' professional identity. *BMC Medical Education*. 2016; 16: 206.

Gattaca. Dir. Andrew Niccol. Perf. Ethan Hawke, Uma Thurman, Jude Law. October 24, 1997.

Grey's Anatomy, 'The Time Warp' Season 6, Episode 15, February 18, 2010.

Grey's Anatomy, 'I Feel the Earth Move' Season 11, Episode 15. March 12, 2015.

Harvard Medical School, '#Study' April 11, 2014.

House, 'Pilot' Season 1, Episode 1, November 16, 2004.

House, 'Resignation' Season 3, Episode 22, May 8, 2007.

House, 'Brave Heart' Season 6, Episode 5, October 19, 2009.

House, 'Softer Side' Season 5, Episode 16, February 23, 2009.

Howe A, Smajdor A, Stockl A. Towards an understanding of resilience and its relevance to medical training. *Medical Education*. 2012; 46: 349–56.

Knocked Up. Dir. Judd Apatow. Perf. Seth Rogen, Katherine Heigl, Paul Rudd. June 1, 2007.

Lapostolle F, Montois S, Alheritiere A, et al. Dr House, TV, and reality. *The American Journal of Medicine*. 2013; 126: 171–3.

M*A*S*H*, 'April Fools' Season 8, Episode 25. March 24, 1980.

M*A*S*H*, 'Trick or Treatment' Season 11, Episode 2, November 1, 1982.

McHarg J, Mattick K, Knight LV. Why people apply to medical school: Implications for widening participation activities. *Medical Education*. 2007; 41: 815–21.

Paul DP, 3rd, Skiba M. Concierge Medicine: A viable business model for (some) physicians of the future? *Health Care Management*. 2016; 35: 3–8.

Primack BA, Roberts T, Fine MJ, Dillman Carpentier FR, Rice KR, Barnato AE. ER vs. ED: a comparison of televised and real-life emergency medicine. *Journal of Emergency Medicine*. 2012; 43: 1160–6.

Scrubs, 'My Fruit Cups' Season 2, Episode 8, November 14, 2002

Scrubs, 'My Fifteen Seconds' Season 3, Episode 7, November 20, 2003.

Scrubs, 'My Full Moon' Season 8, Episode 13, April 1, 2009.

Seinfeld, 'The Package' Season 8, Episode 5, Oct 17, 1996.

Sullivan P. An E.R. that treats you like a V.I.P.: *The New York Times*, April 20, 2018. Available from: www.nytimes.com/2018/04/20/your-money/concierge-emergency-room.html. Last accessed: August 2, 2018.

The Circle. Dir. James Ponsoldt. Perf. Emma Watson, Tom Hanks, John Boyega. April 28, 2017.

The Waiting Room. Dir. Peter Nicks. Perf. Sean Bennett. 2014.

Ye Y, Ward KE. The depiction of illness and related matters in two top-ranked primetime network medical dramas in the United States: A content analysis. *Journal of Health Communication*. 2010; 15: 555–70.

Yellowlees P, Richard Chan S, Burke Parish M. The hybrid doctor–patient relationship in the age of technology: Telepsychiatry consultations and the use of virtual space. *International Review of Psychiatry*. 2015; 27: 476–89.

22

WHO IS THE AUDIENCE FOR THE MEDICAL/HEALTH HUMANITIES?

*Suzy Willson, Pamela Brett-Maclean, and
Bella Eacott*

How do we think about audiences?

Pamela

When I was first presented with the title for this chapter, 'who is the audience for the medical/health humanities?', I realised that I had previously only given superficial thought to this question. We, of course, work hard on promoting our various educational offerings and events, hoping for 'good attendance' (considered variously in relation to numbers, diversity of the audience, engagement, enthusiastic response, etc.). We have done so hoping these tallies will positively reflect on the value of the University of Alberta's Arts and Humanities in Health and Medicine (AHHM) programme in contributing to the faculty, university, and larger community, to help ensure continuing support for the programme. Still, I had not previously given much thought to the importance of audience in relation to what we hope to achieve through our work in the medical/health humanities.

Suzy

In my experience within academia and higher education the idea of 'public engagement with research' is more common than one of 'audience development,' which is so central to the arts and culture industries.

Pamela

Yes, also seemingly more aligned with an empirically based thinking process, beginning with identification of a 'problem,' and steps leading to a particular solution. Nevertheless, over the past decade or so there has been increasing interest in public engagement to promote understanding, and build trust and support for, both the sciences and humanities (Bucchi 2008; Woodward 2009; Bauer and Jensen 2011). Hiram College's 2018 Center for Literature and Medicine Summer Seminar recently focused on new directions for health humanities "by attending to the diverse 'publics' it serves," hoping to open up discussion about "the ethical responsibilities of our field to its 'publics'."

Although I believe these are important concerns and questions, I am not sure that we should assume an equivalency between 'public' and 'audience.' According to Livingstone (2005: 9), the term 'public' refers to a shared collective interest or worldview, or participatory forum in which "understandings, identities, values and interests are recognised or contested." 'Audience' is conceptualised more relationally, referring to those who participate in, encounter, or experience mass media (radio, television, Internet-based media, etc), various artforms (visual art, literature, theatre, music, etc), video games, academic presentations, and so forth. Dayan (2005: 68) has pointed to various publics, inclusive of different kinds of particularly located audiences: (1) an obvious public (e.g., a constituency); (2) pronounced audiences, or "consumer" audiences (passive recipients of unidirectionally shared information); and (3) catalysed, meaning-making audiences, including those that actively contribute to a resulting collective performative text.

It seems that both Clod Ensemble/Performing Medicine and AHHM engage with audiences across all three of these categories of publics in different ways, with a focus primarily on engaging with catalysed, meaning-making audiences.

Bella

The audience engaged and interested in ideas about the body, medicine, and health is potentially huge and diverse—there is a fascination with this subject matter across disciplines. As a performance company, we are always thinking about audiences, but in different ways depending on the context. In this context—a *Handbook of the Medical Humanities*—the first thing to note is that within Clod Ensemble and Performing Medicine we rarely use the term 'medical humanities' when referring to ourselves and to our practice, which in itself says something both about the interdisciplinary nature of medical humanities and then about its audiences. But we also know that our performances, research, and practice draw on research and ideas coming out of medical humanities scholarship and we hope to contribute to it. Our work is practice-based using physical, embodied teaching methods and activities that draw on visual and performing arts and applied arts. This, perhaps, indicates the breadth of health humanities and associated audiences as encompassing a broad conception of 'humanities' and 'arts' beyond academic studies of History, English Literature, Philosophy, and so on.

I think the sense of 'audiences' being a more relational term than 'publics' that Pamela raises is pertinent. As an arts organisation that works with and within universities, hospitals, and cultural venues, we try to embrace a sense of multiple audiences communicating in multiple directions. What this means, when thinking about the audiences for health humanities, is a constant acknowledgement that the ideas, practice, and research with which the health humanities are concerned happen outside of academic settings as well as inside. If we take a contested topic such as 'empathy,' for instance—often addressed within health humanities scholarship—it is important to acknowledge that artists, theatre makers, practitioners, policy makers, schoolteachers, and those working with prison services are also engaging this subject. These ideas and explorations can, and should, feed in all directions; so the audiences for these ideas and practices are just as much those working within the academy as those outside of it.

When thinking and talking about audiences, some active word—usually 'engagement'—comes next. Even though the rhetoric around engagement has moved towards relational 'dialogue' models, it seems difficult to escape 'deficit' models in how we think, speak, and *do* engagement, partly because the people setting up the 'engagement activities' are still universities, researchers in universities, and academic departments (Stilgoe, Lock, and Wilson 2014: 5), which have some kind of final research product to engage our audiences with. The charitable foundation The Wellcome Trust recently published a blog post describing the ways in which they are trying to remind themselves that thinking about problems or issues with other people is part of the process: "discovery isn't something we do before we engage the public—it's a critical first stage of engagement itself" (https://wellcome.ac.uk/news/its-not-what-you-do-public-engagement-its-who-you-do-it). It feels important then to find ways of actively acknowledging the contributions being made to the health humanities by individuals and organisations outside of academia—sharing ideas with audiences in alternative forms, that may not be recognised as 'research,' but rather as arts and practice.

As Pamela says, both Clod Ensemble and AHHM perhaps do primarily engage with audiences through 'catalysed, meaning-making' models. However, I don't think that the style of knowledge transmission through 'pronounced audiences/consumer models' is always problematic in itself. Just as long as the people doing the transmitting and consuming are varied—specifically, that ideas are coming from practice-based settings into the academy, as well as the other way round.

Suzy

Connected to this point about the value of multiple voices being included in the health humanities, we should recognise that these varied voices will also think about audiences differently from the start. As an arts organisation, we are constantly considering who our audiences are. Our work only exists in the presence of others, and to a greater or lesser extent is created through the process of working with audiences or being witnessed by them. Over the last decade there is also an increasing requirement from funding bodies to consider audience engagement and development as central to the organisational mission of arts companies.

Pamela

Suzy, your multi-perspectival insight that different members of our various audiences, including participants and collaborators, will think about audiences differently is intriguing. I wonder if we are generally aware of the times we are viewed as part of an audience by others? I am also reflecting on your observation that "our work only exists in the presence of others." Both are important points, I believe.

Who are our audiences and how can we engage with them?

Suzy

We can identify six key audiences for our work: (1) healthcare professionals at all levels and across disciplines; (2) students; (3) health humanities, arts, and health scholars and practitioners (international); (4) artists and arts audiences; (5) 'general' publics; and (6) senior managers (of hospitals/regulatory bodies and so on) and policy makers. Cross-pollinating these audiences is important to us. Ideas that we address in courses and workshops for medical students may end up feeding into our performance work and vice versa. A single individual might come to a show, end up coming to a talk, and then commission us to provide training for their staff in a hospital.

Pamela

As a humanities programme based in medicine, a guiding focus for AHHM has been to contribute to an enriched interdisciplinary learning environment within the Faculty of Medicine and Dentistry. We have created curricular, co-curricular, and elective offerings and scholarship opportunities to engage students and residents, as well as academic and clinical faculty, who we view both as our primary audiences, and potential collaborators.

Medicine and health, of course, engage the imagination, hopes, and desires of everyone. We are also committed to developing relationships across the university, as well as our larger community, including the public at large and individuals and groups, through multiple means and approaches to engagement. We organise speaker series and various events, such as forum theatre performances, symposia, and exhibitions, and invite those from across, and outside, our university to join us in inquiring into and opening up wide-ranging dialogues about the human side of medicine.

We have invited artists, writers, and performers, such as Christine Borland, Vincent Lam, Brian Lobel, and David Diamond, to visit our programme, as well as medical and health human-ities scholars and educators such as Rita Charon, Arthur Frank, Alan Bleakley, Allan Peterkin, Jonathan Bolton, Arno Kumagai, and William T. Branch, Jr. These events have led to new connections, collaborations, and opportunities, both for those who have participated and for us.

Bella

To build a dialogue and conversation around ideas, we engage with audiences using multiple strategies, at different levels, using varied means. We create situations in which ideas can be accessed in many ways, creating a kind of saturation in order to effect change. We have found at the institutions where we work that, counter-intuitively, there is very little crossover between health humanities and medical education departments; and we have really tried to address that. Often, medical humanities scholarship is taking place in an English or History Department and does not reach medical students. While many people are keen to engage medical students as an audience for health humanities ideas, a major challenge is how to access the students, in the context of often already very overcrowded and pressured curricula.

Pamela

Absolutely, so true. Given curriculum constraints at our medical school our ongoing program-ming is offered primarily through co-curricular and elective offerings. Also, early on, students supported a motion to have an elected AHHM student representative sit on the council for each class, ensuring ongoing communication and collaboration with students across all four years of our undergraduate medical education programme. Our alliance with students has been integral to the success of that programme. Many of our electives have been proposed, or initiated, by our medical students.

Suzy

For us to work with medical students within these pressured curricula we work closely with medical educators to understand what the students' learning needs are, and where there are gaps and opportunities. Sometimes this means finding individuals within the medical school who can help position our work within a particular area of focus, for instance: 'Professionalism,' 'Self Care/Resilience,' or 'Long-Term Conditions.' We try to provide as many access points as possible for students—through compulsory slots in the curriculum, optional modules, extra-curricular events organised with students, and events to which general public are also invited. In addition, we actually rarely talk about arts directly. We focus on the skills the students will learn, rather than lead with the fact that these will be developed through arts-based methods. We have found that this makes it easier to have productive sessions with students and for staff to see their relevance. This also helps to overcome 'us and them'/'science vs arts' dichotomous thinking which can get in the way.

Pamela

Similarly, we often don't focus on the arts methods per se, but have found that clarifying the relevance of arts-based teaching for clinical reasoning and practice enhances engagement and openness to arts-based exploration of difficult and challenging issues in medicine, for example thinking with and through stories and other forms of knowledge.

An approach we have used to inspire interest and engagement has been to point to the vast potential of the medical humanities for supporting inquiry into patient and practitioner experiences of illness and healthcare across different healthcare settings and systems through a wide-ranging, annual programme of events. We have done so with the somewhat unsettling recognition that we are but part of a broader and vital health humanities presence at the University of Alberta.

To address this, we initiated a design–medicine collaboration that resulted in an exhibition called *Insight: Visualizing Health Humanities* that showcased visual, sound, and performance explorations bridging medicine, health sciences, arts, humanities, and social sciences at the University of Alberta. The *Insight* exhibition helped to promote awareness of connections across disciplinary concerns and vocabularies relevant to the health humanities and visualised in the creative works. In addition to the opening reception, a participatory art event and school tour was organised and a book/catalogue and web-based interactive gallery (http://insight. healthhumanities.ca) were published. The following year we extended an open invitation for contributions relating to health humanities and community engagement, which resulted in *InSight 2: Engaging the Health Humanities* (http://insight2.healthhumanities.ca). These exhibitions explicitly recognised the porous, expanding health humanities community that exists across our university, and not just in the Faculty of Medicine and Dentistry.

Currently, an AHHM affiliate structure is being introduced, and an interdisciplinary AHHM Student Committee was recently set up, to help support and recognise engagement of students and faculty across the university in health humanities initiatives. Our newly formed Canadian Association for Health Humanities will also help to promote awareness of the health humanities, both locally and nationally, which will engage new audiences.

Bella

It's brilliant to hear of approaches like these where the electives are proposed, or initiated, by the people they are aimed at. The best way to inspire all the groups of people that we work with is for other individuals in their professional or peer group to act as advocates. When we are programming new courses for healthcare professionals, such as with our Circle of Care programme at Guy's and St Thomas' Hospitals, we have found it invaluable to have a champion from the professions that we are targeting, who can help the programme to relate to the experiences of the audiences we are targeting. We created the Circle of Care framework with colleagues at the hospital in order to better articulate the work we do in an accessible language. It identifies nine skills that support health professionals to remove obstacles in the way of providing compassionate care. This has proved very popular with staff—once these skills are accepted as crucial, it is an easy next step to acknowledge that arts and humanities have a multitude of methods to help develop these skills.

Another strategy we have found helpful in building momentum around particular education programmes we are providing for health professionals is to set up talks, workshops, and performances in high-profile cultural venues in the UK such as Tate Modern or Sadler's Wells, in partnership with medical schools and hospitals. This is with the aim of then helping the health institution to be more outward looking, demonstrating that many people have ideas and opinions about healthcare, and creating platforms for debate and dialogue.

An important part of our work at the moment is to help develop arts in health and health education sectors at a policy level to an audience of policy makers and politicians. In the UK, there is a vibrant debate most recently made clear through the All-Party Parliamentary Group report on Arts, Health and Wellbeing, which we contributed to, about the role of arts to improve health and wellbeing. This area of work is fast gaining momentum and is an important audience to engage.

Why do we want to engage with these audiences?

Pamela

The phrase that comes to mind is 'authentic, collaborative, transformational engagement.' We want to promote positive professional development, and more positive futures for medicine through an expanded sense of community and "future forming" (Gergen 2015) constructive alliances. We are not focused so much on presenting research that bears on *how things are*, but concerned with offering opportunities for deliberating on *where we are* in order to identify ways forward. Here, we are helped by the ideas of Arno Kumagai and Delise Wear (2014), who have proposed that a critical role of the medical humanities is the disruption of "automaticity of thinking." They suggest that "making strange" can help bring habitual assumptions and ways of responding into view "so that one sees the self, others, and the world anew," which may help to orient us and motivate us forward to other opportunities, leading to more positive futures.

Suzy

I like the idea of "making strange." An increasing number of artists in the UK are making work about their experience of illness. By presenting their work in medical schools and health settings we can help to interrupt and disrupt institutionalised ways of thinking, providing a platform for patient stories and experiences.

Pamela

Engaging with audiences aligns with trends towards a democratisation of scholarship and research practice. Inviting multiple perspectives, moving away from elitism to presenting and sharing our ideas and learning from each other, is key, I think. In addition to this, I am recalling how Pattison (2003), in characterising the medical humanities as an emerging interdisciplinary field, noted that the medical humanities *require audiences* as they work to affirm and promote the field and explore its potential, while illuminating insights, understandings, approaches, and practices supportive of human-centred healthcare.

Through all of our performances we hope to effect salient, often disturbing, always memorable and engaging signposts and experiences as starting points for dialogue. Just as we believe or hope that our audiences need us, we also need our audiences. Our engagement with audiences not only helps others to make meaning of things, but also, through processes of ontogenesis, our engagement with our various audiences furthers our own understanding, and enhances our understanding of processes that may lead to more positive possibilities for medicine and health.

Suzy

So perhaps as well as asking 'who is the audience for medical humanities?' we should ask 'who is medical humanities the audience for?' It seems to me that in higher education and research there is an increasing recognition that it takes trans-disciplinary solutions to solve the complex challenges to health and to regulate rapid advances in medical technologies. People working under the umbrella of medical humanities can help to navigate this trans-disciplinary territory, to find ways to articulate, shape, and address challenges within health and wellbeing; and to hold the medical profession to account in ways that support it to change and become fit for practice.

Pamela

What I have come to appreciate is that we are continually performing and exploring the potentials of an ever-evolving medical/health humanities through our relational engagement with audiences of all kinds. The audiences we engage with, the location and settings, and media through which we engage different audiences and our motivation for doing so can be viewed as a matter of identity. This integrally shapes our understanding of the medical/health humanities, what they are about, and our understanding of ourselves as actors in this complex field. Our understanding of our audiences both shapes our practices and influences the directions we follow as we move forward—all of which suggests the need to be mindful of *how* we develop, maintain, and sustain our relationships with our many audiences.

Still, there are so many open questions. For example, given a world in which digital technologies are ever expanding, there would appear to be unlimited potential for extending the reach of the medical/health humanities and connecting with online audiences, both in real time and virtually. Use of the Internet as a platform for audiences to receive, experience, and create media, while also enabling the creation of virtual communities composed of individuals who interact primarily online, is a relatively new frontier for many of us. Our learners, who represent our future, are digital natives—they experience their lives both in-person and online. What might this mean for us in ten, or even five years? How will we come to know our work? Will our work exist in the same way in the presence of 'virtual others'? Will artificial intelligence and big data be used to help us connect with and engage our various in-person and online audiences? If so, what will this mean for the future of the medical/health humanities?

References

Bauer M, Jensen P. The mobilisation of scientists for public engagement. *Public Understanding of Science.* 2011; 20: 3–11.

Bucchi M. 2008. Of deficits, deviations and dialogues: Theories of public communication of science. In: M Bucchi, B Trench (eds.) *Handbook of Public Communication of Science and Technology.* London: Routledge, 57–76.

Dayan D. 2005. Mothers, midwives and abortionists: Genealogy, obstetrics, audiences and publics. In: S Livingstone (ed.) *Audiences and Publics: When Cultural Engagement Matters for the Public Sphere.* Bristol: Intellect Books, 9–16.

Gergen KJ. From mirroring to world-making: Research as future forming. *Journal for the Theory of Social Behaviour.* 2015; 45: 287–310.

Kumagai AK, Wear D. "Making strange": A role for the humanities in medical education. *Academic Medicine.* 2014; 89: 973–77.

Livingstone S. 2005. Introduction. In: S Livingstone (ed.) *Audiences and Publics: When Cultural Engagement Matters for the Public Sphere*. Bristol: Intellect Books, 9–16.

Pattison S. Medical humanities: A vision and some cautionary notes. *Journal of Medical Ethics: Medical Humanities*. 2003; 29: 33–36.

Stilgoe J, Lock SJ, Wilson J. Why should we promote public engagement with science? *Public Understanding of Science*. 2014; 23: 4–15.

Woodward K. The future of the humanities: In the present and in public. *Daedalus*. 2009; 138: 110–23.

Recommended reading

Hadley B. 2017. *Theatre, Social Media, and Meaning Making* (particularly 'Social Media as Cultural Stage: Co-Creation, Audience Collaboration and the Construction of Theatre Cultures,' 169–229). Basingstoke: Palgrave Macmillan.

23

DESIRE IMAGINATION ACTION

Theatre of the Oppressed in medical education

Ravi Ramaswamy and Radha Ramaswamy

The whole art of medicine is in observation . . . to educate the eye to see, the ear
to hear and the finger to feel.

(Sir William Osler)

The problem

A young married woman, complaining of lower abdominal pain, walks into the doctor's consulting room accompanied by her mother-in-law and husband. The doctor, who is male, asks
her questions to ascertain her medical history. All his questions are answered by the mother-in-
law and the husband. The doctor's irritation turns to anger and frustration as all his efforts to
have a conversation with his patient directly are thwarted by her family.

Osler exhorts the doctor "to see . . . to hear and . . . to feel," and these simple words actually sum up the human connection that ideally gets established between a doctor and a patient.
Why is this so difficult to achieve? How can young medical students learn the skills needed to
cope wisely and successfully with situations such as the one described above? Doctors, patients
and caregivers interact in a context that calls for great awareness, sensitivity and multiple skills
for communication, from everyone. Unfortunately, several factors come in the way of free and
genuine interaction between these groups of people. The scene described above highlights the
truth of what Zachariah, Srivatsan and Tharu (2010: preface) describe as the critical factor in
healthcare delivery:

> The mismatch between scientific advance and health care delivery is especially sharp
> in India, where inequality and discrimination exacerbate problems of access to cura-
> tive services. The problem is not only of financial cost—it is also that attempts to cure
> occur in frameworks that are unrelated to the lived reality of the patients. The stress
> and anxiety this results in the doctors, patients and carers have been largely invisible,
> or even ignored.

That there is a huge gap between what doctors need in actual medical practice and what is
taught in our medical schools is widely known. We wish to emphasise here the need to address
this gap in ways that are specific to the context in which the education and training are applied.

In the Indian context, 14-year-old boys and girls start to work long hours, focus on bookish preparation and shut out all 'distractions' in order to obtain a seat in a medical college. Their development as caring and sensitive human beings is deeply impacted by this. During their years of medical training, emotions and feelings again take a beating, as the need to appear calm and 'in control' is stressed, and a doctor's vulnerabilities are not acknowledged. As a refuge from the stresses of medical training, young doctors-to-be often retreat behind 'know-it-all' masks, or develop an indifference to suffering and pain. A student, intern or resident doctor, who probably came into the profession with idealistic dreams, becomes completely mechanised, with Outpatient Departments and ward rounds degenerating into a painful chore rather than the deep and intense learning processes that they can be.

Theatre of the Oppressed and medical humanities

How can we *demechanise* ourselves, and rediscover our potential to be human beings, fully engaging with the world around us? This question came up in a chance conversation between Dr Radha Ramaswamy, educationist turned theatre practitioner and founder of the Centre for Community Dialogue and Change (CCDC), and her friend and schoolmate Dr Ravi Ramakantan, then Head of Radiology at KEM Hospital, Mumbai, and a passionate medical teacher. He introduced her to the field of medical humanities, then little known in India, and thus began CCDC's pioneering work in medical humanities in India.

CCDC is a not-for-profit organisation based in Bangalore, India, working towards individual and social change through the use of Theatre of the Oppressed (TO). TO offers a set of tools, comprising games and exercises that encourage participants to work with their bodies in fun and insightful ways. Accessing deep-seated feelings and emotions through the use of the body, participants experience a liberation of the creative imagination, leading to greater clarity in thinking and enhanced powers of problem solving. TO is a participatory pedagogy created by Brazilian theatre director Augusto Boal and inspired by the work of Paulo Freire. It is widely used all over the world by educators, activists and artists to address a wide range of issues. CCDC's work includes workshops in TO in schools and colleges, an annual six days' training for facilitators, and courses in Pedagogy and TO for undergraduates. We also regularly conduct interactive Forum Theatre performances in different communities in Bangalore. These performances address issues that communities wish to explore, and create dialogue that leads to fresh insights and possibilities for change. A unique feature of Forum Theatre is that actors and audiences collaboratively arrive at these learnings, and the process itself is an exciting demonstration of knowledge creation in democratic ways.

Dr Ramaswamy's initial research into medical humanities threw up an interesting discovery: there is no standard accepted definition of 'medical humanities.' Broadly described as a multidisciplinary field, 'medical humanities' is an umbrella term that includes both a vast range of disciplines drawn from the humanities and the arts, as well as widely different approaches to how these may be used to produce better doctors. Discussions and interviews with medical practitioners, patients and caregivers from across India revealed the need to first hear all the stories and understand the problem in all its detailed complexity. This led to the collection of writings published in a special themed issue of the *Indian Journal of Medical Ethics* on medical humanities, guest edited by Dr Ramaswamy.

The challenges are too many, but we had tasted some success in our first workshop using TO with medical students, and we knew we had definitely entered the field of medical education. Our first workshop in medical humanities was in response to an invitation from Dr Ravi Shankar at KIST Medical College, Nepal, where a voluntary medical humanities model was in place.

We designed a two-day model based on our work with schoolteachers and students. We carefully chose games and exercises that could be adapted to address the needs of medical students. By the end of the second day, we had a powerful glimpse of what TO could accomplish. The games helped the students to connect as a group in no time at all. Without using language, working with their bodies, students created images that told their stories—powerful stories of struggles in relationships, parental pressure, homesickness and loneliness. This was a revelation for us. The problems that were topmost in their minds did not always have to do with issues in medicine. They were human beings first, eager to seize the opportunity to express their very human experiences and feelings of anxiety, hurt or doubt. Out of these shared experiences, short plays were created, which the students performed on the afternoon of the second day for an invited audience that included their teachers and members of the management. The scenes dealt with lack of freedom in the classroom and some ethical dilemmas. When the plays were opened up for interventions from the audience, we could see that the stories had resonated with everyone. The actors and the audience that evening experienced participation and dialogue in the truest sense, and were able to transcend hierarchical barriers and connect on a human level.

Our next TO workshop for medical humanities came out of the publicity that this workshop received in the medical research fraternity. This was at the University College of Medical Sciences, Delhi (UCMS) in 2011, and it was our first medical humanities workshop using TO in India. UCMS was the first medical college in India to start a medical humanities programme, and to introduce TO as a part of their programme. Since then we have returned to UCMS on a few more occasions, and more significantly, three faculty members from the medical education unit of the college travelled to Bangalore to attend CCDC's week-long facilitator training in TO. The team has successfully led several medical humanities programmes outside UCMS, with a prominent part given to TO.

From 2011 to the end of 2017, CCDC conducted workshops in 13 medical colleges. Among them are the All India Institute of Medical Sciences, Bhopal and Jodhpur, JSS Medical College, Mysore, Mahatma Gandhi Institute of Medical Sciences, Wardha and Melaka Manipal Medical College, Manipal. We have continued with the two-day module, sometimes adding an extra day when colleges have wanted a follow-up discussion on the possibilities for including TO in the medical curriculum. Occasionally, as with AIIMS Bhopal, we have conducted workshops for medical faculty. In some colleges, a few members of the faculty, mostly those who are members of the Medical Education Unit, participate in the students' workshop. We have encouraged such faculty participation when we have been convinced that the presence of the faculty would not inhibit the students. In addition to these two-day workshops, we get invited to offer a one-day pre-conference workshop at the annual medical conferences organised by students. These are national conferences, and students from different colleges sign up for the workshops. The TO workshop is usually the only session at the conferences with a 'non-medical' content, and we have been pleased to see the popularity of this workshop.

What happens in TO workshops

The games in the workshop are carefully structured to enable the body to be free and to open the mind to new sensations, leading to a heightened awareness of our feelings. An important element in these workshops is fun. Students experience a sense of aliveness that amazes them and rediscover a part of themselves that had been sidelined and lost in the mad rush of everyday routine. This discovery always leads to a feeling of liberation and great power (see Figure 23.1).

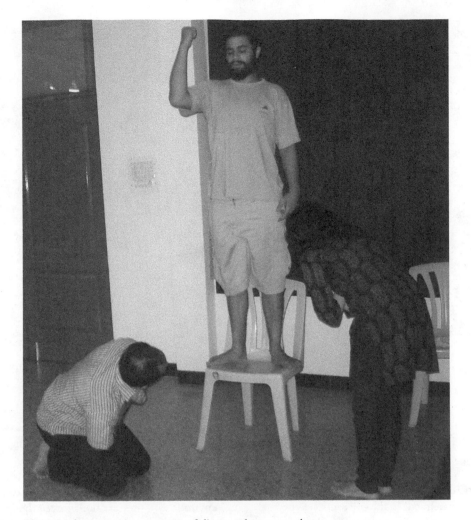

Figure 23.1 Students experience a sense of aliveness that amazes them

The workshops emphasise the power of listening. The games require students to listen deeply to their own bodies as well as to others in the group. Pauses and silences are also experienced as meaningful ways of listening and communicating. When doctors are able to listen to what patients are saying as well as *not saying*, they are able to better understand the realities of the patients. With this heightened awareness, students work through Image Theatre exercises that enable them to dive deeper into the world of hidden feelings and desires and give artistic expression to them. Every voice and every expression is respected and honoured. The images allow us to view ourselves from the outside, triggering new insights and setting off a process of reflection. Often this kindles a desire for change. The artistic distance gives them perspective, and also a greater sense of agency (see Figure 23.2).

Participants then create Forum Theatre—an interactive form of theatre where actors present stories of struggle, and the audience is invited to intervene, and explore multiple solutions to the problem on stage (see Figure 23.3). The games and exercises keep participants moving from

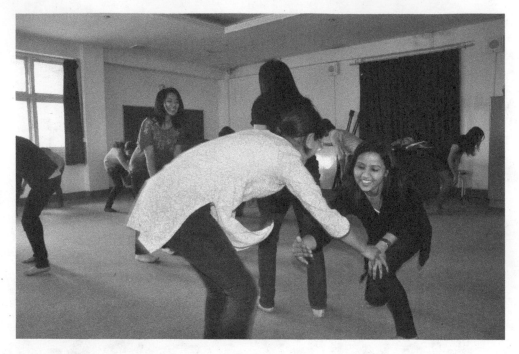

Figure 23.2   Students work through Image Theatre exercises that enable them to dive deeper into the world of hidden feelings and desires and give artistic expression to them

awareness to action and back to awareness in a continuous cycle of self-learning. Such processes ensure that we stay human. In a profession that calls for compassion and sensitivity, the importance of such a process cannot be overemphasised.

A doctor's day is filled with complicated and stressful situations. It is impossible for young doctors to go through their training without facing moments of doubt and confusion, or feeling overwhelmed. In the conventional medical college environment, they are not allowed the space to express their confusions and doubts, but are expected to get on with the job. Fearing that expressing feelings is a sign of weakness and even incompetence as a doctor, as a survival strategy doctors become mechanical in their interactions with patients. The effect of this mechanisation can vary from adopting a mask of confidence (which leads to insincere and artificial communication with patients) to severe depression, leading to attempts at suicide.

TO workshops create the space for doctors to share their stories of vulnerability, without being judged. They are in a position to better understand and have a deep connection with themselves. In this democratic and dialogic environment, they express themselves better, ask questions and are able to know their strengths. They are able to make innovative decisions and look at multiple perspectives to a problem. This awareness and experience of one's own emotions is critical to a doctor's education. Patients come to doctors at a time of great vulnerability and often trust the doctor to fix their illness—to save them, in fact. To deal with this responsibility sensitively, a doctor needs skills beyond what is currently taught in the standard medical curriculum. In an enjoyable way, the workshops put students through a variety of life-like situations, and students acquire confidence in their ability to listen, observe and make quick decisions, and also change and correct their decisions mid-course. This is also extremely valuable training for doctors as no two patients are the same.

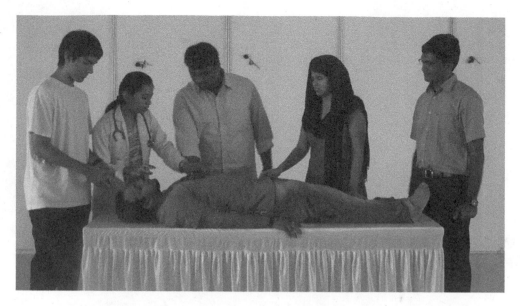

Figure 23.3   The audience is invited to intervene, and explore multiple solutions to the problem on stage

Challenges and reason for hope

We are happy about the responses to our one-day and two-day workshops. We are happy that a few medical colleges believe in this work enough to invite us year after year. But we are aware that the heady experience of the workshops fades quickly. Without reinforcement through repeated and regular workshops, the insights gained have little chance of translating into serious thought and action. The only way to offer this experience in a sustained way is to offer it as part of the regular medical curriculum. What stands in the way is a perception that medical humanities offer a 'soft subject.' In spite of overwhelming positive feedback from students about the workshops, there is a reluctance to see this as an essential part of medical education.

But there are a few colleges with medical humanities programmes, such as UCMS, Delhi, GS Medical College, Mumbai and St John's Medical College, Bangalore, and they offer their students a variety of different programmes, introducing literature, writing programmes, theatre, films and talks on art, etc. These events and activities are offered as voluntary programmes. CCDC is engaged in preliminary discussions with some colleges to collaborate on establishing a medical humanities centre and designing a medical humanities programme. When medicine opens its doors to professionals from the humanities, the arts and the social sciences, we have reason to hope that the core values in medicine will be re-established—doctors and patients connecting as human beings, working towards healing, rather than curing illnesses, and above all, seeing the doctor, patient and caregiver as collaborators in the project of creating wellness for communities.

Note

Images used in this chapter were provided by the authors.

Reference

Zachariah A, Srivatsan R, Tharu S (eds.) 2010. *Towards a Critical Medical Practice: Reflections on the Dilemmas of Medical Culture Today*. New Delhi: Orient BlackSwan Private Limited.

Further reading

Boal A. 2002, 2nd ed. *Games for Actors and Non Actors*. Abingdon: Routledge.
Freire P. 2000, 30th anniversary ed. *Pedagogy of the Oppressed*. London: Bloomsbury.
Ramaswamy R. 2012. Embracing the unknown: introducing medical humanities into the undergraduate medical curriculum in India. *IJME*. Vol. IX No. 3. Available at: http://ijme.in/articles/medical-humanities-for-india/?galley=pdf. Last accessed: 2 August 2018.

24

ZOMBIE SICKNESS

Contagious ideas in performance

Martin O'Brien and Gianna Bouchard

An exchange between Martin and Gianna, reflecting on the figure of the zombie in Martin's live art practice.

Scene 1: Today, 14 March 2018, it has been announced that the world-renowned physicist, Stephen Hawking, has died at the age of 76, outliving his life expectancy by some 53 years. Ian Sample (2018), Science Editor for *The Guardian* newspaper, has written about him that "[t]hose who live in the shadow of death are often those who live most." Diagnosed with motor neurone disease at the age of 21, Hawking was given no more than two years to live. Martin O'Brien (2018: 3), in a similar position of exceeding his life expectancy, puts it thus: "Just a few months ago I outlived my life expectancy as someone with cystic fibrosis. I'm now in the zombie years. I feel a genuine affinity towards the figure of the undead."

Scene 2: This used to be the most optimistic city in the world. Now it's full of darkness illuminated by the fading street lamps. Out of this darkness stumbles life quite different from us. The unwell negotiate this landscape in a way we could not. There is no war in this city, no poverty, no crime, nothing to fear. There is only sickness and this sickness is itself a form of existence, a way of seeing and being, a way of breathing and moving. This is life. They do not fear death because death is already behind them. They are not motivated by material things. To witness the unwell is to understand all of our fears but our fears mean nothing to them. This city used to be our future but now the future belongs to the unwell.

Scene 3: *The Unwell* (2015) is a short experimental zombie film; I (Martin) made it in collaboration with the filmmaker Suhail Ilyas. It was shot over five days in Coventry, a city full of brutalist architecture. The film depicts a city where a zombie apocalypse has already happened. Human life has been wiped out completely and instead the city is occupied by the unwell. They are staggering corpses. I play all 16 of the unwell in the film. They move alone through the empty streets in a city where the sun no longer rises. I dress in badly done zombie make-up, wearing the clothes of commonly used zombie tropes: the bridal zombie, sports zombie, prostitute zombie, chef zombie, patient zombie, banker zombie. There is no drama in the film; it simply documents the activities of these creatures. This is a world where the healthy no longer exist, a place where only the sick can survive (Figures 24.1 and 24.2).

The dystopian aesthetic gives way to a philosophy of existence in which the human is not precious above all else. The new dominant species is the unwell; not a nightmare future, but a development of the human. The only way to survive is to join the unwell. Sickness becomes

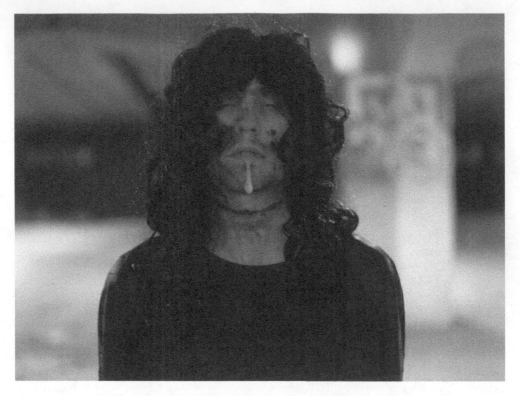

Figure 24.1   Human life has been wiped out completely and instead the city is occupied by the unwell

a desired state of being. It is the only way to survive. Only the sick can survive in this world. Being sick becomes a lifeline, a way to live in a hostile environment. It becomes the only way to be. Sickness becomes life affirming. Paradoxically, it becomes a way of surviving, of enduring, of living. There is no other way; there is no option but to join the unwell. Those who learn to embrace sickness thrive; the rest become prey. The rest are just meat. The rest cannot evade death. Only the sick will survive. Only the sick will survive. Only the sick will survive.

   Scene 4: At the centre of the image is a corpse, delineated by its deathly pallor, the rictus of the mouth in a strange gape and the fixed stare of the eye. Other hands in the picture are fleshy and alive, whereas the hand of the corpse is lifted by forceps grasping a bunch of exposed muscle fibre and tendons. Its forearm and hand have been stripped of the skin, the subcutaneous tissues revealed in their sinewy formation and structure. This is the stripped and pared-down operation of those equivalent functioning and gesturing hands in the painting, made manifest through anatomised visibility. The dissected hand of the corpse is at the centre of the gathering, the raison d'être for the men to be together, as it is lifted, manipulated and gestured over. Tulp, the key figure holding the forceps, seems to be showing and telling, with his parted lips and concentrated expression, whilst the others variously watch and listen to the demonstration. Touch is simultaneously mediated and extended by the forceps that intercept between living and dissected flesh. Here is the opportunity to see how things work, to understand how tissues are connected and animated. This, implicit in the gathered men's postures, needs to be seen and understood for it is interesting, even compelling, and we, as spectators of the image, are invited

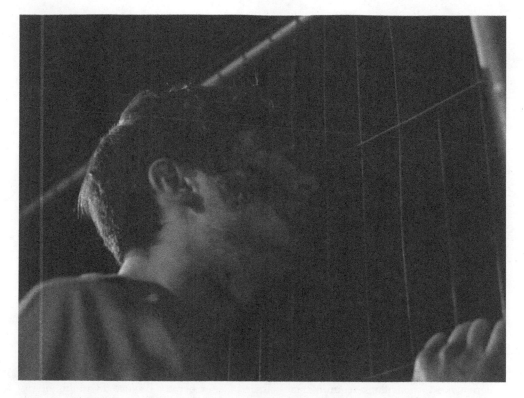

Figure 24.2   This is a world where the healthy no longer exist, a place where only the sick can survive

to partake of this didactic experience. The man at the back of the group looks at us directly and with his hand points down to the body, urging us to look—this is where our gaze should rest, on the object of study and learning. Demonstration is constituted through the object, the flayed flesh, and the combination of gesture and pronouncement is articulated over and above the prop.

This scene re-members the Rembrandt painting *The Anatomy Lesson of Dr Nicolaes Tulp* from 1632. The image honours the once famous Dutch physician, his contribution to medical science and a number of his contemporary surgeon colleagues who are also captured in the moment. It suggests that medicine has long depended on re-animating corpses for its own epistemological and legitimising ends. Using forceps, Tulp manipulates the tendons and ligaments of the forearm to replicate the movement of the hand—in life, undertaken unconsciously, but here, in death, induced mechanically by the doctor. The theatrical notion of the 'as if' operates here, with the dissector guiding specific anatomical features to operate 'as if' alive, animating and infusing these structures through an illusion of organic life and its methods (Phelan 1997: 27). The delivery of effective and constructive medical knowledge is dependent upon such moments of anima-tion and illusory manipulation that can satisfactorily convey information about living processes. The cadaver is consistently enlivened in order to reveal the body as a knowable and curable biological entity. The corpse becomes the re-animated repository of anatomical knowledge and authority, the medicalised zombie at the mercy of the anatomist; a zombie without agency or subjectivity but one that underpins and defines the whole of modern medicine.

These zombie bodies behave as theatrical props in the medical arena, material objects that become animated in the performance space, but they also 'prop up' certain structures of belief and learning—they support specific discourses by appearing in these sites. The medicalised, dissected zombie is then a complex ideological object.

Scene 5: Somewhere else, in Salisbury in the UK, the unwell, the poisoned, have been taken to hospital and remain there in a critical condition. It's March 2018. The bench where they once sat has been vacated, their unconscious bodies removed, and the area sealed off. Since then, the scenes in the town have become increasingly strange: restaurants and shops closed, a car park emptied but for one car, two graves covered with forensic tents in the cemetery, a suburban house with police cars outside, vehicles wrapped in tarpaulins and carried away. Cordons, hazmat suits, gloves, face masks, breathing apparatus and other specialist equipment have separated the living from the threat of death, the public from the expert, the ill from the healthy, the contaminated from the uninfected, the patients from the populace. Control and oversight have passed from one agency to another—the police, the medics, and finally the army. The locals have retreated, staying away from the shops and the market, whilst being advised to wash their clothes and possessions if they were close to the bench or in the restaurant on Sunday. Eleven days later, another village is being disrupted, another scene cordoned off; more people are telling of their fears and worries about contagion.

Scene 6: The Science Museum in London announced in March 2018 that it has commissioned the visual artist, Marc Quinn, to produce a 3.5-metre version of his sculpture 'Self-Conscious Gene' to stand at the entrance to their refurbished medical galleries, which will open in autumn 2019. The work replicates the body and, more importantly, the tattoos of Rick Genest, which were etched all over the surface of his skin and depicted his inner anatomy. Since experiencing a serious illness requiring brain surgery, Genest became fascinated with his internal body and sought to bring it to the surface as a 'living skeleton,' creating an illustrative anatomical atlas mapped onto his skin. Quinn observes that Genest's body "is at the crossroads of popular street culture, deep philosophical meaning, and medicine" (Quinn in Treviño 2018). Genest was known as 'Zombie Boy.' He died on 1 August 2018, in Montreal, Canada, for reasons that are unclear at the time of writing.

Zombies are everywhere, populating our landscape, reminding us of apocalyptic futures—climatic catastrophe, nuclear war, chemical annihilation, post-antibiotic plagues. They perform foreshortened horizons, embodying chronic sickness that consumes, even as it animates and decomposes.

Scene 7: Martin regularly performs as a zombie in popular immersive experiences for thrill-seeking participants across the UK. People pay to be caught up in an imaginary zombie apocalypse, where they have to survive predation by faux corpses, the zombie horde at play across abandoned commercial spaces and wasteland. He adopts the costume, make-up and contact lenses that help to enliven the event and make the fictional world more 'authentic' for the punters; the zombie pretending to be a zombie in zombie clothes. He layers his already sick body with another, a fantastical, imaginary representation that projects and externalises some of his illness experience. The figure of the zombie and his illness intertwine, embodying ideas of contagion and contamination, of quarantine and segregation, of being on the periphery of the healthy, of being a figure of fear and anxiety, of being Other through illness.

This zombie-ism has infected his artistic practice; his 2015 work *Taste of Flesh/Bite Me I'm Yours*, at the White Building, London, for instance, explored 'the fear of contamination associated with the sick body' and explicitly played with the zombie's desire to infect and consume its victims. Staged in a makeshift studio with canvas flooring and plastic sheeting for the walls held up by wooden batons, Martin was tethered and restrained throughout. He was chained to a central pole and wearing a straitjacket, both of which limited his movements and circumscribed his activities. For the first half, he slowly unwound his chain from the central pole by making ever-increasing circles around the space. Wearing a green balaclava, he traced a slow spiral of paint over the floor and walls, as he moved inexorably outwards from the pole, using his head as the paintbrush. This was an agonisingly slow act of making art, restricted as he was to moving on his knees, replenishing his head with paint and shuffling to make the next mark on the canvas. Gradually, Martin and the space became contaminated with the colour of phlegm, the colour of his cystic fibrosis, used as an aesthetic signifier of his illness. It spread outwards and threatened the spectators who were seated around the edge of the studio, just out of reach, for the moment at least.

As Martin reached the limit of his chain, he could start to come into contact with audience members in certain areas of the studio. Here, the figure of the flesh-eating zombie was writ large as he tried to bite spectators who were within his grasp. Initially, the audience tried to escape from him, moving ahead or around him to avoid contact in a playful game. As this went on, some capitulated and even invited this interaction, allowing Martin to bite them, offering themselves to him in this moment of animalistic connection. It was a humorous and mischievous game of hunting, capture and infection, full of expectation, daring and risk that punctured the popular imagery of the terrifying and evil zombie. Through literalising the movement between and across the zombie and victim, the unclean and clean, the contaminated and uncontaminated, Martin's creative practice sought to show, traverse and temporarily close the gap between us—the healthy and the sick.

Scene 8: A fictional town called Roarton in Lancashire, UK. In the TV show *In the Flesh*, the apocalypse has happened, and humans have taken the planet back. The undead are receiving treatment to keep them in a human state. They wear make-up and coloured contact lenses to make them look more human. Zombie-ism in the show is a pathologised condition: it even has a name, Partially Deceased Syndrome (PDS). They take their medication. These are docile bodies, self-governing and submitting to an epistemic authority over both living and dead, and partially dead. The PDS sufferers are medicated in order to contribute to society through work. In his 1951 publication *The Social System* Talcott Parsons outlined a theory he had been developing since the late 1930s. The text draws attention to "medicine as a professional institution engaged in the social control and rectification of a form of deviance and disequilibrium in society: illness" (Thomas 2007: 16). Parsons' theory rests on the notion that 'healthy' people are able to fulfil societal obligations, such as work, whereas sick people are not and thus sickness functions as a form of social deviance, where "their incapacity undermines the social structure" (ibid.: 17). He outlined what he saw as the sick role. This, as he understands it, is a "legitimate status allowing for the suspension of the ill person's normal social roles" (ibid.). Parsons argues that if someone is ill, their social deviance is accepted if they take on the sick role. He notes that "the sick role is also an institutionalized role, which [. . .] involves a relative legitimacy, that is so long as there is an implied 'agreement' to 'pay the price' in accepting certain disabilities and the obligation to get well" (1951: 211). This is a position that has certain obligations attached to it but, in turn, allows the sick person legitimacy. *In the Flesh* seems to point towards structures of living within a society in which medicine is the epistemic authority over the body.

Scene 9: There are those who stop taking the medication and allow themselves to return to the 'rabid' state. They understand the control of bodies and they want to unleash desire—the desire to feast on human flesh. A counter-political movement of zombies who refuse to take their medicine emerges. In other words, the sick choose to stay sick. The politics of this are complicated. Jonathan Metzl (2010: 2) suggests that health "is a desired state, but it is also a prescribed state and an ideological position." Health is, by its very nature, defined in relation to ill health or sickness. The concepts of health and sickness are contingent upon each other to exist. Parsons understands health as a normalising rhetoric. Sick becomes the binary of health and health is understood through its position as the absolute opposite to sickness. Michel Foucault (1973) proposes that health can be understood as a discourse of power. This is enacted in *In the Flesh*. Zombie-ism becomes a way of understanding and unpicking the ideological status of sickness and health. In a world where death can be removed through medical intervention, the undead are simply another sick subject in need of medicine to survive.

Scene 10: Reading illness as philosophically provocative and important, Hari Carel (2016: 208) claims it as a "unique form of philosophizing" that can raise questions about life and underlying assumptions about such things as embodiment, autonomy and health. Illness is "philosophically salient" in its rupture of the everyday and capacity to transform experience, and which brings the taken-for-granted and the overlooked aspects of existence to the fore (ibid.: 212). Martin's work, using live art strategies to explore his experience of CF, demonstrates how such illness philosophy can be made performative and communicated to others through embodied means. Performing a reflective and profound philosophy of illness, his creative practice engages with issues such as breath and breathlessness, contagion, endurance, survival, mortality, death-in-life and regimes of treatment. The zombie acts as a representation of, and a philosophical reflection on, his chronic illness. Removed "from the realm of familiar, predictable, and well-understood experience," he stages and conceptualises his CF as a radical live art practice that resists the normative (ibid.: 210). The zombie captures his relationship to CF and to his status as the unwell; it signals his liminal existence: at the margins, outside of time, beyond life (expectancy) and with a dislocated sense of body and self.

Drawing on the fantasy and iconography of the zombie apocalypse, this intertwining of illness and performance also comments on the imaginary, nightmarish underbelly and endgame of biomedicine and biotechnology—the utter catastrophe of cross-contamination, of genetic interference, of impotent treatments and medicines that slip out of control. The zombie is the abject figure that can no longer be disciplined or contained, beyond anyone's grasp and turning back on itself, an orgy of infected consumption. Bringing the undead into his recent work, Martin conveys and plays with these experiences and insights, drawing attention to the overlapping features of the zombie and the sick. Just as the zombie means reconfiguring the boundaries and exclusions between self and other, so Martin transforms connections between artist and audience, healthy and ill, alive and undead.

Scene 11: It's a sunny Saturday afternoon, 5 August 2017. I arrive at a recently abandoned morgue in South East London. I have a friend who is living there (yes, these are the circles I move in). She doesn't live in the actual morgue but in the offices and, one day, she found a basket of keys and they got her into the morgue. I've organised to use it for a project. I have knots in my stomach. All of my work is physically demanding and takes a huge investment, but this is a bit different. This is the culmination of work over 10 years. I call it a project because it isn't really a performance as there will be no audience. It's a performance for the camera, and with the footage I'm making an installation. The performance (with no audience) will be 30 hours long. It will end at midnight, as Sunday 6 turns into Monday 7. My 30th birthday. My life expectancy. At that point, I imagine I will drop down dead. So, I'm in the morgue in South East London. I've set up. I said this was a culmination of work over 10 years because I was going to use elements from all my work in this. The practice of recycling materials, of repeating the same actions, building a vocabulary, is something I work with a lot. My friend and collaborator Suhail Ilyas is filming the entire thing. I begin. The structure is 30 different actions. One performed every hour on the hour. This 30-hour act of endurance was my 30th birthday celebration. The morgue is dirty and looks as though one day everyone went home and never came back. The tools are still out. The slabs, the body drawers and fridges. Everything is sticky and smells like death. There is a gel over the light, giving everything a green glow. The actions speak of death, partly because they are in this room for the dead. But this meat has life in it yet.

The actions continue into Sunday. Most actions are solo but some are collaborations with other artists. People come and go. I keep going, sleep deprived. I can't stop now—it is my birthday party, after all. Then the final action. A small crowd of friends has come to see this. Even though I told them there's no live audience, it's to the camera. They ignore me and show up; if I'm going to drop dead, they probably want to see it. The final action is simple and not painful. I'm sitting at a desk; the lights are off. On the desk there is a cake and in it a single candle. It's a magical re-lighting candle. I light it, I blow, it goes out and re-lights itself immediately. The room is silent. I blow and blow and blow. It goes on and on. Eventually it burns to the bottom. One final blow and it goes out. We're in complete darkness. Now everything is different. Time is different—this is the beginning of the zombie years.

I should be dead but I'm not. I didn't know but time for me was moving forward towards 30. Towards the end, but now time is different to me. I should be dead but I'm alive. The making of this video work was a rite of passage. Now I'm in a different existence. David Morris talked about chronic time, but I don't think it's even that anymore. This is zombie time. The time of the animated corpse. I feel immortal. Death is behind me, instead of in front. Zombie time is a different relationship to death and life. It's still about survival, but also infecting—creating a horde. It's a form of enduring life when death is no longer the certainty it once was. It is no longer linear; it's full of breaks and ambushes. In zombie time, you keep moving but not towards anything, just for the sake of moving. No goals, only desires. No plans, only reactions. The only constant is the presence of death but not in the way it once was, for the zombie knows death and breathes in death. Death is in me, instead of somewhere else.

Until the last breath is breathed.

References

Carel H. 2016. *Phenomenology of Illness*. Oxford: Oxford University Press.

Foucault M. 1973. *The Birth of the Clinic*. London: Routledge.

Metzl J. 2010. Introduction: Why 'against health'? In: J Metzl, A Kirkland (eds). *Against Health: How Health Became the New Morality*. New York, NY: New York University Press, 1–14.

Morris D. 2008. Diabetes, chronic illness and the bodily roots of ecstatic temporality. *Human Studies: A Journal for Philosophy and the Social Sciences*. 31: 399–421.

O'Brien M. 2018. *A Manifesto for the Political Zombie OR One Sick Queer Artist's Ramblings about How the Zombie Apocalypse Could Save the World*. Unpublished.

Parsons T. 1951. *The Social System*. London: Routledge.

Phelan P. 1997. *Mourning Sex: Performing Public Memories*. London: Routledge.

Sample I. 2018. Stephen Hawking, science's brightest star, dies aged 76. *The Guardian*. Available at: www.theguardian.com/science/2018/mar/14/stephen-hawking-professor-dies-aged-76. Last accessed: 15 July 2018.

Thomas C. 2007. *Sociologies of Disability and Illness: Contested Ideas in Disability Studies and Medical Sociology*. Basingstoke: Palgrave Macmillan.

Treviño J. 2018. Sculpture of 'zombie boy' fleshes out London's Science Museum. *Smithsonian.com*. Available at: www.smithsonianmag.com/smart-news/london-science-museum-commissions-zombie-boy-sculpture-new-medical-gallery-180968470. Last accessed: 15 July 2018.

25

THE MASKS OF UNCERTAINTY

Cara Martin

In an age of Donald Trump, Brexit, and Fake News™, it is difficult to know what in the world you can be certain of. Life and reality television meld; professions are performances. But while we are uncertain of what lies ahead, we live in the most informed of times. With the Internet at our fingertips, we hold access to the entire history of our time as a species on earth. As a collective we are glued to our screens, ravenously gobbling up any and all information to do with whatever our moods fancy. Sometimes, it's trivial: cat videos and arguing in comment sections, taking up swathes of time that we seem to gladly sacrifice. Often, though, it's more serious. We watch with rapt intensity as stories—disasters, terrorist attacks, travesties—unravel before our eyes.

I can remember when the first plane hit the Twin Towers—where I was, what I was doing, and who I was with. I imagine that most people I pass in the street will have a similar story for 9/11 and any of the other, more recent, encompassing tragedies since that fateful day in September. The common denominator, of course, is our insatiable curiosity—a need to know more, to know more of what happened, and who was affected. We are gossip-hunters. But, in contrast, there is this quality of aloofness to it as well. Tragedies run by us without truly being involved, as we hold the event at arm's length, away from personal risk. We've developed strategies that satisfy the need for engagement without events ever touching us too closely, turning events into information rather than experiences.

We often view the future as an intangible, uncertain thing; a blanket of fog (and sometimes dragons) restricting visibility; and when we do see, it's only when it (the dragon) is right in front of our noses, and only then that we understand its meaning, and why it is there in the first place. This defensive detachment—built into our information consumerism—is both protective and damaging. It keeps our fears at bay, allows us to live our daily lives without worrying about the next missile that North Korea is going to fire off, or what country will next fall like dominoes through civil war and unrest. It leaves us totally exposed and ill prepared for the day when we can no longer hide behind distance and detachment: the day that the dragon comes fire-breathing right on our doorstep and we must smell its unfiltered smoky breath.

Such uncertainties—awaiting the dragon's breath—characterise our health and sickness and, in turn, medicine's responses. When we're healthy we can't imagine the day that we won't be—perhaps hooked up to tubes and beeping machines with our loved ones looking on in horror, sick with worry, but leaking unspoken relief that it's you in the bed and not them. The philosophical questions we pose to ourselves are no longer global or wide reaching. Instead we draw in on ourselves, marooned on our tiny islands, the lapping waters rising, in the bubble of the personal. Why me? What is happening to me? Will it maim or kill me? What will happen to my loved ones?

Every patient who walks through the doors of a hospital will experience wired-in similarities in their journeys thanks to the standard, scripted procedures of medicine. All individuals must be turned into population statistics and 'cases.' Although the individual events, and the cumulative endings, differ drastically between people, there is a general format for the journey that is the diagnosis and treatment of what laypersons call 'illness' and medicine calls 'disease.' From presentation and initial consultation to diagnosis and management, there is a general script from which patients and doctors read their cues and move around the stage. Population studies again overshadow the unique presentation.

The walls of a clinic room or ward become those of a theatre, where all the actors involved have their own scripted roles to play. At the centre of the medical drama is the fundamental relationship that directs the scene: patient and doctor, eye to eye. And around, the healthcare professionals with their various but standardised scripts. The characters played do not necessarily align with who these persons are elsewhere. The lines they utter can be very different in quality to those used with spouses, children, fellow workers stacking supermarket shelves, acquaintances made at the food bank, or, for the comfortable, the barista who makes their daily hazelnut latte. For the doctor or medical student-in-training, the projected medical persona acts as a mask signifying to the audience (patients and colleagues) who they are and their involvement in the scene: status, role, general management of impressions, giving off an aura of confidence (even superciliousness), maybe confidently orchestrating a ward round, or meeting the patient's eyes in acknowledgement of human affection.

The doctor's mask may be old and weathered, but smooth with overuse, drawing on well-rehearsed scenes in order to adapt and improvise to the new protagonist. This routine comes as second nature thanks to the years of training and experience under their belts, reinforced by bedside teaching. Their performance isn't one that will draw flocks to Broadway, with hushed excited murmurs that there's a Tony on the horizon. No, these performances are personal, intimate, low key, appropriate for context. They are almost confidential recitals in secluded corners of the hospital—not fully confidential because they have happened so many times before and are now rehearsed and repeatable public engagements such as the low-key 'Grand Round.'

There is almost always a witness to these scenes—the faithful understudy watching from the wings, miming the doctor's words and actions in an effort to make them their own, the small group of medical students almost excluded as the curtains are drawn around the patient's bed to create the stage. Mimicry here really is the best form of flattery, the shadower eventually displacing the shadowed in a standard procession. Medical students are the unspoken audience to the Medical Performance. They observe as the epics, tragedies, comedies (sometimes 'black'), and lyricisms of medicine unfold in real time, much as I did the horrors of 9/11. They are privy to the patient's journey, where, script in hand, we follow patients stage left through the procession of diagnoses, treatments, assessments, and tests. We contemplate the dialogue between them and the doctors who treat them and note how the dialogue is different when the formal exchange is not required, where the doctor is absent. How then the masks shift or melt, based on who is on stage alongside the patient—nurse, physiotherapist, porter, cleaner, family members, and of course students.

We use our time as students to build our own masks, painstakingly gluing together the frame, sculpting the features from papier-mâché, and adding details and colours to represent who we are and what kind of doctor we would like to be. We are halfway between camouflage and the mask of the professional as doctors-in-training and proto-professionals, Company neophytes.

The scenes that we witness aid in this process, showing us features that we should sculpt, or lines we can add to our arsenal (principally, the metaphors of war and conflict shape us, just as they stigmatise and objectify the patient) for the day we move to take on the leading roles. Our freshly completed masks will be rough and ready, and perhaps oversized, or slightly grotesque as we express confidence based on no real knowledge. With time, as we become comfortable in our roles, so too will the fit of our masks improve until they are as worn and smooth on the interior as the masks of those role models around us (some of whom we despised as cruel, arrogant, or unfeeling, and into whose shoes we may step someday).

The masks we wear in medicine allow us to easily transition from behind the curtain to centre stage, giving us a persona to adopt and a preferred dialogue to use during uncomfortable silences or difficult conversations. The mask, heavy at first, but lighter on wearing in (or at least more comfortable), acts as a physical barrier between the patient and us. We adopt a pegged, professional distance to keep our emotions and involvement at bay. Much like our well-loved devouring of information, we don't allow ourselves to get too close, to feel too much, to over-identify. This compartmentalisation affords a safety net, spares us the brunt of the possible heartbreak and burnout after the apex of the identity narrative.

But what happens when the mask on the patient before us is so similar to our own that we glimpse the person beneath and see a reflection of ourselves? Or, we are refracted in the waters of our patients? What happens when we see not the patient, but rather who we could have been had we made different choices, or embraced differing circumstances? We each have patients whose histories strike just that little bit too close to home, each a brush with the stinking dragon's breath that is not our own. For me, it was a mother who had the exact same breast cancer as my own. But her prognosis was much worse—it had metastasised to her lungs, her bones, and, most recently, her brain. Her daughter, of a similar age to me, had dropped out of university to become her full-time carer. Even now, months after our encounter, I find myself thinking of them and considering what could have been had the roles been reversed.

So, when our dragons emerge from the fog, and their pungent, smoky breaths are at your nostrils, the distance our masks provide falls away dramatically, stripped of meaning. Then, do we put the kettle on and twiddle our thumbs? I, for one, would reach for the sword.

PART V

Embodiment and disembodiment

26
NOBODY'S HOME

Susan Bleakley

Susan Bleakley's photographs capture the morgue after hours, when no bodies are at home—the material furnishings rather than the pathologists, mortuary technicians and dead bodies who normally inhabit the space.

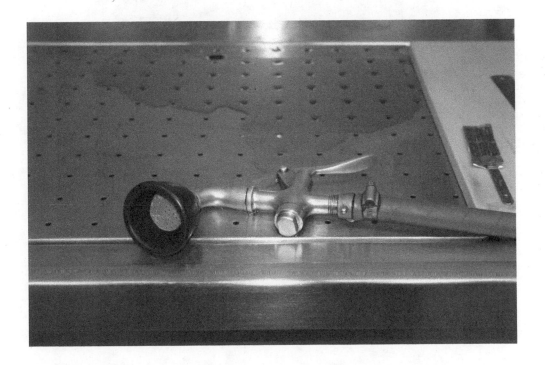

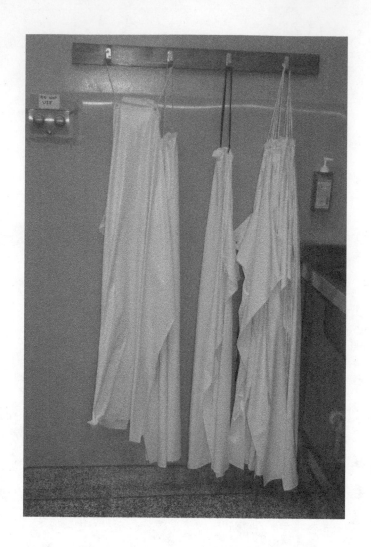

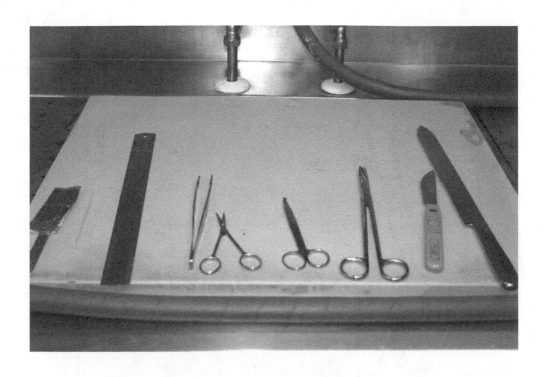

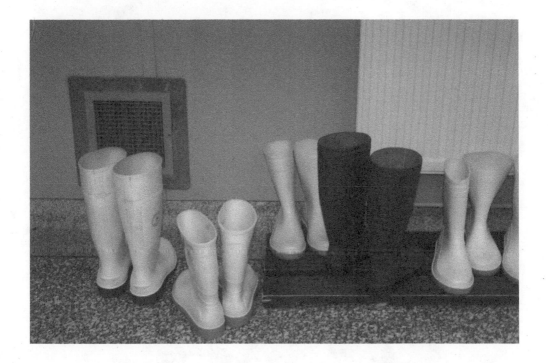

27

ECSTASY

Alphonso Lingis

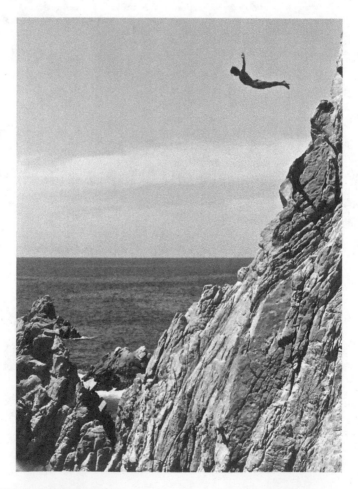

Figure 27.1   Cliff diver in Acapulco. Photograph courtesy of Alphonso Lingis

There are people who actively seek out dangers, heading into lethal situations. Death can appear to be a good compared with a life in which the cause to which one had consecrated oneself without reserve is lost, in which all the goods one aims for are blocked, or with a bleak life in which nothing attracts one.

There are people who readily engage in dangerous activities—reckless speeding in motorcycles or cars, unprotected sex with multiple partners, harmful recreational drugs, unhealthy eating and drink indulgence. They are attached to the pleasures of these things and do not heed the dangers. But perhaps unconsciously they are actively heading into the dangers and into death.

There are government leaders and captains of industry who conduct enterprises of great risk to whole populations and to themselves. They stoke industries that pollute the land and air, they devastate environments and pollute the oceans, they pursue losing wars. Individuals acquiesce in these enterprises out of weakness and inertia.

Sigmund Freud believed that certain behaviours betray a death drive. Soldiers from World War I who suffered grave traumas had dreams that repeatedly brought them back to the scene of the disaster. Freud's patients who had suffered painful experiences that had subsequently been repressed compulsively re-enacted those experiences. Children's play often staged the loss of the mother or of themselves. Freud speculated that all living organisms tend to the quiescence and inertia of inorganic matter.

Maurice Blanchot saw in the active engagement with death the culmination of the value of freedom that characterises Western post-Enlightenment culture. Freedom advances by rejecting the authority of religion and the state and with science and technology delivering humans from bondage to natural and material necessity. Freedom runs up against its ultimate negation in death. Freedom triumphs over this negation by choosing the time and means of one's death. In Dostoyevsky's *Demons* Kirillov dies by his own hand when and how he chooses; his choice of his death is a rejection of the dominion of God.

To know what happens, what is

"We do not know what happens, what is, if we do not know great joys, great pains," Georges Bataille said. That is the conviction, the experience of some people who seek out dangers.

We happen upon unforeseeable objects and events that radiate incalculable excesses of reality. Astonishment and joy open before them. Joy is greeting, acknowledging, affirming the wonder and power of what happens, what is. Joy is the feeling of excess energies surging. Joy is the body affirming itself, saying Yes to itself, overflowing. The joy that breaks forth before an enchanted object or event spreads across the world in which such a wonder is possible. To welcome in joy, the unpredictable marvel, is to say Yes to the zigzag path through confused halts and blind stumblings that brought us there. Joy is the state that opens widest to what happens, what is, what was, what will be.

Joy is the most expansive state; it illuminates the distances and the heights, it opens wide upon what happens, what is. Joy sees the uncertainties and the risks and says Yes to the determinisms and Yes to the chance that composes the world. Joy is the most comprehensive, comprehending state, the most truthful state.

Boredom and sadness, wariness and prudence shrink back from much that reality harbours, they raise up fences and walls, they leave the horizons and the depths in darkness. Scepticism and suspicion narrow down the mind, recoiling from and saying No to things and events; fear peers into the future to say No.

Exposing oneself to the grandeurs and the depths is also vulnerability. We are never so vulnerable, so easily and deeply hurt, as when in love. There are people who understand that to seek fulfilment in the love of one or several people is to close off the love and joy of what the universe lays forth every day. There are people who understand that the body armour of security, status, accoutrements, and possessions walls us off from what is, what happens. Who understand that in vulnerability and exposedness comes ecstasy.

The chosen vulnerability

After Chris McCandless's death, mountaineer and writer Jon Krakauer (2015) recounted his life in *Into the Wild*. Emile Hirsch played him in a film of the same title, directed by Sean Penn (2007) (see also Brown 1993; McCandless 2011; Saverin 2013; McCandless 2015).

Christopher Johnson McCandless was born in 1968 in California and grew up in Annadale, Virginia. His father Walt was an aerospace engineer who worked at NASA and later created his own company. From his first marriage there were six children. Then Walt courted and moved in with Wilhelmina Johnson, called Billie, who worked as a secretary at Hughs Aircraft. Chris was their first child; a daughter Carine was born three years later.

While in high school Chris went to Washington DC and roamed the streets buying hamburgers for homeless men and women. When he finished high school he spent the summer driving his second-hand Datsun south and across Texas to California and back. At Emory University he majored in history and anthropology. He took courses in 'The Food Crisis in Africa' and 'Apartheid and South African History.' The summer between his junior and senior years he drove to Alaska and back. When he graduated in 1990 his parents wanted to buy him a new car and urged him to apply, given his outstanding grades, to Harvard Law School.

He took the remaining $24,292 of his college tuition fund—a bequest from a family friend—and donated it to OXFAM America, to fight hunger. Telling no one, he got in his Datsun and headed West. When asked he said his name was Alexander Supertramp. In July, his car was drenched in a flash flood in Arizona. Removing and hiding the license plates so that it could not be traced, he abandoned the car. He burned the last of his money—$123. He was not seeking risks or death. He cast off the body armour and panoply in order to expose himself, vulnerable, directly to the grandeurs in nature and the individuality in people met at random.

He hitchhiked to Reno, Lake Tahoe, the Sierra Nevada. He fished and scavenged for food. He kept a journal and took photographs. In the fall he hitched and rode freight trains up the Pacific coast to Washington, then east to Montana. In South Dakota he worked for Wayne Westerberg, who operated two grain elevators and combines. In November he hitched to Idaho and down to the Mojave Desert. Everywhere people were drawn to him, his modest charm, his evident intelligence, his enthusiastic storytelling. To some of these people he regularly sent postcards. In a December postcard thanking Westerberg for his hospitality, he wrote,

> Sometimes I wish I hadn't met you though. Tramping is too easy with all this money. My days were more exciting when I was penniless and had to forage around for my next meal . . . I've decided that I'm going to live this life for some time to come. The freedom and simple beauty of it is just too good to pass up.

In Arizona he bought an old canoe and paddled down the Colorado River some 400 miles into Mexico. He paddled down the Mexican coast and camped in a cave, not seeing or speaking to anyone for more than a month. Returning to the US, he worked briefly in Las Vegas and at a McDonald's in Arizona. In January he went back to South Dakota to work for Wayne Westerberg.

He was 24 years old when in April he left for Alaska, to live off the land for the summer. He gave his wristwatch to the last driver who gave him a ride; "I don't want to know what time it is. I don't want to know what day it is or where I am." He headed on foot on a track known as Stampede Trail, with a field guide to the edible and toxic wild plants of south-central Alaska, a light rifle, and 10 pounds of rice. And books—Thoreau, Jack London, Tolstoy, Gogol, Pasternak. Twenty-eight miles down the trail he came upon an old bus that had been left there to serve as a shelter for hunters and trappers and soon made it his base camp. He carved on a board on the bus:

> Two years he walks the earth. No phone, no pool, no pets, no cigarettes. Ultimate freedom. An extremist. An aesthetic voyager whose home is the road. Escaped from Atlanta. Thou shall not return, cause "the West is the best," and now after two rambling years comes the final and greatest adventure. The climactic battle to kill the false being within and victoriously conclude the spiritual revolution! Ten days and nights of freight trains and hitching bring him to the great white north no longer to be poisoned by civilization he flees, and walks alone upon the land to become lost in the wild.

After three months he decided to leave, but found the summer-swollen river impassable and returned to the bus. At the end of July he became violently ill. Subsequent research by Krakauer determined that he was poisoned by a plant that was not identified as toxic in the guide to edible plants he studied. He grew progressively worse and died on the 113th day of his stay in the wild. Hunters discovered his body two and a half weeks later.

Just before he died, he took a photograph of himself standing holding a board on which he had written: "I have had a happy life and Thank the Lord. Goodbye and may God Bless All."

Anxiety and resolve

Philosopher Martin Heidegger explained that our recognition of the possibility of bad luck, the sense of our vulnerability, involves a sense of our being destined to death. We have an inward sense of our vulnerability in anxiety. Anxiety is the sense of being disconnected from the environment, nothing to hold on to, the environment sinking away, the sense of being cast into nothingness. It is an anticipation of dying.

Heidegger distinguishes two responses to our premonition of dying. Anxiety is the feeling of being isolated by the retreat of the environment about one and an intensification of the sense of oneself. Anxiety also intensifies the sense of powers one has and is, and, with them, brings into relief the resources, implements, and possibilities that answer to them. In the perception of one's environment, studded with possibilities, possible for anyone, the brink of nothingness ahead circumscribes a field of possibilities still possible for one. One acquires a vivid sense of possibilities and tasks before one in which to engage the powers one alone has in the limited time one has to live. One resolves to engage the forces that are singularly one's own in the possibilities and tasks in the zone that is circumscribed by the brink of the abyss. One engages and discharges one's forces fully in the tasks at hand. One thereby also intensifies the recognition of risks that may be involved in one's tasks. One becomes an individual agency, empowering one's skills and resources, engaged in tasks that are one's own. One is free, obeying directives of one's own choosing.

But one can shrink back from the abyss ahead, seek to smother the anxiety one feels. One restricts one's view to the day-to-day tasks. One then experiences time as a succession of days, each equivalent to the last and the one to come, without end. It covers over the sense of one's lifetime as a trajectory that is advancing inexorably to its end. One does not feel the approaching total and irreversible impotence. One feels as able to execute the tasks of the day at 50 as when one started, as able to execute them as the 20-year-old the company just hired. This sense of being equivalent and interchangeable with others before tasks that indefinitely recur each day excludes a sense of having powers singularly one's own and tasks addressed to oneself alone in a limited time ahead of one. One does not feel an increasing vulnerability and ageing. One also does not feel intensely risks that may lurk in the familiar day-to-day environment.

There are obscurities in Heidegger's exposition. Heidegger identifies dying as being cast into nothingness. But is the dying that anxiety anticipates rather being cast into the unknown? Or is it sinking into the materiality of nature? The time of my death is unknown. It is not located at a point in the time ahead; it may occur in the next moment; I may slip and fracture my skull; my heart may fail. My death is imminent at any moment. The sense of the imminence of death undermines the vision of a field of possibilities ahead open to me and undercuts initiative.

High-risk leisure

There are people who actively seek out risks. They choose occupations where bodily harm and death are possibilities—fire department, police, regular and mercenary armies. Doctors and nurses go to work in countries torn by civil wars, in refugee camps. Indeed, all doctors and nurses expose themselves to contagious pathogens.

There are people who pursue leisure activities that involve a high risk of serious injury or death. They practise wingsuit flying, BASE jumping, solo rope-free climbing, big wave surfing, creeking, bull riding, cave diving, freeskiing, ice climbing, mountain boarding, skydiving, and parkour. The general public and psychological and sociological researchers often see in them a fascination with danger and with death (Figure 27.2).

Recent studies, admittedly limited, have uncovered more complex motivations. Experienced athletes associate the extreme sports they pursue with positive and life-enhancing experiences. They find the act itself—soaring in a paraglider, catching and surfing a big wave—to be rich and glorious. They find extreme sport experience to be transformational—overcoming and managing fear and anxiety, acquiring mastery and a new identity. They find the extreme sport experience to heal depression, to be therapeutic.

Surfer, writer, and filmmaker Sam Bleakley (Figure 27.3) (2010: 140) writes:

> You wouldn't think it from the way that surfing is represented in contemporary culture—as a get-away-from-it-all form of relaxation, or a beach culture turning its back on the work ethic—but surfing is fundamentally melancholic. It is a 'kind of blue', a strange fascination that becomes an obsession. Not getting in the water makes you blue, but paradoxically, the whole tone of surfing sessions can be like a call and response with the sea that draws sailors' ghosts for company. When you are in your teens, surfing is all funk and strut, but as you get older and test yourself a little, those sea ghosts will try to run you down, and will haunt your nightmares. The top end of ecstasy in the perfect moment—the tube ride, long hang ten or big wave drop—is a small part of surfing's endless grind and challenge in paddling, duck diving, wipeouts, shark anxieties, bodily wear and tear (because the joints and ligaments give way long before the will), and the self-generated insults of extreme-challenge travel. Most surf trips have an underbelly. But I would have it no other way. This is not masochism, but living the blues, improvising life, making meaning.

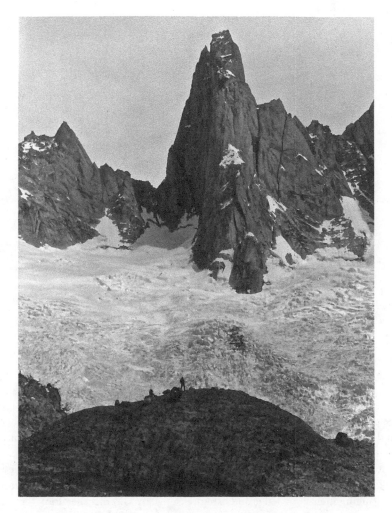

Figure 27.2   "A fascination with danger and with death." Photograph courtesy of Alphonso Lingis

Freeriding is skiing and snowboarding in undeveloped natural spaces. Researchers conducted semi-structured interviews with 40 professional and semi-professional freeriders (Frühauf et al. 2017). They spoke first of valuing challenge, that of encountering new places, overcoming the difficulties of environmental conditions, achieving skill and mastery, and exploring personal limits. They prized the experience of being in nature. Freeriding allowed them to explore and appreciate natural spaces in remote places that are only accessible on skis. Freeriders valued the company of people who share the same passion. Mutual trust when in a risk situation formed unique and deep friendships.

A freerider is forced to be focused and concentrated and completely in the moment. Freeriders contrasted this experience with the rush and turmoil of practical life. They described how skiing calmed them down, leaving them more at ease and relaxed. They don't talk as much about the thrill of pulling off physically challenging feats as about the sense of calm they feel when performing at their peak (Munsey 2006). Freeriding is free from rules and restrictions; freeriders

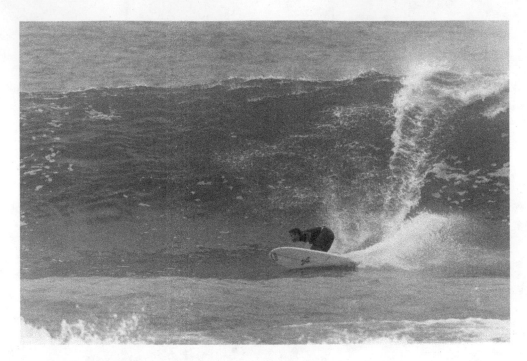

Figure 27.3 Sam Bleakley. Photograph courtesy of Alex Williams

take charge of their own action. They develop individual styles. Freeriders distinguished between positive and negative fear. Positive fear leads to higher awareness, focus, and concentration; negative fear, panic, blocked actions.

None of the respondents reported actively seeking dangerous situations. They strive to manage risk to an acceptable level. They study the weather forecast, snow conditions, terrain conditions, gauging their knowledge and experience. Many said that they look for challenges in everyday life but never take unnecessary risks. Most felt that driving was more dangerous than freeriding and with a less predictable outcome; other people are at risk.

Proximity flying, BASE jumping with a wingsuit where pilots fly close to solid structures, is one of the most extreme of extreme sports; about 90% of the deaths in BASE jumping were wingsuit pilots. A 2006 study of six proximity wingsuit pilots reported that they said that the flying experience yields increased confidence, happiness, enhanced energy, and a realisation that challenges are never too big to resolve (see Arijs et al. 2017; Holmbom et al. 2017). They affirmed that proximity flying had transformed them in profound and positive ways.

Ecstasy

The press and much psychological and sociological literature assume that people practising extreme sports are personality types seeking sensation, seeking thrills, and driven by a death wish. These recent researchers interviewing extreme sport professionals push aside all that and emphasise the experience of mastery of fear, of emotions, of physical skills they recount. But they also neglect the experience of danger in performing the feat itself. There is an ecstatic sense of vulnerability, of mortality quite different from the anxious anticipation of dying that motivates the resolute engagement of our forces in the possibilities and tasks at hand:

> I was stirred by the dark mystery of mortality. I couldn't resist stealing up the edge of doom and peering over the brink. The hint of what was concealed in those shadows terrified me, but I caught sight of something in the glimpse, some forbidden and elemental riddle that was no less compelling than the sweet, forbidden petals of a woman's sex . . . That was a very different thing from wanting to die.
>
> *(Krakauer 2015: 154)*

With reference to mountaineering, Krakauer (2015: 142) writes of pushing oneself to the limits:

> By and by your attention becomes so intensely focused that you no longer notice the raw knuckles, the cramping thighs, the strain of maintaining nonstop concentration. A trancelike state settles over your efforts; the climb becomes a clear-eyed dream. Hours slide by like minutes. The accumulated clutter of day-to-day existence—the lapses of conscience, the unpaid bills, the bungled opportunities, the dust under the couch, the inescapable prison of your genes—all of it is temporarily forgotten, crowded from your thoughts by an overpowering clarity of purpose and by the seriousness of the task at hand. At such moments something resembling happiness actually stirs in your chest.

Philosopher Georges Bataille (1993: 230) focused on all human activities that are not driven by need, that do not issue in contentment simmering over a content appropriated and assimilated. They include laughter, tears, eroticism (individual or not, spiritual or sensual, corrupt, cerebral, or violent, or delicate), the magic of childhood, intoxication, play, dance, combat, music, beauty, poetry, tragedy and comedy, sacrifice, the divine and the diabolical. They include collective feasts, sumptuous dress, jousts, gambling, building monuments and temples, where resources are consumed unproductively. They are releases of excess energy, without appropriation, without requiring the equivalent in return. Laughter is a powerful response to the unintelligible, the unpracticable, the absurd, the peals of laughter holding on to, repeating the moment when the rational breaks off, the utilitarian collapses.

The inner sense of excess energies surging is exhilaration. These forces are not constrained by the limits of the world of work and reason; they plunge beyond those limits. The uncomprehended and unassimilable forces beyond draw us. Anxiety repels; it also spirals in on itself, intensifying itself. In this intensification there pound extreme emotions. We transgress the limits in that compound of anxiety and exhilaration that is ecstasy.

The sense of the sacred is more ancient and more fundamental than the religions of gods and demons, anthropomorphic gods, and abstract God. Bataille studied the accounts of Christian mystics, Zen Buddhism, and Hindu yogis. He found the experience of ecstasy a plunge of the mind and sensibility beyond the limits of the known and knowable, into the outer zone of the uncomprehendable, unapprehendable, also called the impossible, night, nothing. There is oblivion of needs and wants, of concern for status and identity. The experience is both an extreme intensification of life within and an extinction of the acquisitive ego, felt in anguish and bliss.

There are people who establish themselves in the domesticated zone and work to satisfy their needs and wants and minimise all risks. Fire fighters, police, regular and mercenary soldiers, doctors and nurses who have gone to work in countries torn by civil wars, in refugee camps, as well as mountain climbers, BASE jumpers, and surfers, are turned to the outer zone of the unforeseeable and unpossessable. Each in his or her own way plunges into the outer zone where incalculable forces reign that cannot be mastered with reason and labour. The voluptuous abandon in eroticism and the impassioned abandon to nature contract the same diagram of sacred ecstasy (Figure 27.4).

Postscript. I was reviewing what I had written above when the 'phone rang. "You don't remember me," the voice said. "I am Jim, Rob Switzer's son. I am passing through Baltimore and would like to visit you." I recalled that I had last seen him when he was 15. Jim arrived with Amy, on bicycles. Jim is now 30, had been working as an engineer in New York City for the last eight years. Amy is an engineer too, had also worked eight years, in another company. They told me they had just gotten married, and are now starting their honeymoon. Heading south, then West to California, then across the Pacific to Japan and then . . . Had quit their jobs and terminated the leases on their apartments. They are going to honeymoon on their bikes. For a year.

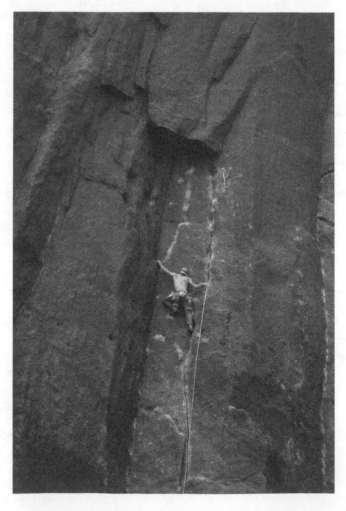

Figure 27.4 "There is an ecstatic sense of vulnerability." Photograph by Hayden Hunt

References

Arijs C, Brymer E, Carless D. 2017. 'Leave your ego at the door': A narrative investigation into effective wingsuit flying. *Frontiers in Psychology*. Available at: www.ncbi.nlm.nih.gov/pmc/articles/PMC5699196. Last accessed: 2 April 2018.

Bataille G. 1993. *The Accursed Share* II and III (trans. Robert Hurley). New York, NY: Zone Books.

Bleakley S. 2010. *Surfing Brilliant Corners*. Penzance: Allison Hodge.

Brown C. 1993. I now walk into the wild. *The New Yorker*, 8 February.

Brown C. 2011. *Christophere McCandless, Back to the Wild*. Indianapolis, IN: Twin Star Press.

Frühauf A, Hardy WAS, Pfoestl D, Hoellen FG, Kopp, M. 2017. A qualitative approach on motives and aspects of risks in freeriding. *Frontiers in Psychology* 8: 1998. Available at: www.frontiersin.org/articles/10.3389/fpsyg.2017.01998. Last accessed: 2 April 2018.

Guthmann, E. 2007. Sean Penn and Emile Hirsch talk about 'Into the Wild.' Available at: www.sfgate.com/entertainment/article/Sean-Penn-and-Emile-Hirsch-talk-about-Into-the-2521050.php. Last accessed: 4 November 2018.

Holmbom M, Brymer E, Schweitzer RD. 2017. Transformations through proximity flying: A phenomenological investigation. *Frontiers in Psychology* 8: 1831.

Krakauer J. 2015. *Into the Wild*. New York, NY: Anchor.

McCandless C. 2011. *Back to the Wild*. Indianapolis, IN: Twin Star Press.

McCandless C. 2015. *The Wild Truth*. New York, NY: Harper One.

Munsey C. 2006. Frisky, but more risky. American Psychological Association. Available at: www.apa.org/monitor/julaug06/frisky.aspx. Last accessed: 2 April 2018.

Penn S. 2007. Director, *Into the Wild* (film).

Saverin D. 2013. The Chris McCandless Obsession problem. *Outside Online*, 18 December. Available at: www.outsideonline.com/1920626/chris-mccandless-obsession-problem Last accessed: 2 April 2018.

28

RELATIONSHIPS THAT MATTER

Embodying absent kinships in the Japanese child welfare system

Kathryn E. Goldfarb

In May 2014, the Tokyo office of Human Rights Watch published a 129-page report entitled 'Without Dreams: Children in Alternative Care in Japan.' The report begins with the words of a 15-year-old girl, who, as a ward of the Japanese state, lives in a child welfare institution: "I don't have any dreams [for the future]" (HRW 2014: 1). The quote is attributed to 'Nozomi M.' 'Nozomi' means 'hope' in Japanese, an irony that Human Rights Watch does not highlight. The report takes an exposé-like tone, illuminating a population that has been referred to in Japan as socially invisible "hidden minorities" (Nishida 2011). Most people in Japan are unaware that around 30,000 children whose parents cannot care for them live in institutions, including over 3,000 newborns and infants. Around 9 per cent of state wards are placed in family-based foster homes. Because average care placements are over four years, many children in state care spend a significant portion of their childhoods in institutions (MHLW 2017).

The HRW report is uniformly critical of the Japanese child welfare system as a whole, which is known in Japanese as 'social care' (*shyakaiteki yōgo*). Critiques focus on the dependency of the system on institutional care that, the report argues, violates children's "universal right to being cared for within a family." Most centrally, the report states that Japan's "system of institutional care may itself be abusive—depriving children of the smaller, family-based care that studies have shown is important for their development and wellbeing" (HRW 2014: 4). This is particularly the case for infants, HRW argues:

> International standards set out that alternative care for young children under three should be, almost without exception, in family-based settings, and many child development specialists suggest that infants are at risk for attachment disorder, developmental delay, and neural atrophy when in institutional care.
>
> *(ibid.)*

The representational logic surrounding very young children focuses predominantly on the neurology of embodied interpersonal relationships. HRW also addresses the life problems of older children being raised within the system, specifically physical and sexual abuse by caregivers and other children, insufficient mechanisms for children to report abuse, and the lack of support once children leave institutional care. This lack of support makes it difficult for young people to obtain higher education and well-paying jobs. Careleavers I know see their own population as vulnerable to homelessness, sexual exploitation, gang involvement, and suicide.

Japan is a welfare state, in which the care of the Japanese people is broadly understood to be the responsibility of family, community, and employer. What happens to children excluded from these networks of support? Despite the fact that adoption for the sake of family continuity—for example, the adoption of someone to continue a family line, inherit a business, or care for ancestors—is a well-established practice in Japan, the adoption of unknown and unrelated children is relatively infrequent. Children disconnected from kin networks, thus, are often cared for in institutional spaces rather than joining a new family through adoption. Critiques of the Japanese child welfare system suggest a brutal contradiction: 'social care' for children—which generally occurs in the non-family spaces of institutions—is 'actually' abuse. If care is something that normatively occurs within family spaces, understood to be private zones separate from the social realm, 'social + care' emerges as an oxymoron. And yet for these children, the family is the central site of maltreatment and neglect that necessitated the involvement of 'social care' to begin with. While one might imagine other ways of receiving care than within a (heteronormative) family, in contemporary Japan, diverse relational possibilities for caregiving and -receiving exist more as social experiments or fringe practices than as recognised forms of social life. ·

Scholars who pay attention to 'social determinants of health,' the ways that social factors impact holistic bodily life, are often attuned to the power of embodied social relationships to impact wellbeing. I suggest here that studying situations where people have been disconnected from kin—and more importantly, disconnected from the possibility of long-term caregiving and receiving relationships—illuminates the ways that social relationships *and their absence* may be represented and experienced as an embodied presence. In this context, the contradictions at the heart of 'social care' in Japan play out in complex ways. Rooted in long-term ethnographic fieldwork in Japan, this chapter examines the stories of people connected to the Japanese child welfare system—people who grew up in child welfare institutions ('orphanages'), activists seeking to reform the system's dependency on institutional care, and caregivers for children removed from their families of origin. I suggest that social relationships *literally* matter in shaping subjectivity and wellbeing, and further, that normative expectations surrounding 'proper' kinship relationships and 'normal,' unmarked embodied subjectivity have unintended and long-lasting consequences. This argument has implications for practitioners and scholars seeking to understand social factors that shape health and wellbeing, and points to an ethical obligation to prioritise lasting social ties in the development and implementation of social welfare services.

Human Rights Watch, along with many Japanese critiques of the nation's child welfare system, focuses on studies that point to institutional care for infants and young children as producing neurological damage and developmental delays, and on studies of child psychology and attachment that indicate the risk for attachment disorders in children cared for in institutional settings. In these representations, social relationships and their absences literally seem inscribed on the brains and bodies of children. In their use of these data, HRW actually echoes the critiques of Japanese scholars and activists well known within the Japanese child welfare system, bringing their oft-articulated (and disregarded by those in power) concerns to international prominence. In so doing, HRW also makes use of the standards set forth in the United Nations Convention on the Rights of the Child, to which Japan became a signatory in 1994, standards that in turn are rooted in studies of neuroscience and child development.[1]

Implicit in these critiques is the understanding that social relationships and their absences shape children physically and emotionally in very material ways.[2] For instance, at a public symposium in December 2009 in Tokyo, where the audience was composed of foster parents and youth who had spent time in institutional care, a keynote speaker commented pointedly on how the institutionalisation of infants and young children prevents them from growing up to be "normal, full-functioning adults." "Because of the lack of physical contact," the speaker told his listeners—many of whom had spent time in baby homes—

> their brains do not develop, the part of the brain for emotional capacity and love . . . Their physical bodies will be smaller than their counterparts. And as they grow older, they will be unable to maintain personal and social relationships with their peers and friends.

During the lunch break after this presentation, the young man to my left, who I will call 'Toshio,' was almost in tears. "I was cared for in a baby home," he said. "The baby home saved me. If there hadn't been baby homes, I probably wouldn't be here." Toshio planned to study child welfare, and his dream, he told those at the table, was to open his own baby home. For Toshio, the symposium speaker's repeated insistence about the harms of baby homes did not accord with his own perceptions, and these arguments drew into question the validity of his personhood, developmental status, and ability to make claims on behalf of his past experiences and future dreams. One intelligent and articulate woman who had lived her entire infancy, childhood, and youth in large child welfare institutions took a few moments to respond when I asked her how it felt to hear institutional care described as irredeemably harmful to physical and neurological development. "It feels . . . unpleasant," she finally replied. "You start to wonder about yourself. I'm short, you know?" she laughed. "Maybe it's because of the baby home."

While there is an abundance of anecdotal evidence—and a smaller amount of statistical and survey data (Tokyo 2011; Futaba 2012)—that exemplifies the problems endemic to Japan's child welfare system, personal, experiential accounts never seem to be the ones with rhetorical clout; it is only by engaging with systems of expert knowledge on brain science, or by representing the system as irredeemably damaging, that reform efforts seem to have any hold. As a cultural anthropologist dedicated to exploring multiple and often contradictory aspects of human relationality, I have been troubled by the ways these discourses of damage and delay are taken up and circulated, and particularly how they represent the personhood of people who have grown up in this system. People become reduced to neuronal connections and stunted bodies, and possibilities for social ties and developmental trajectories remain represented as highly normative.

In contrast, my research shows that the relationship between forms of care in general and child development in particular depends, well, on relationships. Studies of outcomes of formerly institutionalised children indicate that many people raised in institutions have trouble forming interpersonal relationships because of attachment-related, behavioural, and emotional problems. However, according to a survey of data on the harms of institutional care, these problems "were very much a function of the environment that the child had been placed in after institutional care" (Johnson et al. 2006: 48). Literature in child development, psychology, and neuroscience suggests that supportive and caring relationships, even later in life, can have a powerful impact on human development.

Over the course of my ethnographic research, there was one account that I repeatedly returned to because of how it uncannily problematises the very ways that kinship-less neglect is so often represented as durably embodied, and troubles normative expectations for human development. Noriko was the high-school-aged foster daughter of two friends of mine, Masa and Rie. She had been living with them for 18 months and had been raised until then by her mother; she had been neglected for most of her life. Masa and Rie described her socio-emotional development as incredibly stunted, with an affectlessness that they seemed at first to find impenetrable. Masa told me how long it had taken them to coax Noriko to respond even to simple questions, much less begin to express her own preferences and feelings.

In an extended interview, Rie described the changes that Noriko underwent in the months since she had arrived at their house, from her initial unresponsiveness to an emotional volatility that Rie found challenging as a foster parent. However, by the time of our interview, Rie told me, Noriko had "really matured." Then, as though suddenly recalling the most crucial of details, she exclaimed: "It was incredible, suddenly she grew up!" Rie leaned towards me, and in an intense whisper, she said, "Her teeth came in—!!!" "What?!" I asked. Still whispering, Rie explained:

> Until last year, her period was also irregular, but now it's started coming regularly, and her teeth came in. She still had five of her baby teeth! They started to get all wiggly all of a sudden, and I figured they were cavities. "You've got cavities!" I told her, and she was like, "I don't ever remember losing them when I was a kid!" Both Masa and I were like, "No way, you're kidding, you're kidding!" and we took her to a dentist. They took an x-ray, and lo and behold, her baby teeth were still there, and from behind them her grown-up teeth were coming through all of a sudden.

"That is so strange!" I said. "It's totally strange," Rie replied. "Around the time when her teeth started wiggling, her period became regular and—suddenly she got—" Rie put her hands over her own breasts and indicated them becoming larger. "And her frame of mind became totally adult, she became an adult. It was just when I thought, 'This girl has really grown up . . .' when her teeth started to wiggle. In the end, two teeth are still left, but the others all came out, and one by one the adult teeth suddenly came in." Rie laughed. "She got adult teeth. The dentist was so shocked—!"

Later, I commented that Noriko's development might be connected to the good environment Rie and Masa created for her in their home. "Yeah . . ." Rie replied, "She grew up for us." In Japanese, Rie said that Noriko *seichō shite kureta*, which can be translated as: 'Noriko's growing up was done for Rie and Masa,' or, 'Rie and Masa benefited from the favour of Noriko's growing up.' Rie's description contains an important element of reciprocity: in response to something done for her by Rie and Masa, Noriko returned the favour by growing up.

Long after this initial interview, I raised the topic again with Rie. She understood Noriko's growing up as a material expression of her new feelings of safety and security in the foster home. Before she came to their home, Rie told me, Noriko clearly had not been *ready* to be an adult. But in the time she spent with them, she finally became emotionally ready and her body followed suit. "Well," Rie said with a laugh, "you can't see a person's *spirit* (*kokoro*), can you?" In Rie's understanding, the body makes visible and material the status of the spirit, mind, or heart, which otherwise only becomes haltingly knowable as communication skills develop. Rie did not belabour the significance of Noriko's bodily transformations; as surprising as they were, it seemed clear to Rie that Noriko's body and spirit together expressed the emergent relationships in their home and exemplified the surprising and hopeful capacities of caregiving and -receiving.

While Rie's account is particularly striking, she was one of many caregivers I interviewed in Japan who understood the bodies of children and young people in state care to express signs of past histories of interpersonal relationships. Noriko's case makes explicit the potential for transformation and change—in sometimes unexpected ways—quite late in life. I heard accounts from other caregivers about older children who, upon placement in foster homes or institutions where they felt suddenly safe, 'returned to babyhood' (*akachan gaeri*), a term denoting regression, which often involved the child moving rapidly through stages of development; sometimes children curled up in foetal position and then began crawling and pulling to stand, and asked to nurse or drink from baby bottles—all over a period of a few days. One foster parent explained how her developmentally disabled adult foster son suddenly 'returned to babyhood' as he was about to formally 'age out' of the foster care system. Once she explained to him that he would be able to stay in their household, the regression ended. Other caregivers described children's sudden leaps in height and changes in bodily processes like sleep, upon being placed in safe and supportive settings. Overall, caregivers I interviewed described how bodily and emotional transformations of children and youth occurred in thickly relational caregiving spaces, in ways that trouble normative trajectories of development and highlight the importance of substantive relationships between caregivers and those in their care.

One of my interlocutors, a now middle-aged man who was raised in a baby home and then a child welfare institution, likes to say that welfare systems "should not create people who have no one." Studies of child development and neurology, in the context of deprivation and neglect, work to build understandings of how social relationships and their absence get 'under the skin.' My research shows that care rooted in steady social relationships is what matters most, and systems of state care must be constantly attentive to the importance of social ties, and to the critical necessity of social recognition for people raised within the system. Caregivers, service providers, policy makers, and medical professionals must attend to human lives as constantly in flux, emergent, and in transformation—and constantly impacted by social relationships. This orientation requires engaging the people who grew up in non-normative kinship configurations and perhaps deprivation, but in their own terms. It is crucial to be sensitive to the troubles of children who have been removed from their families and placed in state care, but also to avoid deterministic logics regarding the damage of kinship-less neglect. While international child welfare debates centre on the presumably 'universal' right to be cared for, the form that care takes is often highly normative. Activist discourses themselves too quickly pathologise, a representational practice that leaves many people struggling to account for their allegiances, desires, and dreams.

Indeed, both representations of proper caregiving ties and processes of child development express values regarding the types of relationships and attachments viewed as socially desirable. This is particularly true in Japan, where discourses about normative Japanese character tend to revert to statements about the importance of blood relationships in families and the necessity for kin to care for their own. In contrast, perspectives of those who grew up in Japanese state care are highly diverse and, like those mentioned above, complex. Many people who grew up in child welfare institutions later work as staff in institutions and some feel strongly that institutional care—even for babies—is a necessary part of Japan's welfare regime. Some of these people suffered abuse from staff and other children during their time in care (as the HRW report highlights), and some have indeed had significant trouble developing lasting interpersonal relationships, an outcome that is predicted by neuro-developmental research on attachment disorder. But rather than understanding interpersonal difficulties as a problem of brain development, these people often link the experience of abuse in institutional care as cementing a deep distrust for others. These people advocate not abolition, but rather improvement, of institutions. Many feel that their institution is their 'true home' (*jikka* or *furusato*), a place to return and difficult to critique. Some even consider the directors and staff as parents (Hinata Bokko 2009).

For people with experience in state care, discourses surrounding the 'universal right to a family' may fall flat. To those who have family members in their lives, there is nothing idyllic about 'family' per se: it is often the site of conflict or violence. Others may desire relationships with foster families without the pressure to pretend as if these non-kin caregivers were replacement parents. Noriko, for instance, did not consider Rie and Masa to be her parents, but her relationship with them has extended long beyond her official placement in their household. Even young people who prefer institutional care recognise that it is difficult to create durable relationships in an institution, where staff members work in shifts and turnover is high. Indeed, the institutional system in Japan—like the foster care system in many other countries—is generally predicated on short-term relationships between children and caregivers. Toshio's own qualms with the institutional care system in Japan were, he told me in a follow-up interview a year after the symposium mentioned above, that very young children are transferred out of baby homes where they had lived from infancy until age two or three, and moved to institutions for older children, necessitating a break in caregiving relationships. At any institution, staff members frequently burn out, while staff with tenures of longer than three years are considered exceptional. As at my own field site, a child welfare institution outside of Tokyo, the staff members come and go, but the children stay.

My ethnographic research made viscerally evident the long-term difficulties commonly faced by people who grow up in state care. Further, despite differences in the form of state care provided, these difficulties are often similar to those of family foster care alumni in North America, Europe, and Australia. The Human Rights Watch report's title—*Children Without Dreams*—may have been intended to pull at the heartstrings of the public by appealing to a humanitarian rhetoric of vulnerable children being harmed. For some of my interlocutors, however, it contributes to the unrecognisability of children existing outside kinship networks as anything but abject and without agency. The notion of children without dreams places state wards as off-kilter within a temporal logic of kinship, a logic that Danilyn Rutherford calls a "modern rhetoric of descent: a way of talking and writing designed to persuade readers and listeners to follow a particular course of action by locating them in an emerging genealogy" (2013: 261–2), a genealogy that here threatens to point not to continuity but rather, as Rutherford notes, to "potential rupture" (ibid.). Children without dreams index a future without children, and thus a futurelessness for all.

For instance, shortly after the release of the Human Rights Watch report, Al Jazeera posted a 25-minute-long film created by Drew Ambrose, the producer and correspondent for the news outlet's Asia-Pacific current affairs show. The title of Ambrose's mini-film rivalled Human Rights Watch for a lack of subtlety: 'Japan's Throwaway Children.' Ambrose's title speaks to a more intentional objectification and abandonment, a representation in line with Giorgio Agamben's (1998) notion of "bare life," as Lisa Stevenson discusses it: those excluded from community, killed but not sacrificed, cast away and forgotten. These are lives, in Stevenson's (2012: 598) words, "always already exposed to . . . anonymous death"; lives that speak most compellingly to a "'failure of community'" (ibid.). In Ambrose's narrative, this is a community that has chosen to neglect—or has not even considered—the necessity to resituate state wards within alternative relational ties.

None of my interlocutors question the right of a child to receive some kind of care. Yet, rights-based discourses regarding proper care for children contribute to a particular circumscription of the very concept of 'care,' and by extension, a circumscription and re-articulation of normative understandings of kinship. In constant injunctions that proper care for a child occurs within a family, alternative images of intimacy recede ever further from view and 'social care' emerges as a paradox. In the critical rhetoric of child welfare reformers, life outside normative family structures appears to preclude the very possibility for a properly human life. Judith Butler (2000: 23) has articulated this problem as "the question of how it is that kinship secures the conditions of intelligibility by which life becomes livable, by which life also becomes condemned

287

and foreclosed." The imperative that children have the universal 'right' to family does not, in itself, address a broader problem: the fact that situatedness within a culturally legible kinship network is so often the condition for wellbeing. Is there no world we can imagine that considers the desire to "care and be cared for" without prescribing the form of that care (Borneman 1997)? I hope this chapter in some way provokes a more expansive conceptualisation of 'care,' and a more generous notion of the ways relationships—their presences and absences—are embodied. Does the valorisation of family care contribute to the unrecognisability and social exclusion of people whose experiences diverge from this model? My frustration, thinking through the concept of 'social care' in Japan—in which 'care' itself is seen to exist ideally, normatively, and perhaps only within a family setting—is most centrally a frustration levied at a world in which, it seems, we collectively are unable to conceive of 'care' outside of kinship. It may indeed be a failure of community—but it is also a failure of imagination.

Notes

1 A perusal of the UN Convention's periodic responses to Japan's successes and shortfalls in implementing the Convention's suggestions prompts readers to conclude that Japan has a long way to go to meet the Convention's guidelines. See for example UNCRC (2010).
2 Part of the analysis in this section has been previously published as Goldfarb (2015).

References

Agamben G. 1998. *Homo Sacer: Sovereign Power and Bare Life*. Daniel Heller-Roazen, transl. Stanford, CA: Stanford University Press.

Borneman J. Caring and Being Cared For: Displacing Marriage, Kinship, Gender and Sexuality. *International Social Science Journal*. 1997; 49: 573–84.

Butler J. 2000. *Antigone's Claim: Kinship between Life and Death*. New York, NY: Columbia University Press.

Futaba Flat Home. 2012. *Shakaiteki yōgo shisetsu nado oyobi sato oya shushinsha jittai chōsa gaiyō hōkokusho* (Report summary of survey of actual conditions regarding alumni of child welfare institutions and foster families). [online] Ministry of Health, Labour and Welfare. Available at: www.mhlw.go.jp/seisakunitsuite/bunya/kodomo/kodomo_kosodate/syakaiteki_yougo/sonota/dl/120809_01.pdf. Last accessed: 7 May 2015.

Goldfarb K. Developmental Logics: Brain Science, Child Welfare, and the Ethics of Engagement in Japan. *Social Science & Medicine*. 2015; 143: 271–8.

Hinata Bokko. 2009. *Shisetsu de sodatta kodomotachi no ibasyo "Hinata Bokko" to shyakaiteki yōgo* (A place to belong for children who were raised in institutional care: Hinata Bokko and social protective care). Tokyo: Akashi shyoten.

Human Rights Watch. 2014. Without Dreams: Children in Alternative Care in Japan. [online] Human Rights Watch. Available at: www.hrw.org/report/2014/05/01/without-dreams/children-alternative-care-japan. Last accessed: 26 May 2014.

Johnson R, Browne K, Hamilton-Giachritsis C. Young Children in Institutional Care at Risk of Harm. *Trauma, Violence & Abuse*. 2006; 7: 34–60.

Ministry of Health, Labour and Welfare (MHLW). 2017. *Shyakaiteki yōgo no genjyō ni tsuite* (Present Conditions in Social Protective Care). [online] Ministry of Health, Labour and Welfare. Available at: www.mhlw.go.jp/file/06-Seisakujouhou-11900000-Koyoukintoujidoukateikyoku/0000172986.pdf. Last accessed: 30 November 2017.

Nishida Y. 2011. *Jidō yōgo shisetsu to shyakaiteki haijyo* (Children's homes and social exclusion). Osaka: Kaiho shyuppannsya.

Rutherford D. 2013. Kinship and Catastrophe: Global Warming and the Rhetoric of Descent. In: S McKinnon, F Cannell (eds.) *Vital Relations: Modernity and the Persistent Life of Kinship*. Santa Fe, NM: School for Advanced Research Press, pp. 261–82.

Stevenson L. The Psychic Life of Biopolitics: Survival, Cooperation, and Inuit Community. *American Ethnologist*. 2012; 39: 592–613.

Tokyo Metropolitan Government Social Welfare and Public Health Bureau. 2011. *Tōkyōto ni okeru jidō yōgo shisetsu nado taishosha e no ankēto chōsa hōkokusho* (A survey of Tokyo Metropolis careleavers from institutional and foster care). [online] Tokyo Metropolitan Government Social Welfare and Public Health Bureau. Available at: www.fukushihoken.metro.tokyo.jp/joho/soshiki/syoushi/ikusei/oshirase/H27taisyosyatyousa.files/H22taisyosyatyousa.pdf. Last accessed: 22 September 2011.

UNCRC Committee on the Rights of the Child. 2010. Consideration of Reports Submitted by States Parties under Article 44 of the Convention: Convention on the Rights of the Child: Concluding Observations: Japan. CRC/C/JPN/CO/3, 20 June. [online] Available at: www.unhcr.org/refworld/docid/4c32dea52.html. Last accessed: 4 July 2011.

29

STILL ALICE?

Ethical aspects of conceptualising selfhood in dementia

Lisa Folkmarson Käll and Kristin Zeiler

The 2014 film *Still Alice* depicts the prominent linguistics professor Alice Howland who at the age of 50 is diagnosed with early onset familial Alzheimer's Disease (hereafter AD). The film follows Alice from her first experiences of disorientation and forgetting of words through the progression of her condition that eventually leaves her unable to care for herself. It depicts how Alice's mode of being and interacting with others gradually changes, how these changes unfold, affect, and are affected by her intimate social relations, and how her lived situation as a whole helps shape and delimit her as a subject. Alice is happily married to John, an equally successful physician and researcher, with whom she has three grown children. Together they are portrayed as the poster family of (rationality and) success, with the only exception of the youngest daughter Lydia whose career path as a struggling actress is pictured as irresponsible and incomprehensible in the eyes of her mother and older sister Anna.

This chapter turns to the film *Still Alice* in order to discuss frameworks for conceptualising subjectivity in relation to dementia, and particularly AD. We juxtapose our reading of the film—that centres on the themes of altered experience of space and time, recognition of lived experience and the conditions for subject formation, and responsibility—with a discussion of what we identify as two interrelated tendencies characterising current debates about dementia. First, there is an increase in screening or early tests for dementia, aiming for early diagnosis with the possibility of treatment and a slowing down of the progression of decline, coupled with debates about the uncertainty of the effects of screening (Boustani et al. 2003; Eichler et al. 2015). Second, there is a strong move away from descriptions of dementia in terms of loss of abilities and ultimately loss of selfhood to formulations that focus on the role of remaining abilities and what individuals with dementia still can do, in relation with others (Kitwood 1997, 2007; Hughes et al. 2006; Örulv 2008; Hughes 2011; Hydén, Lindemann, and Brockmeier 2014; Zeiler 2014; Hydén and Antelius 2017). Without explicit intention of scholars addressing the role of remaining abilities, the first tendency can also feed into the second one. This can be the case if early screening and testing, followed by prompt diagnosis and treatment to slow down decline, come to function as a promise of continuous control of one's bodily self, and one's bodily future, despite loss of cognitive functions, through mobilisation of social relations and networks and through development of dementia-friendly environments—if this feeds into the emphasis on remaining abilities. Furthermore, we understand these two tendencies as underpinned by or expressive of specific conceptualisations of subjectivity.

Albeit seriously questioned, the dominating view of subjectivity in relation to dementia has long been that conditions of dementia lead to a loss of self and that subjectivity deteriorates with the deterioration of cognitive abilities. Such a view was popularised in Donna Cohen and Carl Eisdorfer's 1986 book *The Loss of Self* and still recurs in the cultural consciousness of the Western world (Van Gorp and Vercruysse 2011). In response to such a 'loss-of-self' paradigm, research has demonstrated and argued for the survival of subjectivity throughout cognitive decline, focusing, as mentioned above, on remaining abilities. This growing bulk of literature is heterogeneous, and our focus within this chapter is on a *specific version* of this remaining-abilities-remaining subjectivity understanding, where subjectivity is not equated with cognitive functions of the brain but emphasis, instead, is on the role of social interaction, but where *the emphasis on social interaction seems to come at the cost of an acknowledgement of loss as an integral part of human existence*. These ideas seem to underpin Steven Sabat's (2002: 26) reasoning, when he argues that loss in aspects of selfhood, in moderate to severe forms of AD, can be traced to "dysfunctional social interactions," and that such loss can be seen as stemming from how persons without Alzheimer's limit those living with Alzheimer's, through their way of interacting. Dysfunctional social interaction, in this reasoning, is seen as resulting in a loss of self, and a more functional social interaction a way to remedy loss—and loss becomes understood as preventable and unfortunate rather than as a continuous dimension of subjectivity.

Even though the loss-of-self conceptualisation of subjectivity in dementia and this specific remaining-abilities-remaining-subjectivity conceptualisation operate with different understandings of selfhood, one focusing on the cognitive capacity of the brain, the other focusing on social interaction, they nevertheless seem to share what might be called a subtractive conception of loss (Käll 2017), according to which loss entails a subtraction of a part from something whole, leaving that whole incomplete, reduced, or diminished. In the first case, claiming cognitive loss as loss of subjectivity, that whole is the brain. In the second case where claims are made regarding the survival of subjectivity throughout the development of dementia, there is at times at play an idea of an original wholeness and stability that *withstands loss through withstanding change*. As an example, this is the case if social interaction is seen as a way to inhibit changes in selfhood that may be brought about by cognitive decline, through the maintenance of abilities and sense of identity and self-worth by, for instance, engaging in joint activities and offering affirmation of known abilities and features of a person's identity, and *if such inhibition of changes would also imply a stop to any loss of self*.

While not denying the significant value of not conceptualising the person with dementia solely in terms of loss or diminishment, we argue that we need to problematise the very terms in which conceptions of loss and subjectivity are articulated. Our point of departure is an understanding of subjectivity—understood as the first-person lived perspective of oneself as a self, including one's sense of self, even on a very minimal level of sensing one's own body, for instance one's heartbeat or respiration (Zahavi 2005)—as *dynamic* and *in continuous becoming through processes of alteration which in themselves incorporate continuous loss*. Loss is here taken to be an integral element of subjectivity insofar as subjectivity is finite through its embodiment, situatedness, and relatedness with others. Finitude is not understood simply in terms of death, but also in the important sense that there is an element of subjectivity that continuously escapes description from outside perspectives (Bernet 1996). Further, understanding subjectivity in terms of alteration, where the self is shaped in relations with others, entails recognition of subjectivity as elusive, refusing simple ideas of neat borders (Weiss 1999; Zeiler 2018). The understanding of subjectivity we are proposing can "serve to de-stigmatise the deep forgetfulness that accompanies the onset of dementia and to establish a sense of continuity between that which passes unmarked as 'normal' subjectivity and that which is marked and pathologised as the subjectivity of dementia" (Käll 2017: 25). However, the alterations of self and self-experience involved in conditions of dementia are at the same time radically and qualitatively different from the alterations involved in the continuous becoming of subjectivity, insofar as they entail drastic alterations in the experience of space, time, and relations to others.

In the remainder of this chapter, we engage the film *Still Alice* in order to think through conditions for subjectivity formation and for approaching possible meanings of responsibility and recognition in framing the formation of subjectivity. Following what Thomas Wartenberg (2011: 10) terms the "cinematic philosophy thesis," we see film as actually being capable of doing or being philosophy in similar ways to written or spoken discourse. Our focus is not on the film as empirical material for analysis, but instead on how the narrative of the film and the portrayal of the different characters and their relations to each other can aid us in theorising meanings of responsibility and recognition in relation to subjectivity formation.

Our analysis focuses on the conceptual triad subjectivity-recognition-responsibility, along the lines of a long tradition of continental philosophy. We ask how these three interrelated concepts form one another in different ways, taking on different meanings and setting conditions for what it means to be a subject in the world and in relation with others. The meanings of responsibility and recognition help shape the framework for conceptualising subjectivity and, in turn, given conceptualisations of subjectivity, help shape the framework for how we come to understand responsibility and recognition. As an example, conceptualising subjectivity solely in terms of cognition, in the hyperbolic sense characterising what Stephen Post (2000) terms "hypercognitive culture," sets limits for how we conceptualise abilities to take responsibility for oneself and to recognise oneself and others as subjects. Framing subjectivity solely and simply in terms of cognition has especially grave consequences for cases in which cognitive functions deteriorate, such as cases of dementia disorders.

Recognition

Dementia is a term encompassing several different conditions, but is usually used to signify AD. The cognitive decline involved in AD, and other forms of dementia, affects most commonly memory, spatial, and temporal orientation and self-experience. All of these aspects are portrayed in *Still Alice* where the viewer is brought straight into Alice's perspective, showing alterations, in the form of gaps and discontinuities, in her experience of space and time and her experience of herself in space and time as well as in relation to others. The gaps and discontinuities in Alice's experience are portrayed mostly through the surrounding characters' reactions to her actions, comments, and questions, which also offer a normalising perspective for the viewer.

In one scene Alice wakes up in the middle of the night distressed that her phone is missing and in the next scene her husband finds it in the freezer in the kitchen. Here the viewer is under the illusion that the second scene, coming straight after the first, portrays the next morning, as Alice says "I was looking for that last night" but then John reveals that a month has passed. In this scene, the film first brings the viewer into Alice's temporality and then suddenly brings us back to objectively 'real' temporality, a temporality we supposedly share, through the comment of her husband that a month has passed. John's comment is not intended for Alice but is instead directed to their oldest daughter Anna; John keeps his voice low and neither John nor Anna make any attempt to correct Alice; they say nothing to her about the lapse of time, thereby letting her continue living in her temporality, enabling her to stay in an 'illusion' that gives her world meaning. Here, we see how Alice is recognised to be physically present by her husband and her oldest daughter Anna, who tolerate her changing world and self-experience without letting it interfere with (their) normality and who do their best to compensate for her failing capacities.

Relatedly, a moment earlier John is on the phone and when Alice asks 'who called,' and John answers that it was 'The Mayo Clinic,' Alice looks worried and asks if anyone is sick, connecting the talk of a clinic with possible illness rather than with the research position her husband is about to accept. Also, in this interchange, John and Anna let Alice stay in the 'illusion' that is her reality. Here, it becomes even clearer how the two worlds are kept in separation, and how John and Anna's recognition is not in fact a recognition of Alice's subjectivity and ability to interact, but instead a tolerance of her being outside and parallel to normality. When Alice responds, asking if someone is sick, her response is to a common understanding of the meaning of the word 'clinic.' John gently dismisses Alice's response, saying that no one is sick and for her not to worry. His comment is well meaning but upholds the parallel worlds. In the specific scene in the film, he makes no attempt to include Alice in the conversation (however, the viewer is not given any clue as to whether John has indeed already made such attempts).

What becomes apparent in this interchange between John and Alice is a lack of communication in the sense of taking the perspective of the other seriously as expressing subjectivity. There appears to be no genuine interaction taking place, but instead parallel positions, and this has consequences for the very conditions of subject formation. The conditions for Alice's subject formation are shaped—and limited—by John's refusal to allow her into the conversation on her own terms, and this also limits the conditions for his own subject formation (Käll and Zeiler 2014). As Merleau-Ponty (1973: 20) states in his account of the relation between self and other, being extended out into the world and intentionally directed towards others is to be open to alterity and to allow oneself "to be pulled down and rebuilt again by the other," who in turn is pulled down and rebuilt again by the self. Self and other draw towards one another and only become who they are through this process of being drawn out of oneself, towards the other, and back to oneself. According to this account, subject formation is thus at core a matter of alteration and of continuously allowing encounters with others to form one's own subjectivity. In the interaction between Alice and John, there seems to be an absence of recognition of the conditions for subjectivity formation in terms of alteration, in the sense that the far-reaching implications of everyday encounters for subjectivity are not recognised, and the level of the efforts to understand and engage with each other can in this sense be said to be rather low. Rather than engaging with Alice as the person he knows and with the history he in part shares, John engages with Alice as a person with AD, letting the condition set the tone and limits for the interaction. In this respect his response to Alice is a perfect illustration of the idea of "malignant social psychology" (Kitwood 1997), insofar as the way John treats Alice appears to be without malicious intent but still results in her being depersonalised, invalidated, and treated more as a disease than as a person.

In the above scene, the only reason for the viewer to be brought back to 'normal' time is the knowledge of Alice's condition. John and Anna's reactions to Alice serve to exclude her in part from 'normal' reality while in one sense accepting her norms of perception by silently letting them be. The acceptance protects her from the distress of having her own sense of reality invalidated through any corrective move, and could thereby also be read in terms of respecting her reality and recognising it as valid to her. Acceptance of Alice's norms of perception could, however, also be seen as a way of not letting these norms disturb or risk 'normality,' while recognised as valid to her. Further, this acceptance of her norms of perception as existing parallel to normal continuity makes them appear all the more manifest from an outside perspective as discontinuous with normal continuity, and in that sense as the very opposite to normality. On the one hand, as said above, John and Anna, representing 'normal' temporality, are in no way trying to force Alice back into their way of viewing the world, nor do they appear to simply dismiss her way of seeing the world; instead they respond on her conditions, letting her world and experience co-exist with theirs. On the other hand, and at the same time, there are clear boundaries and limitations for how far this 'altered' way of being in the world can be carried out. As Alice shows signs of anxiety, or of reflecting on her altered way of perceiving and being in the world as strange or no longer falling within the bounds of normality—simply as 'wrong'—this way of being becomes a disturbing element that must be negotiated. When the limitations of peaceful co-existence become manifest, it also becomes clear that peaceful co-existence in fact happens under certain conditions and on specific terms.

In contrast to John, the youngest daughter Lydia (who throughout the film is portrayed as a disruptive voice that questions the assumptions of what a successful life should look like) shows little interest in diagnostics. Instead, she shows genuine concern for Alice's experience of altered perceptions of herself and of reality. In one powerful scene, Lydia asks Alice what it is like, what it feels like, and when Alice responds that on bad days it is like she cannot find herself and does not know who she is, Lydia's simple response of recognition is that it sounds horrible. Alice responds by thanking Lydia for asking; no explanations or diagnostics are needed, nor will they help in any way to take away the experience of horror of disorientation and sense of loss. In asking for Alice's experience of her situation, Lydia recognises the validity of that experience regardless of how it can be explained through diagnostic criteria. She also recognises Alice as a subject in her own right, able to tell her own story and answer questions related to her own experience. In her interaction with Alice, Lydia faces the risk that her mother might break apart simply by being asked this question; but she also recognises that she will not get any answer at all without asking the question, thereby exposing them both to the risk of interaction and communication. Within our conceptualisation of subjectivity, such interaction and communication is inherent to subject formation, where there is risk involved in being pulled down and rebuilt again by each other.

A scene precedes the interaction between Alice and Lydia where Alice asks her daughter questions, revealing that she has read Lydia's personal diary. Lydia quite naturally gets upset with her mother but then approaches her to say she is sorry, recognising that Alice in fact did not realise that she was reading Lydia's journal. Alice in turn apologises to Lydia, thereby holding herself accountable for not knowing or remembering that she has inadvertently violated her daughter's privacy, and trusting Lydia to have the knowledge and memory she herself is missing. Here, there is recognition on Alice's part of Lydia's account of events, taking this seriously—thereby also taking seriously, and validating, Lydia's subjectivity.

Asking for someone's experience is to recognise that someone as a *subject* who is able to give an account of herself. This recognition in the case of dementia is essential, as it involves recognition of a continuity of life and abilities through the discontinuities implied by cognitive decline and loss of abilities. At the same time, however, asking for someone's experience is never done in a complete vacuum, but is conditioned by the limitations of how experience can be expressed, and what experience is deemed as recognisable, acceptable, and intelligible. Being able to read or carry on a conversation both qualify as abilities. But while those may be lost with the onset and development of dementia, the fundamental ability to answer the question of how one experiences one's own self through the progression of cognitive decline may remain in advanced stages (Eustach et al. 2013), yet it is perhaps rarely brought into focus as an 'ability.' It is precisely this ability that Lydia recognises in Alice, resting on the assumption that her mother is a self-reflecting subject throughout the progression of her condition. With her question, Lydia is not testing her mother to see whether she is still a self-reflecting subject, but, rather, her continuous conversations with her rest on this assumption as part of their interaction. By engaging with her mother in this way, Lydia allows herself to be pulled down and then rebuilt in the interaction with her mother. Here, she becomes a self in relation to her mother (and allows the same for her mother in relation to herself). While the parallel co-existence that John and Anna accept does not invite such mutual co-constitution or forming of one another, still, this co-constitution will nevertheless take place, whether we welcome or seek to refute it.

Responsibility

One of the central questions raised by *Still Alice* is that of the meaning of acting responsibly in relation to one's health and life, a question that generates different responses depending on how subjectivity is conceptualised. Alice early on, as she experiences memory lapses and disorientation, acts responsibly by seeking medical help. In her conversation with her doctor, it becomes clear that she is the archetype of the responsible subject, understood in a context where "controlling or appearing to control one's health has become a sign of being a responsible individual" (Harjunen 2016: 68). Alice takes a multivitamin, flaxseed oil, and iron supplements, she is an avid runner, keeping in shape, and she listens to small changes and symptoms, seeking medical help before they grow out of control. In spite of her precautions, however, she is subjected to the genes of familial AD, which she did not know she carried and which she has had no reason to look for.

As Alice goes through the process of medical assessment and receives her diagnosis, she also subjects herself to systematic self-testing. She memorises words and sets a series of questions to herself on her phone, which she answers regularly every day. She makes the decision that when she fails to answer the questions, it is time for her to end her life and she records a video message for her future self with instructions to swallow a bottle of sleeping pills hidden in her bedroom, and go to sleep without telling anyone about it, assuming that her future self would no longer be able to assess her situation and take (responsible) action. Her action of recording the video demonstrates the ideal of taking responsibility for oneself, protecting one's autonomy, and not burdening others to assume responsibility. After a Skype call with Lydia, months later, Alice accidently opens the video from her past self and starts to follow the instructions, walking up the stairs to her bedroom only to find that once upstairs she has forgotten why she is there. After having walked up and down the stairs a number of times, replaying the video with her instructions to herself, she eventually walks up the stairs carrying her laptop with her. She finds the pills and is about to swallow them but instead drops them on the floor when startled by the arrival of her care assistant downstairs and then forgets what she was doing.

Responsibility, however, can be conceptualised in different terms. As Alice and John tell their children of the diagnosis, Lydia decides against taking a genetic test to determine the risk of developing the disease. However, the two elder siblings Anna, a lawyer, and Tom, a physician like his father, take the test. Anna, who is in the process of going through IVF-treatment, tests positive for having the gene and makes sure her embryos are also tested prior to her next treatment. At the end of the film, Anna gives birth to twins who are not carriers of the specific Alzheimer's gene and who thereby will not risk passing on the condition through genetic inheritance. By taking the test and making sure that her children will not carry on the gene, Anna takes responsibility for future generations. However, it could also be argued, given a specific understanding of responsibility, that the responsible course of action for her would be not to have children at all as she herself is a carrier of the gene and, the film tells us, has a 50% risk of developing early onset Alzheimer's. Her character in that respect could be interpreted as recognising a level of unpredictability of life.

Alice's husband John takes up a position in Minnesota, far from their home in NYC, and Lydia moves back home from California to care for Alice. Here, John takes a form of breadwinner responsibility, providing the material means to hire a caretaker and for Alice to continue living at home as well as for Lydia to move back and care for her mother. Lydia takes responsibility in a different sense and comes to represent in the film the ethical position, by stating clearly that she knows she needs to be with Alice. At this point, the responsibility of John and Lydia also intertwine, in the sense that Lydia's staying with Alice is only possible given a certain privileged economic setting, where John's income makes this a possible choice at all.

Even so, Lydia's response that she knows she needs to be with her mother could be understood as reflecting a minimal sense of responsibility in terms of giving a response to a situation one finds oneself in. This is different from the ideal of taking responsibility for oneself in several ways, among them in the way that it is not a matter of responsibility *either* for oneself *or* for others. In our analysis of the film, Lydia's response is not immediately a response to her mother, but *rather to their shared situation involving the present of her mother's condition, the choices of others, and a shared past.* Her response should, in this sense, be understood not as an occurrence to a one-time event, or as set apart from that of others. Instead, as established in phenomenological philosophy, responding to our being-in-situation is something we do *by being situated in relation with others.* Relatedly, it is not specific situations of crisis that generate response to begin with, but instead such situations make manifest that we always respond as part of our existence, and call upon us to respond in specific ways and of making ourselves aware of the necessity (inescapability) to respond.

The understanding of the situatedness of subjectivity as a matter of continuously responding to our situation and others has in some thinkers, such as Levinas, Løgstrup, and Butler, been developed in ethical terms of responsibility. If we understand responsibility in a minimal sense in terms of responding to the situation one finds oneself in, and if we understand this minimal sense of responsibility as integral to an understanding of the self as relational in the sense of alteration, then discussions of ethics and questions of how we *should* act in response to specific situations must be reframed. Responsibility, here, can come to be understood in terms close to that of Løgstrup (1921). For Løgstrup, human existence is always already entangled with other human beings, this entanglement is ontologically prior to our constitution as individuals, and because of this entanglement we always hold (some part of) the other person's life in our hands: (some part of) the other person's life depends on how we act, and interact, in the concrete shared situation. This very entanglement creates an ethical demand: not only are we situated as response-able, but we should act in ways that express care for (the parts of) the life of the other that we hold in our hands (Holm 2001).

This conceptualisation of responsibility is far from the conception that centres on the self as neatly demarcated from others, and where the responsible thing to do, when living with dementia, is to not burden others, and for this reason to prepare for oneself to end one's life. If used as a lens when engaging with *Still Alice*, this minimal conception of Løgstrup, as an example, instead allows for the understanding of Alice herself as responsible, for example when responding to Lydia's upset reaction—even if Alice does not understand that she has read Lydia's diary, she takes responsibility for what Lydia tells her, responding to her by apologising. Furthermore, because this conception of responsibility starts in an understanding of subjectivity as dynamically entangled with others, it seems compatible with our conceptualisation of subjectivity in terms of continuous alteration, through and in relation with others.

Rethinking the two tendencies via *Still Alice*

To return to where we started, we see two tendencies in current discussions about dementia: first, an increasing emphasis on the benefits of early detection of dementia via early cognitive tests for dementia or screening; and second, an emphasis on remaining abilities when living with dementia.

The first tendency to increase early testing for dementia fits well with a biomedical imperative to detect, and if possible prevent, the onset and development of cognitive decline, in a reasoning where loss of cognitive function equals loss of self, and where early testing can come to be understood as a way to enable subjectivity to remain intact. It can be seen as a response to a loss-of-self paradigm, by attempting to catch the "mysterious thief" of dementia before robbing its victim "of the very thing that makes human beings unique" (Khachaturian 1997: 21). The second tendency to focus on remaining abilities is heterogeneous. We acknowledge that the larger field of remaining-abilities-remaining-subjectivity conceptualisations reflects a multifaceted reaction against a reductive cognitive framework and an imperative to recognise the survival of subjectivity or selfhood beyond the deterioration of cognitive faculties. And our concern rests with an emphasis on remaining abilities at the *expense* of an acknowledgement of loss as an integral and continuous part of subject formation. Neither the first nor this second (more specific) approach draw on an understanding of subjectivity as formed in relation with others—continuously—where loss is an integral part and parcel of the formation of subjectivity as such, and not just when living with dementia.

In contrast to these conceptualisations of subjectivity, we suggest that we need not only critically respond to a dominating loss-of-self paradigm, in which subjectivity is easily reduced to cognitive functions of the brain, but we must also question the ontological foundation that makes such an understanding of subjectivity possible. A response that simply shifts focus to social interaction as central to selfhood and subjectivity without addressing its ontological foundation is, then, not enough.

Throughout this chapter, we have engaged with the alternative understanding of subjectivity as dynamic, relational, and continuously formed in relation with its surroundings and other people. This formation of subjectivity cannot be reduced to a level of social interaction, which might risk making both loss and survival primarily a matter of social relations, but instead it is an ontological formation of subjectivity in terms of alteration, where loss is incorporated as a constitutive feature. Returning to the portrayal of Alice in the film, the alterations in her experience of space and time, given our understanding of subjectivity, cannot be understood in any simple sense of subtraction but are instead qualitative shifts in experience. These types of qualitative shifts in the experience of oneself in the world are *not necessarily radical breaks* with an understanding of oneself as a subject, but *rather precisely qualitatively different ways of being in the world as a subject*. In that respect such shifts in self-experience may be experiences of an urgent presence of oneself experiencing one's altered self, perhaps in terms of loss, but not reducible to loss (Käll 2017). This does not imply that the experience itself is not taken seriously in its radically qualitative difference. Quite the contrary, it is recognition of the *seriousness of qualitative shifts*. An understanding of disorientation as loss of orientation in subtractive terms risks not taking seriously the qualitative difference in experiences of disorientation.

Furthermore, specific conceptualisations of subjectivity fit with specific understandings of responsibility. If subjectivity is conceptualised as atomistic in terms of cognition and self-sufficiency, this can harmonise with the idea of fixed boundaries also of responsibility, where responsibility for oneself only extends to oneself and should not be imposed as a burden on another. By contrast, a conceptualisation of subjectivity in terms of social interaction also implicates boundaries of responsibility, but these focus instead on how responsibility extends also to others who are no longer able to care, or take responsibility, for themselves. The understanding of subjectivity in terms of alterations, where loss is an integral part, encourages understandings of the *implications* of such continuous formation. In contrast to the idea of responsibility for oneself as only extending to oneself—where not being a burden becomes a matter of responsibility— this understanding of subjectivity aligns itself with an understanding where self and other always contribute to forming each other, and hence always respond to each other, and are thereby always responsible for each other in the minimal sense discussed earlier. The issue, then, is not to ensure that one is not a burden to others, but how one's mode of responding not only allows for but also recognises, and acknowledges, the mutual co-formation (Örulv 2014).

Taking seriously the conceptualisation of subjectivity in terms of alteration, and the related conceptions of recognition and responsibility, implies specific, critical entrance-points for the two tendencies in debates about dementia. These conceptualisations invite a questioning of the logic of early detection in order to enable control of oneself. They do so in a specific sense: while acknowledging that early detection can have positive effects if enabling adequate treatment, it questions a narrow focus on cognitive loss and control of oneself. This conceptualisation also acknowledges how subjectivity is continuously shaped not only in relation to other persons, but also in relation to a situational whole, including objects. As a consequence, such conceptualisation invites questions of how the very cognitive tests help shape subjectivity— sometimes in ways that are experienced as positive by the person being tested, and sometimes in more troubling ways—*because* of this thorough acknowledgement of subjectivity as continuously and dynamically shaped in relation with others, things, and one's socio-material world. It takes this uncertainty of the results of early testing seriously, and is capable of doing so because of the acknowledgement of how subjects continuously are pulled down and built up again in relation to others, and to a surrounding world of objects and meaning. Early testing, then, is nothing to be performed lightly, since it can help shape subjectivity.

On the one hand, the understanding of subjectivity in terms of alteration is compatible with the view that social interaction can enable persons with dementia to engage in everyday activities that may otherwise not have been possible. On the other hand, it helps recognise loss, also within such interactions, not as primarily, or only, due to dysfunctional interaction, but also as integral to subjectivity. This reasoning can help transform the understanding of subjectivity when living with dementia, and can help shape how we talk about life with dementia. It can also underpin dementia care practices that, through social interaction, seek to enable persons with dementia to engage in everyday activities. For this reason, on a surface level, the dementia care practice may seem to be the same irrespective of whether it is based on the conception of subjectivity in terms of alterations and loss, or the understanding of subjectivity where social interaction fills in the gaps and restores the self to an initial whole. Yet these conceptions are starkly different. From within the conceptualisation that we have argued for, dysfunctional social interactions can indeed be limiting for the subject, but because subjectivity is shaped through alterations, there is also room for, and an analytic acknowledgement of, different altered experiences of space, time, oneself, and others, and the qualitatively different alterations when living with dementia.

Finally, to return to our approach of engaging a film in our philosophical discussion: as with any cultural representation, film, or other narrative, there are limitations as to how content is represented, which sets boundaries and directs the viewer in certain ways, making some readings possible and more probable than others. However, by presenting us with a limited universe or closed circuit, a fictional narrative, such as *Still Alice*, makes it possible to ask specific questions and closely interrogate these within a given framework while also highlighting and problematising precisely the limitations of such frameworks.

Acknowledgement

The Swedish Research Foundation (the project: A Feminist Approach to Medical Screening) supported parts of this research.

References

Bernet R. 1996. 'The Other in Myself'. In: S Critchley, P Dews (eds.) *Deconstructive Subjectivities*. Albany, NY: SUNY Press, 169–84.

Boustani M, Peterson B, Hanson L, et al. Screening for Dementia in Primary Care: A Summary of the Evidence for the U.S. Preventive Services Task Force. *Annals of Internal Medicine*. 2003; 138: 927–37.

Cohen D, Eisdorfer C. 1986. *The Loss of Self: A Family Resource for the Care of Alzheimer's Disease and Related Disorders*. New York, NY: New American Library.

Eichler T, Thyrian JR, Hertel J, et al. Rates of Formal Diagnosis of Dementia in Primary Care: The Effect of Screening. *Alzheimer's & Dementia*. 2015; 1: 87–93.

Eustach et al. Sense of Identity in Advanced Alzheimer's Dementia: A Cognitive Dissociation between Sameness and Selfhood. *Consciousness and Cognition*. 2013; 22: 1456–67.

Glatzer R, Westmoreland W. 2014. *Still Alice*. Killer Films.

Harjunen H. 2016. *Neoliberal Bodies and the Gendered Fat Body*. London: Routledge.

Holm, S. The Phenomenological Ethics of KE Løgstrup: A Resource for Health Care Ethics and Philosophy? *Nursing Philosophy*. 2001; 2: 26–33.

Hughes J. 2011. *Thinking Through Dementia*. Oxford: Oxford University Press.

Hughes J, Louw S, Sabat S. 2006. Seeing Whole. In: J Hughes, S Louw, S Sabat (eds.) *Dementia: Mind, Meaning and the Person*. Oxford: Oxford University Press, 1–40.

Hydén L-C, Antelius E (eds.) 2017. *Living with Dementia: Relations, Responses and Agency in Everyday Life*. Basingstoke: Palgrave Macmillan.

Hydén L-C, Lindemann H, Brockmeier J (eds.) 2014. *Beyond Loss: Dementia, Identity, Personhood*. Oxford: Oxford University Press.

Käll LF, Zeiler K. Bodily Relational Autonomy. *Journal of Consciousness Studies*. 2014; 21: 100–20.

Käll LF. 2017. Toward a Phenomenological Conception of the Subjectivity of Dementia. In: L-C. Hydén & E. Antelius (eds.) *Living with Dementia: Relations, Responses and Agency in Everyday Life*. Basingstoke: Palgrave Macmillan, 14–28.

Khachaturian Z. Plundered Memories. *The Sciences*. 1997; 37: 20–5.

Kitwood T. 1997. *Dementia Reconsidered: The Person Comes First*. New York, NY: Open University Press.

Kitwood T. 2007. *Tom Kitwood on Dementia: A Reader and Critical Commentary*, C Baldwin, A Capstick (eds.). New York, NY: Open University Press.

Løgstrup K. 1994 [1921]. *Det etiska kravet*. Gothenburg: Daidalos.

Lorentz W, Scanlan J, S Borson. Brief Screening Tests for Dementia. *Canadian Journal of Psychiatry*. 2002; 47: 723–33.

Merleau-Ponty M. 1973. *The Prose of the World*. Evanston, IL: Northwestern University Press.

Örulv L. 2008. *Fragile Identities, Patched-Up Worlds: Dementia and Meaning-Making in Social Interaction*. Linköping: Linköping University.

Örulv L. 2014. The Subjectivity of Disorientation. In: L-C Hydén, H Lindemann, J Brockmeier (eds.) *Beyond Loss*. Oxford: Oxford University Press, 191–207.

Post S. 2000. *The Moral Challenge of Alzheimer's Disease*. Baltimore, MD: The Johns Hopkins University Press.

Sabat SR. Surviving Manifestations of Selfhood in Alzheimer's Disease. *Dementia*. 2002; 1: 25–36.

Sabat S. 2005. The Self in Dementia. In: V Bengtson, P Coleman, T Kirkwood (authors) and M Johnson (ed.) *The Cambridge Handbook of Age and Ageing*. Cambridge: Cambridge University Press, 332–7.

Van Gorp B, Vercruysse T. Frames and Counter-Frames Giving Meaning to Dementia: A Framing Analysis of Media Content. *Social Science and Medicine*. 2011; 74: 1274–81.

Wartenberg T. 2011. On the Possibility of Cinematic Philosophy. In: H Carel, G Tuck (eds.) *New Takes in Film-Philosophy*. Basingstoke: Palgrave Macmillan, 9–24.

Weiss G. 1999. *Body Images: Embodiment as Intercorporeality*. London: Routledge.

Yokomizo JE, Simon SS, de Campos Bottino CM. Cognitive Screening for Dementia in Primary Care: A Systematic Review. *International Psychogeriatrics*. 2014; 26: 1783–804.

Zahavi D. 2005. *Subjectivity and Selfhood*. Cambridge, MA: The MIT Press.

Zeiler K. A Philosophical Defense of the Idea That We Can Hold Each Other in Personhood: Intercorporeal Personhood in Dementia Care. *Medicine, Health Care and Philosophy*. 2014; 17: 131–41.

Zeiler K. 2018. On the Autós of Autonomous Decision-Making: Intercorporeality, Temporality and Enacted Normativities in Transplantation Medicine. In: K Aho (ed.) *Existential Medicine. Essays on Health and Illness*. London: Rowman and Littlefield International, 81–100.

30

BODY MAPS

Reframing embodied experiences through ethnography and art

Cari Costanzo

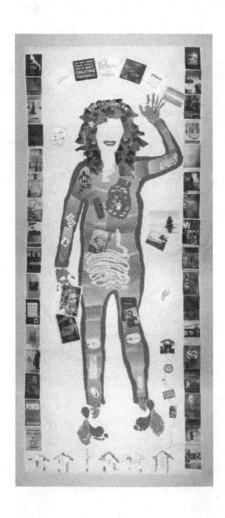

Figure 30.1 Body Map

I felt out of place during most of my college experience. The only times I actually felt like I fit in were the quarters where I went abroad, where I was living in cities that were more multicultural or had more economic diversity. I am a black female, and the colour of my skin stands out here. And on top of that, I am from a low-income family. On this campus, when I look out I see white and I see privilege. I participated in service learning programmes here as a way to find other diverse spaces, but even then the assumption was that all the students in the programme should feel a great distance from the people we served in the next town over. But I didn't feel distance. I just can't escape being physically out of place here. Ironically, when I was on the overseas programmes though . . . being an American while abroad, well suddenly that put me into a new category . . . the category of privilege myself. Here in the U.S. as a child of parents from Ethiopia, I feel like people treat me with less respect than they would if I were white. Or wealthy. Or both. But when I was studying abroad in Cape Town [South Africa], in the eyes of the people I worked with there I was 'American,' so I was seen as someone with privilege. In some ways, I felt more at ease there too. Happier. Less anxious. I don't know, I guess my body—this same body—can mean two very different things in different places: 'disadvantaged' here, and 'advantaged' there.

(Anonymous; Stanford University student—
reproduced with permission)

Introduction

Embodiment is a powerful concept. It helps us think about the ways that our lived experiences are perceived and felt, not just inside our minds, but also within our physical bodies. As the above ethnographic narrative suggests, our views about our bodies are shaped in large part by the expectations of the cultural norms established and continually reconstituted within the social, political, and economic environments in which we live (Murphy 1990; Freedman and D'Emilio 2012; Aldersey-Williams 2013; Shilling 2016; Gay 2017). In this chapter, I engage the idea of embodiment through an anthropological lens, casting light on the ways that culturally constructed norms around race, class, gender, and sexuality inform our understanding of our own bodies, sometimes disempowering or undervaluing our sense of personhood. I then propose that anthropology's critical ethnographic examination of the production and reproduction of identity hierarchies around the world allows for a richer understanding of the concept of embodiment. Finally, I close with a discussion of Body Mapping, a creative tool that has been used as a research method, a therapeutic intervention, and an instrument for community development and social change. I suggest that Body Mapping workshops create space for self-reflection and inspiration, and can be used as a tool to promote health and wellness in the workplace, schools, or communities at large. Body Mapping can also be used to help individuals reframe and reclaim the personal sense of empowerment that certain cultural and social norms threaten to strip away, especially for people whose identities exist on the margins of society. The workshops I run—guiding participants through the creation of their own 'ethnographic body map'—are designed to locate the cultural landscape(s) that both positively and negatively shape our views of our bodies, creating a space for active awareness and empowerment.

We are all embodied beings

As humans, we may make meaning out of our lives, contribute to the development of society, or earn a living through the many ideas we generate in our minds, but our minds are not simply floating around various social spheres, producing ideas or creating meaning. Likewise, when we engage in spiritual or contemplative practices, our 'souls' are not drifting about, attempting to connect to a higher consciousness. Our minds, our consciousness, our souls are all contained in a tangible vessel—the marvellous human body. In this sense, we are all 'embodied beings.'

Modern and classical philosophers alike have posed myriad questions about what it means to be an embodied being. Within the Western tradition, Plato and Aristotle in the fourth century BC examined the relationship between the body and the soul (Holmes 2017: 19; Lang 2017: 52). Later, René Descartes pushed forward the work of early Greek philosophers, focusing on the oppositional nature of the body and the mind (Strathern and Stewart 2011: 388; Peterman 2017: 215). Twentieth-century French phenomenological philosopher Merleau-Ponty argued that we cannot rely on our minds to perceive reality, and therefore the body, rather than consciousness, must be the true site of primary knowledge in the world (Merleau-Ponty 1962 [1945]). Jewish philosophers have examined the contradictory needs of the body and the soul, asking whether the human body has a determining effect on character, or whether human character has a physical expression (Meyrav 2017: 126–7).

Philosophical theories about embodiment run a wide gamut, and are of course constituted by wider intellectual, social, political, economic, and religious traditions at particular moments in history. Likewise, just as intellectual ideas evolve within specific cultural spaces and at precise historical moments, so have our ideas about the body. Our tendency, however, is to think of the entire human body as one absolute biological fact. While factual knowledge around the structure and function of the human body has expanded over time and continues to evolve at the molecular and genetic levels—leading to significant advances in science and medicine (Reich 2018)—our views about our bodies are never entirely objective; they are shaped through the lens of culture at particular moments in history (Martin 2007). And history is marked by an incessant contest for power—power to control the means of production, markets, governments, political ideals, religious narratives, cultural values, and so on.

Much of the ethnographic work within the field of anthropology highlights the fact that humans have constructed or redefined for political purposes the very categories over which power is contested. Classifications around race, gender, and sexuality, for example, have been imbued with salient political meanings that naturalise power differentials and have real, lived consequences (Omi and Winant 1986; Butler 1990; Yanagisako and Delaney 1995; Freedman and D'Emilio 2012). As American anthropologist Clifford Geertz (1973: 5) points out, "Man is suspended in webs of significance he himself has spun." In other words, there are not necessarily biological facts or inherent truths that make some groups of people or sets of ideas more powerful than others; there are only human beings—in search of power—who have decided it should be so. Sometimes brute force is used to subjugate people or to silence alternative historical narratives in an effort to maintain power differences (Trouillot 1995), while at other times cultural hegemony is used subtly and artfully to maintain control over entire classes of people (Gramsci and Buttigieg 2011; Crehan 2016). Rhetoric that situates one group of people above another group is deeply experienced in the bodies of *both* groups. Narratives around skin colour in the U.S., for example, influence where, how, and when an individual with dark skin might walk along a city street, resulting in a kind of racial embodiment (Fassin 2011: 420). This is true for individuals in the same city whose skin is white—in socio-economically advantaged areas they will experience a freedom of movement that defines a different kind of racial embodiment, one typically marked by privilege rather than surveillance. These very distinct and asymmetrical forms of racial embodiment can lead to vastly different opportunities and obstacles in life, as well as different ways of valuing the 'self.'

Sometimes we inhabit our bodies in ways that may appear to have little or no connection to discourses of domination or subjugation. For example, religious doctrine that seeks to separate the sacred from the profane (Douglas 1966) may filter down into the secular world, determining that the majority of any given population is destined to use the right hand over the left (Holder 1997; Hertz 2007: 31). There are countless examples of how our collective body memory shapes the way we physically experience the world:

> Human Bodies are similar all over the world, but their habits, postures, and comportment are to a large extent shaped by culture. Cultures preordain and suggest certain ways of sitting, standing, walking, gazing, eating, praying, hugging, washing, and so on. In so doing, they induce certain dispositions and frames of mind associated with these bodily states and behaviors: for example, attitudes of dominance and submission, approximation and distance, appreciation and devaluation, benevolence and resentment, and the like. Cultural practices, rituals, roles, and rules shape the individual's *techniques of the body*, as Mauss (1935) termed them, and the resulting way the body moves and comports itself is one of the main carriers of cultural tradition.
>
> *(Fuchs 2017: 333)*

The discipline of anthropology—and specifically the anthropology of experience—has evolved as a means of addressing conceptually the body, embodiment, and personhood, offering a holistic way of thinking about how mind, body, and experience come together to govern people's lives (Strathern and Stewart 2011: 388). The intersection of one's multiple identities—race, socioeconomic class, gender, and sexual orientation, for example—can have a profound influence on how one physically experiences life, just as the reproduction of cultural *habitus* (Bourdieu 1977) governs how individuals comport their bodies in both public and private spaces. Given the always already shifting cultural landscape in which we live, anthropology helps us understand the various ways our sense of embodiment is shaped not so much by biological truths or facts, but by mere cultural constructions. This, of course, is an empowering principle.

Embodiment and ethnography

> Embodiment is not the same as 'the body.' Embodiment refers to patterns of behavior inscribed on the body or enacted by people that find their expression in bodily form. It thus bridges over from the body as a source of perception into the realms of agency, practice, feeling, custom, the exercise of skills, performance, and in the case of rituals performativity.
>
> *(Strathern and Stewart 2011: 389)*

Anthropology—and its main research methodology, ethnography—provides a lens through which we can analyse and assess shifting cultural norms around the human body, from racial stereotypes generated during the colonial era (Stoler 1995; Burke 1996; Gupta and Ferguson 1999) to 'naturalised' gender hierarchies aimed at disempowering women (Yanagisako and Delaney 1995). Shifting cultural norms influence the way we think about every aspect of the body—from skin colour, to hair texture, body shape, age, gender, and more. Narratives around such physical characteristics directly influence our sense of embodiment and result in the creation of oppositional dyads, such as 'weak/strong,' 'normal/abnormal,' 'beautiful/ugly,' and 'exotic/familiar' (Murphy 1990; Lutz and Collins 1993; Desmond 1999).

Ethnographies that focus specifically on the cultural construction of identities, and the way various identities intersect in our lives in complex ways, give us insight into the historical roots of our own contemporary sense of embodiment, allowing us to ask such questions as:

- How are our various identities situated politically in the world, and how has that shaped the obstacles and opportunities with which we—and others with similar identities—have been met?
- How might we reflect on our 'life story,' recognising the many identities we simultaneously inhabit, and the ways we must negotiate those identities in our everyday lives?
- How does an 'anthropological lens' allow us to re-envision meaningful events from our past, ultimately empowering our future?
- How can we—each with our own unique body and embodied experiences—find deeper meaning in our identities, whether or not those identities are met with social and cultural acceptance?
- How can we heal from painful experiences rooted in the rejection or violation of our bodies or our identities?
- How can we approach human diversity and difference with greater compassion and empathy?

Reading the body

The desire to work through these questions in a meaningful way was the catalyst behind an undergraduate course I co-developed for Stanford's 'Thinking Matters' programme. All Stanford students are required to take one Thinking Matters course in their first year of study. There are 22 courses from which to choose—with provocative titles like *Rules of War, What is Love*, and *Evil*. The course I co-teach with physician and Stanford University Professor of Medicine Dr Abraham Verghese is interdisciplinary, combining themes and theories from both anthropology and medicine. Our course—*Reading the Body*—offers a tripartite approach, looking at the body as a specimen, a spectacle, and a patient (Jones 2011). In so doing, we attempt to provide students with a more nuanced lens through which to examine the ways we have come to perceive our own bodies, and the bodies of others. As viewed through the lens of medicine, the body is a text that offers clues to health and illness—in other words, we can actually 'read' the body. But even the way the body is clinically 'read' is never entirely objective; it is shaped through the lens of culture at particular moments in history. Culture therefore informs and distorts how we discern, accept, reject, and analyse our bodies. It affects the ways we experience illness, gendered and racial identities, perceptions of beauty, and our rights (or lack thereof) to control our own bodies.

Themes from the final week of the course, centring on end-of-life care, death, and the disposal of the body, can be deeply divisive subjects, but they also illustrate well the inseparability of culture from medicine. While the journey we offer through medicine, anthropology, history, art, and literature hopefully leaves students with new understandings of the human body in the context of cultural norms, we know well that lessons emerging from the medical humanities are often self-contained within academic circles—in the classroom and in publications that are consumed mostly by scholars and practitioners. Interventions are needed that allow individuals in a range of communities to reflect, reclaim, and reframe their own embodied experiences, outside of an academic or medical context. Body Mapping is one such intervention.[1]

History of Body Mapping

Body Maps—life-sized drawings or other artistic representations that result in a visual depiction of one's physical body and life experiences—have been used for thousands of years by people searching for a better understanding of their bodies and their place in the world (Solomon 2002: 2). The first published scientific study that integrated Body Mapping as part of its research methodology was a 1987 cross-cultural exploration of fertility among rural Jamaican women and women in the United Kingdom (MacCormack and Draper 1987). The use of self-drawn body maps among participants highlighted several findings, including the ways that fertility gave Jamaican women immediate adult status in their communities, as well as the fact that different levels of awareness existed in each culture around participants' understanding of their reproductive systems (MacCormack and Draper 1987). While the information obtained was highly useful to the researchers, the study was not aimed at assessing the impact of the actual Body Mapping process for participants themselves.

In 2002, however, a therapeutic Body Mapping project was launched in South Africa, proving to be a cathartic experience for women living with HIV/AIDS. Efforts to combine artistic expression with self-reflection among people living with HIV/AIDS began at the University of Cape Town—not at first with Body Mapping specifically, but rather with clinical psychologist Jonathan Morgan's Memory Box Project (Solomon 2002: 1). The goal of the Memory Box Project was to provide psychosocial support for people living with HIV/AIDS in a group therapy setting. At this time, only 25,000 of the 4.7 million people living with HIV/AIDS in South Africa had access to life-saving medications, and approximately 600 South Africans were dying of HIV/AIDS every day (Solomon 2002: 1). The Memory Box Project was a therapeutic way for women with HIV/AIDS to record their stories and provide a keepsake for their loved ones in a handmade 'memory box.' At the end of the project, participants wanted to share their stories about hope for a treatment with a wider audience, beyond the recipients of their memory boxes. This prompted art facilitator Jane Solomon to assist the group with the development of an advocacy book called *Long Life: Positive HIV Stories*. Solomon found that Body Mapping was an ideal tool to help participants tell their life stories through the lens of their felt, physical experience of living with the stigma of HIV/AIDS. Solomon's Body Mapping project not only gave public voice to participants living with HIV/AIDS, it also helped to decrease the stigma of living with HIV/AIDS, as well as bolster community efforts to advocate for anti-retroviral medication (de Jager et al. 2016).

The success of the South Africa project contributed to the growth of Body Mapping as a research tool, a therapeutic process, and force for change. As Gauntlett and Holzwarth (2006: 8) suggest,

> we need research which is able to get a full sense of how people think about their own lives and identities, and what influences them and what tools they use in that thinking, because those things are the building blocks of social change.

In 2007, a Canadian-based Body Mapping project with strong social justice roots was piloted and redefined two years later to assess the impact of social exclusion and working conditions on undocumented Latin American workers living in Toronto. Denise Gastaldo and Lilian Magalhaes used Body Mapping to explore the intersection of health, migration, gender, and other factors that influence the wellbeing of undocumented workers (Gastaldo et al. 2012: 8). Fearing deportation, participants wanted to remain anonymous throughout the research. As Gastaldo et al. (2012: 9) write,

> Body Mapping also seemed to be an ethically-appropriate method for data generation given that body maps help maintain anonymity by not exposing the individual, while at the same time making participants visible as full human beings engaged in society, by showing their hidden trajectories through art.

Body Mapping is growing as an important research methodology, and should therefore be recognised as a "knowledge translation strategy" that both produces and disseminates empirical research (de Jager et al. 2016). Body Mapping also has the power to increase inclusion and respect, and build cultures of health and wellness in the workplace, schools, and communities at large. Last year, in an effort to inspire physical and emotional wellbeing, I began a series of workshops aimed at creating personal 'ethnographic body maps.' These workshops—designed to locate the cultural landscape(s) that both positively and negatively shape our views of our bodies, creating space for active awareness and empowerment—grew into what is now a 10-week undergraduate seminar on Ethnographic Body Mapping which I teach every Winter Quarter at Stanford University.

Ethnographic Body Maps

Ethnographic Body Mapping is a creative tool that combines self-reflection with artistic expression to develop a visual 'map' of one's life story in the context of the social and cultural norms in which we live. As Jonathan Gottschall (2012: xiii) writes in *The Storytelling Animal*, "Tens of thousands of years ago, when the human mind was young and our numbers were few, we were telling one another stories." It is widely understood that we can deepen our lives through our own storytelling. Reflecting on our life experiences is a way to make sense of our past while visualising our goals for the future. And while storytelling began as an oral tradition, one could argue that cave drawings found in Australia, South Africa, France, and Spain were in fact the first attempts at a kind of pictorial storytelling, perhaps even an early form of depicting the body's lived experiences.

In the Ethnographic Body Mapping course I teach, and in the independent Body Mapping workshops I design for a range of organisations, I encourage participants to externalise and reframe bodily and emotional experiences, viewing them through an anthropological lens—a lens that casts light on the ways that cultural constructions have shaped deeply held ideas about our bodies. My goal is to help individuals reframe and reclaim the personal sense of empowerment that certain cultural and social norms can threaten to strip away. In my classes and workshops, individuals are paired so that one partner can trace an outline of the other's body onto a life-size canvas or paper, and vice versa. Guided by meditations designed to honour a person's past, present, and future, participants use paint, photos, words, collage, and other craft or materials to represent visually the central embodied experiences of their lives. Integrating contemplative practices that embrace mindfulness and self-reflection, I encourage individuals to locate the cultural landscape(s) that either positively or negatively shape their own views of their bodies. This form of Body Mapping allows participants to create their own personal, felt view of their body, while challenging any negative assumptions or stigma about identities they embrace, or conditions with which they live. Shaped by the need to develop more creative tools to enhance health and wellness, my workshops focus on "the art of stillness" (Iyer 2014)—offering a space in which one can retreat, reflect, and create.

According to the Global Wellness Institute, wellness is now a $3.7 trillion industry. Global workplace wellness specifically has grown 6.4% from 2013 to 2015, as employers responded to the health and wellness needs of a workforce that is often burned out, disillusioned, or uninspired. Such is the case in the medical profession, where physician burnout is reaching epidemic proportions (O'Rourke 2014; Shanafelt et al. 2017). I have written with colleagues elsewhere about how rituals such as the physical exam strengthen the physician–patient relationship and add meaning and joy to the practice of medicine (Verghese et al. 2011; Costanzo and Verghese 2018). Likewise, Body Mapping can be embraced as a ritual or practice that allows individuals to find deeper meaning in their lived experiences.

In *The Power of Moments: Why Certain Experiences Have Extraordinary Impact*, Chip Heath and Dan Heath argue that we must create defining moments in order to enrich our lives, connect with others, and improve experiences for customers, patients, clients, and employees. One important finding in their research within the health care industry is that health care providers cannot deliver positive experiences to patients if they are not first offering significant experiences to their own employees (Heath and Heath 2017: 206). Recognising that in order to offer valuable services, those offering such services have first to be valued themselves is an important step towards making available more tools for reflection, wellness, and inspiration across a range of industries, organisations, and workplaces. Helping people reflect upon their embodied experiences—personally, professionally, and in community—can be a healing and empowering process that imparts voice and value to all individuals.

Note

1 Many thanks to our 2017 Teaching Fellows, Dr Tara Dosumu Diener, Dr Erin Johnston, and Dr Stephen Spiess. And especially to Reading the Body Teaching Fellow Dr Risa Cromer, who developed the lesson plan and course materials to guide our undergraduates through the first iteration of an in-class Body Mapping exercise.

References

Aldersey-Williams H. 2013. *Anatomies: A Cultural History of the Human Body*. New York, NY: W.W. Norton and Company.

Bourdieu P. 1977. *Outline of a Theory of Practice*. Cambridge: Cambridge University Press.

Burke T. 1996. *Lifebuoy Men, Lux Women: Commodification, Consumption, and Cleanliness in Modern Zimbabwe*. Durham, NC: Duke University Press.

Butler, J. 1990. *Gender Trouble: Feminism and the Subversion of Identity*. New York, NY: Routledge.

Costanzo C, Verghese A. The Physical Examination as Ritual: Social Sciences and Embodiment in the Context of the Physical Examination. *Medical Clinics of North America*. 2018; 102: 425–31.

Crehan K. 2016. *Gramsci's Common Sense: Inequality and Its Narratives*. Durham, NC: Duke University Press.

de Jager A, Tewson A, Ludlow B, Boydell K. Embodied Ways of Storying the Self: A Systematic Review of Body-Mapping. *Qualitative Social Research*. 2016; 17: 22. Available at: www.qualitative-research.net/index.php/fqs/article/view/2526/3986. Last accessed: 28 March 2018.

Desmond J. 1999. *Staging Tourism: Bodies on Display from Waikiki to Sea World*. Chicago, IL: University of Chicago Press.

Douglas M. 1966. *Purity and Danger: An Analysis of Concepts of Pollution and Taboo*. London: Routledge.

Fassin D. 2011. Racialization: How to Do Races with Bodies. In: FE Mascia-Lees (ed.) *A Companion to the Anthropology of the Body and Embodiment*. Malden, MA: Wiley-Blackwell, 419–34.

Freedman E, D'Emilio J. 2012. *Intimate Matters: A History of Sexuality in America*. Chicago, IL: University of Chicago Press.

Fuchs T. 2017. Collective Body Memories. In: C Durt, T Fuchs, C Tewes (eds.) *Embodiment, Enaction, and Culture*. Cambridge, MA: MIT Press, 333–52.

Gastaldo D, Magalhães L, Carrasco C, Davy C. 2012. Body-Map Storytelling as Research. Methodological Considerations for Telling the Stories of Undocumented Workers through Body Mapping. *Facilitator Guide*. Available at: www.migrationhealth.ca/undocumented-workers-ontario/body-mapping. Last accessed: 28 March 2018.

Gauntlett D, Holzwarth P. Creative and Visual Methods for Exploring Identities. *Visual Studies*. 2006; 21: 82–91.

Gay R. 2017. *Hunger: A Memoir of (My) Body*. New York, NY: Harper Perennial.

Geertz C. 1973. *The Interpretation of Cultures*. New York, NY: Basic Books.

Gottschall J. 2012. *The Storytelling Animal*. Boston, MA: Houghton Mifflin Harcourt.

Gramsci A, Buttigieg J (eds.) 2011. *Prison Notebooks, Volumes 1–3*. New York, NY: Columbia.

Gupta A, Ferguson J. 1999. Beyond 'Culture': Space, Identity and the Politics of Difference. In: *Culture, Power, Place: Explorations in Critical Anthropology*. Durham, NC: Duke University Press, 33–51.

Heath C, Heath D. 2017. *The Power of Moments: Why Certain Experiences Have Extraordinary Impact*. New York, NY: Simon & Schuster.

Hertz R. 2007. The Pre-Eminence of the Right Hand: A Study in Religious Polarity. In: M Lock, J Farquhar (eds.) *Beyond the Body Proper: Reading the Anthropology of Material Life*, Durham, NC: Duke University Press, 30–40n.

Holder MK. 1997. Why Are More People Right-Handed? *Scientific American*. 18 August. Available at: www.scientificamerican.com/article/why-are-more-people-right. Last accessed: 28 March 2018.

Holmes B. 2017. The Body of Western Embodiment: Classical Antiquity and the Early History of a Problem. In: Smith JEH (ed.) *Embodiment, A History*. Oxford: Oxford University Press, 17–49.

Iyer P. 2014. *The Art of Stillness*. New York, NY: Simon & Shuster.

Jones N. 2011. Embodied Ethics: From the Body as Specimen and Spectacle to the Body as Patient. In: FE Mascia-Lees (ed.) *A Companion to the Anthropology of the Body and Embodiment*. Malden, MA: Wiley-Blackwell, 72–85.

Lang H. 2017. Embodied or Ensouled: Aristotle on the Relation of Soul and Body. In: JEH Smith (ed.) *Embodiment, A History*. Oxford: Oxford University Press, 51–68.

Lutz C, Collins J. 1993. *Reading National Geographic*. Chicago, IL: University of Chicago Press.

MacCormack CP, Draper A. 1987. Social and Cognitive Aspects of Female Sexuality in Jamaica. In: P Caplan (ed.) *The Cultural Construction of Sexuality*. London: Routledge, 143–65.

Martin E. 2007. The Egg and the Sperm: How Science Has Constructed A Romance Based on Stereotypical Male-Female Roles. In: M Lock, J Farquhar (eds.) *Beyond the Body Proper: Reading the Anthropology of Material Life*. Durham, NC: Duke University Press, 417–27.

Mauss M. Les techniques du corps. *Journal fur Psychologie*. 1935; 32: 271–93.

Merleau-Ponty M. (1962 [1945]). *Phenomenology of Perception* (transl. by C. Smith). London: Routledge & Kegan Paul.

Meyrav Y. 2017. Medieval Jewish Philosophers and the Human Body. In JEH Smith (ed.) *Embodiment, A History*. Oxford: Oxford University Press, 109–42.

Murphy R. 1990. *The Body Silent: The Different World of the Disabled*. New York, NY: W.W. Norton and Company.

Omi M, Winant H. 1986. *Racial Formation in the United States: From the Sixties to the Nineties*. New York, NY: Routledge.

O'Rourke M. November 2014. "Doctors Tell All—and It's Bad." In: *The Atlantic*. Available at: www.theatlantic.com/magazine/archive/2014/11/doctors-tell-all-and-its-bad/380785. Last accessed: 28 March 2018.

Peterman A. 2017. Descartes and Spinoza: Two Approaches to Embodiment. In: JEH Smith (ed.) *Embodiment, A History*. Oxford, Oxford University Press, 215–40.

Reich D. 2018. How Genetics is Changing Our Understanding of Race. In: Gray Matter, Science and Society, *The New York Times*. 23 March 2018. Available at: www.nytimes.com/2018/03/23/opinion/sunday/genetics-race.html. Last accessed: 28 March 2018.

Shanafelt T, Dyrbyr L, West C. Addressing Physician Burnout. The Way Forward. *JAMA*. 2017; 317: 901–2.

Shilling C. 2016. *The Body: A Very Short Introduction*. Oxford: Oxford University Press.

Solomon J. 2002. "Living with X": A Body Mapping Journey in the Time of HIV and AIDS. Facilitator's Guide. Psychosocial Wellbeing Series. Johannesburg: REPSSI (the Regional Psychosocial Support Initiative). Available at: http://repssi.org/index.php?option=com_content&view=article&id=46&Itemid=37. Last accessed: 28 March 2018.

Stoler AL. 1995. *Race and the Education of Desire*. Durham, NC: Duke University Press (Chapter 4: Cultivating Bourgeois Bodies and Racial Selves).

Strathern AJ, Stewart PJ. 2011. Personhood: Embodiment and Personhood. In: FE Mascia-Lees (ed.) *A Companion to the Anthropology of the Body and Embodiment*. Malden, MA: Wiley-Blackwell, 388–402.

Trouillot, M-R. 1995. *Silencing the Past: Power and the Production of History*. Boston, MA. Beacon Press, Chapters 1–2.

Verghese A, Brady E, Costanzo [Kapur] C, Horwitz R. 2011. Bedside Exam: Ritual and Reason. *Annals of Internal Medicine*. 2011; 155: 550–3.

Yanagisako S, Delaney C. 1995. Naturalizing Power. In: S Yanagisako, C Delaney (eds.) *Naturalizing Power: Essays in Feminist Cultural Analysis*. New York, NY: Routledge, 1–22.

31

PERSPECTIVES ON OLFACTION IN MEDICAL CULTURE

Crispian Neill

The value of smell in assisting medical diagnosis is a staple of medical culture, and has attracted extensive critical commentary. Laurence Totelin (in Bradley 2015: 17–29) describes the significance accorded to olfaction by classical medical practitioners such as Galen, Celsus and Dioscorides of Anazarbus. As Richard Palmer (in Bynum and Porter 2004: 67) observes, these early writers proposed an influential and enduring linkage between stenches and illness: "At the most basic level bad smells deriving from the body or its products were symptoms of disease requiring investigation." This association between malodour and illness was lent theoretical credence by treatises such as Galen's *The Olfactory Organ*. His account of olfactory sensation, although by no means universally accepted, ascribes substance to odours: "Moreover that the head is at, once made painful and made heavy when filled by strong odours and sometimes the patients are seized with delirium is a sign that some of the material itself is carried into the brain" (Wright 1924: 11). The appealing logic of this assertion—that odours admit the substance of diseases into the body—is echoed in medieval theories of olfaction and disease and their indebtedness to classical precedent. Plagues, as Constance Classen suggests, were a frequent feature of medieval Europe, and were invariably attributed to malodour: "By far the most widely accepted cause of the plague, however, was foul odour caused by putrefaction" (Classen 1994: 59). Belief in the miasma theory of disease, and its correlation of foul-smelling air and epidemics, persisted into the nineteenth century, and inspired a range of sanitary reforms, epitomised by the Public Health Act of 1848 (Noble Tesh 1996: 30).

Throughout this period, Katherine Ott suggests, the diagnostic utility of olfaction remained intact: "Skin diseases activated the diagnosticians' senses like the food that excited the patricians' senses at a Roman feast. The viscous crusts of favus, for example, smelled to high heaven. Physicians likened the odour to cat urine or mice nests" (Serlin 2010: 94). A process of olfactory training was, a nineteenth-century manual of diagnosis advised, an obligatory stage in the professional development of the aspiring clinician: "The uneducated nose may recognize the genus stink, but has no power of analysis; as it may recognize fragrance, and have no pleasure from it" (Scudder 1874: 37). The value of olfaction as an aid to assisting diagnosis remains intact in the modern era, despite innovations and improvements in hygiene, and their assumed consequent neutralising effect on bodily derived malodours. However, representations of olfactory diagnosis are elegiac, suggesting a vanishing body of experiential knowledge. As 'Smelling Out Disease' laments in 1928:

The medical profession at the present time pays little attention to the matter, and does not attempt to use the olfactory organs as it should. In this day of laboratory diagnosis, a good many of the older bedside helps have been sidetracked, and among them the use of smelling.

(Anon. 1928: 24)

Despite this apparent decline, Andrew Bomback (2006: 327), writing in 'The Physical Exam and the Sense of Smell' in 2006, stresses the continuing relevance of olfaction for clinicians:

I have come to appreciate one part of the physical exam that cannot be replaced by blood draws and x-rays [. . .] This part often doesn't make it into my official histories or daily progress notes, but its prognostic implications can be as important as those of the white-cell count or costophrenic angles. I am referring to a patient's smell.

A neglected feature of the re-education of the senses entailed by medical training is, I argue, the repression of sensory disgust inspired by malodour. The layman, *Specific Diagnosis* declares, is characterised by their non-discriminatory olfactory abilities; the odours of all diseases are designated as a general 'stink.' To the uninitiated, the olfactory signatures of a range of diseases merely smell 'to high heaven.' To publicly register such smells *as* offensive, is, however, symptomatic of unprofessionalism, regardless of their powerfully emotional effects. As Sameena Mulla (in Hamilton et al. 2017: 195–214) suggests, citing a nurse in *Sensing Law*: "If the smells ever bother you, please don't go out in the hallway to regain your composure. Be prepared, because bad smells happen." Clinicians undoubtedly encounter a range of distressing sensory experiences throughout their careers, including harrowing sights and sounds. Yet the placement of smell within Western culture suggests that olfaction possesses a visceral immediacy unmatched by rival sense modalities. The belief, *qua* Galen, that olfaction is characterised by incorporation—the smelling subject absorbs part of the source of an odour—is echoed by Kant (2006: 50):

Filth seems to arouse nausea not so much through what is repugnant to the eyes and tongue as through the stench that we presume it has. For taking something in through smell (in the lungs) is even more intimate than taking something in through the absorptive vessels of the mouth or throat.

For Kant, and for post-Enlightenment commentators on properties of olfactory experience, smell is emblematic of an unwanted intimacy occasioned by the erasure of the division between subject and object. A qualitative difference between olfactory and visual experience is pithily described by the Frankfurt School philosophers Max Horkheimer and Theodor W. Adorno: "When we see we remain who we are, when we smell we are absorbed entirely" (Horkheimer et al. 2002: 151).

However, there is an asymmetry between the affective power of (mal)odours—their immediacy and mnemonic associations—and their literary representation. An obvious and unavoidable example is Patrick Süskind's (1985) novel *Perfume: The Story of a Murderer*, and Proust's (1919–27) evocation of the recollective power of olfaction in *À la recherche du temps perdu* has been assimilated to the point where he has been credited with an eponymous psychological phenomenon—the Proust Effect (Toffolo et al. 2012: 83). Odour's lack of representation as an object of literary interest is, in part, attributable to the cultural placement of olfaction inherited from classical and Enlightenment precedents. These writers—from Plato to John

Locke—provide an influential modelling of odour based upon binary oppositions; the subordination of olfaction in relation to the 'higher' sense modalities of vision and hearing, and the categorisation of odours as either foul or fragrant. An undeniable plurality of odours is offset by an inadequate vocabulary available for their evocation, as noted by Locke (1768: 86): "The variety of smells, which are as many almost, if not more than species of bodies in the world, do most of them want names." In addition, following Kant's (2006: 50) diminution of smell as "the most ungrateful and also [. . .] the most dispensable," olfaction has been persistently classed as a primitive sense modality, a position epitomised within Freudian psychoanalytic discourse. Although Freud's pronouncements on smell are meagre—limited to an incidental feature in a number of case histories and a footnote supporting a broader argument—they are undoubtedly influential. Olfaction, proposes Freud, is a relict sense modality, transcended by the advent of civilisation, a development described in *Civilization and Its Discontents* (1930): "The diminution of olfactory stimuli seems itself to be a consequence of man's raising himself from the ground, of his assumption of an upright gait; this made his genitals, which were previously concealed, visible" (Freud 2001a: 99).

Attempts to culturally rehabilitate olfaction within the Western sensorium, demonstrated in such initiatives as the creation of the Smell Society in 1935, have foundered on the intransigence of odours (Anon. 1936: 8). Smells are difficult to describe, and, unlike visual and audial impressions, are resistant to mechanical capture, reproduction and transmission. While osphresiologists such as Joseph-Hippolyte Cloquet, Septimus Piesse, Hendrik Zwaardemaker and Hans Henning proposed taxonomies of odours which adhered to prismatic and musical models, a satisfactory classification of odours remains lacking, at least when compared with the exactitude offered by musical notes or the Pantone Matching System. Moreover, the exact operation of the sense of smell remains undetermined by science, a lacuna reiterated throughout the osphresiological literature published in the modern period and noted by Dan McKenzie (1923: 99): "To the physiologist [. . .] olfaction is the most mysterious of all the senses." All current theories of odour perception hinge upon the perception of scent molecules; stereochemical theory suggests that smell is ordained by the shape of molecules, whereas other theorists have proposed primary odours, which operate in a similar manner to the colour spectrum in vision. A radical—and contested—theory proposed by Luca Turin suggests that the vibration of odorant molecules detected by smell receptors signals odours. Even the sensitivity of the human nose in relation to the detection of odours is currently a source of debate. A previous estimate of a range of 10,000 odours is derived from research carried out in the 1920s that proposed four classes of odour: fragrant, acid, burnt and caprylic. However, more recent research has questioned the findings of Crocker and Henderson, suggesting that human olfactory acuity may be far more sensitive than previously recognised, with a suggested upper limit of one trillion olfactory stimuli (Bushdid et al. 2014).

This brief survey of the cultural categorisation of the sense of smell has important, and overlooked, implications when considered in the context of medical training, and in the maintenance of the professional identity of clinicians. The binary pairing of physician and patient is a foundational construct of medical culture, and is dependent upon the maintenance of an appropriate professional division. What, then, of a class of sensory experience which threatens to transcend this demarcation by inspiring an apparently irresistible reaction from a trainee clinician? And, interrelatedly, what of the strategies employed by medical students to surmount this difficulty, and the psychological and emotional consequences of succeeding in the repression or neutralisation of physical disgust inspired by malodour? Furthermore, if a patient is perceived as malodorous due to their medical condition—that is, productive of an unavoidable response of disgust—what implications does this have for patient care and safety? Patient testimony—literary and archival—suggests the powerfully stigmatising effects associated with malodour, or more precisely, of being a source of malodour. For example, Aleksandr Solzhenitsyn, writing in *Cancer Ward* (1969), describes the experience of Sibgatov: "because he felt ashamed of the foul smell from his back [he] chose to stay out in the hall, even though he had been in the hospital longer than all the other residents" (Solzhenitsyn 1969: 26). Sibgatov's self-disgust is echoed by the more recent account of a colostomy patient:

> I don't think I will ever get used to it. It doesn't hurt anymore—if anything I am start-ing to feel better for the first time in ages. It just smells. That's the bit I hate: it smells all the time. I can tell that other people don't like it too. Even the nurses pull faces when they change it.
>
> *(Freshwater 2003: 45)*

Despite the ostensible decoupling of odour from the transmission of disease inspired by the advent of germ theory, odour's capacity to signify the discreditable and potentially dangerous remains intact. More pertinently, the presence of personal, patient-derived malodour suggests (however unfairly) culpability. Unlike, for example, facial disfigurement, which might provoke a similarly affective response, malodour is at least notionally amenable to control or banishment through the exercise of hygiene. This stigmatisation of patient malodour is, in part, informed by the emergence of a mode of pseudo-medicalised discourse at the beginning of the twentieth century. This development—calculated to inspire social discomfort as a response to non-patho-logical yet socially discomforting conditions—was epitomised by the marketing of Listerine by Lambert Pharmacal as a cure for halitosis. The rhetoric of Listerine's advertising—'even your closest friends won't tell you'—transformed public conceptions of halitosis from a personal complaint to a medical condition, but more relevantly placed bad breath (and by extension, *all* personal malodour) under personal jurisdiction.

However illogical and undesirable this perception, its influence is acknowledged in rep-resentations of the development of the trainee clinician. To be repulsed by stenches is an understandable human reaction, but although almost irresistible, it must be transcended by the doctor, in the same way that healthcare professionals must guard against exhibiting inappropriate reactions of fear, guilt and other negative emotions. This ability to repress or screen an invol-untary response to malodour is, George Kazantzidis argues, a prevalent feature of Hippocratic medical writings:

> None of these texts mention disgust, nor do they contain the faintest hint at the dif-ficulties that a doctor is facing when, during clinical examination, he must taste for instance, the blood or bile in a sick person's vomit [. . .] the words used to indicate that something, for instance, smells bad reveal a clinical attitude that often avoids the use of charged vocabulary.
>
> *(Lateiner and Spatharas 2017: 56)*

Conversely, more recent medico-literary texts have frankly admitted the traumatic effects of olfactory experience. For example, Danielle Ofri's *What Doctors Feel* (2013) vividly describes the challenge of suppressing a negative reaction to malodour. She recounts her experience of 'the chaos of ER' as a trainee clinician, during which she is confronted with a "clearly home-less" woman, "with shaggy, matted hair and dirt-encrusted clothing of indeterminate color." Ofri's visually inspired evocation is determinedly neutral, a stance that crumbles when she draws within smelling distance: "As I drew closer, a pungent odor enveloped me, the fetid smell of an unwashed body and moldering clothes [. . .] I stood frozen, my stomach clenching to keep its contents in place" (Ofri 2013: 8–9). Despite Ofri's appeal to ideal standards of clinical behaviour—"The Hippocratic oath, the oath of Maimonides"—she is incapacitated by an overwhelming physical reaction: "my body refused to move. The revolting smell [. . .] was simply too much for me [. . .] all I could do was cringe behind the desk, gutlessly pretending to examine paperwork" (ibid.).

Given the force of this reaction—and Ofri's account does not suggest an unusual squeamishness—it is surprising that comparable olfactory episodes are relatively lacking in comparable medico-literary texts. The obligation of such texts to represent negative aspects of medical culture is a staple of the genre. Arthur Conan Doyle, for example, writing in his introduction to *Round The Red Lamp*, suggested that:

> If you deal with this life at all, however, and if you are anxious to make your doctors something more than marionettes, it is quite essential that you should paint the darker side, since it is that which is principally presented to the surgeon or physician.
>
> *(Conan Doyle 1894: iii)*

Yet despite Conan Doyle's stipulation, fictional (or fictionalised) accounts of the olfactory experiences of clinicians are outweighed by representations of the sights and sounds of hospitals and doctor/patient encounters. Such an omission is not surprising, given the foundational difficulties in describing odours outlined above—in part, this omission merely rehearses the lack of available descriptors for smells and the placement of olfaction in the Western hierarchy of the senses. After all, *qua* Wittgenstein, we may be obliged to pass over in silence that which we cannot describe. In addition, the (Western) cultural history of olfaction suggest that odour tests the politic limits of what can and cannot be represented in literary discourse. A rich history of representations of odour within medico-literary texts may be lacking because of established conventions of propriety, a tendency recognised in an early review of James Joyce's *A Portrait of the Artist as a Young Man* (1916): "You can write about what you see that you don't like, what you touch, taste and hear; but you can't write about what you smell; if you do you are accused of using nasty words" (Heap 1917: 8). Certainly, Joyce's critical designation as an exemplar of olfactory representation among literary modernists has been accompanied by the imputation that his evocations of odour are evidence of an underlying authorial paraphilia (Neill 2016: 116). This designation invites reference, again, to Freud's influential disparagement of odour, and his accompanying linkage between olfaction and sexual deviance. Commenting on the appeal of "dirty and evil-smelling feet" as fetish objects, Freud further notes: "Psycho-analysis has cleared up one of the remaining gaps in our understanding of fetishism. It has shown the importance, as regards the choice of a fetish, of a coprophilic pleasure in smelling which has disappeared owing to repression" (Freud 2001b: 155).

Freud's pathologisation of olfaction is shared by early sexologists such as Richard von Krafft-Ebing, Alfred Binet, Havelock Ellis and Iwan Bloch, all of whom identify a fascination with odour as connotative of a retreat from civilisation. As Bloch counsels, "we must regard any excessive attention to, or cultivation of, the olfactory sense today as a sort of atavism" (Bloch 2006: 264). This framing of olfaction—even allowing for the hyperbole of Bloch's pronouncement—suggests an implicit conflict between two rival understandings of olfaction, at least when viewed within the context of medicine. Olfaction is at once retrograde, suggestive of a primitive past transcended by the advent of (deodorised) Western civilisation. Yet this devaluing runs counter to the close interrelationship of medicine and olfaction described above, which advances the propriety of olfaction as a diagnostic sense modality comparable to that of vision and audition, when sanctioned by appropriate medical training and experience. That which is symptomatic of paraphilia in a layman—that is, a heightened interest in, and engagement with, bodily odours—is permissible when expressed within a professional context.

In one sense, this merely reiterates a fundamental feature of clinical practice. Healthcare professionals are, after all, routinely confronted with the body as a disordered entity, and are permitted, as a consequence of their occupation, to handle and inspect otherwise taboo areas of the body. Yet, I argue, olfactory experience not only offers a particular challenge to this kind of obligatory professional demarcation, but also tracks a shift in the representation of medicine, and indeed, in the self-representation of clinicians via such literary forms as the medical memoir and medical fiction. Improvements in hygiene have, as Liz Haggard and Sarah Hosking suggest, diminished the potency of the hospital as a source of malodours: "Modern continence products and care mean that the unwelcome urine and faecal smells should be a smell of the past, providing sensible choices are made about floor coverings and cleaning is regular and thorough" (Hosking and Haggard 1999: 166). They further argue that the modern hospital is an ideally odour-neutral space, in which even hedonic odours are absent: "Pleasant smells are difficult to introduce because the pollen of any scented plant can aggravate respiratory complaints" (ibid.).

This association of deodorisation with progress echoes the linkage proposed by Freud between the diminution of olfaction and the advance of civilisation, but also inevitably invites a further correspondence between the hospital as an orderly entity and the ideally functioning body. Disorderly hospitals and unruly bodies stink, the logic of this association suggests, a congruence that is illustrated by inquiries into the Mid Staffs hospital scandal. Patient testimonies asserts a powerful correlation between the breakdown in the administration of the hospital and the emergence of malodour:

> They put these pads on the bed to prevent the soiling of the mattress, and like we went in on visiting times, and you walked into the room, you just could not stop in the room. The smell was appalling [. . .] it became apparent that the smell was coming from one of the foot-operated metal bins that is actually in the room. And the soiled bed pads were just put in there.
>
> *(Mid Staffordshire NHS Foundation Trust Inquiry et al. 2010: 105)*

Tellingly, a further patient testimony recounts an incident in which the failure of appropriate standards of clinical care is directly identified with olfactory experience: "[two nurses] had just come out of the ward and were laughing and saying about the smell in there, and they were talking in general [. . .] they were actually taking the mickey out of the patients" (ibid.: 157). In this instance, olfactory experience exactly exemplifies an inappropriate reaction to patients— a reaction customarily screened from healthcare recipients signifies a wider disintegration of appropriate standards of professional behaviour. Even more suggestive, in light of odour's established cultural encoding as emblematic of the instinctual and irrational, is the use of olfactory terminology in further reports investigating the Mid Staffs crisis. Here, the limited repertory of adequate descriptors to evoke olfactory experience evokes that which can be recognised but resists authoritative description. As a 2013 Government response into the Independent Mid Staffs Inquiry argues, when speaking of the difficulty of assessing the culture of a hospital, "culture is easier 'to smell' than it is to measure" (Great Britain et al. 2013: 33).

The ubiquity of smell-related objections in patient accounts of the culture of Mid Staffs suggests the continuity of a rival counter narrative to idealised conceptions of the doctor, patient and hospital as unconcerned with, and unaffected by, olfactory experience. This dissident reaction to odour by clinicians finds expression, as discussed, within the context of the medical memoir, or through unguarded comments by healthcare providers—spaces in which ideal standards of professional rectitude are either interrogated, or less laudably, disregarded. If, then, the articulation of negative olfactory experience—distinct from the dispassionate assessment of odours for diagnostic purposes—represents that which cannot normally be described, what is the significance of its representation into medico-literary fiction? As noted, the evocation of malodour in literature has been constrained by shifting conceptions of propriety. Modernist representations of smell—such as those by Joyce—offer a franker, and more scatologically determined evocation, than those of literary predecessors. More recent representations of malodour in a medical context—exemplified by Danielle Ofri's *What Doctors Feel*—offer even more visceral details. However, it is appropriate to conclude by highlighting a further point of divergence between olfaction and the culturally dominant senses of vision and hearing. Olfactory experience remains unamenable to mechanical capture and transmission, unlike sight and sound, which have been mastered by a range of technologies. Cinema, television, radio, photography and text support an extension of what can be seen and heard through the application of technology, but more significantly, habituate their recipients to the artificiality of their production. By contrast, olfactory experience remains powerfully suggestive, in the early twenty-first century, of that which is *real*, or more pertinently, that which is indicative of directly lived experience. Television representations of medicine, whether categorised as drama or documentary, faithfully convey (albeit in edited, attenuated form) visual details of clinical practice and patient care, but the affective power of olfactory power remains insubmissible to technological mastery, and therefore exempt from representation in cinema, television and photography.

Conversely, although text logically cannot *be* that which it represents, literature offers a means of announcing that which remains excluded from visual and sonic representations of medical experience. Framed in this way, literary representations of olfactory experience, at least within the context of our current discussion, serve a strongly authorising function—reifying the authenticity of the text as reflective of the genuine details of medical culture, by revealing aspects of it hitherto alien and inaccessible to the layman. As discussed, these features of clinical practice include negative, transgressive emotions epitomised by impermissible reactions to malodour. For example, Jed Mercurio's *Bodies* enacts a deliberate attempt to humanise the figure of the doctor by describing the fallibilities of healthcare practitioners, as human, rather than exalted figures. A key (and persuasive) feature of Mercurio's pessimistic and revisionist evocation of hospital culture is the authorising presence of biographical details—he worked as a junior doctor prior to embracing a literary career (Chohan 2002). *Bodies* is, therefore, permeated with sensory vignettes which suggest the authenticity of experience, rather than fancy—epitomised, of course, by the agency of smell. Here, olfactory impressions serve a conventionally accepted diagnostic function, but also blur the distinction between the physician as an emotive human being, and as a sensorily disciplined professional. The narrator dispassionately notes the olfactory signature of a female patient seconds before he is assaulted by her: "The woman strides towards me and I smell alcohol and urine and vaginal secretions before she hurls a slap across my cheek" (Mercurio 2004: 97). Later, olfaction is harnessed for more directly diagnostic effect, as the narrator explains the value of smell for an uninitiated layman: "There's a strange sweet smell [. . .] You might be able to smell it. It's a substance called acetone. Sometimes it's a sign of a blood-sugar problem" (ibid.: 164) or diabetes. More revealing, however, are instances of olfactory evocation which recruit odour as a master-conceit for that which cannot be fully articulated, whether generally resistant to description, or excluded from 'appropriate' cultural conceptions of medicine. As the narrator becomes increasingly disillusioned with clinical practice, olfactory experience is mobilised to suggest that which is detectable and undesirable in medical culture, but which is screened from patients in the interest of propriety: "like dishwater dribbling from a sink [. . .] the stinking black swirl won't budge but stays there so every time you come to run water you smell it and have to look down in disgust: pressure that builds like silence" (ibid.: 124). Odour's characteristic reliance upon analogue to suggest its presence—a smell *of*, a smell *like*—is here inverted, as olfaction becomes a metaphor for the darker side of clinical practice, but tellingly is always already associated with the 'real,' and with the emotive and incommunicable, rather than the objective and rational.

References

Anon. 1928. Smelling Out Disease. 99: 24.

Anon. 1936. Smell Society's Objects. *Western Daily Press and Bristol Mirror*, 8.

Bloch I. 2006. *Odoratus Sexualis*. Whitefish, MT: Kessinger Publishing.

Bomback A. The Physical Exam and the Sense of Smell. *New England Journal of Medicine*. 2006; 354: 327–29.

Bradley M. (ed.) 2015. *Smell and the Ancient Senses*. Abingdon: Routledge.

Bushdid C, Magnasco MO, Vosshall LB, Keller A. Humans Can Discriminate More than 1 Trillion Olfactory Stimuli. *Science*. 2014; 343: 1370–72.

Bynum WF, Porter R (eds.) 2004. *Medicine and the Five Senses*. Cambridge: Cambridge University Press.

Chohan N. 'Bodies' by Jed Mercurio. *BMJ: British Medical Journal*. 2002; 324: 682.

Classen C. 1994. *Aroma: The Cultural History of Smell*. London: Routledge.

Conan Doyle A. 1894. *Round the Red Lamp: Being Facts and Fancies Of Medical Life*. New York, NY: D Appleton and Company.

Freshwater D. 2003. *Counselling Skills for Nurses, Midwives and Health Visitors*. Maidenhead: Open University Press.

Freud S. 2001a. Civilization and Its Discontents. In: *The Standard Edition of the Complete Psychological Works of Sigmund Freud*. London: Vintage; The Hogarth Press and the Institute of Psycho-Analysis.

Freud S. 2001b. *The Standard Edition of the Complete Psychological Works of Sigmund Freud*. London: Vintage; The Hogarth Press and the Institute of Psycho-Analysis.

Great Britain, Department of Health, Great Britain and Parliament 2013. *Patients First and Foremost: The Initial Government Response to the Report of the Mid Staffordshire NHS Foundation Trust Public Inquiry*. London: Stationery Office.

Hamilton S, Majury D, Moore D, et al. (eds.) 2017. *Sensing Law*. Oxford: Routledge.

Heap J. James Joyce. *The Little Review*. 1917; 3: 8–9.

Horkheimer M, Adorno TW, Noerr GS. 2002. *Dialectic of Enlightenment: Philosophical Fragments*. Stanford, CA: Stanford University Press.

Hosking S, Haggard L. 1999. *Healing the Hospital Environment: Design, Management, and Maintenance of Healthcare Premises*. London: E & FN Spon.

Kant I. 2006. *Anthropology from a Pragmatic Point of View*. Cambridge: Cambridge University Press.

Lateiner D, Spatharas DG (eds.). 2017. *The Ancient Emotion of Disgust*. New York, NY: Oxford University Press.

Locke J. 1768. *An Essay Concerning Human Understanding in Four Books*. London.

McKenzie D. 1923. *Aromatics and the Soul*. London: Heinemann.

Mercurio J. 2004. *Bodies*. London: Vintage.

Mid Staffordshire NHS Foundation Trust Inquiry, Great Britain, Parliament and House of Commons 2010. *Return to an Address of the Honourable the House of Commons dated 24 February 2010: Independent Inquiry into care provided by Mid Staffordshire NHS Foundation Trust January 2005–March 2009*. London: Stationery Office.

Mulla S. 2017. Sensing Sexual Assault: Evidencing Truth Claims in the Forensic Sensorium. In: SN Hamilton, D Majury, D Moore et al. (eds.) *Sensing Law*. Oxford: Routledge, 195–214.

Neill C. The Afflatus of Flatus: James Joyce and the Writing of Odor. *James Joyce Quarterly*. 2016; 53: 115–34.

Noble Tesh S. 1996. *Hidden Arguments: Political Ideology and Disease Prevention Policy*. New Jersey, NJ: Rutgers University Press.

Ofri D. 2013. *What Doctors Feel: How Emotions Affect the Practice of Medicine*. Boston, MA: Beacon Press.

Palmer R. 2004. In Bad Odour: Smell and Its Significance in Medicine from Antiquity to the Seventeenth Century. In: WF Bynum and R Porter (eds.) *Medicine and the Five Senses*. Cambridge: Cambridge University Press, 61–68.

Scudder JM. 1874. *Specific Diagnosis: A Study of Disease with Special Reference to the Administration of Remedies*. Cincinnati, OH: Wilstach, Baldwin & Co.

Serlin D. 2010. *Imagining Illness: Public Health and Visual Culture*. Minneapolis, MN: University of Minnesota Press.

Solzhenitsyn A. 1969. *Cancer Ward*. New York, NY: Farrar, Straus and Giroux.

Toffolo MBJ, Smeets MAM, van den Hout MA. Proust Revisited: Odours as Triggers of Aversive Memories. *Cognition & Emotion*. 2012; 26: 83–92.

Totelin L. 2015. Smell as sign and cure in ancient medicine. In: M Bradley (ed.) *Smell and the Ancient Senses*. Abingdon: Routledge, 17–29.

Wright J. The Organ of Smell. *The Laryngoscope*. 1924; 34: 1–11.

PART VI

The medical humanities in medical education

32

THE 'AWE-FULL' FASCINATION OF PATHOLOGY

Quentin Eichbaum, Leonard White,
Gwinyai Masukume, and Gil Pena

In two hands you carry yourself to doctors,
offering up the body on a metal table, a steel shelf, a plate.
You lay out the thing sick and invisible,
and they look at you like you're beautiful.
'The Paper House'

(The Anatomy Theater: Nadine Sabra Meyer)

Medical pathology as a human science

Pathology is a beautiful science. As pathologists and anatomists, we devote most of our time to looking at histological slides or cytological preparations, carefully stained with different colour dyes. Even the most aggressive and malignant cancers can present themselves as beautiful pictures under a microscope. To the pathologist, they are not abstract art, but a concrete manifestation of disease, a specific cellular disorder that in many cases can be confidently diagnosed, sometimes leading to devastating consequences for the person harbouring the pathologic diagnosis.

Working so close to death, in the living person and in the deceased body, we practise a wonderful, if not an 'awe-full,' medical specialty. How can we account for such a medical, scientific, and profoundly human enterprise that is the practice of pathology? It seems appropriate to us to respond in poetic voice (see Box below, 'The awe-full fascination of pathology'). To situate this practice, it is worth noting that pathology arose as a discipline in the morgue. We question the corpse, the nature of the disease, reconstructing the course of events from the very early inception of the disease until death. As pathologists entered the world of microscopy, they characterised the cell as the unit of life. How 'awesome/awe-full' it must have been to look at the first slides on a microscope! How to make sense of that myriad of findings, the complex multitude of different cells, awaiting discovery and understanding? Today, we look at slide specimens routinely stained in haematoxylin and eosin. But in those early days, multiple different dyes would have been tried and the pathology researcher likely had an aesthetic sensibility to choose one for a routine use. Beyond routine stains, an array of special stains has been developed with specific purposes.

Our modern understanding of the brain was founded in the late nineteenth century with the tireless efforts of one such pioneering histopathologist, Camillo Golgi, who developed his 'black reaction,' laying the foundation for the first accurate descriptions of neural circuits, their constituent nerve cells, and the bewildering array of protoplasmic processes (dendrites and axons) by which neural circuits and systems are constructed (Mazzarello 2010).

The awe-full fascination of pathology

Pieces of human beings lay on the macroscopy bench
What you deal with is the magic
To deal with the person
Bones, soft tissues, viscera, on the bench
Examine, section, sample, process, soak, embed them!
Paraffin block, candle, wax. Microtome.
Micron is the measurement of what you see.
Organelles, details, structures within the structures, cell, microcosms.
Awe.
People come to you in their tissue. Awe-full!
Observe, interpret it! Formulate diagnostic settings
Labyrinth of life, glimpsed doors
Hope always aiming to divert the last exit. Law of nature
Mirror the lives you care for
In the fragments you analyse, draw maps, chart pathways
Diagnose, do not determine
Decipher, do not designate
No judgement, no prosecution
Law of nature, always keep hope, the possibility of the unexpected
Open doors, as long as the last one does not close
The impossible, the miracle, locked in the improbable. Magic
Law of nature, to go through the last door, to go, to leave
Nobody immune or exempt
Humans, all the same, we die.

Preparation of pathologic specimens—microscopic and macroscopic—leads to images and ultimately to pictures that illustrate books, journal publications, and presentations. The more we know about a disease, the more we are able to perceive in the cases we examine (Fleck 1986). We ask the slide images questions and they give us answers. Such a perceptual apprenticeship between the pathologist and the pathologic image is largely based on the appreciation of cases, an activity pathologists frequently share with each other in case meetings and slide seminars where it is not uncommon to hear from pathologists as well as non-pathologists in the audience: 'That is a beautiful case!'

How can that be? The patient is suffering from a disease, and yet pathologists delight when looking at diagnostic images in examining the case. The disease the patient suffers from is not, however, the disease the pathologist deals with. We must contrast the disease (or, rather, illness) as a personal experience of the affected person and the disease as an object of study of the pathologist. Pathologists love morphology. And behind the pathologist's brain, one ultimately finds a dedicated heart (Bussolati 2006). Through pathologists' diagnostic interventions, it is sometimes possible to change the course of disease; the diagnosis changes the horizon of disease, opening the way to the control of disease and, in some cases, cure (Pena 2010).

Awe-full metaphors in pathology

The fascination that pathology exerts amongst its practitioners is registered in the variety of metaphors pathologists use to describe and name their diagnostic findings. The search for beauty in chaos, the search for hope in despair, the search for the familiar in the unfamiliar may be what propelled biomedical pioneers often to appreciate and name the appearances of certain diseases as images of beauty. Two centuries ago, gazing at cells under the microscope, the researcher observing a particular cancer of the immune cells, Burkitt lymphoma, must have marvelled that its microscopic appearance was reminiscent of a starry night ('starry-sky pattern'). For millennia women and men gazing at the night sky must have marvelled and pondered about the great beauty and mystery that lay yonder. Nonetheless fear of the unknown must also have coloured their sentiments. Nowadays the celestial realm still inspires immense awe—so much so that humanity envisages settling on other planets within a generation. 'The Starry Night,' a painting by Vincent Van Gogh, is the quintessential celebration of this great beauty and mystery (Andrade-Filho 2014).

An opposite perspective, the grasp of the disease plot by its destructive nature, can also be seen among pathologists, as when, hurtling through the blood stream, a detached mass of cancerous cells lodges in the lung, eventually destroying it; death ensues, like a cannon ball flying through the air and striking its target, reducing it to rubble, also creating death. It is no surprise then that these cancerous lesions in the lung, which originate from elsewhere in the body, are called *cannon ball lesions* (Agarwal et al. 2015). Each of these examples (and many more) bear metaphorical names that reflect the association of specific pathological manifestations with the human experience of the commonplace, the natural world, and even the intrusive and sometimes violent actions of human beings inflicting suffering on one another (Bleakley 2017a).

Metaphors and analogies in pathology associated with everyday living are frequently derived from food and drink—no surprise, as even pathologists eat and drink! It is interesting that such pleasant activities like eating and drinking are associated with pathology, given its Greek root *pathos* (suffering). Despite the enormous progress made in bioscience—for instance, in the form of monoclonal antibodies, robotic surgery, and telemedicine—something as primal and seemingly basic as food metaphors continues to appear in prestigious biomedical journals (see Table 32.1). Such conventions in medical nomenclature and pathological terminology would seem to reflect the grounding of phenomenological and social dimensions of cognition in the operations of biological systems for perception and action in the contingent world we share (Barsalou 2008; Masukume and Zumla 2012; Masukume 2012; Kipersztok and Masukume 2014; Bleakley 2017a). In some curious turn of hedonic aestheticism, pathologists, and perhaps other disciplines in the anatomical and health professions, seem to have a tendency to readily associate even the most horrific transformations of healthy bodily tissue with the beauty and harmony experienced and observed in the natural world. In this sense, the 'awe-full' fascination with the pathological would seem to engender a profound reflection of the human experience—even of encounters with beauty and sublimity (Burke 1757).

Table 32.1 Some food-derived medical terms

Term	Author (year)	Journal
Rice water stool—Cholera	Alexakis (2017)	*Pan African Medical Journal*
	Clemens et al. (2017)	*The Lancet*
Blueberry muffin rash—Langerhans cell histiocytosis	Schmitt et al. (2017)	*The Lancet*
Salt-and-pepper skin changes—Scleroderma	Giberson et al. (2017)	*New England Journal of Medicine*
The afternoon tea technique—Ultrasound probe stabilisation	McMenamin et al. (2017)	*Journal of the Intensive Care Society*
Strawberry gingivitis in granulomatosis with polyangiitis	Ghiasi (2017)	*New England Journal of Medicine*

Studying and celebrating the humanities in medicine enriches healers and enhances the age-old art of healing. Medicine has been compared to a war, and illness to a battle. Viruses and other pathogens are seen as enemies; the immune system, including 'soldiers' known as 'killer cells,' is a defensive system capable of destroying 'invaders.' The human body is no longer seen as 'flesh and bone,' but as a machine: 'the brain is computer' and the 'heart is a pump' (Bleakley 2017b). Cultures and practices of medicine change as new metaphors emerge, and metaphors change as new cultures and practices of medicine emerge. Which new metaphors will emerge, as we advance a humanistic culture and practice of medicine?

The meta/neurocognitive perspective

Cognitive complexity and diversity

The human brain is an organ of cosmic capacity and complexity. Nearly a hundred billion interconnected neurones (and about the same number of glial cells) communicate through trillions of synapses at speeds of a one-thousandth of a second to create an organ of stupendous individual diversity. No two brains on the planet now or at any time past are/were identical, nor are any two hemispheres from the same brain. Even the most conserved and stereotyped of all cortical convolutions, the pre- and post-central gyri, which harbour the primary somatic motor and somatic sensory cortices, can be strikingly dissimilar when the left and right hemispheres of the same brain are closely compared (White et al. 1997). We humans are all unique in our identities, personalities, perspectives, and beliefs. Appreciating this uniqueness and diversity should instil in us not only a humbling sense of awe, but also tolerance and empathy towards others.

But such complexity can also be a source of cognitive and emotional dissonance, leading to us 'being wrong,' to inherent bias, mistakes, and diagnostic errors. In short, we can get our 'wires crossed.' Perhaps it would be more consistent with modern neurobiology to assert that our brains evolved 'cross-wired,' with richly associative networks facilitating the integration of explicit and implicit processing by which we generate dynamic, flexible models of the perceived world that guide behaviour. The human brain is a fallible organ prone to misjudgement, misinterpretation, and probabilistic error. Reaching a diagnosis in pathology, as the Polish bacteriologist Ludwik Fleck noted, is a complex process involving an array of intersecting cognitive and emotional attributes rather than proceeding along a clear linear path of reasoning (Fleck 1986).

To understand how pathologists reach a diagnosis—and how we can even come to speak about an 'awe-full fascination of pathology'—demands a grasp of the intricacies of mind, or "how the mind works," as cognitive psychologist Steven Pinker (1997) puts it.

Four metacognitive lenses

In this section, we will look at this 'awe-full' mind in pathology through four metacognitive lenses—*reflection, empathy, perception*, and *attention*. Metacognition, in brief, refers to the cognitive skills of 'thinking about thinking and emotion' (Flavell 1976; Eichbaum 2014). Whether metacognition is a unique human capacity or extends also to other primates (and even non-human primates) is not fully known; but it seems likely that the ability to engage, monitor, and regulate our thinking and emotion evolved with survival advantages as we became humans living in communities.

Reflection is a form of mental processing that the mind can engage in either without specific purpose (*being reflective*), or purposefully to achieve an anticipated outcome (*reflecting*). Donald Schön, author of the seminal book *The Reflective Practitioner* (Schön 1984), coined the terms *reflection-in-action* (being reflective) and *reflection-on-action* (reflecting) to connote these modes of reflection. The pathologist looking through the microscope would appear to engage in both forms of reflection: reflection without purpose while being absorbed in looking at the image of a specimen on a slide, and purposeful reflection which may be engaged while reaching a diagnosis. The latter, purposeful, form of reflection is metacognitive in essence as it entails 'thinking about thinking (and emotion).' Metacognitive reflection may be implicated not only in deciding on an accurate medical diagnosis, but also more contemplatively in considering how this image can be at once 'beautiful,' but also may entail a 'horrific' diagnosis for the patient. Thus the pathologic image can be at once awe-full (full of awe, inspiring awe) and awful (terrible, horrific).

In neurobiological terms, this concurrent duality of awe-full and awful in the mind of the pathologist suggests conjoint modulations of competing neural networks. The brain's saliency or attentional network (see below) would be engaged by the close inspection of the histopathological, especially the visual details that support particular pathological diagnoses (Fox et al. 2005; Rosenberg et al. 2017). The so-called 'default mode network' is typically engaged when mentalising and reflecting internally (e.g., when 'mind wandering') (Fox et al. 2005; Mittner et al. 2016). Elements of this network—situated mainly on the medial face of the cerebral hemisphere and deep inside the temporal lobe—would be expected to underlie the subjective, affective, and phenomenological appraisals that inspire awe in the mind of the pathologist.

Empathy is a second metacognitive lens through which to understand the 'awe-full' mind where the spin-off of our cognitive diversity is empathy. Appreciating our 'awesome' cognitive complexity and individual uniqueness should render us more compassionate and imbue us with empathy towards one another. Science has also now determined some of the biological underpinnings of empathy—such as mirror neurons and hormones like oxytocin—that serve as the social 'glue' for our species.

For example, consider the proposed contributions of mirror neurons to social cognition. Such neurons, which are localised to the lateral aspects of the inferior frontal lobe and the junction of the temporal and inferior parietal lobes, would seem to encode the intention of movement (Rizzolatti et al. 1996; Rizzolatti and Sinigaglia 2016). Thus, a subset of neurones in these cortical regions shows increased activity—not just in preparation for the execution of particular movements, such as a visually guided reach to an object of interest or an intentional gesture—but also when the very same action is simply *observed* passively. Some mirror motor neurones show suppression of firing during action observation, even if the same neurones fire during action execution; this physiological behaviour is thought to contribute to the suppression of imitation (Rizzolatti and Sinigaglia 2016).

Taken together, these findings suggest that the mirror motor system is involved in encoding the intention to make a specific movement based on the observation of the behaviourally relevant actions of others. They are also taken to suggest that this neuronal system may contribute not just to motor control, motor learning, and mimesis, but also to more complex brain functions such as social communication, language, theory of mind, and empathy (Lamm and Majdandžić 2015). Although these ideas remain subject to active and vociferous debate, the grounding of such critical behaviours—that promote social cohesion in the operations of sensory and motor networks in the mammalian brain—has been a powerful provocateur of much productive research and theorising in cognitive neuroscience, and in fields as diverse as evolutionary anthropology, behavioural economics, literature, the performing arts, and even the practice of medicine.

For the pathologist, we would suggest that empathy is a cognitive and emotional attribute that may come into play when viewing a prepared specimen that heralds an awful diagnosis. The realisation that a beautiful slide image has a horrible diagnosis may be tinged with dissonance and guilt for the pathologist. Little in their current training helps pathologists deal with such humanistic ambiguities and uncertainties. Empathy for this pathologist may present a unique conundrum because only the inanimate glass slide as a laboratory result—and not the patient-in-person—is present for the 'empathetic' encounter. The 'ghostly' absence of the implicated patient to 'humanise' the diagnostic encounter can be 'awful' for the pathologist.

Perception: anatomic pathology is a visual discipline demanding of the pathologist accuracy in seeing and perceiving in order to reach the right diagnosis. Seeing and perceiving are, however, fraught statements from a neurocognitive perspective. A common misconception is that we 'see with our eyes.' The eye is itself little more than an organ for mediating the passage of light through the lens and a complex array of rods and cone cells in the retina before it reaches the brain for image interpretation (Ramachandran 2012). Seeing is more complex than the reduction to physiology, involving social elements, or linked brains.

Another misconception is that what we see is projected as an inverted image on the back of the retina. This is known as the *homunculus fallacy* and is false because it would entail an infinite inversion and re-inversion of the image on the retina. Understanding that 'seeing' does not create a camera-like image on the retina but instead entails an act of perceptual judgement in the brain (Purves and Lotto 2011; Ramachandran 2012) is a sobering and humbling consideration for the pathologist in trying to avoid diagnostic error. Indeed, even the retina—a relatively simple structure anatomically and physiologically—is an embryological derivative of the brain itself and therefore is involved in active construction, neural computation, and synaptic plasticity. The creation of perceptual imagery thus begins in the retina and is elaborated in more posterior divisions of the brain, with roughly half of the cerebral cortex in each hemisphere contributing to the generation of percepts that guide behaviour and become the substance of other metacognitive operations. The practice of microscopic pathology is inherently perilous from a perceptual perspective, given the critical dependence of the practice on visual analysis, entailing cognitive appraisals based on the perception of form, texture, and colour—all of which are subject to profound ambiguities relative to the transmission of photos through thin slices of stained tissue on a glass slide that in turn collide with photopigments in the back of the retina, setting in motion the complex neural reactions by which the visual brain generates imagery. Realising how fraught perception is—with the constant potential for error—the practice of pathology is, or should be, likewise an 'awe-full' experience. A second opinion from another expert immediately makes the context of judgement more complex—not additive (one brain + one brain), but multiplicative (one brain x one brain).

Attention: reaching a diagnosis in pathology in an accurate and timely manner requires the metacognitive capacity of attention. The underlying components of attention involve efficiently allocating motor and perceptual resources for spatial scanning, feature selection and object recognition (Summerfield and Egner 2016). Striking a balance between 'soft' ('wandering') and 'hard' (focused, feature-based) attention is a quality pathologists need to cultivate to remain at once open-minded and to mitigate bias, and to be efficiently focused to reach an accurate and timely diagnosis. It is not clear how the cognitive attribute of 'fascination' might mediate this balance between soft and hard attention, but again, the competing operations of saliency/attentional and default mode networks in the brain must be involved. Fascination could either effectively focus attention or distract attention if the fascination becomes too intent; in effect, the default mode network could out-compete the saliency network with the content of consciousness wandering from the object of attention. Studies have shown that radiologists who spend too much time on an image increase their error rate (Groopman 2007), but it is not understood if this is due to hyper-focused attention, or to loss of attention.

The 'awe-full' dualities of the human brain

The awe-full fascination with pathology thus begs a profound neurocognitive question that underlies who we are as human beings: how is it that we can be at once captivated/'fascinated' by the beauty of a pathologic image and by the 'horror' of the patient's grave diagnosis?

Analogously, why are we at once arguably the most empathetic of species and evidently the most destructive and violent? These uncharted dualities present a conundrum to our understanding of who we are as moral, thinking, and spiritual beings. These dualities are moreover of relevance in the practice of medicine where physicians (especially pathologists) are daily confronted with the sublime visual and cognitive 'beauty' of diagnoses and disease (e.g. a fascinating case or beautifully stained microscopic specimens) that may portend the horror of terminal illness and untimely death.

According to neuro-philosopher Heidi Ravven, the reason that we can be at once empathetic and violent is that the neuroplasticity of our brains has left them extremely flexible, and susceptible to being influenced by belief systems and interpretations (Ravven 2013). We look at the world through cognitive frames. These frames are set through the evolutionary provenance of our species, the idiosyncratic experiences that have shaped our belief systems, as well as the biologically grounded biases emanating from the depths of our limbic forebrain to which we are all susceptible. Neuroplasticity, Ravven argues, is thus both a blessing and curse. This awe-full duality must surely have biological correlates in the brain. Cognitive neuroscientists, physiologists, and psychologists are describing with ever-increasing precision the means by which emotional experience and even the origins of appraisals of beauty and sublimity are generated in body and brain (Ishizu and Zeki 2014; Kragel and LaBar 2016). The implications for our systems of general and discipline-specific ethics and for our systems of medical education are only just beginning to be explored.

Engendering awe-full fascination in medical education

In recent years, one of us (LW) has begun to consider the implications of the 'awe-full' for the education of future physicians in the early phase of medical education. In particular, we have sought to challenge medical learners with an opportunity to slow their pace of learning and explore the awe-fullness of neurological pathology through artistic visualisation and representation of human brain structure. These experiences happen as optional evening sessions (including a dinner for orientation and preliminary discussion) during a blocked, one-month-long, accelerated course on neurophysiology, clinical neuroanatomy, and the biological foundations of human behaviour in the Duke University School of Medicine ('Brain and Behavior'). Our primary goal has been simply to invite medical learners to see the human brain through their metacognitive lenses. Secondarily, our aspirational goal has been to bring learners to a place where imagination and subjectivity can engage with objectivity in the creation of visual representation of brain structure and function. Learners are encouraged to engage the human brain specimens as objects worthy of 'close reading' and re-presentation in artistic form. Media are provided for the creation of visual art, including charcoal, pastel chalks, acrylic and watercolour paints, and a variety of paper stocks.

In at least one such evening session (among 2–4 sessions) during the fast-paced month of 'Brain and Behavior,' learners are challenged to engage with the brain in more humanistic terms. Specimens from individuals who died with grossly visible pathologic alterations in the brain are examined and represented, with encouragement to reflect deeply and imaginatively on the human impact of brain injury and neurological disability. Thus, in these sessions with pathology, the brains are not merely objects of 'awe-full' fascination. They are that; but they are also the means by which learners engage the depth and meaning of human experience contextualised by pathological transformation of brain structure and function. Two representative examples of specimens (coronal slabs through the human forebrain) and artistic renderings by novice first-year medical students are presented in Figure 32.1. It is our hope that such creative encounters with the 'awe-fullness' inherent in biomedical education will contribute in some small but formative way to a deepening appreciation of the necessity of metacognitive proficiencies for the humanistic practice of medicine.

Summary

To us, and for many similar practitioners of the anatomical sciences, pathology remains a beautiful science. To engage medically, scientifically, and creatively with histopathological specimens is fundamentally a human enterprise subject to all the capacities and limitations of the practitioners. We believe that such a practice requires full recognition and deep engagement of the meta/neurocognitive lenses through which we see the specimens before us and the people afflicted with disease and injury from which samples were obtained. Nevertheless, our consideration of the 'awe-fullness' of this enterprise leaves several questions unanswered awaiting further reflection, scholarship, and investigation. While the pathologist may quietly revel in the awe-full fascination of pathology, how do such appraisals of the histopathological reshape the meta/neurocognitive lenses of the clinician? Does such meta/neurocognitive plasticity impact our understanding of human suffering and our capacity for empathy? In what ways is the experience of the awe-full distinguished in the minds of expert pathologists in comparison to the minds of novice observers, such as medical learners? How will emergent technologies, the globalisation of medical practice, and the advance of a humanistic culture in the practice of medicine birth new metaphors for understanding health, wellness, and the medical armamentarium for combatting disease?

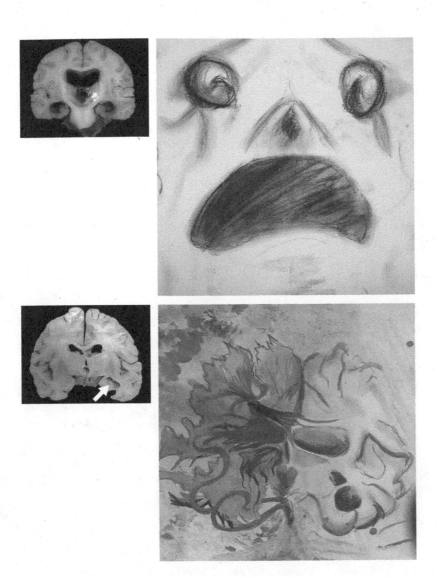

Figure 32.1 Creative representations of 'awe–full' neuropathology by first-year medical students. During a course on 'Brain and Behavior' in a first-year medical school curriculum, students interacted with human brain specimens from individuals who died with visible pathological conditions. In the upper row, a student created a charcoal sketch of the coronal slab shown (upper left). The student reflected upon the presumed suffering of the individual who experienced a haemorrhagic stroke and represented the slab in an inverted orientation with the enlarged, blood-filled ventricles drawn to resemble a human face (recalling the famous 1893 painting, 'The Scream,' by the Norwegian expressionist, Edvard Munch). In the lower row, a student represented the coronal slab shown (lower left), which lacks the left amygdala (white arrow) explained presumably by a past focal stroke. The student's illustration in water colour of this slab itself represents a duality, with the right side of the illustration representing the slab as a visual object and the left side evoking a more fanciful representation of living life without an amygdala—a brain structure that serves to detect threat and increase vigilance.
[Upper illustration courtesy of Raeann Whitney; lower illustration courtesy of Rebecca Fabbro; photographs of brain slabs courtesy of Leonard White]

References

Agarwal R, Mukhopadhyay J, Lahiri D, et al. Cannon-ball pulmonary metastases as a presenting feature of stomach cancer. *Lung India: Official Organ of Indian Chest Society.* 2015; 32: 300–2.

Alexakis LC. Cholera: 'Rice water stools.' *The Pan African Medical Journal.* 2017; 26: 147.

Andrade-Filho Jde S. Analogies in medicine: Starry-sky appearance. *Revista do Instituto de Medicina Tropical de Sao Paulo.* 2014; 56: 541–2.

Barsalou LW. Grounded cognition. *Annual Review of Psychology.* 2008; 59: 617–45.

Bleakley A. 2017a. Functions of resemblances in medicine: 'Food for thought'. Chapter in: *Thinking with Metaphors in Medicine: The State of the Art.* Abingdon: Routledge.

Bleakley A. 2017b. 'Medicine as war' and other didactic metaphors. Chapter in: *Thinking with Metaphors in Medicine: The State of the Art.* Abingdon: Routledge.

Burke E. 1757. *A Philosophical Enquiry into the Origin of Our Ideas of the Sublime and Beautiful.* London: Dodsley.

Bussolati G. Dissecting the pathologist's brain: Mental processes that lead to pathological diagnoses. *Virchows Archiv.* 2006; 448: 739–43.

Clemens JD, Nair GB, Ahmed T, et al. Cholera. *Lancet.* 2017; 390: 1539–49.

Eichbaum QG. Thinking about thinking and emotion: The metacognitive approach to the medical humanities that integrates the basic and clinical sciences. *The Permanente Journal.* 2014; 18: 64–75.

Flavell JH. 1976. Metacognitive aspects of problem solving. In: LB Resnick (ed.) *The Nature of Intelligence.* Hillsdale, NJ: Lawrence Erlbaum, 231–5.

Fleck L. 1986. To look, to see, to know [1947]. In: RS Cohen, T Schnelle (eds.) *Cognition and Fact: Materials on Ludwik Fleck.* Dordrecht: Reidel, 129–51.

Fox MD, Snyder AZ, Vincent JL, et al. The human brain is intrinsically organized into dynamic, anticor-related function networks. *Proceedings of the National Academy of Sciences, USA.* 2005; 102: 9673–8.

Ghiasi M. Strawberry gingivitis in granulomatosis with polyangiitis. *The New England Journal of Medicine.* 2017; 377: 2073.

Giberson M, Brassard A. Salt-and-pepper skin changes. *The New England Journal of Medicine.* 2017; 377: 173.

Groopman J. 2007. *How Doctors Think.* Boston, MA: Houghton Mifflin.

Ishizu T, Zeki S. A neurobiological inquiry into the origins of our experience of the sublime and beautiful. *Frontiers in Human Neuroscience.* 2014; 8: Article 891.

Kipersztok L, Masukume G. Food for thought: Palatable eponyms from pediatrics. *Malta Medical Journal.* 2014; 26: 46–50.

Kragel PA, LaBar KS. Decoding the nature of emotion in the brain. *Trends in Cognitive Sciences.* 2016; 20: 444–55.

Lamm C, Majdandžić J. The role of shared neural activations, mirror neurons, and morality in empathy: A critical comment. *Neuroscience Research.* 2015; 90: 15–24.

Masukume G. Food for thought. *Croatian Medical Journal.* 2012; 53: 77–9.

Masukume G, Zumla A. Analogies and metaphors in clinical medicine. *Clinical Medicine (London).* 2012; 12: 55–6.

Mazzarello P. 2010. *Golgi: A Biography of the Founder of Modern Neuroscience.* New York, NY: Oxford University Press.

McMenamin L, Wolstenhulme S, Hunt M, et al. Ultrasound probe grip: The afternoon tea technique. *Journal of the Intensive Care Society.* 2017; 18: 258–60.

Meyer NA. 2006. *The Anatomy Theater.* New York, NY: Harper Collins.

Mittner M, Hawkins GE, Boekel W, Forstmann BU. A neural model of mind wandering. *Trends in Cognitive Sciences.* 2016; 20: 570–78.

Pena GP. O relato de caso como situação gnosiológica: reflexões sobre a prática diagnóstica em patologia a partir de um caso de abetalipoproteinemia. *Revista Brasileira de Educação Médica.* 2010; 34: 622–6.

Pinker S. 1997. *How the Mind Works.* New York, NY: WW Norton & Co.

Purves D. Lotto RB. 2011. *Why We See What We Do Redux: A Wholly Empirical Theory of Vision.* Sunderland, MA: Sinauer Assoc., Inc.

Ramachandran VS. 2012. *The Tell-Tale Brain: A Neuroscientist's Quest for What Makes Us Human.* New York, NY: WW Norton & Co.

Ravven H. 2013. *The Self Beyond Itself: An Alternative History of Ethics, the New Brain Sciences, and the Myth of Free Will.* New York, NY: The New Press.

Rizzolatti G, Sinigaglia C. The mirror mechanism: A basic principle of brain function. *Nature Reviews Neuroscience*. 2016; 17: 757–65.

Rizzolatti G, Fadiga L, Gallese V, Fogassi L. Premotor cortex and the recognition of motor actions. *Cognitive Brain Research*. 1996; 3; 131–41.

Rosenberg MD, Finn ES, Scheinost D, et al. Characterizing attention with predictive network models. *Trends in Cognitive Sciences*, 2017; 21: 290–302.

Schmitt AR, Wetter DA, Camilleri MJ, et al. Langerhans cell histiocytosis presenting as a blueberry muffin rash. *Lancet*. 2017; 390: 155.

Schön DA. 1984. *The Reflective Practitioner: How Professionals Think in Action*. New York, NY: Basic Books.

Summerfield C, Egner,T. Feature-based attention and feature-based expectation. *Trends in Cognitive Sciences*. 2016; 20: 401–4.

White LE, Andrews TJ, Hulette C, et al. Structure of the human sensorimotor system. I: Morphology and cytoarchitecture of the central sulcus. *Cerebral Cortex*. 1997; 7: 18–30.

33

BIOMEDICAL ETHICS AND THE MEDICAL HUMANITIES

Sensing the aesthetic

Paul Macneill

Introduction

Biomedical ethics and the medical humanities are fields of study and practice with both conventional and competing approaches. In this chapter, I bracket and critically appraise conventional approaches to biomedical ethics and the medical humanities. I then consider more radical accounts and look for commonalities between two of those more radical approaches. Commonly accepted understandings of biomedical ethics and the medical humanities could be seen as sedimented—'settled' as usual understandings. To extend the metaphor, further up the cliff face is a second stratum comprising more unusual crystallisations of ethics and the humanities, some of which are still under study and have yet to gain wide acceptance. Of those more radical accounts, I am particularly interested in representations of biomedical ethics and the medical humanities as aesthetic practices.

My focus is on understanding a productive relationship between the medical humanities and biomedical ethics. How that relationship is developed depends upon what we understand by both the 'medical humanities' and 'biomedical ethics.' Conventional accounts in both fields merely offer add-ons to 'business-as-usual.' They may assist in augmenting healthcare education and delivery, but only to a limited extent. Medical education and healthcare are predominantly hierarchical institutions with allegiances to scientific 'objectivity' as a 'biomedical model' that currently shapes much of medical education and practice. Neither biomedical ethics nor the medical humanities fit comfortably in such a conservative configuration, nor are they well translated into healthcare practices.

The two radical approaches considered below are explorations of biomedical ethics and the medical humanities as *aesthetic* practices. The word 'aesthetic,' in its original sense, refers to the experiences of sensing and feeling. This offers a broader political challenge to understandings of healthcare itself, and to practices within healthcare and healthcare education. The value of these more provocative accounts is that each of them could reframe healthcare with a potential to change practices in ways that would be beneficial to participants in the healthcare industry, including patients and staff at all levels. A further benefit of a reframing of this kind is that biomedical ethics and the medical humanities would have more in common with one another.

Biomedical ethics and medical humanities understood conventionally

The conventional view of biomedical ethics is normative. Most commentators identify widely held values and apply these as principles of biomedical ethics to particular ethical problems in healthcare—an approach typified by 'principlism.' Such principles are drawn from a broad consensus of values, applied through reason to particular circumstances. Kagan (2018: 2) describes *normative ethics* as involving "substantive proposals concerning how to act, how to live, or what kind of person to be . . . and attempts to state and defend the most basic principles governing these matters." For example, reasoning from the importance of individuality and autonomy—values supported by a broad consensus—defends the proposal that 'healthcare workers should respect patients' rights to decide for themselves.' What is missing from this normative account is recognition of a *purpose* for ethics. In this postmodern age, talk of purpose and ultimate ends is much denigrated. Nevertheless, I contend that there is something more than 'normative ethics.' In health practice and in bioethics, we are aiming for some-*thing*—which of course is not a 'thing.' The Greeks called it *telos*. The OED defines *telos* as "end, purpose, ultimate object or aim." Defined in that way, as "an achievable finished state, an end point," *telos* is eminently suspect as it promises closure in open-ended, complex processes (Bleakley 2018). I propose, however, that *telos* is not an end point but indeed a process—one of *reaching for an ideal*, a verb rather than a noun. Although we may glimpse the goal we are striving for, we may not be able to specify it—at least in words. It is aiming for an 'horizon.'

A conventional account of biomedical ethics is provided by Hedgecoe (2004: 122) who includes those discourses and practices that fall within 'medical ethics,' 'clinical ethics,' 'research ethics,' and 'bioethics.' I also accept Green's (1990) descriptive account of

> both medical ethics and the somewhat broader field of 'bioethics' [as involving] the self-critical application of modes of moral reasoning, in the form of ethical theory or fundamental moral principles, to the new range of questions raised by the biomedical sciences.

Although Green himself criticises this approach for its lack of "strenuous moral analysis . . . and its disturbing tendency to pass over difficult but vital questions," his description is nevertheless apt. I have been critical of such an emphasis on moral reasoning (Macneill 2017, 2010). While accepting that reason is a good thing, "it becomes a problem when bioethics is founded primarily on reason, and rational justification is its *raison d'être*" (ibid.). Others (e.g. Murray 2007) have expressed similar concerns about 'medical ethics' constructed on the basis of what Hoffmaster (1994) describes as "a rationally justified system of norms."

Yet, teaching biomedical ethics, at least in all three medical schools where I've been on staff, typically fits Green's (1990) account in its focus on *moral reasoning* based on a system of norms. Teaching ethics is invariably accompanied by teaching of some health law—another normative discipline relying primarily on reason. Ethics and law are applied to a range of issues in medicine and healthcare, many of which arise from new biomedical technologies, commonly as a juridical approach to ethics that focuses on achieving normative standards rather than aiming for an ideal (Hope et al. 2008; Tsai and Harasym 2010; Page 2012; Kerridge et al. 2013; Gillam et al. 2014). It is a view of biomedical ethics that is ubiquitous, represented by Beauchamp and Childress's (2013) influential *Principles of Biomedical Ethics*—now in its seventh edition.

Having made a claim for its hegemony, however, I also acknowledge that biomedical ethics is a contested field both conceptually and in terms of how it could be taught and practised.

To some extent, these contestations affirm the predominant view.[1] Here, I challenge the hegemony of biomedical ethics as a normative, consensual approach. One ground for challenge is that consensus marginalises dissenting voices, resulting in negative repercussions—both theoretical and practical.

The medical humanities

A conventional definition of the medical humanities is that they comprise an interdisciplinary field in which the arts, humanities, and aspects of the social sciences are applied to healthcare education and practice. A common justification for doing so is that the medical humanities broaden the education of healthcare workers, for example by encouraging medical students to read novels relating to healthcare, or to study the history of medicine, on the assumption that these exposures 'humanise' students and trainees as a counterbalance to the predominant biomedical model. These justifications amount to supporting medicine to achieve its own humanistic goals. Warner (2011) observes that influential physicians, including Sir William Osler, advanced arguments for the medical humanities, "precisely [at] the moment when modern biomedicine became ascendant." The assumption that the medical humanities were capable of 'humanising' medical students and countering the reductionist tendencies of medical education provided arguments to sustain claims for space for the humanities in medical schools' curricula (and subsequently the curricula of nursing and allied health schools).

Having gained some traction, the medical humanities are anxious not to rock the boat, as they maintain a benign and servile relation to medicine and the health professions (Macneill 2011). This is an approach typified by the early views of Downie and Macnaughton (2007) where the medical humanities afford a valuable supplement to healthcare education. It is, however, a weak justification that leaves the medical humanities as an 'optional extra'—a charge which Downie and Macnaughton appear to have accepted (Bustillos 2009). Of more concern is that the value of any supplementary role is brought into question by Warner's (2011) historical (and critical) account of the way in which the medical humanities were promoted from the end of the 19th century as a means for attaining the "ideal of the 'gentleman-physician' well versed in the classic liberal arts."

Alan Bleakley (2015: 40) has characterised this conventional approach as the 'first wave' of the medical humanities which he terms "naïve and celebratory." Bleakley is dismissive of this 'first wave,' describing it as "characteristically 'lite' educationally—a supplement within the curriculum, as optional learning, as light relief from biomedical science and even conceived as 'edutainment'" (ibid.: 47). Unsurprisingly, the 'second wave' of the medical humanities is more critical and reflexive (ibid.: 40).

Commonalities between biomedical ethics and medical humanities understood conventionally

Even as conventionally understood, however, there are commonalities between biomedical ethics and the medical humanities. Both accounts are typically normative in that they identify predominant values: for example, autonomy in biomedical ethics, and the 'humanising' value of medical humanities. The assumption in biomedical ethics is that medical students *should be* more ethically informed and aware; and, in the medical humanities, that they *should be* 'humanised,' as paradoxical imperatives. Of more significance is the claim that the humanities have a capacity to achieve ethical goals: such as broadening students' understanding of moral issues, and the contexts in which they arise. There is a certain 'face validity' in this assumption. Many novels do in fact raise concerns of an ethical kind—and so literature is an obvious resource within the humanities to look for overlap with ethics.

Biomedical ethics and the medical humanities are both construed as 'patient-centred' and focused on 'the person.' In ethics, there has been an emphasis on the patient *as a person*, in opposition to the 'medical gaze' on disease and symptoms. The medical humanities are seen as a means for reinforcing and giving persuasive power to the experience of patients—whether through novels such as *Faces in the Water*—a fictionalised account by Janet Frame of her incarceration in a mental hospital; or in movies such as *The Doctor* (played by William Hurt) in which trainees were ordered by him to change into pyjamas and undergo medical tests typically suffered by patients. Those are just two of many possible choices from literature (Nussbaum 1990; John and Lopes 2004) and film (Colt et al. 2011; Teays 2012) that provide relevant narrative accounts of patients' experiences in medical treatment and give a human experiential dimension to abstract ethical issues.

Biomedical ethics and the medical humanities are both regarded as 'soft' in relation to the 'hard' medical sciences and clinical training. In a large measure this is because of priorities within medical schools that are shared by both staff and students. Students can be failed, and ejected from the course, for not meeting knowledge standards in biomedical science subjects, and for identified inadequacies in clinical assessments. Conversely, few medical schools are willing to eject students for failures in biomedical ethics or in medical humanities courses (in the rare cases where medical humanities are formally assessed). My experience, in examination committees in medical schools in which I have been on faculty, is that most staff from medical sciences and clinical courses are comfortable with failing students and requiring them to repeat a year, but very reluctant to require the same of a student who is failing badly in biomedical ethics.[2]

The assumption that teaching medical, nursing, and allied health students in this manner is effective can, however, be questioned on a number of different grounds. One critique derives from consistent findings of a decrease in empathy in medical students and medical trainees as they progress. Bleakley (2015: 78–99) provides a rich commentary on these studies, and criticises the 'empathy scales' on which these studies rely. Nevertheless, to the extent that there is a decrease in empathy, it indicates systemic problems in medical education. Conventional approaches to biomedical ethics or the medical humanities do not overcome such systemic issues but may be seen to add to them.

This concern about systemic failures is supported by a growing recognition of 'the hidden curriculum' in medicine—a term which indicates how a curriculum can be subverted by what occurs 'on the wards.' This amounts to what people *do*, rather than what they *say*. The term is attributed to Hafferty and Franks (1994). In their 1994 paper about the teaching of medical ethics, the authors also advanced the broader idea that "the critical determinants of physician identity operate not within the formal curriculum but in a more subtle, less officially recognized 'hidden curriculum.'" They went on to characterise the "overall process of medical education" as "a form of moral training of which formal instruction in ethics constitutes only one small piece." Their point was to "acknowledge the broader cultural milieu within which [a] curriculum must function." In his Report on medical professionalism, 'A Flag in the Wind,' Inui (2003, emphasis in the original) assessed Hafferty's (and others') writing on 'the hidden curriculum' and came to the alarming conclusion that in "noting the difference between what we *say* and what we *do*, students learn that medicine *is* a profession in which you say one thing and do another, a profession of cynics."

Another ground for questioning the assumptions inherent in teaching biomedical ethics and the medical humanities in the conventional manner is that proponents for both approaches have emphasised the importance of these subjects as providing knowledge needed by healthcare trainees. This inevitably places these subjects in a doomed competitive relationship with the biomedical sciences and clinical knowledge. What is missed, in characterising biomedical ethics and the medical humanities as 'necessary knowledge,' is a recognition that they are constituted by different kinds of knowledge. As far back as 1945, philosopher Gilbert Ryle (1946 [1971]) proposed distinct kinds of knowledge in terms of 'knowing how' and 'knowing that,' where: "knowledge-how cannot be defined in terms of knowledge-that and further, that knowledge-how is a concept logically prior to the concept of knowledge-that" (Ryle 1945). More recent commentary proposes that 'knowing how' emphasises practical application, but that these two kinds of knowledge work together rather than in opposition (Fantl 2017). The distinction remains useful and important, yet continues to be overlooked.

The difficulty with emphasising '*knowing that*'—defined in terms of factual and propositional knowledge—is that biomedical ethics and the medical humanities then have to compete with claims of importance of biomedical science and clinical knowledge (as discussed above). This leads to ethics and the humanities being marginalised by placing them early in degree courses and characterising them as 'pre-clinical.' If ethics and the humanities were to be reconstrued as '*knowing how*,' this would shift the emphasis to practical application and to the importance of relating *with* patients in both an ethical and richly informed manner. Those qualities are more readily perceived as relevant in clinical practice.

A further ground for questioning the assumptions inherent in teaching biomedical ethics and the medical humanities in the conventional manner is that—given the assumptions discussed above, and the apparent disdain towards subjects conceived by clinicians as 'soft'—students (understandably) identify with the attitudes of the members of the profession they seek to join. What is needed is a different approach that demonstrates the relevance of ethics and the medical humanities in relating to patients.

Another concern relates particularly to ethics. Conventional biomedical ethics is normative (as discussed above). However, 'normative' has two senses: as 'prescriptive' and as "derived from a norm" (OED). By definition, *norms* have their basis in *consensus*. The difficulty that arises is that consensus is attained by ignoring or placating dissenting voices. This leads to a number of other difficulties, both in theory and in practice. Normative ethics has difficulty in respond-ing effectively to conflicting views and resolving them because it is based on a 'predominant' norm.[3] To give a specific example, when teaching biomedical ethics in the National University of Singapore Medical School, I became aware that Singaporean clinicians typically withheld information about serious conditions from their patients. Withholding information about a seri-ous condition from (say) an elderly parent is regarded as appropriate in many Chinese-Malay families (who are in the majority in the Singaporean population). This is a view that is supported by patients themselves. Quite understandably, clinicians were reluctant to challenge this cultural norm. Yet this is in opposition to Western biomedical principles of ethics that give priority to autonomy and the patient's 'right to know'—the principle we were innocently teaching Singaporean medical students and trainee doctors.[4]

An alternative, and (in my view) healthier, approach is offered by Jacques Rancière (Rancière and Corcoran 2010), who recognises that ethics is a *political* process (one of power differentials) in which differing values are in tension within communities. Indeed, communities are constituted by those with differing views. Recognising this reality, and respecting tensions between these views, is to give value to 'dissensus.' However, presenting a community in terms of *consensus* is an abstraction that denies that political reality, and excludes those with differ-ing views. As Rancière and Corcoran (2010: 188) expresses this idea: "consensus . . . defines a mode of symbolic structuration of the community that evacuates the political core constituting it, namely dissensus." In other words, the process of identifying 'consensus' (which is implicit in normative ethics) obviates dissenting voices and so conceals (or evacuates) the political nature of ethics. This analysis presents an inescapable challenge to the conventional approach to biomedical ethics.

A similar issue is apparent within the medical humanities in which the conventional approach is criticised by Hooker and Noonan (2011: 79) as predominantly "expressive of Western cultural values." They propose that the medical humanities need "to reflect . . . cultural diversification" and "come to celebrate and question culture, and difference." To do so is to "foster productive encounters with cultural difference by practical and inclusive measures," acknowledging a political dimension within the medical humanities also, and celebrating 'dissensus.' As with biomedical ethics, accepting cultural diversity is a challenge to conventional approaches to the medical humanities with their foundations in predominantly Western cultural values and Western canonical works of art and literature.

Biomedical ethics and medical humanities understood as aesthetic practices

I am particularly interested in representations of biomedical ethics and the medical humanities as aesthetic practices: as being about sensing and feeling. In part this relates to Ryle's distinction between 'knowing how' and 'knowing that,' discussed above. 'Knowing how,' in this context, is to know how biomedical ethics and the medical humanities can contribute to healthcare practice. An aesthetic approach to both biomedical ethics and to the medical humanities draws on 'knowing how' in supporting healthcare practised with qualitative discrimination and sensitivity.

Aesthetics

'Aesthetics' has a convoluted history. It was brought back into currency in the 18th century by Baumgarten to mean: "things perceived by the aesthetic understanding." Immanuel Kant took this further, describing a "science dealing with the principles of perception by the senses." These days (according to the OED) the word is most often used to mean "philosophy of the beautiful or of art."[5] However, I am not using the word 'aesthetic' in any of the senses above. Rather, I want to return aesthetics to its original meaning.

'Aesthetic' can be traced back to the ancient Greek αἰσθητικός (*aisthitikos*) meaning 'sense perception,' and has its root in the verb 'to perceive.' If we track far enough back to Sanskrit *āviš* it has the sense of 'manifestly;' and, in another form—through Old Church Slavonic *avě*—it means 'openly' (OED). These meanings are fully conveyed by noting its opposite: *anaesthetic*. When we are anaesthetised, we are unconscious. An *aesthetic* response is to be *fully conscious* and *perceptually aware*, a state of mind in which we are open to manifest sensory and perceptual experience.

Both medical ethics and medical humanities find their commonality at this deeper level: at a level of sensory perception and openness to experience—hard to specify because it is *not primarily* cognitive. It is an *appreciation* of something felt and sensed. In claiming that biomedical ethics includes the aesthetic, I am attending to the relevance of perception (as sensory awareness), emotion, and feeling in ethical healthcare practice. Similarly, in highlighting the aesthetic in the medical humanities, I am drawing attention to the capacity of the humanities and the arts (both in appreciating the arts and in participating in the arts) to open us to an aesthetic—that is, sensory and felt—experience.

Biomedical ethics as an aesthetic

In a previous publication, I argued that bioethics would be more balanced, in theory and in practice, if it gave greater weight to the aesthetic (Macneill 2017). The aesthetic was defined in terms of sensory perception, emotion, and feeling, elaborated as a *non-cognitive capacity*. Taken together, these three aspects comprise aesthetic sensitivity and responsiveness. 'Perception,' 'emotion,' and 'feeling' have many different meanings. In defining 'perception' I draw on a distinction that David Hume (1888/2000) made between "impressions arising from sensation" and "impressions as ideas arising from reflexion" (Jeffery 2014: 80). I follow Hume in "focussing on perceptions 'as they make their first appearance' in consciousness; and in distinguishing perception from abstract ideas, thinking, and reasoning as such" (Macneill 2017). In relation to 'emotion,' I am aware of the debate in the literature that emotion comprises both cognitive and affective components (Jeffery 2014: 126). However, I take 'emotion' to be primarily a somatic response (a movement of energy—literally *e-motion*) that is, for most of us, an important signifier "of an emotion as distinct from thoughts pure and simple" (Macneill 2017). This is emotion in the sense of a visceral experience.

I also distinguish *emotion* from *feeling* along a line that separates between the "calm and the violent" impressions as Hume refers to them (Hume 1888: 276). The 'violent impressions,' or 'the passions,' include hatred, envy, jealousy, fear, guilt, disgust, and grief—and could well include surprise, and outbreaks of joy and happiness. These are emotions (and *e-motive*) in their corporeal immediacy and power. They have what Nussbaum (2001: 64) refers to as "tumult or arousal."

The calm impressions are experienced quite differently. They are much less tumultuous. Feelings include contentment, joy, sadness, remorse, love, and gratitude. I am not proposing a hard and fast line between emotions and feelings but, rather, a distinction between the immediacy and upheaval of a passionate somatic response (on the one hand), and the quietude of a reflective feeling (on the other). This experiential distinction between emotion and feeling is also supported by neurological findings indicating that different areas of our cortex and hormonal systems are activated by emotions as distinguished from feelings (Damásio 1994, 2003; Macneill 2017). More importantly, there is a practical reason for distinguishing between them. When I am 'in the grip' of a tumultuous emotion, there may be little I can do, other than recognise the experience, sit with it, and allow the emotion to pass. Feelings, however, can more readily provide insight and constructive solutions. Gillam et al. (2014) claim that emotions can potentially "enhance ethical decision-making." That is even more true of feelings as distinct from an overpowering emotion. Feelings may not provide a sufficient guide on their own, but the insight we gain from them has the potential to enhance our ethical understanding and responsiveness.

These aesthetic qualities are always in play and influential, although not always recognised (Macneill 2017). Sensory perceptions, emotive responses, and feelings are constants in interactions between people, including between healthcare professionals and their patients. Furthermore, these are 'in play' in an ethical sense. For example, when a healthcare professional does something well (or badly), we have both an aesthetic response and may, quite separately, make a cognitive judgement about the ethics of what was done. Biomedical ethics has focused on the latter and has given little attention to our aesthetic responsiveness. Whilst this aesthetic dimension may not be easily specified, my contention is that biomedical ethics is given depth and purpose when the aesthetic dimension is acknowledged. Indeed, neurologist Damásio (2003: 159–60) argues that the capacity to discriminate between good and bad depends on emotion and feeling. This capacity is especially relevant to ethics, given that ethics is primarily about doing good and avoiding harm.

One of the justifications for arguing that bioethics should be balanced 'by sensing the aesthetic' is that bioethics inextricably relies on aesthetic distinctions. This is to appeal to one of Bleakley's (2006) aspects of 'aesthetic medicine' that he terms *sensibility*, and defines as "close noticing." Noticing means paying close attention to actual circumstances. This could mean, for example, paying close attention to an individual's symptoms, as well as to her posture and facial expressions, idiosyncratic needs, and desires. It allows the possibility of adjusting clinical protocols to better serve that person. A recognition that human beings are capable of these qualitative discriminations, and that this capacity potentially adds depth and understanding to ethically relevant situations within healthcare, supports my case for 'balancing bioethics by sensing the aesthetic.'

The medical humanities as an aesthetic

Bleakley (2015) proposes "an aesthetic challenge" to the culture of medicine. He claims that "sensibility and sensitivity" should be developed in trainees, as opposed to current medical education that fosters "a kind of numbing or insensitivity" (ibid.: 5). Bleakley, Marshall, and Brömer (2006: 197) define "sensibility and sensitivity" as the elements of "aesthetic medicine" and elaborate them in terms of "three main foci":

> first, fine or discriminatory use of the senses, as close noticing in diagnosis and prognosis; second, as bodily discourse in learning varieties of the clinical gaze, where the conditions of possibility for expert use of the senses in diagnostic judgement are established; and third, as sensitivity towards both patients and colleagues (another kind of noticing) where aesthetic medicine is practised ethically and configured as a narrative activity.

'Sensibility and sensitivity' also link biomedical ethics and aesthetics in that Bleakley et al. (ibid.) regard 'sensitivity' as essential to biomedical ethics and related to 'sensibility' as an aesthetic quality.

Bleakley (2015: 33) introduces and champions "the development of the 'critical' medical humanities in medical education" as a political challenge to the forces which lead to "numbing and insensitivity" in medical trainees. Medical humanities, as conventionally understood ('first wave' medical humanities), are not capable of mounting such a challenge. To the contrary, they may well have had the unintended consequence of producing insensibility (ibid.: 26). In part this is because of the acquiescence of the medical humanities as a "handmaiden to normative medicine" and in supporting medicine in its pursuit of "health," "happiness," and "wellbeing" (ibid.: 2, 26). The alternative would be to take "a more active role within medical education by challenging the assumptions and myths of the predominant biomedical model" (Macneill 2011).

Bleakley (2015: 32–4) further recognises that 'critical' medical humanities is unlikely to be a "stable interdisciplinary field" and may (at least to some observers) be seen as anarchic. Nevertheless, he promotes a more radical medical humanities as having the potential to resist the "production of insensibility" and to offer a "political call to democratize medical practice with an aesthetic call to promote education of the sensible, or sensibility" (ibid.: 60). This is a political challenge to the "dominant discourses and habits of practice" and to existing power structures within medical education (ibid.: 60–1). He draws on a number of commentators, including Foucault and Rancière, to demonstrate that these "dominant discourses and habits of practice" are enculturated, to the extent that the capacity to sense, and patterns of sensing—what we are sensitive to—is controlled and produced by power structures within the culture. In medical culture, for example, the result is habitual patterns of noticing, and conversely, habitual patterns of *insensibility*—the inhibition of sensitivity. Medical education produces *insensibilities* by, for example, 'objectifying the patient.' These patterns remain "largely unexamined" (ibid.: 62–3). There is a potential, through arts and the humanities, to challenge those patterns and to educate for sensitive and compassionate medical practice (ibid.: 60).

Bleakley (ibid.: 67) draws in particular on Jacques Rancière who takes a political, Marxist approach, in commenting on the lack of "fair distribution of aesthetic and emotional capital":

> Rancière notes that the 'sensible' in life—what is worth noticing and appreciating and the processes by which sensing, noting and appreciating are socially legitimated—does not simply occur as a transparent or natural process. Rather, what is considered worth noticing and, more importantly, who is given the privilege to notice and appreciate, is determined socially.

This brings us back to a recognition of the power of those who determine what is 'worth noticing.' What is required is resistance or (in Rancière's term) 'dissensus'—"a political process that resists . . . by confronting the established framework of perception, thought, and action" (ibid.: 69). Bleakley takes the view that "[t]ampering with this system will not change it . . . the processes of production and distribution of the capital of sensibility and sensitivity, the system of medical education needs root and branch changes." He argues that "the medical humanities may provide the vehicle for such a fundamental redistribution of the sensible" but that this "requires a revolution in medical education" (ibid.: 71). Obviously, this is beyond the capacities of 'first wave' conventional medical humanities. It entails an overhaul of the fundamental premises of medical education in its commitment to biomedical objectivity, and a challenge to the hierarchical power structures within medicine. The challenge is to 'democratise' medicine and to promote an alternative *raison d'être* for education in which 'the aesthetic' is valued as highly as 'the objective.' Within a revolutionary approach such as this, the critical medical humanities could play a part in promoting 'sensibility and sensitivity.'

Bleakley's approach is to take 'aesthetic medicine' (in terms of 'sense and sensitivity') and give it a political dimension as "the politics of aesthetics."[6] This political recognition follows from acknowledging that simply recognising 'the aesthetic,' without challenging associated power structures and "dominant discourses and habits of practice," is insufficient to bring about change.

Conclusion

Conventional biomedical ethics is a normative discipline based on a consensus about what is ethically acceptable in healthcare practice. Similarly, the medical humanities, conventionally understood, are justified by the view that exposure to the medical humanities provides a 'humanistic' counterbalance to the objectifying approach of biomedicine. Consensus, in both fields, is problematic. Biomedical ethics, as consensus, suppresses conflicting views and effectively 'evacuates' the political processes that are inherent in conflicts about morality and ethics. The medical humanities, based on an assumption of their effectiveness in counterbalancing 'the biomedical model,' and aiding medicine to achieve its goals, are complicit in maintaining a benign and servile relation to medicine and the health professions. This is consensus of a different kind: one that 'defangs' the potential of the humanities to play a critical role in medical education and practice (Macneill 2011). Conventional accounts, in both fields, are add-ons to 'business-as-usual.' They may assist in augmenting healthcare education and delivery, but only to a limited extent.

In this chapter, I have argued for an approach to ethics that focuses on its purpose (or *telos*). This is an art, beyond science. Ethics is understood as an activity that includes reaching for a goal—something we experience as authentic, true, extraordinary, and beyond consensual norms. An account of this kind necessarily brings qualitative and aesthetic attributes into considerations of ethical healthcare. Taking this approach is to enter the second level (or stratum) I referred to in the introduction and to seriously consider biomedical ethics and the medical humanities as linked aesthetic practices. Biomedical ethics and the medical humanities find their commonality at a level of sensory perception and openness to experience. I have drawn attention to the capacity of the humanities and the arts to open us to an aesthetic—that is, sensory and felt—experience. I claim further that this is needed if we are to do more than practise ethics as the application of normative principles and rules. It is also needed if we are to be open to a broad range of medical humanities offerings. An aesthetic approach would assist in developing 'sensibility and sensitivity' and a compassionate regard for patients in healthcare education. To achieve these goals, biomedical ethics and medical humanities would be reformulated as practices of dissensus that require political action to establish an authentic 'aesthetic medicine.'

Biomedical ethics and the medical humanities, reframed in aesthetic terms and as radical practices, draw attention to the commonality between them, and provide an approach that is practical and more readily applicable in healthcare education and healthcare practice. An aesthetic approach to both biomedical ethics and to the medical humanities also enriches our understanding and appreciation of healthcare, promoting healthcare as a democratic practice in support of patients and staff. Such aesthetic, and more politically provocative, accounts have the potential to reframe healthcare in ways that benefit all participants.

Notes

1 Hedgecoe (2004: 123) notes that the "very fact that these [alternative] approaches have appeared as challengers confirms principalism [*sic*] as the dominant way of doing bioethics, in the US at least."
2 It is only when ethics and law have been incorporated within medical professional courses that failure has become more accepted (Parker et al. 2008).
3 This difficulty is added to by a fear expressed in the bioethics literature—that if a concession is made on an important principle like patient autonomy, then ethics becomes *relativistic*.
4 Whilst I have treated Western and East Asian approaches to autonomy as opposing, Fan (1997) has tried (I believe unsuccessfully) to reconcile them.
5 This reference to beauty needs to be nuanced in recognising that the aesthetic may refer to beauty, and to the pleasure we take in beauty. However, the aesthetic also includes the visceral responses we have to other qualities that move us, including our experiences of horror and repugnance (Eaton 2004: 73; Macneill 2017: 638).
6 As Rancière himself has acknowledged, "The politics of aesthetics would more accurately be named as a meta-politics: the politics without *dēmos*, and attempt to accomplish—better than politics, in the place of politics—the task of configuring a new community by leaving the superficial stage of democratic dissensus and reframing instead of the concrete forms of sensory experience and everyday life all" (Rockhill and Watts 2009, in an afterword by Rancière, note 8).

References

Beauchamp TL, Childress JF. 2013. *Principles of biomedical ethics* (7th ed.). New York, NY: Oxford University Press.
Bleakley A. A common body of care: the ethics and politics of teamwork in the operating theater are inseparable. *The Journal of Medicine and Philosophy*. 2006; 31: 305–22.
Bleakley A. 2015. *Medical humanities and medical education: How the medical humanities can shape better doctors*. Abingdon: Routledge.
Bleakley A. Bad faith, medical education, and post-truth. *Perspectives on Medical Education*. 2018; 7: 3–4.

Bleakley A, Marshall R, Brömer R. 2006. Toward an aesthetic medicine: developing a core medical humanities undergraduate curriculum. *Journal of Medical Humanities*. 2006; 27: 197–213.

Bustillos D. Review of R. S. Downie and Jane Macnaughton, *Bioethics and the humanities: Attitudes and perceptions*. *The American Journal of Bioethics*. 2009; 9: 64–6.

Colt HG, Quadrelli S, Friedman LD. 2011. *The picture of health: Medical ethics and the movies*. New York, NY: Oxford University Press.

Damásio AR. 1994. *Descartes' error: Emotion, reason, and the human brain*. New York, NY: GP Putnam.

Damásio AR. 2003. *Looking for Spinoza: Joy, sorrow, and the feeling brain*. London: Heinemann.

Downie RS, Macnaughton J. 2007. *Bioethics and the humanities: Attitudes and perceptions*. Abingdon: Routledge-Cavendish.

Eaton MM. 2004. Art and the aesthetic. In: P Kivy (ed.) *The Blackwell guide to aesthetics*. Oxford: Blackwell Publishing, 63–77.

Fan R. Self-determination vs. family-determination: two incommensurable principles of autonomy. *Bioethics*. 1997; 11: 309–22.

Fantl J. 2017. Knowledge how. In: EN Zalta (ed.) *Stanford Encyclopedia of Philosophy* (Fall ed.). Palo Alto, CA: Stanford University Press.

Gillam L, Delany C, Guillemin M, Warmington S. The role of emotions in health professional ethics teaching. *Journal of Medical Ethics*. 2014; 40: 331–5.

Green RM. Method in bioethics: a troubled assessment. *Journal of Medicine and Philosophy*. 1990; 15: 179–97.

Hafferty FW, Franks R. The hidden curriculum, ethics teaching, and the structure of medical education. *Academic Medicine*. 1994: 69: 861–71.

Hedgecoe AM. Critical bioethics: beyond the social science critique of applied ethics. *Bioethics*. 2004; 18: 120–43.

Hoffmaster B. The forms and limits of medical ethics. *Social Science & Medicine*. 1994; 39: 1155–64.

Hooker C, Noonan E. Medical humanities as expressive of Western culture. *Medical Humanities*. 2011; 37: 79–84.

Hope R, Savulescu J, Hendrick J. 2008. *Medical ethics and law: The core curriculum*. Edinburgh: Elsevier Health Sciences.

Hume D, Selby-Bigge LAS. 1888. *A treatise of human nature*. Oxford: Clarendon Press.

Hume D, Norton DF, Norton MJ. 2000. *A treatise of human nature*. Oxford: Oxford University Press.

Inui TS. 2003. *A flag in the wind: Educating for professionalism in medicine*. Available at: https://members.aamc.org/eweb/upload/A%20Flag%20in%20the%20Wind%20Report.pdf. Last accessed: 21 June 2018.

Jeffery R. 2014. *Reason and emotion in international ethics*. Cambridge: Cambridge University Press.

John E, Lopes D (eds.) 2004. *Philosophy of literature: Contemporary and classic readings—An anthology*. Malden, MA: Blackwell.

Kagan S. 2018 [1998]. *Normative ethics*. New York, NY: Routledge.

Kerridge IH, Lowe M, Stewart C. 2013. *Ethics and law for the health professions* (4th ed.). Annandale, NSW: Federation Press.

Macneill P. Balancing ethical reasoning and emotional sensibility. *Medical Education*. 2010; 44: 851–2.

Macneill P. The arts and medicine: a challenging relationship. *Medical Humanities*. 2011; 37: 85–90.

Macneill P. Balancing bioethics by sensing the aesthetic. *Bioethics*. 2017; 31: 631–43.

Murray SJ. Care and the self: biotechnology, reproduction, and the good life. *Philosophy, Ethics, and Humanities in Medicine*. 2007; 2: 6.

Nussbaum M. 1990. *Love's knowledge: Essays on philosophy and literature*. London: Oxford University Press.

Nussbaum MC. 2001. *Upheavals of thought: The intelligence of emotions*. New York, NY: Cambridge University Press.

Page K. The four principles: can they be measured and do they predict ethical decision making? *BMC Medical Ethics*. 2012; 13: 8.

Parker M, Luke H, Zhang J, et al. The 'pyramid of professionalism': seven years of experience with an integrated program of teaching, developing, and assessing professionalism among medical students. *Academic Medicine*. 2008; 83: 733–41.

Rancière J, Corcoran S. 2010. *Dissensus: On politics and aesthetics*. New York, NY: Continuum.

Rockhill G, Watts P (eds.) 2009. *Jacques Rancière: History, politics, aesthetics*. Durham, NC: Duke University Press.

Ryle G. Knowing how and knowing that: the presidential address. *Proceedings of the Aristotelian Society*. 1945; 46: 1–16.

Ryle G. 1946/1971. *Knowing how and knowing that: Collected papers (Vol. 2).* New York, NY: Barnes and Nobles, 212–25.

Teays W. 2012. *Seeing the light exploring ethics through movies.* Malden, MA: Wiley-Blackwell.

Tsai TC, Harasym PH. A medical ethical reasoning model and its contributions to medical education. *Medical Education.* 2010; 44: 864–73.

Warner JH. The humanising power of medical history: responses to biomedicine in the 20th century United States. *Medical Humanities.* 2011; 37: 91–6.

34

MEDICAL HUMANITIES ONLINE

Experiences from South Africa

Steve Reid and Susan Levine

The part of the MOOC that I enjoy the most is the asynchronous discussion that happens at the end of the first module entitled 'The Heart of the Matter: A Matter of the Heart.' Having spent most of this first week presenting different ideas of what the heart is, including perspectives from a cardiac surgeon, a poet, and a transplant recipient, I ask the innocent question: 'what keeps *you* alive?' It is a discussion that rolled on around different understandings of the heart as being more than just a pump and also, actually, the centre of our being, as Peter Anderson explained it, and the sense of temporality that he unpacked for us. Off we go, every time, on an extraordinarily deep and very meaningful series of reflections, from a hugely diverse group of people from all over the world. The medical student from Mexico responds to the retired nurse in New Zealand, and an African researcher gently chides the cynic from the UK. And it rolls on sometimes for weeks after the main cohort of participants has left that week behind and got on to other topics. Somehow this question, partly existential, partly academic, partly clarifying assumptions, hooks people into a very rich discussion. I've reflected a lot on that discussion. I think it exemplifies what we are trying to do in the medical humanities.

(Steve Reid, reflecting on the MOOC in the final week)

Introduction

'Medicine and the Arts: Humanising Healthcare' is a free introductory Massive Open Online Course (MOOC) offered by the University of Cape Town (UCT) in the interdisciplinary field of the medical humanities. It was created and is presented by Associate Professor Susan Levine, a medical anthropologist in the School of African and Gender Studies, Anthropology and Linguistics in the Faculty of Humanities, and Professor Steve Reid, Head of the Primary Health Care Directorate in the Faculty of Health Sciences (Table 34.1).

The six-week course is hosted on the FutureLearn online platform and has 17 presenters in addition to the two lead educators. In each week of the course, a trio of disciplinary experts is assembled from across disciplines in the health sciences, social sciences AND the arts to bring their perspectives into dialogue on a specific health-care topic. The course aims to facilitate exploration and engagement of the interdisciplinary space between health sciences, social sciences and

Table 34.1 Programme content

Week 1: The Heart of the Matter: A Matter of the Heart
Week 2: Children's Voices and Healing
Week 3: Mind, Art and Play
Week 4: Reproduction and Innovation
Week 5: At the Edge: Madness and Medicine
Week 6: Death and the Corpse

the arts. Each week investigates a new aspect of the human life course from the perspective of the body, of social life and of the imagination (Figure 34.1).

The motivation for 'going online'

Inspired to explore what the medical humanities might mean in a South African context, we designed a Master's-level course called *Medicine and the Arts* in 2013, and offered it to a

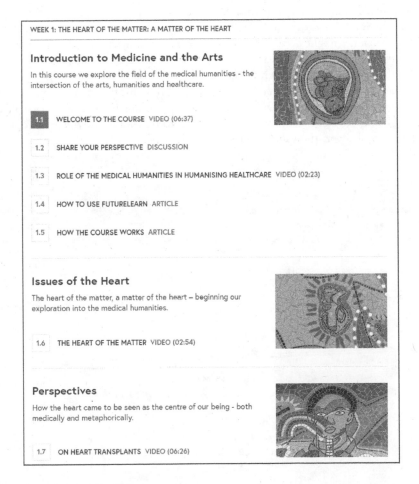

Figure 34.1 Example of a screen from Week 1

maximum of 20 students in 2014 for the first time. The standard MA-level course includes 36 lecturers drawn from the arts, health sciences and social science faculties at UCT, focusing on the human life cycle from the perspectives of artists, social scientists and health practitioners. The curriculum explores themes of reproductive health, paediatric oncology, heart disease, mental health, traditional medicine, empathy and care, death and the corpse. The course helps students to develop skills in critical thinking and instils the value of collaboration in producing new knowledge to face the significant challenges of 21st-century health care in Africa. Our aim is to explore how inter- and trans-disciplinary problem solving and creative engagement might advance ideas for humanising health care and medical education. To distinguish it from the MOOC, we have recently retitled the MA course *Critical Medical Humanities in Africa*.

In 2014, the Vice Chancellor of UCT invited us to reproduce this course as a MOOC. We were hopeful that an online platform for critical enquiry would help to generate a conceptual framework for social justice in the context of deep health-care inequity. In our original course proposal we stated that this would be "an opportunity to develop an academic project in the medical humanities in Africa and globally" (Czerniewicz et al. 2017a) (Figure 34.2).

The basis of this course is to question how we think, speak and act in relation to health, medicine, the body and healing. The idea for the online version arose out of both an interest in building the medical humanities in Africa and as part of the bigger project of developing 'theory from the global South.' We were interested in thinking about how this trans-disciplinary space of medical humanities might be understood as both a local project, with local actors, agendas and perspectives, and as part of a broader global effort to bring together fields of experience and knowledge that have historically been forced apart.

Part of the journey of this particular course is to discover what the medical humanities mean for Africa and in particular South Africa. So much theory making in medical sociology, medical anthropology and the health sciences comes from the North. And we now have an opportunity to introduce, to discover, the value of producing theory in the South. So we've selected six

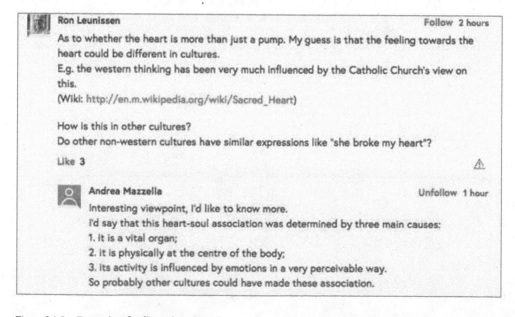

Figure 34.2 Example of a discussion thread

critical issues to do with life, with what it means to be human or mortal, locating these in a South African context, but hoping that you'll translate those or interpret them into your own context (Susan Levine, in the introduction to the MOOC).

Transforming a face-to-face course into an online format

It was not as straightforward as we initially imagined to translate the lectures and ideas from the face-to-face course into an interactive online learning space, but it was a creative process. In this we were fortunate in having an excellent technical support team in the Centre for Innovation in Learning and Teaching (CILT) at UCT, who created the framework for us to populate with the content.

First of all, we had to choose 'six of the best' topics for the online version of the course out of the 13 weeks of the MA course, as the standard length of a MOOC is six weeks. This was a difficult process as it meant excluding certain issues which some felt were 'core' knowledge in favour of others that would be more appealing to an online audience. Secondly, the venues that we used for the face-to-face course—which included a laboratory, a pathology museum and a community health centre—were unsuitable for filming so we lost much of the contextual richness of the real experience.

The process of filming each of the lecturers was interesting, as the online experts told us that the attention span for any online lecture is only seven minutes, so they had to condense what they wanted to say down to the absolute essentials. Drawing on our colleagues across faculties and departments at UCT, we invited them to be part of the online (ad)venture. Some lecturers refused to 'dumb down' their lectures, as they put it, and thereby excluded themselves from the process. But we maintained that a good lecturer is able to put her ideas across succinctly in language that is accessible and engaging, and seven minutes should be enough to do that. Many had to script their lectures and some used a teleprompt, which gave a more contrived feel to the delivery.

The interdisciplinary space that brought medical scientists and practitioners, artists and social scientists together around issues of common concern generated a curiosity and genuine interest in one another's fields, requiring a degree of interdisciplinary generosity and reciprocal humility in traversing the languages and assumptions of diverse areas of expertise. The performance of epistemic generosity offered a welcome break from the more familiar reality of 'epistemic violence,' with science often assuming a 'higher' authority than that of the social sciences and the arts (Spivak 1988). Our colleagues who have presented their work on the MOOC have found it to be a useful vehicle for public engagement with their field of expertise. The more difficult aspect was getting an interaction between the lecturers and students going in a discussion that could be authentically captured on camera. For this we came to rely on the asynchronous discussion threads that online participants can contribute to over the ensuing week, in response to a topic raised by a lecture, or a particular question that we articulated. This is supplemented by quizzes, assignments and opportunities for participants to share their own experiences and perspectives. In all of this, our colleagues in CILT were invaluable in suggesting different formats, rescripting and redesigning some sections, and adapting the context technically to suit the online space. Judging by the feedback, they have been unusually successful, as the course was judged as one of the 'Top 50 MOOCs of All Time' in 2016 by Class Central, and there has been encouraging student feedback and reviews (Vernon 2015).

Two technical points are worth mentioning. The first is that excluding the cost of paying for academic staff, maintenance of the site and developing new content, the technical cost for producing the MOOC in 2015 was ZAR200,000 (£12,000). In the context of austerity measures in South African Higher Education, this amount is rather exorbitant for a free access course. The value of the course lies not in financial gain, but in terms of relational objectives and our desire to build a critical global platform for thinking through knowledge production in the South. The second point is that MOOCs are hosted on publicly accessible web-based platforms, and the enrolment for these online courses is open and free. The running of the courses is largely automated so there is no limit to enrolment numbers, which enables thousands to participate. Publishers generally copyright scholarly articles and only those with a paid subscription can typically access published articles, such as through a university library, with a small number being downloaded for a fee. In the cases where publishers give free/open access to copyrighted articles, these have often been released under a creative commons license and involved the author paying for the publishing costs directly or indirectly. Ideally, academic MOOCs would provide access to published materials, reaching beyond the traditional university audience. We needed to identify free/open access articles. All the material created for this open online course was then released with a creative common license to encourage re-use, since one of the goals of the UCT MOOCs project is to make knowledge accessible to a wider audience.

The experience of online learning

Putting anything online attracts an amazingly diverse group of people from all over the world. Registering for the course implies some degree of commitment even though it is free, so the MOOC format invites them to interact with one another in a particular space of expectant learning. The spread of countries is interesting, with predominance in the UK, since FutureLearn is a private company wholly owned by The Open University (Figure 34.3).

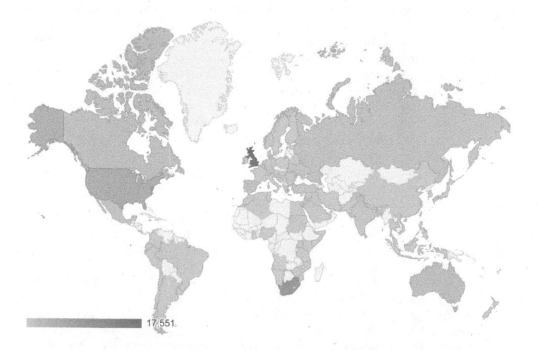

17,551

Figure 34.3   A world map of enrolments in first run of 'Medicine and the Arts'

Another of the extraordinary features of online learning is the numbers and the metrics, which can be tracked in enormous detail ('down to the last keystroke'). So when our first run of the MOOC in 2015 attracted almost 10,000 initial registrations, we felt overwhelmed. But it was short-lived: the standard pattern for all MOOCs is for less than 10% of 'joiners' to become 'learners' who actively engage with the material and each other over time (Table 34.2). Still fewer see every MOOC through to completion. But we had our hands full with 300 active learners on each iteration of the course, and had to engage a few of our 'real' MA students to act as online mentors as we were not able to interact with every participant constantly. Initially developed as a practical intervention to cope with the numbers of online students, the practice has become a pedagogical hallmark of the flipped classroom model, where online and face-to-face students have the chance to share insights drawn from the course. Our online learners, through the mentorship of our students, come to deepen their understanding of the local context, while our students benefit from taking 'ownership' of the course, by which I mean a sense of being responsible for translating ideas to others from around the world.

The 'cohort effect' of starting a course on a particular date and running it over six weeks stimulates a learning environment from the beginning. While all six weeks' material is available for viewing from the time of registration, and some zip through the whole course in a day or two, participants quickly realise the value of interactions with fellow learners through responses to their own comments or from commenting on others' ideas, so the cohort amplifies learning on each topic. It also became a rehearsal space to play with ideas before submitting assignments. Unlike other courses where the content is 'owned' by the expert lecturer, this learning space is much more egalitarian, and therefore more suited to the medical humanities as a democratising process (Bleakley 2015). As convenors, we soon became learners alongside everyone else, as we marvelled at the diversity and richness in the response to our initial ideas from the literally hundreds of different life situations and worldviews of the participants. The contribution by participants of resources, links and cross-references related to the topic under discussion was also a strong feature of this format, as they offered other websites, images, essays and poems that enhanced the learning experience way beyond the readings that we had chosen.

The online space is unexpectedly personal: online learners felt liberated to share personal stories of affliction and of healing in the context of the medical humanities in a much greater way than students on our face-to-face course. The virtual anonymity of being an online learner offered a kind of 'permission' for the vulnerable observer to emerge and invite the kind of affective learning that we had imagined as only possible in 'actual' classroom contexts. By affective learning we simply mean, in Brian Massumi's (2015) terms, "the capacity to affect and to be affected." In fact, the classroom environment may be intimidating to many students, involving various levels of perceived judgement. Although participants do reveal their names, where they are from and as much detail as they would like to share, it is possible that the anonymity afforded by the MOOC platform nevertheless gives people enough cover to share relatively intimate stories and reflections on their lives, their values and the ideas about health. It is a fascinating meeting space:

Table 34.2 Participation rates over time

Participation measure	Total for the first 6 runs
Joiners	26,651
Learners	12,822
Fully participating learners	1,773
Learners with ≥ 90% step completion	688

I have been heartened (!) by the depth of your engagement with the ideas and presentations, and fascinated by the diversity of people contributing to the course. It seems to have struck a need, particularly amongst health practitioners but also for those who have been patients or close to those who have experienced illness, to rethink medical practices. The online space is a new and exciting one, with the strangeness of never meeting most of you physically, but it allows us to have a series of extraordinary conversations, that are located precisely in that inter-disciplinary space that we were aiming for. I have really enjoyed reading your comments; please continue to share your insights and stories. With the online course process, there is the sense that, because it is online and we do not meet in the flesh, it is 'unreal.' However the online discussions and responses are strikingly authentic and personal, and in some ways are more real than the somewhat contrived presentations in the videos, since they are dealing with your real experiences in hundreds of different situations. And this is what I find absolutely fascinating—that is, how our somewhat parochial ideas and conversations here in Cape Town find resonance, like Peter's idea of concentricity, in your multitude of diverse experiences all over the world. That is the most exciting part of this massive online course experience for me.

(Steve Reid, note to participants at the end of week 1)

The interaction of online and face-to-face courses

The intention to wrap the MOOC with face-to-face classroom teaching came from the original design proposal. The intention was to make possible more classroom discussion in a so-called 'flipped classroom' mode (Baker 2000). The Master's course has weekly seminars on campus (see Figure 34.4), with the MOOC material matching six of these weeks and public lectures four other weeks. In each case, the students get to engage with experts on a topic before they have their seminars.

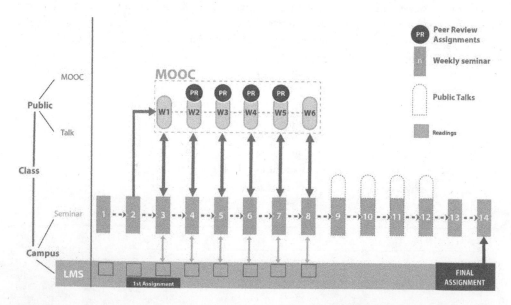

Figure 34.4 Wrapping of the 'Medicine and the Arts' MOOC into a Master's course

We found that the wrapping into the Master's course allowed for more discussion in the seminars. Another unanticipated impact of changing the course pedagogy was to bring youthful graduate students into dialogue with a wide range of participants that included doctors, nurses, healers and artists who offered "a wealth of knowledge and who could then bring that back into conversations and into an environment which was not prejudiced along age lines, race lines or gender lines" (Czerniewicz et al. 2017a). Students reported positive experiences from engaging with the course content outside of the more traditional academic paradigm of the postgraduate seminar space. Participating alongside many others—not obviously identified as experts and without many of the social status identifiers—allowed students more freedom to rehearse their ideas around the topics before seminars.

What is the role of online education in medical humanities?

Online learning experiences can be offered as add-on electives to medical education, or integrated into core components around case studies, using the 'flipped classroom' approach. To offset the tendency in medical education towards a tightly structured curriculum, online learning has the potential to restore creative passions that rigorous medical training often excludes, by offering alternative ways of thinking. The trouble arises when the pressures of teaching medicine emerge as students move from one module to the next, without time for extra courses that are seen as peripheral or non-essential. This is where online learning offers a potential solution for students and faculty members who desire to work beyond the microscope and recover something that might have been lost in the process of becoming health practitioners in the modern age of medical science.

Emerging opportunities within the medical humanities offer health science students a space to pause and reflect on their training as constituted within a cultural paradigm that reproduces very specific demands while undermining the practice of self-reflection and awareness, self-care, and the role of the arts in health. This reduces education to 'training.' While this paring away of the self gives rise to efficient and focused health professionals skilled in the work of diagnosing and treating illness, that very self might suffer under the pressures of exam stress, exhaustion and the weight of enormous responsibility. In South Africa there are the additional pressures of uneven access to health care.

Medical historians, bio-ethicists, medical anthropologists, medical sociologists, novelists, artists, filmmakers, songwriters and musicians have largely been excluded from the formal medical curriculum, and yet all have the potential to transform the experience and outcome of medical education from the perspectives of practitioners and patients. Feedback on the MOOC from medical students and other health science students bears this out: many articulate the experience of having rediscovered their 'lost' passion through the online interactions.

Another attribute of the MOOC is that its content constitutes a 'living archive,' which students and presenters can revisit for the purpose of research (Hamilton and Leibhammer 2017). In particular, we would like our students to access those segments of the MOOC that could generate new interdisciplinary research projects.

Is online learning a feasible and suitable medium for promoting the field more broadly?

The reach of free online platforms such as FutureLearn, edX and Coursera is flexible enough to embrace a range of presentation styles from formal lectures to dialogic community-building chat rooms. The designers of MOOCs can play with the vital relationships between sound, text and image, using montage and bricolage to communicate complex ideas. New technologies in online learning can include not only pre-recorded lectures or even operas as the case might be (see week 5 of 'Medicine and the Arts'), but also include spaces for live updates in the form of video uploading and the means to build the discipline of the medical humanities by drawing on the multiple sources that online students bring with them. Because online students come from all walks of life and from all over the world, they bring rich life experiences and examples to the course. The chat rooms become sites of sharing literature or sharing personal stories of illness and disease from the perspectives of patients and doctors. Situated at this time historically, where social media are everyday for a younger generation glued to their smart devices, online platforms are suitable for promoting the field of the medical humanities widely, with the additional flexibility of speed and the circulation of knowledge in the field (Figure 34.5).

Medical humanities in the 'global North' appear to be largely text-based and disembodied, embedded in ethics, history, philosophy and English literature. By contrast, the 'global South' expression of medical humanities could be seen as more interdisciplinary and embodied, rooted in the arts such as oral narrative, song, dance and movement rather than exclusively in text. Rendering these forms of understanding accessible to students and other learners is a challenge, and online formats including video and audio could extend the field beyond the fortunate few who make it into a classroom. Czerniewicz et al. (2017b) recently emphasised the issue of accessibility in an article about making education more open through MOOCs:

> Pressing educational challenges prevalent in the Global South include the need for high quality and accessible education. The Open Education movement, centred on the adoption of Open Educational Resources (OER), is purported to be part of a possible solution, where the creation and sharing of OER ignites the possibility of lower cost education, efficiency and pedagogical innovation.

Conclusion

One of the conditions that we set when we started the course was that we would only continue as long as we were having fun ourselves! And this has proved to be a useful indicator, with

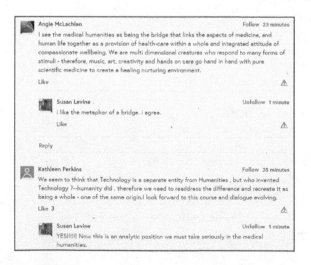

Figure 34.5 Online exchanges

curious and openhearted interdisciplinarity at its core. The issues of medical humanities are fascinating at both academic and emotional levels (head and heart), and the online space leads to a way of constructing new knowledge together with an extraordinarily diverse group of people that does not get stale: it is fresh and inspiring every time we run the course. Feedback from online students offers ideas for future iterations of the course including the themes of end-of-life care, nursing and traditional healing in South Africa.

#WatchThisSpace! www.futurelearn.com/courses/medicine-and-the-arts

References

Baker JW. 2000. The "classroom flip": Using web course management tools to become the guide by the side. In: Selected Papers from the 11th International Conference on College Teaching and Learning: 9–17. Available online: http://works.bepress.com/j_wesley_baker/21. Last accessed: 8 April 2018.

Bleakley A. 2015. *Medical Humanities and Medical Education: How the Medical Humanities Can Shape Better Doctors*. London: Routledge.

Czerniewicz L, Deacon A, Small J, Walji S. Developing world MOOCs: A curriculum view of the MOOC landscape. *Journal of Global Literacies, Technologies, and Emerging Pedagogies*. 2014; 2. Available at: https://open.uct.ac.za/handle/11427/19562. Last accessed: 8 April 2018.

Czerniewicz L, Deacon A, Walji S, Glover M. 2017a. Chapter 10: OER in and as MOOCs. In: C Hodgkinson-Williams, PB Arinto (eds.) *Adoption and Impact of OER in the Global South*. Available at: http://roer4d.org/edited-volume-2. Last accessed: 8 April 2018.

Czerniewicz L, Deacon A, Glover M, et al. MOOC-making and open educational practices. *Journal of Computing in Higher Education*. 2017b; 29: 81. Available at: https://doi-org.ezproxy.uct.ac.za/10.1007/s12528-016-9128-7. Last accessed: 10 April 2018.

Gardner SK. 2013. Paradigmatic differences, power, and status: A qualitative investigation of faculty in one interdisciplinary research collaboration on sustainability science. *Sustainability Science*. 2013; 8: 241. Available at: https://doi-org.ezproxy.uct.ac.za/10.1007/s11625-012-0182-4. Last accessed: 12 April 2018.

Hamilton C, Leibhammer N (eds.) 2017. *Tribing and Untribing the Archive: Volumes 1 and 2*. Durban: University of KwaZulu Natal Press.

Levine S. How online courses can bring the world into Africa's classrooms. *The Conversation*, 2016; 18 August 2016. Available at: https://theconversation.com/how-online-courses-can-bring-the-world-into-africas-classrooms-63773. Last accessed: 12 April 2018.

Massumi B. 2015. *Politics of Affect*. Cambridge: Polity Press.

Spivak GC. 1988. *Can the Subaltern Speak?* Basingstoke: Macmillan.

Vernon J. 2015. My love of learning thrilled by some of the online courses with FutureLearn: Medicine and the Arts review. *Mindbursts*. Available at: https://mindbursts.com/2015/04/30/my-love-of-learning-thrilled-by-some-of-the-online-courses-with-futurelearn. Last accessed: 12 April 2018.

35

'YOUR EFFORT WAS GREAT/YOU CARRIED ME NINE MONTHS'

The birth of medical humanities in Ethiopia

Ian Fussell and Robert Marshall

PART I: 'YOUR EFFORT WAS GREAT'

Ian Fussell

When I Hear Your Name

My thought is with you mum.
How can I imagine all your love?
I cannot guess all your love.
Time cannot determine it.
You gave birth to me
With great labour;
Your favour for me is countless.
I will pay you in my life.

Your effort was great
You carried me nine months
Then carried me long after,
Grew me well
Fed me food
Fed me your breast

I saw light through you mum.
Thank you for that.
You are a mirror for me
And for the whole world.

You encouraged me,
You taught me life.
Now I have learned and
Grown through your labour.

I am thinking of you
I am thinking of my country
When I hear your name,
I feel at ease
I feel at home.
> *(Demith Daniel (Ethiopia))*

When I hear your name

I sit nervously in a huge, freshly painted auditorium in the University of Wollega, Nekemte, Ethiopia. You'll struggle to find it on a map—it's not on the tourist trail. I witnessed this building's construction: the poorest women binding eucalyptus trees together into makeshift scaffolding and pushing creaking, battered wheelbarrows over parched, uneven ground over-filled with gravel. I never believed the building would be finished, and yet here I sit, the only white westerner among a sea of black, beautiful faces. Despite the women toiling at construct-ing the scaffolding, the audience is all men, wearing dowdy, ill-fitting suits and dour ties in the blistering heat, from the best universities and medical schools in the country. I concentrate on the key presentation. The 'Road Map for the University' sounds ambitious—to become one of the top 30 universities in Africa within five years. Maybe it could happen. The long and detailed feedback from the floor to the presenter is delivered mainly in the Amharic lan-guage with smatterings of English. We are in Oromia, but nobody speaks Oromo at this event.

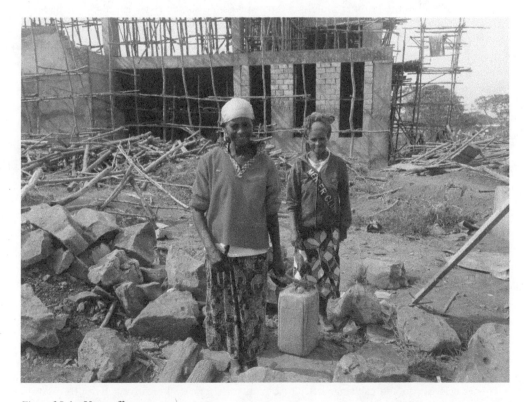

Figure 35.1 Your effort was great

We had already felt the close pressure of the complex politics of the region, and later that week Nekemte descended into violence and chaos under our noses.

From our Truro (Cornwall, UK) outpost, Dr Robert Marshall, Dr Julie Thacker and I have evolved a regular cycle of visits to Wollega, with some of our medical students in attendance. Our link with an Ethiopian medical school is part of the bigger rising tide of global exchanges within medical education.[1] But ours is possibly unique in putting emphasis on the value of the medical humanities. My parent school, Exeter University Medical School, was once part of the progressive Peninsula Medical School that pioneered a core, integrated and assessed medical humanities programme within the undergraduate curriculum, led by Alan Bleakley and Rob Marshall.

I work as a doctor and am Associate Dean of Education at the University of Exeter Medical School, and here in Nekemte I am about to give a lecture on the importance of arts and humanities in medical education. I will then give all students and faculty a book of poetry written in Oromo by Ethiopian students and translated into English (see header poem to this chapter). For someone from a poorly performing inner city comprehensive school in Bristol who was brought up on a housing estate, was bullied, abused and somehow managed to escape by going to medical school, I feel rather proud and privileged at this moment. The medical humanities have helped me to get where I am, and this is how . . .

While at school in the 70s, I joined the drama club and landed the lead in the school play. I played Harry in 'Zigger Zagger'—a troubled lad who decided against a life of football hooliganism and crime for one of education and work. I was 13. This didn't help the bullying, but cut me out as different. In the Sixth Form the drama club members helped a local amateur dramatics society by providing extras for their summer plays. We travelled to the Minack Theatre in Porthcurno in West Cornwall in the summer months and our minds blossomed as we gazed out at the wide Atlantic sea with nothing between the wild Cornish coast and Nova Scotia, Canada (Figure 35.2).

At medical school, I organised and performed in Medic Reviews and on qualification as a doctor chose to move to the closest hospital to the Minack that I could find in the phone book, West Cornwall Hospital in Penzance. In 1994, I qualified as a General Practitioner and not wishing to end my personal development and ambition, continued to look for opportunities and openings. I became a member of the local Primary Care Trust in 2008. They needed an Education Lead, so I volunteered and persuaded them that they should support me to study for a Postgraduate Certificate in Education (PGCE) to inform this role. I was shocked that established GP educationalists behaved in an unsupportive and unkind way towards me at that time. I had spotted that there was a strong possibility of a new medical school opening in the South West region and I wanted to be a part of it. After a number of roles in the medical school I landed the Community Sub Dean Role and the Clinical Special Study Unit Lead. Responsibilities included overseeing and managing medical humanities in the curriculum. I was elected to the Committee for the UK Association of Medical Humanities, began to present my own work, and encouraged medical students to present their work, at international conferences.

My work in Ethiopia started over three years ago. The University of Wollega Medical School is a new school and part of a National Programme to increase the number of medical schools and doctors across Ethiopia. I am in a team that has visited the university many times over this period to help deliver the curriculum, develop the teachers and the faculty and quality assure their procedures. It seemed ridiculous to us at the time, but Dr Rob Marshall and I thought it would be interesting to explore the introduction of medical humanities to the new school. We were certain that this had never been attempted before and so agreed to run an event—a celebration and exchange of culture with some practical creative activity thrown in. We contacted the Head of the Faculty of Arts and Humanities, Dr Zeleke Tesome, and made

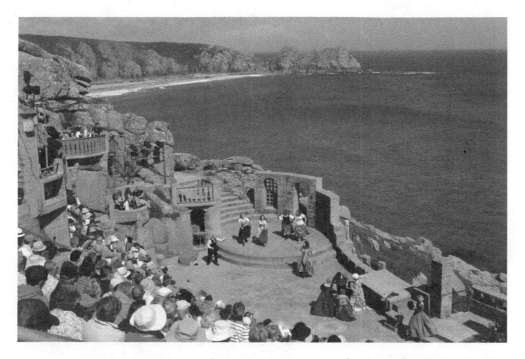

Figure 35.2   The Minack Theatre, Porthcurno

a plan. We invited all of the humanities students who were studying English, drama, art and music, and also the medical students in the University of Wollega. We also included the UK students who had ventured out with us. On the morning of the event, a room crammed full of happy, funny and excited students greeted us enthusiastically.

All the humanities faculty staff members were in attendance and we felt very much out of our comfort zones and wondered what lay ahead of us. I opened the event with a welcome in the Oromo language: *baga nagaan dhuftan* ('welcome'); *maganke* ('my name is') Ian. The cheers were reassuring. My lecture on medical humanities was translated in real time by the Head of Drama, and included reflections on the work of the surgeon and writer Atul Gawande, and artists Grayson Perry and Frida Kahlo for their impact on medical education. I stood back and wondered how the students would receive this—students who were living in extremely difficult conditions with barely enough money for a biro. I needn't have worried. The response was phenomenal. The lecturers were really excited and were downloading articles to show me, while the students were clapping and buzzing. The day was off to a good start.

The Humanities department had been tasked to provide us with a piece of drama incorporating a medical angle. The play they had written and rehearsed explored physical and sexual abuse of women. We were not expecting that. We experienced and witnessed a completely different view of the young Ethiopians, particularly the women. They behaved completely unlike the medical students that we had previously been working with, who were shy and unconfident. These students were amazing; they were intelligent, confrontational, boisterous and assertive. They were prepared to talk about difficult issues and in subsequent events the pieces of drama addressed HIV infection, promiscuity, unwanted pregnancy and abuse of elder people. Emotive stuff. Our medical students could learn a lot from this bunch. I recalled that at Peninsula we had brought in drama and performance students from Falmouth University to run very successful workshops with our medical students on 'managing identity.' Years before, Rob Marshall, then head of postgraduate education at Royal Cornwall Hospital Truro, had brought in the Education Officer from the Royal Shakespeare Company to work with senior doctors on 'self-presentation.'

Our last exercise with the students, and we included our own medical students who had travelled with us, was a poetry workshop. We gave them the first line—'when I hear your name'—and set them off to write. It was all eyes down and the 100 or so students in the room got busy. After 20 minutes we gathered together and the Ethiopian tutors selected students to stand up to read their work in Oromo. Again, the Head of Drama translated this into English in real time. We witnessed students crying while they read, supporting each other and enjoying themselves. Dr Zeleke subsequently told me that this was the greatest day of his academic career. We decided there and then that we would collect the poems, translate them properly and publish the first Oromo-English poetry book (Figure 35.3).

We repeated these sessions and presented the humanities in medical education lectures again at the first ever Medical Conference held at the University of Wollega Medical School. I stand nervously on the stage of this huge, impressive building that can hold in excess of 2000 people. The building that I had seen a few years back, looking as though it would never be finished, is now an icon for the University of Wollega. In front of me are educators from around the country, Vice Chancellors of the top universities, representation from the Ethiopian Government and delegates from neighbouring countries; and I am going to give my lecture again and give them the poetry collection as a gift.

The talk is well received, there were no giggles when Frida Kahlo's half-naked self-portrait filled the screen. The astonished reaction to the book, which looks beautiful, was incredible

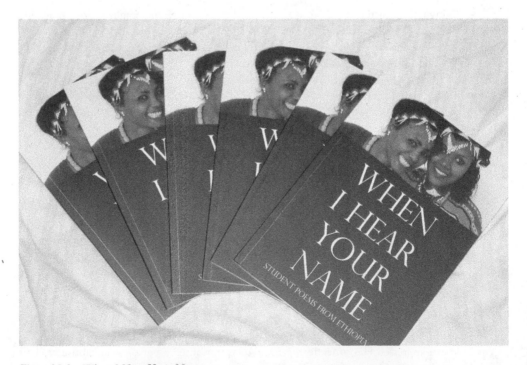

Figure 35.3 When I Hear Your Name

to observe. How could these people from the UK have invested time, energy and money into producing such a thing and to validate our young oppressed people in this way? Is this another colonialist gesture, following the Italians' long involvement in our land and culture? We certainly had no intentions of exporting our Western medical education ideals to Nekemte. But it is so hard to get out of your national skin and Robert Marshall's piece following this raises some of those tensions. Importantly, we sowed the seeds of the medical humanities and perhaps that venture will flower over the years according to Ethiopian will.

PART II: SPICES AND HARD QUESTIONS[2]

Robert Marshall

In 2013, a partnership was formed between the medical schools of the University of Exeter in the UK and Wollega in Ethiopia (see Ian Fussell's essay above). At first, the president and vice-president of Wollega asked us to help with teaching, in particular teaching their teachers to teach. Almost the entire faculty, including the Dean, was two or three years post-qualification and, like most medics, they thought that they knew how to teach and did not need any help, thank you. But as our help extended to teaching clinical skills, they joined in with greater enthusiasm. We have tried to visit twice a year. Our groups now are of about six to ten people—faculty and students—and the trips are staggered over four to six weeks.

Their vice-president has been a great support from the start and enthuses about every project we suggest. We wanted to introduce the medical humanities into medical studies, using the personnel and facilities of their humanities department. We also planned a project to bring clean water and clean lavatories to the local schools. The heads of the humanities and engineering departments were summoned, and we discussed how to take the projects forward for an hour or so. The Exeter end of the link consists of student and faculty volunteers from the campus in Truro, Cornwall in the far southwest of the UK, where we have invested strongly in the value and importance of the arts and humanities in medical education (including throughout one's postgraduate career). It seemed only natural to us therefore to introduce the medical humanities into the curriculum in Wollega. Although I was instrumental, with Alan Bleakley, in setting up the medical humanities in Exeter medical school's first incarnation (as Peninsula Medical School, and later as Peninsula College of Medicine and Dentistry), I did not know how to best set about this curriculum intervention in Wollega. What might the 'medical humanities' mean in the Ethiopian setting?

When I return from visits to Wollega, they assume a dreamlike quality. The events that follow all happened, probably not during the same visit, and bear directly on the issue of the 'global' medical humanities (as invented and exported by the affluent cosmopolitan West).

As I leave the hotel in the morning to get the bus to 'Campus,' I have to step over a young woman with a baby in her arms lying in the gutter. She looks near to death. Several times since I have been visiting, there have been bodies lying in just this spot, male and female, and usually young (the old prefer the opposite corner where there is a larger area of pavement for them to beg, if they are able, or sit quietly and die, if they are not).

What should I do with the dying mother? This is one of the busiest corners of the town and hundreds of local people are walking over and around her without a glance. Is it the right question—'what should I do with' her? Why not 'do about' or 'do for'? In English, these phrasal verbs carry different meanings, but also important nuance, as in this case. 'Do about' has a managerial ring; she is a problem to be sorted. Indeed, to step back and take a detached view may be right. After all, I have said this is not the only time it has happened, and it makes sense to organise help such that we would know what to do next time and that might operate in our absence. 'Do with her' is a question that answers itself, I suspect. It is the question asked by countless exasperated parents, as their child is brought back from yet another foray with illegality. 'What am I going to do with you?' Answer: nothing, because you are beyond my limited skills and I have no idea what to do. 'What should I do for her?' puts the questioner in an awkward spot, because it implies, as 'do with' and 'do about' do not, that I actually care, that I feel emotionally engaged with this sick person. It makes it more difficult to walk away, which is probably why my subconscious used 'with.'

In practice, what I do is nothing. I look at her, because to pretend I haven't even noticed her would be wrong. I consider if there is anything practical to be done. I could stop any one of the other pedestrians, whose English is likely to be limited, and ask if we can get her to hospital; I could phone one of our local medical contacts for advice; I could go back to the hotel and ask one of our group to help me load her into a bajaj, the tiny, local three-wheeled taxis, to take her to the hospital. In practice, I join the throng walking around her and don't think of any of these possibilities until later. I need to hurry to the medical school, where 50 or so students will either have been waiting for an hour or more, or will simply not be there—on strike, on vacation, turning up tomorrow. I have a German friend who worked in Zimbabwe for seven years. One of the first things he told me, when I briefly worked with him there, was that we were in Africa and we must think African, think and work at African pace and in African style; it was their country. It is a knack I have yet to master.

The students are there and we start a long session on brain pathology. After an hour, I realise that I am going to have to open my bowels within the next 20 minutes. This is a serious issue, because the only facility I am aware of is a hut with eight cubicles in the centre of the university, overlooked by several of its departments. I have been to a few low-income countries and to several European countries in the 1960s, and regard myself as something of a lavatory connoisseur. This one is the worst I have come across, and I try to organise my day's activities so that I never need to use it. I suspect that I am one of the more feeble of our group in this respect, as others seem to battle through bouts of diarrhoea and continue with their teaching. We don't talk about the issue much, which seems to me odd for a group of medics, but typical for a group of British. The subject should be included in all books on medical humanities, because it is a fundamental that affects human behaviour. I find I am in good company with the Duchess of Orleans, writing in 1694 to the Electress of Hanover from Fontainbleau, worried less by the quality of the lavatory than the fact that it is open to the public gaze and all manner of people pass by—men, women, children and, a nice touch, Swiss Guards.[3] Her worry is less to do with public defecation than with having to bare her bottom in public. In Wollega too, it is not just a matter of aesthetics. Girls miss a good deal of education if lavatories are mixed sex and poorly constructed. One of our UK students has just completed a brief survey of menstruation in Wollega—knowledge about, preparation for, facilities for dealing with—and the results are depressing.

My own problem is sorted by sending the students off for a coffee and taking a quick walk to a hotel about a mile away, where there is actually something to sit on. It makes for a long mid-morning break.

When I return to our hotel in the late afternoon, the sick woman and her baby are gone. I sit and have a cup of tea in the courtyard of the hotel and prepare the next day's lecture. This is one of the pleasantest parts of the day. The vice-president, who has taken good care of us from the start, arrives unexpectedly for an update. He seems preoccupied and asks if I would like to come to a meeting that he must go to. I think it would be interesting to see how faculty discussions are handled and agree.

As we walk, it occurs to me that his remit is university wide, he is not medical, and the meeting is unlikely to be about the medical faculty; still it will be interesting. Then I realise we are walking away from the university and ask what sort of meeting this is. He explains that it is to honour the memory of a senior ruling party official, who controlled a large area of our locality. Given that the Oromo region where we work is vigorously and sometimes violently opposed to the government, it seems unwise for me to go. But I suspect I am making too much of it and anyway, we are late and will slip quietly to the back. We enter an enormous hall, dating from the Soviet era, and my colleague walks to the front row and sits us in the centre. All of us in the front are given a thin candle about a metre long, which is lit for us. A young man is delivering a long speech and, about halfway through, I realise that there is a cadence and rhythmicity to it that suggests it is poetry. I may be witnessing the end of a long tradition of African praise-poems for great leaders. I try to work out the scansion scheme that underlies the poem but am distracted by the candle, which has burned quickly and is now threatening my fingers and to cause an incident. My colleague solves the problem by throwing his on the floor; I follow suit; damage to the carpet is minimal.

At the back of the stage on which the poet is performing, I notice television cameras recording the event, and wonder if those in the front row will be conspicuous on this evening's news: 'Visiting British doctor-academic shows support for ruling party.' The eulogies go on for a long time, and I finally make my apologies and slip away.

The head of the 'humanities department' is a good contact to have made. Actually, the department doesn't go by that name, but 'humanities' seems to cover all artistic endeavours—fine art, music, dance, drama and more. The students lack most practical materials, instruments to play, crayons and paints for their art, but do what they can. It is right to hold one's tongue, particularly about subjects of which one is so ignorant. We visit an art class where a few students are copying a painting of a man's face (not a very good painting)—copying a simulacrum. I am actually standing at the back of Plato's cave. How inspiring the students would find a nude and a good teacher.

A colleague and I organise a poetry workshop for the medical students. I think how much my wife, a proper poet, would disapprove of this blind leading the blind, and worry that the students will not engage. But once they understand what is asked, they think and write in an atmosphere of terrific concentration. I ask them to continue from the first line: 'When I hear your name.' They write in Afan Oromo, the local language, and the head of department—a good English speaker—translates their poems. They write mostly about parents, nearly always their mothers:

'When I hear your name,
The goodness of your character,
Your wisdom in your home,
The love deep-rooted in your heart,
The sweet sound of your voice
Make me choked with tears.
I cannot tell the measure of your love.
I remember your advice that day
Of shade, cool air, and encouragement.
You give happiness, give light to others;
You hurt yourself but strengthen others.
I will forget you never;
In my whole life, I will forget you never,
My friend, my comfort.'

They often write about the region of Oromo, their homeland:

'When I hear your name,
Beautiful Oromia,
Land of milk and honey,
All of us belong to you,
My country Oromia, more than money,
Place of my birth,
I will not leave you till I die.
Oromia wide, land of animals and forest,
You live for us, for us you are a gift.'

We have been privileged to attend several performances of dance and drama by the students. At one, our group is put in the front row of a room filled with the students and teachers who are not performing. The play was written by the students and is a 'rags to riches' story about a young man, born in poverty to a single mother, who achieves wealth and status by study and hard work. It starts before his birth with his mother bemoaning her hard life. A wealthy man enters, spots her, drags her into the bushes off-stage and, from noises off, we are clearly to understand that he rapes her. He returns on-stage, buttoning his flies and goes off the other side; she staggers back on and exits at the back of the stage, allowing us to see that the back of her dress is covered in blood. Worse things have been done on the London stage. What amazes us Brits about this performance is how amused the audience is by the rape; there are smiles and chuckles as the rapist returns to the stage, reaching a crescendo as we see the woman's bloodstained dress. This is not a gender-related issue as most of the audience is young women; nor is it age-related as the elderly academic next to me and another teacher are chuckling away. What can have been funny about that scene? We were seated in a slight curve in the front row, so that I could see the reaction of our own students, one of whom, sitting at the far end, was a caricature of shock and disbelief.

There are official documents in the UK acknowledging that links such as ours benefit the visitors as much as the country visited. This has been our belief from the start. The teaching has developed into an activity relatively straightforwardly and the digging of wells for clean water raises only practical problems. Dip your presumptuous toe into humanities' water and you are likely to have it grasped by a crab. One of the poems from the workshop makes little sense, at least not to me:

'They was you with blood day and night
When they attempt to convince you, but you hesitate
But . . .
My thought couldn't be avoided from your mind
But exists in yokes dipped into your bone
Your garnet do not lose me
And disconnected your hand from me
Disliking our meeting each other
They made me out of your sight
Dogs are guarding your compound
So how do I come to your surround?
But don't hesitate my existence
I didn't forget my promise
Though you have no relatives I am your relative.'

'Yokes dipped into your bone' is good stuff, but what on earth does it mean? A mis-spelling? 'Yolks' also makes no sense, though equally graphic. A mistranslation? But the translator's English is good. A student that needs help? Then so does another whose mother is starving, and another . . . It troubles you when you get home. Like the funny rape.

Notes

1 Since 2007, the University of Texas Health Science Center (The Center for Medical Humanities and Ethics) has been running a programme—'Ethiopia Outreach'—for medical students to work in Ethiopia. However, the programme appears to involve community health and medical interventions and not the medical humanities (www.texashumanities.org/Ethiopia-Outreach). The University of Toronto has set up a major collaboration with Addis Ababa University focused on improving and expanding the latter's post-qualification health professions education programmes (www.utoronto.ca/news/transforming-health-care-ethiopia-u-t-s-collaboration-addis-ababa-university-takes-centre-stage).
2 From the account in the Bible of the Queen of Sheba's visit to King Solomon. 1 Kings 10. 1–10.
3 Quoted in: Laporte D. 2000. *History of Shit*. Cambridge, MA: The MIT Press.

36

MEDICAL HUMANITIES IN CANADIAN MEDICAL SCHOOLS

Progress, challenges and opportunities

Allan Peterkin, Natalie Beausoleil, Monica Kidd,
Bahar Orang, Hesam Noroozi and Pamela Brett-Maclean

Introduction

Kidd and Connor (2008) documented a diversity of views as to what constitutes the 'medical humanities' (hereafter 'MH')—now also widely termed 'health humanities' (Atkinson et al. 2015)—noting a lack of consensus regarding associated best practice teaching approaches in Canadian medical schools. Appendix A summarises information obtained in 2005–2006 from key informants in their study. They described the field as having marginalised status, where a biomedical and evidence-based medicine model has dominated since the 1990s (Mykhalovskiy and Weir 2004). Recognising the heterogeneity and fluidity of the developing field (Hurwitz 2013; Bleakley 2015), we define MH as *a field embracing perspectives and approaches across the arts, humanities and social sciences focused on educational goals concerned with the human side of medicine.* We note Kidd and Connor's (2008: 47) definition of MH as inclusive of content and approaches that encourage "reflection and critical thinking about the human body and mind" and related systems.

Over the past decade, significant advances in medical education have occurred including enhanced emphasis on humanism and professional identity formation (Cruess et al. 2014; Branch 2015; Wald et al. 2015). A shift towards social accountability as a core mandate for medical education was also introduced by the 2010 'Future of Medical Education in Canada' report (AFMC 2009). A recent study of medical school websites and course databases also found evidence of increasing integration of MH teaching in Canadian undergraduate medical programmes (Lam et al. 2015).

In light of these developments, this chapter provides an update regarding the status of MH in Canadian medical schools, and, we hope, will serve as a template for others seeking to survey a similar field in other geographical locations.

Methods

Setting and participants

Key informants at all 17 Canadian medical schools known to have expert knowledge regarding MH offerings at their medical school, or recommended by their medical school dean, participated in this study. In turn, our research team advertised a wide range of (inter)disciplinary expertise.

Data collection

In mid-2014, we conducted a virtual consultation via various medical/health humanities listserves (such as the Arts, Humanities, Social Sciences and Medicine e-listserve) and asked colleagues to suggest questions they believed were relevant to both characterising and understanding MH teaching and learning in medical education. We considered both frequently nominated questions and those most relevant to Canadian medical education. Questions involving brief or closed-ended responses were included in an online survey. Open-ended questions were included in a semi-structured interview guide.

Our survey covered: admission policies, MH disciplines and approaches used in the curriculum, inter-professional learning, co-curricular (or extra-curricular) opportunities, assessment, disciplinary backgrounds of those involved in MH teaching, faculty development, funding and MH website texts. Key informants were also asked about contributing to a centralised Canadian MH resource. Finally, respondents were invited to participate in a 20-minute-long interview about experiences of MH teaching and learning. Data collection occurred over a period of 10 months (beginning 09/2014). Interviews were audiotaped and transcribed. The Mount Sinai Hospital Research Ethics Board (Toronto) approved our research protocol.

Data analysis

We used a mixed-methods approach. We considered survey and interview responses to characterise curricular and co-curricular MH offerings at each school, and summarised these in tables. We used the constant comparative method (Glaser and Strauss 1967) to identify key themes in interview transcripts. In interpreting data we adopted a critical analysis approach, reflexively articulating and exploring our emerging understandings through dialogue (Russell and Kelly 2002; Alvesson and Sköldberg 2009; Green and Thorogood 2013).

Findings

We obtained survey responses from 26 faculty (Kidd and Connor 2008) members at all 17 medical schools, and conducted telephone or in-person interviews with informants at 10 medical schools (nine with those who had also completed the survey, where one person responded to survey questions when they were interviewed and subsequently confirmed our tabulated summary). Although we hoped to connect with at least two representatives from each medical school, due to scheduling and time constraints, this was not possible. We recorded all positive responses when key informants from the same school differed in their survey responses (we used an asterisk [*] to indicate responses provided by only one of two key informants in our summary tables). We assumed that key informants had knowledge of different educational offerings at their medical school.

The lay of the land: key survey findings

Appendix B (Table A36.2) provides an overview of admissions policies and provision of MH teaching at all 17 Canadian medical schools. Thirteen schools considered applicants from a broad range of disciplines (see 'Open admission'). In relation to curriculum exposure, all schools included MH teaching in the first year, while nine offered MH opportunities in all years of the MD programme.

Twelve schools reported inclusion of arts, humanities and social sciences teaching in the curriculum, and/or as elective offerings (see Appendix B—Table A36.2: 'MH disciplines, content'—A, H and SS listings). Additional MH-related curricular content and electives were reported for five schools. With respect to arts-based disciplines and approaches, literature/narrative and/or reflective exercises were included in all MD programmes. All schools also included content related to bioethics/philosophy, and 15 covered history of medicine topics. Social science (medical anthropology and/or sociology) perspectives were also included in curriculum offerings at 12 schools.

MH teaching was integrated in the core curriculum via mandatory and optional lectures, seminars, small group sessions, activities and assignments (Appendix B—Table A36.2). Stand-alone and longitudinal elective courses were offered at 13 schools. MH curricular material was also used in inter-professional learning initiatives at 15 schools. A variety of approaches were used to assess learning, including: pass/fail (based on attendance), examination (frequently described in relation to bioethics teaching), feedback and production of scholarly, reflective and creative work.

In 15 schools, MD faculty with an interest, and some who had a degree, in the humanities were involved in MH teaching. In all schools, clinical faculty in other health professions, PhD scholars and artists were involved. MH-related faculty development was offered at 11 schools (see Appendix B—Table A36.2).

A variety of funding sources supported MH teaching (Appendix B—Table A36.2). At all schools, internal University Medical Education (UME) funding supported mandatory MH teaching such as bioethics. At a few schools, faculty positions and infrastructure supporting humanities teaching and related activities had been secured through internal, and/or endowed funding. Several informants shared that they struggled to obtain funding for elective and other curricular and co-curricular offerings (several reported donating their own funds). Many, including those with more established infrastructure in place, described the need to fundraise and secure external research and programme grants.

Appendix C (Table A36.3) summarises co-curricular MH opportunities that our key informants identified at their medical schools. These included: ongoing interest/study groups (n=14 schools), research opportunities and awards/contests (n=13), lectures, workshops and conferences (n=12), student blogs, publications (n=10), and performances, art shows, etc. (n=7).

Twenty-three out of 26 of our key informants indicated they would be interested in contributing to a centralised Canadian MH teaching repository.

At the heart of it: tales from the field

Key informants who were interviewed agreed that MH teaching is important in educating effective and caring physicians, resulting in better patient outcomes, though their views differed regarding the extent to which this occurred 'intrinsically' (promotion and protection of empathy) or 'extrinsically' (enhanced analytical ability and capacity for critical reflection). Additional MH contributions were suggested, including enhanced understanding of marginalised or vulnerable patients and communities, development of the senses/close noticing (e.g., visual literacy), enhanced capacity for critical reflection, enhanced understanding of the history and culture of medicine and the provisional nature of knowledge, increased creative problem-solving, tolerance of ambiguity, broadening perspective/worldview, recognition of professional challenges and better self-care.

Other themes identified across key-informant interviews are described below.

Theme 1: successes and challenges

Key informants viewed the introduction of enhanced MH curricular offerings and contributions over the past decade as an important accomplishment. Examples include: introduction of reflective portfolios, creation of humanities certificates, contributions to curricular reform, introduction of MH curricular themes, inter-professional learning opportunities and faculty development. Increasing engagement with the broader community was also viewed as an important advance.

Successful introduction of small-scale MH innovations, which were valued by others, and viewed as benefitting the medical school, was associated with the expansion of MH teaching. One participant shared: "We believe our work facilitated the successful accreditation process at our school!" Another shared that MH offerings at the school were profiled when prospective students came for admission interviews.

The support of students, as well as faculty champions and curriculum leads who understood the contribution of humanities teaching, was noted as integral to the uptake and expansion of MH offerings. A number of interviewees shared that creation of dedicated MH faculty positions and programmes had helped to expand MH networks and curricular offerings at their school.

Annual conferences and leadership fora in the humanities and social sciences, including the 'Creating Space' pre-symposia at the Canadian Conference on Medical Education (CCME) since 2011, were considered a significant advance. A number of interviewees mentioned the 'White Coat, Warm Art' juried art exhibit (Courneya 2011) at the annual CCME meeting as an important accomplishment.

Documentation of successful MH innovations included: creation of new course materials, formal and informal student evaluations, certificates of distinction and teaching awards, annual reports, media coverage, successful funding applications, scholarly presentations and published papers (by both students and faculty).

Challenges included: ongoing perceptions of marginalisation, lack of consensus regarding the MH field, competition for curricular time, limited funding and unrealistic expectations of humanities-based scholarship. Additional challenges included geographic distance between medical schools and arts and humanities faculties (at some universities), lack of recognition of humanities contributions in academic promotion, turf wars between disciplines and the lack of a central repository of educational modules and resources.

Theme 2: medical students and medical humanities teaching

Medical student involvement and leadership in this area were emphasised. When asked how medical students at her school responded to MH teaching, one key informant responded: "Enthusiastically. And the reason I say that is almost every time we have introduced something new on the horizon of arts and humanities in medicine, we've been overwhelmed with the response." One respondent made reference to the bell curve: "15% love it, 15% hate it and 70% are open to seeing the value." Another informant hypothesised that the few students who provide strongly negative evaluations to humanities exercises were likely those most challenged by it.

Many key informants shared examples of medical students who were active in advocating for humanities teaching, and creating MH resources and curricular and co-curricular offerings. One shared that students at his school were starting a "student-run 'Arts and Humanities' journal. They have their first call for submissions out. They've invited students from the schools of nursing and pharmacy and human genetics . . . I'm quite excited."

Theme 3: moving forward

Key informants were keen to share their ideas for promoting MH teaching in the curriculum. Some favoured a 'soft' approach—enticing students with content they love:

With medical students. . . if you've got a core group who say this is not completely crazy, they can be highly influential with their peers . . . Students are a powerful motivator. They can be your best advocates more than you can ever be as an individual.

Advocating a proactive approach, another informant shared:

You have to get onto the curriculum committee . . . and you have to be persistent. You might very well be told no the first time, but you go around and you get it later by a different route. You have to keep working hard to get stuff in the curriculum, and then once you've got it in, you've got to defend it.

Recognising the broad network of influences involved in curriculum innovation and change, most advocated a flexible approach, making use of different strategies depending on the situation. One key informant shared the following example:

We had the portfolio course first and then a monthly narrative medicine group for faculty, and they energised each other. Really engaged portfolio mentors came from that study group. This led to paying attention to the patient voice and organising a community event/partnership at the public library about that.

As for advancing MH teaching, continued opportunities to meet with others at national and local medical education meetings were viewed as vital. Increasing collaboration between humanities scholars with 'critical depth' and physicians who have 'clinical insight to make it relevant to medical students' was also recommended.

Interpretation

Our review contributes to earlier articles published in the *Canadian Medical Association Journal* (Van Wyck 1951; Bates 1971; Squires 1985; Peterkin 2008) and elsewhere on humanities in Canadian medical education and practice. Information presented in Appendix A (Table A36.1) compared with Appendices B (Table A36.2) and C (Table A36.3) suggests significant change in the field. Our findings suggest a positive evolution in MH in medical education, including enhanced exposure to MH disciplines and approaches across more, and in some cases all, undergraduate medical educational programme years.

Most Canadian medical schools have admission policies that welcome students across a range of disciplines, not exclusively science majors. We note that MH offerings currently encompass a wide range of disciplines. All schools include MH teaching in the first year, while over half include MH offerings across the MD programme. Bioethics/philosophy, history, literature/narrative and reflection were most common (reflecting, at least in part, current accreditation requirements and also showing that more traditional subject areas within MH 'stick'). Along with associated challenges (Ellaway et al. 2014), this evolution of MH in medical education suggests a broadened view. Enhanced MH offerings likely reflect emergent curriculum needs and opportunities and, as originally suggested by Kidd and Connor (2008), the varied disciplines and interests of those involved. Most schools profiled the presence of MH offerings via URLs included within, or associated with, their medical school website.

Our key informants associated progress in this area with a number of factors including the skill, creativity and persistence of faculty and students, supportive 'champions' (Nisker 2014) and faculty development opportunities (Boudreau, Liben and Fuks 2012). Successful introduction of MH offerings was viewed as not only contributing to the educational mandate of MD programmes, but also benefitting the school in relation to recruitment (Hall et al. 2014) and accreditation (Zimmerman and Marfuggi 2012). While a shift 'from the margins' was described, many informants described ongoing tensions in relation to hegemonic biomedical discourses (Whitehead 2013) resulting in emphasis on behavioural and clinical competencies (Whitehead et al. 2014), as well as legitimacy concerns in relation to both assessment (Kuper 2006; Holmboe 2016) and MH-related research/inquiry practices (Albert, Paradis and Kuper 2015). While acknowledging challenges, many described being proud of the growing community and success of Canadian MH educators and scholars. The importance of collaborating within and across medical schools, working with both students and humanities colleagues, was emphasised. There were also key successes in public engagement through, for example, art exhibitions (Courneya 2011).

There are a number of limitations to our study. We cannot ensure the accuracy or completeness of the data we collected (particularly in relation to MH teaching across MD programmes and sites at larger medical schools). Key informants were not asked to refer to a curriculum database when responding to our survey, nor did we require back-up documentation or detailed information about the MH teaching they described. It is likely that knowledge of MH offerings varied across informants both within and between medical schools. Some may question the disciplines we listed in our survey as inadequately reflecting the scope of the MH (we included history of medicine and bioethics, but did not include health law, or psychology, or design studies, for example). We did not systematically inquire into the existence of MH working groups or committees, or curriculum representatives at each school (an unfortunate oversight). We recognise that our update is probably already out of date. The perpetual refinement and evolution of MD programmes makes it likely that some curricular contributions are no longer offered, and other MH offerings have been introduced (D'eon and Crawford 2005). While we asked about inter-professional learning opportunities, this review does not cover health humanities (Atkinson et al. 2015) in non-medical health profession educational programmes in Canada. Most importantly, we collected descriptive data that does not relate to factors of quality of provision. For example, in what sense does MH provision at each school lead students to 'think otherwise' or think creatively through appropriate challenge? Also, we did not ask if MH provision might be counterproductive or have unintentional consequences, such as engendering varieties of imperialism, where the MH simply serve the medical enterprise, or reinforce unproductive hierarchies.

Despite these limitations, our review provides an important update on MH teaching at all 17 medical schools in Canada. What implications follow from it? Our findings offer a point of reference for development of the MH globally. What is happening in medical schools worldwide and do MH provisions have local flavours and biases? Our survey offers a template for similar research, for example across medical schools in the USA (143 schools), or in the UK (33 schools with five new schools planned to open by 2021). Importantly, our findings offer a starting point for dialogue, curriculum planning and inquiry by proponents committed to ensuring that medical students are able to provide effective and compassionate care to patients and their families. We recognise the wide diversity of views regarding the MH field (Atkinson et al. 2015; Bleakley 2015), as well as diverse views regarding what might be considered substantive teaching contributions in this area linked to a variety of ways of learning, including the favoured work-based experience. While the former may be considered a strength (Pattison 2003; Campo 2005; Kidd and Connor 2008; Bleakley 2015), we believe it would be helpful to engage in dialogue about 'best practices' to ensure the clarity, purpose and quality of MH education. Given the lack of specificity of our findings, development of a centralised Canadian MH teaching repository (including objectives, outcomes, assessment and related faculty development opportunities) might be pursued to enable MH educators to share the curricula they have developed. Almost all of our informants indicated that they would be interested in contributing to such a database. We also recommend that medical schools consider developing a centralised MH web presence at their school. Reviews by Lam et al. (2015) and others (Brandon 2008; Pask and Brett-Maclean 2011) attest to the level of Canadian student interest in MH teaching.

Increasing critical scholarly activity in this area (Bates, Bleakley and Goodman 2013; Cole, Carlin and Carson 2014; Jones, Wear and Friedman 2014; Bleakley 2015; Whitehead, Woods and Atkinson 2016; Bleakley 2019—this Handbook) suggests the emergence of a burgeoning field with fault-lines. For example, one school of 'critical' medical humanities admits that it is not concerned with applications to medical education, but only with the study of medical culture (Whitehead et al. 2016). While it is difficult to predict how MH pedagogy and scholarship will evolve over the coming years, we anticipate that our findings will be helpful to those involved in advancing the MH globally. We recognise the value of national and international networking, dialogue and formal collaboration.

Delese Wear (2006) has described the contributions of the medical/health humanities in relation to the development of self and sensibility, as learners "move through an increasingly complex life in medicine, examining themselves, their patients, their profession, and the culture in which they serve." Given increasing adoption of a spiral approach (Bruner 1960) to curriculum planning in medical education, involving the "iterative revisiting of topics, subjects or themes . . . with each successive encounter building on the previous one" (Harden and Stamper 1999: 141), we would also encourage inquiry into best practices in creating coordinated, developmental MH curricula that support future practitioners from their pre-medical studies through graduation (Bleakley, Marshall and Brömer 2006)—and beyond.

Acknowledgements

We extend our thanks to all key informants for their time and thoughtful contributions to this review. We also thank all those who have 'gone before us' for their contributions in developing the diverse field of MH.

References

Albert M, Paradis E, Kuper A. Interdisciplinary promises versus practices in medicine: The decoupled experiences of social sciences and humanities scholars. *Social Science & Medicine*. 2015; 126: 17–25.
Alvesson M, Sköldberg K. 2009. *Reflexive methodology: New vistas for qualitative research*. London: Sage.
Association of Faculties of Medicine of Canada. The Future of Medical Education in Canada (FMEC): A collective vision for MD education; 2009. Available at: www.afmc.ca/pdf/fmec/FMEC-MD-2010.pdf. Last accessed March 21, 2016.
Atkinson S, Evans B, Woods A, Kearns R. The 'medical' and 'health' in a critical medical humanities. *Journal of Medical Humanities*. 2015; 36: 71–81.

Bates DG. Humanism in undergraduate medical education. *Canadian Medical Association Journal.* 1971; 105: 258.

Bates V, Bleakley A, Goodman S. 2013. *Medicine, health and the arts: Approaches to the medical humanities.* London: Routledge.

Bleakley A. 2015. *Medical humanities and medical education: How the medical humanities can shape better doctors.* London: Routledge.

Bleakley A, Marshall R, Brömer R. Toward an aesthetic medicine: Developing a core medical humanities undergraduate curriculum. *Journal of Medical Humanities.* 2006; 27: 197–213.

Boudreau JD, Liben S, Fuks A. A faculty development workshop in narrative-based reflective writing. *Perspectives on Medical Education.* 2012; 1: 143–54.

Branch WT. Teaching professional and humanistic values: Suggestion for a practical and theoretical model. *Patient Education and Counseling.* 2015; 98: 162–7.

Brandon N. Reading more into the medical curriculum: The history of literature and medicine teaching in undergraduate medical education at American and Canadian medical schools. 2008. Available at: www.med.uottawa.ca/historyofmedicine/hetenyi/brandon.html#09. Last accessed April 19, 2016.

Bruner JS. 1960. *The process of education.* Cambridge, MA: Harvard University Press.

Campo R. 'The medical humanities,' for lack of a better term. *Journal of the American Medical Association.* 2005; 294: 1009–11.

Cole TR, Carlin NS, Carson RA. 2014. *Medical humanities: An introduction.* Cambridge: Cambridge University Press.

Courneya CA. White coat, warm art. *Ars Medica.* 2011; 8: 81–185.

Cruess RL, Cruess SR, Boudreau JD, et al. Reframing medical education to support professional identity formation. *Academic Medicine.* 2014; 89: 1446–51.

D'eon M, Crawford R. The elusive content of the medical school curriculum: A method to the madness. *Medical Teacher.* 2005; 27: 699–703.

Ellaway RH, Bates A, Girard S, et al. Exploring the consequences of combining medical students with and without a background in biomedical sciences. *Medical Education.* 2014; 48: 674–86.

Glaser BS, Strauss A. 1967. *The discovery of grounded theory: Strategies for qualitative research.* London: Weidenfeld and Nicolson.

Green J, Thorogood N. 2013. *Qualitative methods for health research.* London: Sage.

Harden R, Stamper N. What is a spiral curriculum? *Medical Teacher.* 1999, 21: 141–3.

Holmboe E. Bench to bedside: Medical humanities education and assessment as a translational challenge. *Medical Education.* 2016; 50: 275–8.

Hurwitz B. Medical humanities: Lineage, excursionary sketch and rationale. *Journal of Medical Ethics.* 2013; 39: 672–4.

Jones T, Wear D, Friedman LD. 2014. *Health Humanities Reader.* New Brunswick, NJ: Rutgers University Press.

Kidd MG, Connor JT. Striving to do good things: Teaching humanities in Canadian medical schools. *Journal of Medical Humanities.* 2008; 29: 45–54.

Kuper A. Literature and medicine: A problem of assessment. *Academic Medicine.* 2006; 81: S128–37.

Lam M, Lechner B, Chow R, et al. A review of medical humanities curriculum in medical schools. *Journal of Pain Management.* 2015; 8: 289.

Mykhalovskiy E, Weir L. The problem of evidence-based medicine: Directions for social science. *Social Science & Medicine.* 2004; 59: 1059–69.

Nisker J. There for the grace of our deans go we. Canadian Association for Medical Education (CAME) ACEM Newsletter, Special Conference Edition. 2014; 20: 8–9.

Pask C, Brett-Maclean P. Arts, humanities and social sciences-related activities in Canadian medical schools: A web-based directory listing. Poster presentation, Canadian Conference on Medical Education (CCME), Toronto, ON. 2011, May. (Available from phrett@ualberta.ca).

Pattison S. Medical humanities: A vision and some cautionary notes. *Medical Humanities.* 2003; 29: 33–6.

Peterkin A. Medical humanities for what ails us. *Canadian Medical Association Journal.* 2008; 178: 648.

Russell GM, Kelly NH. Research as an interactive dialogic process: Implications for reflexivity. In Forum Qualitative Sozialforschung/Forum: *Qualitative Social Research.* 2002, Sep. 30 (Vol. 3, No. 3).

Squires BP. The humanities in the general professional education of the physician: Can Canadian schools meet the challenge? *Canadian Medical Association Journal.* 1985; 132: 1000.

Van Wyck HB. The role of the humanities in medical education. *Canadian Medical Association Journal*. 1951; 64: 254–60.

Wald HS, Anthony D, Hutchinson TA, et al. Professional identity formation in medical education for humanistic, resilient physicians: Pedagogic strategies for bridging theory to practice. *Academic Medicine*. 2015; 90: 753–60.

Wear D. Viewpoint: Trends and transitions in the medical humanities. AAMC Reporter: October 2006. Available at: www.aamc.org/newsroom/reporter/oct06/viewpoint.htm. Last accessed August 21, 2018.

Whitehead C. Scientist or science-stuffed? Discourses of science in North American medical education. *Medical Education*. 2013; 47: 26–32.

Whitehead C, Selleger V, Kreeke J, Hodges B. The 'missing person' in roles-based competency models: A historical, cross-national, contrastive case study. *Medical Education*. 2014; 48: 785–95.

Whitehead A, Woods A, Atkinson S (eds.) 2016. *The Edinburgh companion to the critical medical humanities*. Edinburgh: Edinburgh University Press.

Zimmerman T, Marfuggi R. Medical humanities role in medical education. *World Medical & Health Policy*. 2012; 4: 1–11.

Additional recommended reading

Arntfield SL, Slesar K, Dickson J, Charon R. Narrative medicine as a means of training medical students toward residency competencies. *Patient Education and Counseling*. 2013; 91: 280–6.

Boudreau JD, Fuks A. The humanities in medical education: Ways of knowing, doing and being. *Journal of Medical Humanities*. 2015; 36: 321–36.

Brett-Maclean P, Cave MT. Text and context: Involving faculty panelists as models for reflection in a film-based narrative reflective practice module in undergraduate medical education. *Reflective Practice*. 2014; 15: 540–9.

Cox SM, Brett-Maclean P, Courneya CA. My turbinado sugar: Art-making, well-being and professional identity in medical education. *Arts & Health*. 2015; 14: 1–7.

D'Alessandro PR, Frager G. Theatre: An innovative teaching tool integrated into core undergraduate medical curriculum. *Arts & Health*. 2014; 6: 191–204.

de Leeuw S, Parkes MW, Thien D. Questioning medicine's discipline: The art of emotions in undergraduate medical education. *Emotion, Space & Society*. 2014; 11: 43–51.

Dennhardt S, Apramian T, Lingard L, et al. Rethinking research in the medical humanities: A scoping review and narrative synthesis of quantitative outcome studies. *Medical Education*. 2016; 50: 285–99.

Frank C, Martin RE. Humanities and geriatric education: A strategy for recruitment? *Canadian Geriatrics Journal*. 2015; 18: 37.

Hall P, Brajtman S, Weaver L, et al. Learning collaborative teamwork: An argument for incorporating the humanities. *Journal of Interprofessional Care*. 2014; 28: 519–25.

Hazelton L, Delva N. Exploring the intersection of mental health and humanities: The Dalhousie psychiatry student writing competition. *Academic Psychiatry*. 2015; 30: 1–2.

Jones DS, Greene JA, Duffin J, Warner JH. Making the case for history in medical education. *Journal of the History of Medicine and Allied Sciences*. 2015: 70: 623–52.

Kidd M, Nixon L, Rosenal T, et al. Using visual art and collaborative reflection to explore medical attitudes toward vulnerable persons. *Canadian Medical Education Journal*. 2016; 7: 22–30.

Kuper A. The intersubjective and the intrasubjective in the patient–physician dyad: Implications for medical humanities education. *Medical Humanities*. 2007; 33: 75–80.

Kuper A, D'Eon M. Rethinking the basis of medical knowledge. *Medical Education*. 2011; 45: 36–43.

Leichner P, Wieler C. Maladjusted: Participatory theatre about human-centred care. *Arts & Health*. 2015; 7: 75–85.

Martimianakis MA, Michalec B, Lam J, et al. Humanism, the hidden curriculum, and educational reform: A scoping review and thematic analysis. *Academic Medicine*. 2015; 90: S5-13.

McNaughton N. Discourse(s) of emotion within medical education: The ever-present absence. *Medical Education*. 2013; 47: 71–9.

Peterkin A. Curating the medical humanities curriculum: Twelve tips. *Medical Humanities*. 2016; 42: 147–8.

Peterkin A, Brett-Maclean P (eds.) 2016. *Keeping reflection fresh: A practical guide*. Kent, OH: Kent State University Press.

Razack S, Lessard D, Hodges BD, et al. The more it changes, the more it remains the same: A Foucauldian analysis of Canadian policy documents relevant to student selection for medical school. *Advances in Health Sciences Education*. 2014; 19: 161–81.

Ritz SA, Beatty K, Ellaway RH. Accounting for social accountability: Developing critiques of social accountability within medical education. *Education for Health*. 2014; 27: 152.

Whitehead C, Kuper A, Freeman R, et al. Compassionate care? A critical discourse analysis of accreditation standards. *Medical Education*. 2014; 48: 632–43.

Wong A, Trollope-Kumar K. Reflections: An inquiry into medical students' professional identity formation. *Medical Education*. 2014; 48: 489–501.

Zazulak J, Halgren C, Tan M, Grierson LE. The impact of an arts-based programme on the affective and cognitive components of empathic development. *Medical Humanities*. 2015: 41: 69–74.

Appendices

Appendix A

Table A36.1 Medical humanities curricular and co-curricular offerings, by Canadian medical school (2005–2006)[1]

Medical school[2]	MH curricular exposure, by YR[a]	MH disciplines/content[b,c]	Curriculum integration[d]
Alberta, University of	1,2,3,4	Arts—✓ Hum—✓ SS—✓	Required Optional Co-curricular
Calgary, University of[5]	1	Hum—H	Optional Co-curricular
Dalhousie University	?,?,?,?	Arts—✓ Hum—B/P SS—✓	Required Optional
Manitoba, University of	?,?,?,?	Hum—B/P, H SS—HL (1)	Required
McGill University	4	Arts—✓ Hum—✓ SS—✓	Required
McMaster University[3]	?,?,?	Arts—✓ Hum—✓ SS—✓	Required *("but unstructured and tutor-dependent")*
Memorial University of Newfoundland	1,2	Arts—F, L/N Hum—B/P, H SS—HL	Required
Northern Ontario School of Medicine[4]	"Still unfolding"	Hum—H	[Required] [Optional]
Ottawa, University of	1,2	Hum—H	Required Optional
Queen's University	1,2	Arts—L/N Hum—B/P, H SS—HL, HE	· Required Optional
Saskatchewan, University of	1	Hum—B/P SS—✓	Required

(continued)

Table A36.1 (continued)

Medical school[2]	MH curricular exposure, by YR[a]	MH disciplines/content[b,c]	Curriculum integration[d]
British Columbia, University of	1,2	Hum—B/P SS—A	Required
Toronto, University of	1,2	Hum—B/P SS—HL Other—"The Healer's Art" elective	Required Optional
Western University	1,2,4	Arts—CW, F, L/N, T/P Hum—B/P SS—HL	Required Optional

Notes

[1]Extracted from Kidd and Connor's (2008) Table 1, 'Brief program descriptions'; NB: content that did not easily fit within a humanities discipline (e.g., sexual medicine, palliative care) was not included in this summary.

[2]Only 14 medical schools responded to Kidd and Connor's (2008) key informant survey (Université Laval, Université de Sherbrooke and Université de Montréal did not respond).

[3]The University of Calgary and McMaster University have three-year undergraduate medical degree programmes.

[4]The Northern Ontario Medical School had just enrolled its first cohort of students in 2005; Kidd and Connor conducted their interviews between 07/2005 and 01/2006.

Legend

[a]? denotes that while inclusion of medical humanities content was described, it was unclear in which year(s) this occurred.

[b]MH disciplines/course content: (1) Arts—CW: Creative Writing, F: Film, L/N: Literature/Narrative, T/P: Theatre/Performance; (2) Hum (Humanities)—B/P: Bioethics/Philosophy, H: History; (3) SS (Social Sciences)—A: Anthropology, HL: Health Law, HE: Health Economics; ✓ used to denote a global reference to "medical humanities," or "arts, humanities and social sciences."

[c]Curricular integration: Required (courses, lectures, activities); Optional (lectures, electives, activities); Co-curricular (interest/discussion groups, lectures).

Appendix B

Table A36.2 Admissions and medical/health humanities curriculum characteristics by medical school (2014/2015)

Medical school	Open admission?[a]	Curricular exposure[z] by YR	MH disciplines/content[b]	Curriculum integration[c]	Interprof'l learning?	Assessment[d]	Who teaches?	Faculty dev't?	Funding[e]	Website(s) (2016)[f]
Alberta, University of (n=2 respondents)[1]	Yes	1,2,3,4	Arts—CW, F, L/N, R, T/P, VA; Hum—B/P, H, S; SS—A, S; Other—White Coat Ceremony, Health Design	Core Curriculum—M, O; Elective—S, L	Yes	Production Feedback T/Exam Attendance	MDs, Other health professionals, PhDs, Artists, Other—Patients	Yes	Internal External Donations, volunteers	www.med.ualberta.ca/programs/ahhm www.bioethics.ualberta.ca www.med.ualberta.ca/communities/hom
Calgary, University of[2] (n=2)	Yes	1,2*,4	Arts—CW, F, L/N, R, T/P, VA*; Hum—B/P, H; SS—A*, S*	Core Curriculum—M, O; Elective—S; Other—Guide to humanities teaching resource	Yes	Production Feedback Attendance	MDs, Other health professionals, PhDs, Artists	Yes	Internal Donations, volunteers*	www.ucalgary.ca/healthhumanities https://hom.ucalgary.ca
Dalhousie University (n=1)	Yes	1	Arts—L/N, T/P; Hum—B/P, H	Core Curriculum—M, O; Elective—S	Yes	Production T/Exam Attendance	MDs, Artists	No	External	http://humanities.medicine.dal.ca
Laval, Université[3] (n=1)	No	1,2	Arts—L/N, R, VA; Hum—B/P	Core Curriculum—M, O; Elective—S	No	Production Feedback	MDs, PhDs	No	. . . None reported	
Manitoba, University of (n=1)	Yes	1,2,3,4	Arts—F, L/N, R, VA; Hum—B/P, H, S; SS—S	Core Curriculum—M	Yes	Production Feedback Attendance	MDs, Artists	Yes	Internal Donations, volunteers	
McGill University[3] (n=2)[d]	Yes	1,2,3,4	Arts—L/N*, R; Hum—B/P*, H*; SS—A*, S	Core Curriculum—M, O*; Elective—S*	Yes*	Production T/Exam Attendance	MDs, PhDs	Yes	Internal* Donations, volunteers*	www.mcgill.ca/ssom
McMaster University[2] (n=2)	Yes*	1,2*	Arts—CW*, L/N, R, T/P*, VA*; Hum—B/P, H*, S*; SS—A*	Core Curriculum—M; Electives—S*, L*	Yes*	Feedback Attendance*	MDs, Other health professionals,* PhDs*	Yes	Internal* Donations, volunteers*	
Memorial University of Neufoundland (n=2)	Yes	1,2,3*	Arts—F*, L/N, R, T/P*, VA*; Hum—B/P*, H; SS—S*; Other—White Coat Ceremony	Core Curriculum—M, O*; Elective—S*	Yes	Production* Feedback Attendance*	PhDs, Artists*	No	External	www.med.mun.ca/CommunityHealth

(continued)

Table A36.2 (continued)

Medical school	Open admission?[a]	Curricular exposure,[a] by YR	MH disciplines/content[b]	Curriculum integration[c]	Interprof'l learning?	Assessment[d]	Who teaches?	Faculty dev't?	Funding[e]	Website(s) [2016][f]
Montréal, Université de[3] (n=1)	Yes	1,2,3,4	Arts—R, Hum—B/P, H, SS—S, Other—Mindfulness	Core Curriculum—M, O; Elective—S	Yes	Feedback, T/Exam, Attendance	MDs, Other health professionals, Other—Patients	Yes	. . . None reported	http://medecine.umontreal.ca/faculte/direction-collaboration-partenariat-patient http://medecine.umontreal.ca/faculte/medecine/bureau-de-lethique-clinique
Northern Ontario School of Medicine (n=1)	Yes	1,2,3,4	Hum—B/P, H,S, SS—A, S	Core Curriculum—M, O	Yes	Production, T/Exam, Feedback, Attendance	MDs, Other health professionals, PhDs, Other—Patients, Elders	Unknown	Unknown	
Ottawa, University of (n=2)	Yes	1,2,3,4*	Arts—CW*, D*, F, L/N, M*, R*, VA; Hum—B/P, H; SS—S*; Other—Mindfulness*	Core Curriculum—M, O*; Electives—S, L; Other—Certificate option	Yes	Production*, Feedback, T/Exam*, Attendance	MDs, Other health professionals, PhDs,* Artists	Yes	Internal	http://med.uottawa.ca/department-innovation/education-and-training/medicine-and-humanities-program
Queen's University (n=2)	Yes	1,2*,3*,4*	Arts—CW*, F*, L/N, M*, R, T/P*, VA*; Hum—B/P, H, S; SS—S*; Other—Health Law*	Core Curriculum—M, O*; Electives—S, L*	Yes*	Production, Feedback, T/Exam, Attendance*	MDs, PhDs*, Other*—Lawyers, Librarian	Yes*	Internal, External*, Donations, volunteers*	http://meds.queensu.ca/medicine/histm/core.html http://post.queensu.ca/~forsdyke/john_austin_society.htm
Saskatchewan, University of (n=1)	Yes*	1	Arts—CW, L/N, M, R*, T/P, VA (6); Hum—B/P, H, S*; SS—A*, S*	Core Curriculum—M	Yes	Production, Feedback*, Attendance*	MDs, PhDs, Artists*	No	Internal	https://medicine.usask.ca/department/clinical/surgery-pages/surgicalhumanities.php
Sherbrooke, Université de[3] (n=1)	No	1,2,3,4	Arts—R, Hum—B/P, H	Core Curriculum—M	Yes	Feedback, T/Exam	MDs, Other health professionals	Yes	Internal	
British Columbia, University of (n=1)	Yes	1,2,4	Arts—L/N, R, VA; Hum—B/P, H, S	Core Curriculum—M, O; Electives—S	Yes	Feedback, T/Exam, Attendance	MDs, Other health professionals, PhDs, Artists	No	External	http://heartfelt.med.ubc.ca

School	Open admission[a]		MH discipline/course content[b]	Curricular integration[c]	Assessment[d]		People		Funding[e]	Website(s)[f]
Toronto, University of (n=2)	No	1,2,3,4	Arts—CW, F, L/N, M*, R, T/P, VA Hum—B/P, H, S* SS—A*, S	Core Curriculum—M*, O Electives—S*, L Other—*Certificate option; curated narrative medicine content (upon request)*	Yes	Production* Feedback T/Exam* Attendance	MDs, Other health professionals, Artists	Yes	Internal	http://health-humanities.com
Western University (n=2)	Yes	1,2,3,4	Arts—F*, L/N, R Hum—B/P, H*	Core Curriculum—M Electives—S*	Yes	Production Feedback T/Exam* Attendance	MDs, Other health professionals*, PhDs*	Yes	Internal *External*	http://narrativemedicineatwestern.ca

Notes

[1] n=2 faculty members collaboratively responded to, and submitted a single survey.

[2] The University of Calgary and McMaster University have three-year undergraduate medical degree programmes.

[3] In Quebec, students can apply to medical school directly after completing CEGEP (undergraduate study in science or another area of study is not required).

[4] When two faculty members from the same medical school completed separate online surveys, all positive endorsements were recorded (it was assumed that key informants would likely have knowledge of different educational offerings at their medical school); the symbol * denotes a positive response endorsed by only one of the key informants in these cases.

Legend

[a] Open admission: 'Yes' indicates the key informant(s) described policies and procedures at their medical school which supported admission of students across a range of disciplines (and not exclusively those who majored in science).

[b] MH discipline/course content codes: (1) Arts—CW: Creative Writing, D: Dance, F: Film, L/N: Literature/Narrative, M: Music, R: Reflective Exercises, T/P: Theatre/Performance, VA: Visual Art; (2) Hum (Humanities)—B/P: Bioethics/Philosophy, H: History, S: Spirituality; (3) SS (Social Sciences)—A: Anthropology, S: Sociology.

[c] Curricular integration: (1) Core Curriculum—M: Mandatory, or O: Optional (lectures, seminars, small group sessions, assignment or activity); (2) Elective—S: Stand-alone (time-limited/one-off); L: Longitudinal.

[d] Assessment: *1) Attendance—pass/fail based on attendance; (2) T/Exam—tests/examination: to assess recall of facts/concepts; (3) Feedback—via evaluation forms, rubrics, written feedback and discussion (including peer assessment): to assess understanding, directed to enhancing skill/ability in applying understanding in new situations; (4) Production—submission of creative work, essays, portfolios, presentations, etc.: providing evidence of application of, or opportunity to extend learning (new insights).

[e] Funding: (1) Internal—dedicated and ad hoc, via UME programme or course funding (in support of humanities programming, faculty leads, etc.); (2) External—endowed grants, research funding; (3) Donations, Volunteers—including active fundraising and fund development efforts.

[f] Website(s): Several key informants described plans for introducing an online presence within or linked to their medical school's website, when they responded to this survey question. MH-related URLs listed in this column include both those provided by key informants (n=9), as well as eight additional URLs we identified when we subsequently scanned the websites of all 17 medical schools in April 2016 (the latter set included URLs associated with both new as well as long-established websites).

Appendix C

Table A36.3 Medical/health humanities co-curricular opportunities by medical school (2014/2015)

Medical school	Interest/study groups[a]	Performances, art shows, etc.[b]	Blogs, Websites, publications	Lectures, workshops[c]	Conferences	Research	Awards/contests
Alberta, University of (n=2 respondents)[1]	✓	✓	✓	✓	✓	✓	✓
Calgary, University of (n=2)	✓*,[2]		✓	✓	✓	✓	✓*
Dalhousie University (n=1)			✓	✓		✓	✓
Laval, Université (n=1)	✓				✓		
Manitoba, University of (n=1)	✓	✓					✓
McGill University (n=2)[d]	✓*					✓	✓*
McMaster University (n=2)	✓				✓*		
Memorial University of Newfoundland (n=2)	✓	✓*	✓	✓	✓*	✓	✓*
Montréal, Université de (n=1)						✓	

Medical School						
Northern Ontario School of Medicine (n=1)			✓	✓		✓
Ottawa, University of (n=2)	✓*	✓*	✓	✓		✓
Queen's University (n=2)	✓*	✓*	✓*	✓*	✓*	✓*
Saskatchewan, University of (n=1)	✓*	✓*	✓*	✓	✓*	✓
Sherbrooke, Université de (n=1)	✓	✓	✓		✓	✓
British Columbia, University of (n=1)			✓	✓	✓	✓
Toronto, University of (n=2)	✓*	✓	✓	✓	✓	✓*
Western University (n=2)	✓*	✓	✓*	✓*	✓*	✓*

Notes

[1] n=2 faculty members collaboratively responded to and submitted a single survey.

[2] When two faculty members from the same medical school completed separate online surveys, all positive endorsements were recorded (it was assumed that key informants would likely have knowledge of different educational offerings at their medical school); the symbol * denotes a positive response endorsed by only one of the key informants in these cases.

Legend

[a] Includes ongoing groups, including, book and journal clubs, etc.

[b] Includes art shows, musical/theatrical performances (choirs/bands), literary readings, spoken word events, etc.

[c] Stand-alone, optional; workshops including content focused on visual, literary and other MH-related topics.

PART VII

The patient will see you now

37

CAN WE MAKE EMPATHY MORE INTELLIGENT? TRY SOCIAL EMPATHY!

Caroline Wellbery

In his essay 'The woman in the mirror,' Frank Huyler (2013) describes his encounter with a hostile patient in the emergency room. The patient is drunk, homeless, and seriously ill—the kind of patient health care professionals receive with dread. Empathy for the patient, the supposed lubricant of medical interactions, is glaringly absent. And yet, this should not limit the physician's ability to act. There are times, Huyler concludes, when we must provide the best possible care even when we feel no empathy whatsoever. Although Huyler makes no mention in his essay of Paul Bloom (2016), Jesse Prinz (2011) or social psychologists, moral philosophers and others who have written critically of empathy, he is tapping into an intriguing 'anti-empathy' discourse that has recently flared in the popular press as well as in the academic literature.

The notion of being 'against empathy' is provocative, to say the least, but all that is meant (to sum up Bloom's argument in a nutshell) is that empathy is just another vehicle for bias, and may be particularly dangerous because it encourages us to feel good about ourselves while flagrantly and unfairly favouring the individuals or groups we prefer. The converse, dismissing those with whom we cannot identify, is equally a manifestation of empathy's distortions. In its starkest form, this bias manifests as a national crisis when a blonde teenager is kidnapped in Aruba, and, when empathy is absent, as relative indifference to a gang shooting in a societally neglected part of town. Empathy, insofar as it is defined as imagining 'walking in another person's shoes,' Bloom and others argue, so often goes terribly awry: it is parochial, tribal and irrational. Imagining ourselves in another's shoes has its limits. As human beings we are unable in fact to imagine very much, for example the encampment experience of thousands of refugees, or even the specific sufferings of an aged heroin addict in downtown Detroit. We are much more likely to empathise with someone we know, recognise and love; someone who is just like us. Empathy, therefore, is not a helpful way to achieve social justice.

Might Bloom's perspective on empathy be different as it applies to medicine? After all, the literature in medical journals abounds with studies, reflections and exhortations, all focused on empathy (Decety and Fotopoulou 2014). Further, regardless of how empathy is operationalised, it does seem that empathy has an important role in caring for both the engaged clinician and her patients (Mercer and Reynolds 2002; Rakel et al. 2009; Hojat et al. 2011; Lown 2016; Derksen et al. 2013). Empathy in fact is regarded as a healing modality in its own right, not just as a means of facilitating practical outcomes such as the patient's acceptance of, say, complex, difficult or unpleasant therapies (Kelley et al. 2014; Decety and Fotopoulou 2014).

I argue that the limitations of empathy Bloom and others describe are relevant to medical education insofar as clinical practice has typically focused on individual care, whereas now, in a volatile, changing global environment, both education and practice are facing new, societally challenging, morally engulfing and health threatening realities (Westerhaus et al. 2015; Kasper et al. 2016). So, while much has been written on the beneficial effects of empathy, its tribal and prejudicial tendencies need to be acknowledged and addressed. Being *against* empathy in the medical setting may seem like madness, but understanding what is wrong with empathy at least can force us to rethink empathy in the context of social and global turmoil. The argument for an empathic expansion of empathy for the greater good is not new (Frazer 2010). Given medical educators' increasing awareness of health disparities and interest in population health (Sklar 2018), it is time for medical educators to inquire into whether fostering *social* empathy might counteract the implicit and explicit biases of *individual* empathy.

But precisely what is empathy? Empathy is as often defined within a cluster of closely allied but distinct concepts such as compassion, sympathy, empathic concern and emotional contagion (Bloom 2016; Jeffrey 2016; Perez-Bret et al. 2016; Segal et al. 2017). It overlaps with 'kindness' and 'love.' Each of these is defined (often inconsistently across the literature) along a spectrum of emotion, cognitive apprehension and even behaviour, sometimes including all three dimensions (Mercer and Reynolds 2002; Marshall and Bleakley 2009; Sulzer et al. 2016).

Most frequently applied is this definition from Hojat: "Empathy in the context of patient care is . . . a predominantly cognitive attribute that involves an understanding of the patient's experiences, *concerns*, and perspectives, combined with a capacity to communicate this understanding *and an intention to help*" (Hojat 2016) [the italicised text refers to additions to an early 2002 definition (Hojat et al. 2002); in that definition the modifier 'inner' describing the 'patient's experience' was removed]. Empathy has also been characterised as a "resonance" (Shapiro 2011), "compassionate solidarity" (Misra-Hebert et al. 2012) and the capacity to be moved by another's experiences (Halpern 2003). In yet another definition, empathy is described as an engaged act in which "the physician must draw closer to the patient, putting the interests of other above those of self, even at some sacrifice to oneself" (Shapiro 2008).

What's not to like about these generous impulses? None of the definitions I have cited overcome Bloom's argument that empathy is innumerate, racist, sexist and otherwise biased. It is therefore quite possible that, even in medicine, empathy is subject to such distortions. In the medical literature, empathy has typically focused on the self-contained dyad between doctor and patient (Prinz 2011). Clinical empathy is not designed to integrate the unrecognised contextual circumstances of the encounter that inform our biases. And this leads potentially to preferential treatments for certain kinds of patients.

Richard McCann, an early recipient of a liver transplant at Georgetown University Medical Center, has spoken eloquently of keeping himself well informed about his illness, deliberately so, in order to ensure his doctor's full engagement with his particular case. McCann describes himself as wearing a silver medical alert bracelet so that in the event of an emergency, he will be perceived as someone who values himself enough to convey more than just medical information. This fine bracelet will alert his rescuers to his character, one worthy of saving if found in a coma (McCann, personal communication 2006). All McCann's self-conscious observations are geared towards eliciting empathy because, as a patient, McCann knows that empathy is necessary in order to stoke his doctor's commitment and thereby to motivate her to meet his medical and psychological needs. And no wonder, as any patient stuck with illness can attest, the pain of irrelevance to one's physician is often equal to the pain of ill health itself.

This is precisely where Bloom and colleagues locate empathy's flaws. McCann's charming manipulations show an acute awareness that empathy is biased: it is biased towards those who are 'the same' (McCann's stuffing himself with medical knowledge so that he can present himself as someone almost akin to a medical peer) and those with shared social status (McCann's silver bracelet connoting both economic worthiness and self-respect). But when it comes to individuals who do not meet those standards, individuals who smell bad, who are incontinent of their emotions, who have no resources—these individuals are at risk of garnering less respect, less attention, less effort. They might even generate, in Huyler's words, "no empathy whatsoever."

The problem of empathy may be, as Paul Bloom (2016) flat-out states, that it is stupid. "My Christ, they are dumb," Sharon Olds says of her breasts, still singing for the husband who abandoned her; "They do not even know they are mortal" (Olds 1999). Empathy, in other words, does not reflect on where it comes from. In spite of its apparent focus on the individual, it reflects moral, social and political biases, often channelled without self-reflection to produce the identifications or aversions just described. But if one recasts empathy as a social phenomenon, one that is complexly informed by group norms and societal values, perhaps it is possible to educate empathy, to make it less stupid while retaining those qualities of connectedness so important to medical practice. Of note, this infusion of consciousness may push empathy into another definitional domain. Educating empathy may, once it is made sufficiently self-aware, find itself transformed into something else altogether (Decety and Cowell 2014; Morgan 2017).

Empathy that incorporates social knowledge engages reason to determine what the morally justified plan of action might be. This "human capacity of enlarged sympathy" (*Internet Encyclopedia of Philosophy* 2018) has been variously incorporated into definitions of cognitive empathy, social empathy and even reaches towards anti-empathy's bastion of hope, 'moral reasoning' (*Stanford Encyclopedia of Philosophy* 2013; Bloom 2016; Segal et al. 2017).

An educated empathy not only recognises the forces that shape it, but also those that prevent it from achieving its purported well-intentioned aims. We cannot understand the limitations of empathy without understanding its systematic subversion by our medical institutions. On the one hand, there may be (but no guarantees) the caring doctor who expresses empathy in Hojat's nuanced definition cited above. On the other, the bureaucratic, impenetrable sprawl of institutional medicine threatens to engulf even the most empathic caregiver.

Take McCann's experience during his initial intake in 1991 as a candidate for a then experimental protocol used to treat hepatitis C (McCann 2005). The study nurse asks his age, occupation, HIV status and family history. "Then," McCann states, "she asked the question that I'd already known to dread: 'What were my known risk factors for HCV?'" After some embarrassed hemming and hawing, he reluctantly admits having once used intravenous drugs. "Recreationally," he quickly adds. Then he goes on to say:

> The nurse looked at me, then looked down at her desk, picked up a rubber stamp and stamped both sides of my folder in red ink: IVDU (intravenous drug user). At that moment I realised I was no longer a university professor, I was no longer the gentleman known as Richard McCann, I was no longer a writer, I was no longer even the most broadest of categories, a white male. I was IVDU. And she gave me the folder and told me to report upstairs to the gastroenterologists' suite. And as I rose in the elevator floor after floor holding my folder, I saw people looking at it. '*Who's he,*' they thought. 'Oh, IVDU, IVDU.'

Nothing, in my mind more poignantly illustrates the codified empathy antagonism inscribed in institutional protocols. To be sure, such practices as the one proclaiming McCann as an illicit drug user were ultimately banned. But one could argue that one bureaucratic solution merely generates another, equally bureaucratic, problem. For example, the new HIPAA rules

(Health Insurance Portability and Accountability Act—itself a bureaucratic mouthful), instituted in 1996 to protect patients' personal information, levelled a new strike against institutional empathy, at least metaphorically speaking, in that HIPAA isolates each patient within the protective walls of his or her privacy bubble.[1]

The anti-empathy movement, then, may not be so much against empathy but against the morally questionable exclusions of empathy. Those exclusions erasures occur both individually and institutionally, but are most dangerous, or at best most unpalatable, when institutional practices swallow up or suppress empathy's 'intentions to help.' My position is that, as healthcare educators, to educate empathy—that is, make empathy less stupid—we must address it at the structural level (Kumagai 2008; Pedersen and Pope 2010; Sharma et al. 2018). We must integrate our benevolence towards individuals within a benevolent institutional framework; that is, situate empathy within a framework of institutional values that support the pursuit of social justice on a larger scale.

The medical humanities are in this respect a fruitful and necessary, if not sufficient, starting point (Decety and Yoder 2016). In using the term 'medical humanities' I include the very chapter I am writing, but by virtue of my education, I am actually most interested in the humanities' less discursive products: literature, visual art, performance and the like, that may be mobilised in an educational setting to encourage open-ended reflection on the practice of medicine, including, literally, the practice of empathy. I single out the arts because, as theorists have long noted, the arts represent the general through the particular, and thus model empathy's full potential by providing an opportunity to extrapolate from concrete experience to its broader contexts.

Literature and the arts provide more than an educational lesson; they are experiential, often in an oddly communal way. The arts illuminate larger meanings by creating amongst spectators (or readers) a bonding experience. The *New York Times* recently referenced an unpublished study that purportedly showed the synchronisation of heartbeats amongst audience members during a live theatre performance, citing the study's investigator, Joe Devlin: "Experiencing the live theater performance was extraordinary enough to overcome group differences and produces a common physiological experience" (Akhtar 2017). Well prior to Theodor Lipps' exploration of *Einfühlung* (*Stanford Encyclopedia of Philosophy* 2013), the German word for empathy that means variably to 'feel as one' or to feel 'within' the other, the German dramatist G.E. Lessing wrestled down the term *Mitleid* (based on Aristotle's terms 'pity' and 'fear'), to mean a 'feeling' and an 'awareness' that had the power to unite people through shared experience, allowing them to recognise themselves as part of an 'ultimate' human community (Böhler 1975). Lessing's concept of *Mitleid*—as he applied it to tragedy—may invoke the days following the real-life tragedy of 9/11, truly implicating large swathes of the US population in a collective experience of fear and commiseration. One subjective piece of evidence for this: for days after the catastrophe, traffic slowed, no drivers honked horns at the other, no one ran a red light.

Of course, Lessing was not thinking directly about the capacity of real-life catastrophes to bring people together. But he was hoping for such an effect through dramatic performance. Literature and the arts, in other words, are most fascinatingly suited to bridging the gap between individual experience and social empathy. Specifically, pictures, stories and performances project the imagined self into the locus of indignities, suffering and marginalisation of social groups, societies and even nations. There is plenty of evidence for this. For example, according to a recent study on journalistic writing, narratives used to communicate news stories were more effective in engaging subjects compared with non-narrative modalities, where: "Narrative-formatted stories produce more compassion toward the individuals in the story, more favorable attitudes toward the group, more beneficial behavioral intentions, and more information-seeking behavior" (Oliver 2012: 205).

Susan Sontag's extraordinary treatise regarding the pain of others, while warning of voyeur-ism and jadedness associated with story-telling news images, makes a powerful case for the latter's undeniable, politically game-changing impact (Sontag 2003). More particularly focused on medical science, Meisel and Karlawish (2011) argue that narratives should be an integral part of scientific communication, citing studies showing their positive effect on health behaviour and persuasiveness in "overcoming preconceived beliefs and cognitive biases." The mechanism of this persuasiveness sounds suspiciously like empathy, and indeed, Kidd and Castano's (2013) seminal study shows that reading literature increases empathy. But I would like to chime in with Meisel and Karlawish (2011) by suggesting that artistic works and performances engage empathy while doing something more—that is, interrogating the context in which empathy arises. This context includes the societal conditions that define the perimeter of empathy itself, which I call the 'edges of empathy.'

A medical humanities teaching agenda focused on the 'edges of empathy' should begin with an investigation of the complexities of individual empathy. Artistic sources that thema-tise empathy as a challenge include Fildes' iconic painting 'The doctor' which, when taught in conjunction with John Stone's poem, 'Talking to the family,' allows students to compare conventional, sentimentalised gestures (leaning forward) with more ambiguous ones (donning vs. removing a white coat) and to extract nuanced definitions of empathy within the frame-work of emotion, duty and uncertainty. Observing Bruno Perillo's painting 'Hoping for Plan C' can lead to a useful exploration of empathy as the superposition of different agendas—in the case of Perillo's painting, the artist conflates the different perspectives of a man and a woman in response to an unwanted pregnancy, as indicated by the emergency contraception packet in the subject's left hand (Wellbery 2010). The resulting image of a blended transgendered figure holding a card that says 'Plan B' then evokes *reductio ad absurdum* the desire for a plan C that alternatively undermines or supports the supposed empathic compromise.

'Edges of empathy' should also incorporate the medical humanities in order to examine precisely in what ways empathy exerts social constraints, facilitates conversations, consolidates individual or tribal interests, or lends itself to moral regulation. For example, students reading Patrick Süskind's (1991) novel *Perfume* can explore the margins of empathy, its absence and its excesses, in defining societal belonging. Empathy, metaphorically represented through human scent, is configured as a highly restrictive socialising force. Yet without the human perfume (manufactured by the novel's central character from cheese, cat excrement and vinegar) the individual remains a marginalised, animal-like non-entity. Another fictional work, *Two Old Women*, also explores the social volatility of empathy, which is no longer useful when it exceeds the utilitarian interests of the group (Wallis 1993). Anticipating a harsh winter, an Alaskan tribe abandons two of its members to fend for themselves. Furious at being abandoned, the two women resolve to fight for their lives. Together they make it through the miserable winter and are reunited with their tribe in the spring. Their fellows are overjoyed to see them, but that does not negate the fact that the two women were rejected as an 'out-group' threatening 'in-group' survival. As another parable, this story shows that tribal empathy quickly gives rise to exclusions when the integrity of the whole is under threat. In both of these literary examples, empathy is a tool that carves out a narrow space between social integration and disintegration.

These examples support a reflective approach to empathy that should be pursued in the con-text of philosophical, historical and psychological readings (including from the anti-empathy court) of empathy. In order to stick, this interdisciplinary approach is best woven into the institutional culture not only through reflective exercise, seminar, conference or lecture series, but also through institutional actions that include top-down interventions, bringing in, for example, storytellers from marginalised groups, or sponsoring workshops on public narratives

(Ganz 2008). Medical schools might portray images in communal spaces representing all walks of life (Wellbery and Mishori, submitted) and incorporate reflection-provoking exercises in basic and clinical sciences courses.

Activities such as these converge on the premise that the pursuit of empathy—insofar as empathy remains a usable, well-examined term—must be grounded in social values. If 'putting oneself in another's shoes' is no longer sufficient for today's complex, global and unstable society, then perhaps we should contemplate shoes in their plurality, for example Gyula Pauer's and Can Toga's bronze cast 'Shoes on the Danube,' representing Jews in Budapest executed by firing squad before being thrown into the river (Shoes on the Danube Bank 2018). The idea of a 'social empathy' that connects individual empathy reflectively to a larger context, although not new, is now surely ripe for renewal.

And for this to occur, we need to confront the anti-empathy discourse, which emphasises not only the neural basis of pro-social behaviour but also its purely rational (as opposed to empathic) underpinnings. According to some neuro-imaging evidence, distinct cognitively associated regions in the brain are implicated in perceptions of social justice (Decety and Yoder 2016; Jordan et al. 2016). I prefer to distance myself somewhat from these efforts to correlate socially observed phenomena with anatomical sites, akin to searches for the exact location of the soul. Instead, I favour a more dynamic bio-metaphorical model. The different components of empathy are both independent and interdependent (Kanske et al. 2016). It is not as though these different regions in the brain do not talk to each other; they are connected networks. In other words, the neuro-biological circuitry becomes a metaphorical representation of what we experience rather imperfectly as we struggle through our various definitions of empathy, and their complex relationships with morality (Singer and Lamm 2009).

No one has done more to translate these bio-metaphorical neural networks into an orderly progression than Elizabeth Segal, who makes clear distinctions among the different components of empathy, and shows how social empathy builds on individual empathy. Her work presents a highly nuanced step-wise, multi-modal definition of individual empathy, including at its most primitive level an affective response, and at its most refined level emotional regulation (Segal et al. 2017). She then goes on to coin, define and operationalise the term "social empathy," composed of two categories: "contextual understanding" and "macro self-other awareness/perspective-taking" (Segal et al. 2017).

In a recent study combining a survey and a reflective essay assignment, we explored the interconnection of Segal's individual and social empathy categories. We found that students linked personally experienced emotional empathy to a broader concern for social groups, suggesting that emotional empathy, insofar as it becomes the object of reflection, can lead to social empathy, with its open lens (Wellbery et al. 2017). At the same time, the students' essays also characterised individual and social empathy as independent entities, making room for a distinction between affective affinity for one person and moral obligation towards a broader social group.

More importantly, the quantitative portion of our study determined that social empathy can be taught. Despite high initial social empathy scores in response to Segal's survey instrument, the Social Empathy Index (Segal et al. 2012), we still found a statistically significant increase in one of the two aforementioned social empathy domains after the students had undergone a course on the social determinants of health. This finding coincides with published evidence on the malleability of empathy generally. One excellent summary of a sequential series of studies shows subjects' ability to increase their empathy based on whether they believe empathy is learnable (Schumann et al. 2014). Further work on the feasibility and durability of teaching social empathy has become an urgent (and resurgent) challenge of our times (Baernstein 2006; Batt-Rawden et al. 2013; Chen and Forbes 2014).

Finally, I need to highlight and clarify a few points. Dyadic clinical empathy is important. This is because besides being sacrosanct as a value, the doctor–patient relationship has been shown to be emotionally powerful and healing, as mentioned earlier. Indeed, "there is solid and accumulative evidence that all facets of empathy play an important role in medical practice and have an impact on both the patient and his/her physician" (Decety and Fotopoulou 2014). Still, without critical self-reflection, individual empathy risks being not just tendentious, but somewhat self-deceiving, as Jane MacNaughton (2009: 1940) explains in 'The dangerous practice of empathy':

> I can be close to tears with a patient, but 10 minutes later engage in a light-hearted conversation with a colleague over coffee. The sadness, or fear, or whatever feeling I have experienced is not sustained, and is so different from what the patient is feeling that it seems disrespectful to suggest that I somehow participate in his or her experience.

This same idea—of honouring another's experience without laying hegemonic claim to understanding—surfaces in a student's succinct comment noted in our study: "While medicine does stress empathizing with patients, sometimes it is impossible to understand what some people have gone through and who am I to judge?" (Wellbery et al. 2017). Recognising the limits of one's own emotional response may be the way forward in embracing the possibilities of a more rationally guided, morally informed compassion. This is why the multi-component laddered definitions of empathy and the incorporation of social empathy are so important.

But even with skilful parsing of all the dimensions of empathy, as in the work of Segal and her predecessors, the self-conscious progressive integration of reflection and rationality that I advocate here may itself not be a panacea. Institutions must embody the values they purport to embrace, but who decides what these values are? Bloom (2016) assumes that we all know what is fair—unbiased, egalitarian—and that such fairness can be (better) achieved when we leave our empathic impulses behind. I am concerned that this may be just another means of 'kicking the can down the road.' I am not a moral philosopher, but as an observer of our society in its current divisive state, it seems clear that the values espoused by different institutions and even within institutions are as variable as constructs of empathy.

In his TED talk Robert Willer (2016) suggests that: "the political divide in our country is undergirded by an underlying moral divide." Drawing on the work of Jon Haidt and Jesse Graham, Willer argues that while liberals are concerned with equality, fairness, care and protection, conservatives are driven by values such as loyalty, authority and moral purity. Such arguments are potentially just as tribal as emotions, which represent among individuals the same deeply held beliefs as that of their political affiliates. As Willer says: "People are willing to fight and die for their values"; that is, to sacrifice the individual self for a larger principle. It seems to me that in the anti-empathy discourse, this intertwining of emotions, beliefs, values and moral arguments is insufficiently addressed. Bloom (2016) makes a fatal error in his crusade for rationalism by claiming that his solution concerns only what individuals can reasonably control, while his entire argument against empathy has relied on an attack against empathy's inability or uneducable unwillingness to countenance the very unfairness in the world about which we can do little or nothing.

My own argument remains that we should not get rid of empathy but make it smarter. Social empathy means explicitly exploring the roots of partisanship and identifying proven methods of broadening medical learners' moral compasses. These might include strategies for moral enhancement. Interestingly, some approaches to moral enhancement, rather than attempting to augment appreciation of others, suggest *diminishing* self-interest (Ahlskog 2017) and *reducing* empathy for one's own in-group (Weisz and Zaki 2018). These sorts of strategies may be consistent with Buddhist-based mindfulness modalities emphasising 'lovingkindness' and 'not-self,' whisking us away, once more, from the individual as fulcrum of empathy to something both more dissolving and encompassing.

For moral enhancement interventions to be successful, some sort of preparatory intervention would presumably be necessary, such as education on the malleability (teachability) of social empathy, building on previous studies focused on teaching individual empathy but more fundamentally on those connecting empathy theory, empathic effort and empathic change (Schumann et al. 2014). An important argument for the meaningfulness (and fairness, if that word can even any longer be used fairly, given its politicisation) of institutional conversations involving differently positioned participants is that they take place in public forums, thus transcending the monadic limitations of individual empathy (Ganz 2008). The medical humanities have enormous potential to generate just such ecumenical discussions, as the reflective essay portion of our social empathy study showed, but this potential requires more explicit emphasis on how experience at the granular, individual level is embedded in a social context.

In summary, while empathy manifested in the context of the traditional doctor–patient dyad is subject to the argument that empathy potentiates bias, a reasoned, socially mediated recasting of empathy may yield new possibilities for today's trainees. For those interested in the medical humanities, the role of narratives and other arts modalities as a means of incubating social empathy is gaining traction, at least at our institution where the medical humanities have increasingly found their home in our office of diversity and inclusion. The arts and humanities, in the context of other teaching, have the power to foster a broader, more socially responsible and socially conscious awareness, and if they are housed in an institutionally sanctioned programme, their message diffuses into the culture; conversely, they can be a means of clarifying the culture's message in dynamic attunement to institutional change.

Note

1 With reams of electronic safeguards decreasing access to all but the most tech-savvy patients, we are a far cry from what my colleague Jay Siwek experienced during a three-month sabbatical in the UK to study geriatrics in the mid-1980s (personal communication). In his tour of hospitals, he noted that:

- many of the patients were on open wards, with maybe 20 beds in two rows of 10 in a very large ward/room/space.
- most of the patients were dressed in their street clothes.
- most were not in bed; they were sitting in a chair, or milling about.
- there were mementos, newspapers, etc.
- when tea was served in the late afternoon, everything would stop: the nurse would push the tea cart between the rows of beds, and dispense tea and biscuits to all; the medical staff would stop and participate.
- the atmosphere/feeling was a lot more personal and equal, rather than hierarchical.

References

Ahlskog R. Moral Enhancement Should Target Self-Interest and Cognitive Capacity. *Neuroethics*. 2017; 10: 363–73.

Akhtar A. An Antidote to Digital Dehumanization? Live Theater. *New York Times*. 29 December 2017. Available at: www.nytimes.com/2017/12/29/theater/ayad-akhtar-steinberg-award-digital-dehumanization-live-theater.html. Last accessed: 13 February 2018.

Baernstein SK. Educating for Empathy. *Journal of General Internal Medicine*. 2006; 21: 524–30.

Batt-Rawden SA, et al. Teaching Empathy to Medical Students: An Updated, Systematic Review. *Academic Medicine*. 2013; 88: 1171–7.

Bloom P. 2016. *Against Empathy*. New York, NY: Harper-Collins.

Böhler M. 1975. Mitleid als sozialisierungsaffekt. In: *Soziale Rolle und aesthetische Vermittlung. Studien zur Literaturtheorie von Baumgarten bis F. Schiller*. Verlag Herbert Lang: Bern, Frankfurt, 166–84.

Chen S, Forbes C. Reflective Writing and Its Impact on Empathy in Medical Education: Systematic Review. *Journal of Educational Evaluation for Health Professions*. 2014; 11: 20.

Coulehan J. Compassionate Solidarity: Suffering, Poetry, and Medicine. *Perspectives in Biology and Medicine*. 2009; 52: 585–603.

Decety J, Cowell JM. The Complex Relation between Morality and Empathy. *Trends in Cognitive Sciences*. 2014; 18: 337–9.

Decety J, Fotopoulou A. Why Empathy Has a Beneficial Impact on Others in Medicine: Unifying Theories. *Frontiers in Behavioral Neuroscience*. 2014; 8: 457.

Decety, Yoder KJ. Empathy and Motivation for Justice: Cognitive Empathy and Concern, but Not Emotional Empathy, Predict Sensitivity to Injustice for Others. *Society for Neuroscience*. 2016; 11: 1–14.

Derksen F, Bensing J, Lagro-Janssen A. Effectiveness of Empathy in General Practice: A Systematic Review. *British Journal of General Practice*. 2013; 63: e76–84.

Frazer M. 2010. *The Enlightenment of Sympathy: Justice and the Moral Sentiments in the Eighteenth Century and Today*. Oxford: Oxford University Press.

Ganz M. 2008. What Is Public Narrative? Available at: https://comm-org.wisc.edu/syllabi/ganz/Whatis PublicNarrative5.19.08.htm. Last accessed: 12 February 2018.

Halpern J. What is clinical empathy? *Journal of General Internal Medicine*. 2003; 18: 670–4.

Hojat M. 2016. A Definition and Key Features of Empathy in Patient Care. In: *Empathy in Health Professions Education and Patient Care*. Dordrecht: Springer International Publishing, 83–128.

Hojat M, et al. Physician Empathy: Definition, Components, Measurement, and Relationship to Gender and Specialty. *The American Journal of Psychiatry*. 2002; 159: 1563–9.

Hojat M, et al. Physicians' Empathy and Clinical Outcomes for Diabetic Patients. *Academic Medicine*. 2011; 86: 359–64.

Huyler F. The Woman in the Mirror: Humanities in Medicine. *Academic Medicine*. 2013; 88: 918–20.

Internet Encyclopedia of Philosophy. "Human capacity of enlarged sympathy." Available at: www.iep. utm.edu/mill-eth. Last accessed: 12 February 2018.

Jeffrey D. Empathy, Sympathy and Compassion in Healthcare: Is There a Problem? Is There a Difference? Does It Matter? *Journal of the Royal Society of Medicine*. 2016; 109: 446–52.

Jordan MR, Amir D, Bloom P. Are Empathy and Concern Psychologically Distinct? *Emotion*. 2016; 16: 1107–16.

Kanske et al. Are Strong Empathizers Better Mentalizers? Evidence for Independence and Interaction between the Routes of Social Cognition. *Social Cognitive and Affective Neuroscience*. 2016; 11: 1383–92.

Kasper J, et al. All Health Is Global Health, All Medicine Is Social Medicine: Integrating the Social Sciences into the Preclinical Curriculum. *Academic Medicine*. 2016; 91: 628–32.

Kelley J, et al. The Influence of the Patient–Clinician Relationship on Healthcare Outcomes: A Systematic Review and Meta-Analysis of Randomized Controlled Trials. *PLoS One*. 2014; 9: e94207.

Kidd DC, Castano E. Reading Literary Fiction Improves Theory of Mind. *Science*. 2013; 342: 377–80.

Kumagai AK. A Conceptual Framework for the Use of Illness Narratives in Medical Education. *Academic Medicine*. 2008; 83: 653–8.

Lown B. A Social Neuroscience-Informed Model for Teaching and Practising Compassion in Health Care. *Medical Education*. 2016; 50: 332–42.

MacNaughton J. The Dangerous Practice of Empathy. *Lancet*. 2009; 373: 1940–1.

Marshall R, Bleakley A. The Death of Hector: Pity in Homer, Empathy in Medical Education. *Journal of Medical Humanities*. 2009; 35: 7–12.

McCann R. 2005. Interview transcript. Available at: https://sites.google.com/a/georgetown.edu/mdarts/ units/unit-5/section-2/video-hipaa. Last accessed: 12 February 2018.

Meisel ZF, Karlawish J. Narrative vs evidence-Based Medicine: And, not Or. *JAMA*. 2011; 306: 2022–3.

Mercer SW, Reynolds WJ. Empathy and Quality of Care. *British Journal of General Practice*. 2002; 52(Suppl): S9–13.

Misra-Hebert AD, Isaacson JH, Kohn M, et al. Improving empathy of physicians through guided reflective writing. *International Journal of Medical Education*. 2012; 3: 71–7.

Morgan A. Against Compassion: In Defence of a 'Hybrid' Concept of Empathy. *Nursing Philosophy*. 2017; 18.

Olds S. Poem for the Breasts. In: *Ploughshares*, ed. Mark Doty. Spring 1999, Emerson College, 25. p. 23.

Oliver MB. The Effect of Narrative News Format on Empathy for Stigmatized Groups. *Journalism & Mass Communication Quarterly*. 2012; 89, 2: 205–24.

Pedersen PB, Pope M. Inclusive Cultural Empathy for Successful Global Leadership. *American Psychologist*. 2010; 65: 841–54.

Perez-Bret E, Altisent R, Rocafort J. Definition of Compassion in Healthcare: A Systematic Literature Review. *International Journal of Palliative Nursing*. 2016; 22: 599–606.

Prinz J. Against Empathy. *The Southern Journal of Philosophy*. 2011; 49: 214–33.

Rakel DP, et al. Practitioner Empathy and the Duration of the Common Cold. *Family Medicine*. 2009; 41: 494–501.

Schumann, K. Jamil Zaki, J, Dweck C. Addressing the Empathy Deficit: Beliefs About the Malleability of Empathy Predict Effortful Responses When Empathy Is Challenging. *Journal of Personality and Social Psychology*. 2014; 107: 475–93.

Segal EA, Wagaman MA, Gerdes KE. Developing the Social Empathy Index: An Exploratory Factor Analysis. *Advances in Social Work*. 2012; 13: 541–60.

Segal E, et al. 2017. *Assessing Empathy*. New York, NY: Columbia University Press.

Shapiro J. Walking a Mile in Their Patients' Shoes: Empathy and Othering in Medical Students' Education. *Philosophy, Ethics, and Humanities in Medicine*. 2008; 3: 10.

Shapiro J. Perspective: Does Medical Education Promote Professional Alexithymia? A Call for Attending to the Emotions of Patients and Self in Medical Training. *Academic Medicine*. 2011; 3: 326–32.

Sharma M. Pinto AD, Kumagai AK. Teaching the Social Determinants of Health: A Path to Equity or a Road to Nowhere? *Academic Medicine*. 2018; 93: 25–30.

Shoes on the Danube Bank. 2018. Available at: https://en.wikipedia.org/wiki/Shoes_on_the_Danube_Bank. Last accessed: 12 February 2018.

Singer T, Lamm C. The Social Neuroscience of Empathy. *Annals of the New York Academy of Sciences*. 2009; 1156: 81–96.

Sklar D. Disparities, Health Inequities, and Vulnerable Populations: Will Academic Medicine Meet the Challenge? *Academic Medicine*. 2018; 93: 1–3.

Sontag S. 2003. *Regarding the Pain of Others*. New York, NY: Farrar, Straus and Giroux.

Stanford Encyclopedia of Philosophy, updated 2013. Available at: https://plato.stanford.edu/entries/empathy. Last accessed: 12 February 2018.

Sulzer SH, Feinstein NW, Wendland CL. Assessing Empathy Development in Medical Education: A Systematic Review. *Medical Education*. 2016; 50: 300–10.

Süskind P. 1991. *Perfume: The Story of a Murderer*. New York, NY: Pocket Books.

Wallis V. 1993. *Two Old Women*. Fairbanks/Seattle, WA: Epicenter Press.

Weisz, E, Zaki J. 2018. The Case for Less Solidarity: The Surprising Effects of Reducing Empathy for Your Own Ingroup. Available at: http://nautil.us/issue/48/chaos/the-case-for-less-solidarity. Last accessed: 12 February 2018.

Wellbery C. The Value of Medical Uncertainty? *Lancet*. 2010; 375: 1686–7.

Wellbery C, Mishori R. Deck the Halls with (Minority and Female) Portraits. Submitted to *Family Medicine*. 2018.

Wellbery C, et al. Medical Students' Empathy for Vulnerable Groups: Results from a Survey and Reflective Writing Assignment. *Academic Medicine*. 2017; 92: 1709–14.

Westerhaus M, et al. The Necessity of Social Medicine in Medical Education *Academic Medicine*. 2015: 90; 565–8.

Willer R. 2016. How to Have Better Political Conversations. Available at: www.ted.com/talks/robb_willer_how_to_have_better_political_conversations. Last accessed: 12 February 2018.

38

A LETTER FROM MARIJKE BOUCHERIE TO ALAN BLEAKLEY

Marijke Boucherie

Rana, 23rd March 2018

Dear Alan

In October 2017, you sent me an e-mail asking me to write a chapter for a book to be edited by you and published by Routledge in 2019: *Handbook of the Medical Humanities*. You even suggested a title 'The non-verbal as shared language in clinical encounters' planned as chapter 34 in part 6 of the book: 'Performativity and performance.'

I was surprised by the invitation but grateful.

In November 2017, I sent you an abstract of my contribution, changing the title to: 'The non-verbal as (non) shared language in clinical encounters.'

I am supposed to submit the first draft on 31st of March 2018. Today is the 23rd and here I am to tell you that I haven't written the chapter and cannot write it. I am too ashamed even to say that I am sorry.

The fact is that I do not really feel sorry. I deeply regret failing with my commitment towards your project and the project of all those who contribute to it. I never have, in my now 70-years-long life, failed with a professional obligation. As a Flemish living in Portugal, I used to be laughed at in a good-mannered way by my Portuguese fellow students because I always handed in my assignments on schedule unaware that my colleagues had manoeuvred a new deadline out of the professor. And when it was my turn to supervise a thesis and was adamant that the candidate hand in his or her work on time, I learned again that others had managed an extension. At least, the anger that this incident provoked gave me the courage to defend the thesis.

When one is not living in one's own culture, things become interesting.

I arrived in Portugal in 1968 to join a Portuguese student I had met at the University of Leuven. I followed him to Africa and in the next six years, three sons were born, the oldest two in Angola, the youngest in Mozambique, countries that were, at that time, colonies of Portugal. In April 1974 the 'revolution of the carnations' broke out in Portugal and war raged in Portuguese Africa. We left and some months later, the whole family was settled again in a town in the north of Portugal.

It was here that our youngest son—I shall call him Ben—began showing strange behaviour. I loved his stubbornness at first but soon became alarmed at a persistent waywardness that could not be ignored. The doctors were elusive and spoke of the danger of labelling; one even suggested that we put Ben in an institution and forget about him. And then finally, a child psychiatrist from Belgium I had consulted by letter (this was the time before the internet) wrote to me using the word 'autism.'

She also sent a list of features of 'autism' drawn up by Lorna Wing, the doctor whose work on the syndrome is pioneering (Wing 1972). Reading the list, I had the impression that someone had closely observed Ben and then issued a detailed description of him.

Autistic: I was happy with the word (no one, at that time, spoke of the 'autism spectrum' or used the word 'Asperger'). My son's special behaviour had a name, which meant that he had a condition that could be addressed and perhaps treated. But I soon found out that the doctors we consulted held different opinions about what the word autism might entail: was it a psychosis, a form of child schizophrenia, a syndrome? They did not take kindly to 'autism,' a diagnosis coming 'from abroad.' We even moved to Lisbon in order to have a wider choice of child psychiatrists. They were kind, careful and never used the word 'autism' themselves. But they were adamant: my child could not be treated. The person to be treated was the mother.

The books I consulted told me the rest: children with autism lived in empty fortresses (Bettelheim 1967)—they fled into safety from their cold mothers who rejected them. Mothers with an academic degree were prime suspects.

I was kindly invited to lie down on the couch—I more than willingly complied. The sooner I came in touch with the unconscious rejection of my child, the sooner he could be cured. Because *he could be cured*: that is what one of the doctors assured. He was the head of the team that followed the evolution of our son in monthly follow-up sessions. I was 'swept off my feet' with his prognosis, so much so that I did not notice that many people besides him were always present in his office, that my son and I were food for a seminar. I did not notice because I did not want to notice. I was very young. I only heard the good news: Ben can be cured. Moreover, in the very traditional culture where I grew up (and thought I had put behind me), doctors know best. The behaviour of people in authority was not to be questioned.

My happiness—my husband was older, wiser and remained aloof—lasted four weeks, the exact time between the follow-up sessions. This time, however, the doctor wanted to see me alone. I now felt so confident that I took with me the thick file where I had recorded Ben's funny sayings, the drawings he asked for, and photos of the compositions he made with orange peel or stones.

Ben was then four years old and almost two years had passed since the diagnosis. I had always asked myself why doctors were not interested in my child. They never asked what kind of person he was, the things he did, or the things he did not do. Why was no one interested in him as a person?

I wanted to tell the doctors about Ben sitting on my arm, his head on my shoulder, dancing to the music of children's songs, always the same record, over and over again. I would have liked to tell them that we do this every day when I come home from my classes, and how it appeases him, how it appeases me, how happy we are.

How do I tell the doctor of Ben's walks with his father, Ben pointing at each street lamp, my husband imitating his gesture, me spying on them—loving to look at their silhouettes outlined against the sky? Ben calls the street lamps 'sidi,' a non-existent word that means much to him. Still today, half a century after his father's death, we visit the 'sidi'-lights of the place where we first lived.

When do I tell them that, when we go for a walk, he wants me to keep a distance of about five metres, Ben leading, me following? Arriving at the old football field, I sit down on a stone and read my book (guiltily) and Ben walks up and down the field gathering sticks and old bits and pieces. He screams when I try to roll a ball in his direction.

And when, really when, can I speak of Ben's brothers, playing at civil war (Klaas is a communist and Koen is right wing—this is post-revolutionary Portugal and strife is in the air)? They battle with sharp sticks and self-made swords because we are modern parents and do not buy toy guns for our children. Ben wiggles himself between his brothers, apparently without noticing them, although he does. He eventually picks up their interest in Heavy Metal, so that today Ben may well be the greatest Heavy Metal expert in Portugal and has established close friendships with various Metal shopkeepers in Portugal and abroad.

So now, after three seminar sessions, when the doctor asks me to come and see him on my own, I hope to be able to interest him in my son's 'being' (as Ben himself today speaks of some-one's personality: 'what is his or her being?'); perhaps I can show him the file with the texts and the drawings and the photos.

I show the doctor a photo of one of Ben's doings: a composition of stones, spread out in a curved line on our porch. It looks like an installation.

"Did you take the picture?" the doctor asks.

I am happy to answer: "Yes, I did."

The doctor looks at me; he wipes the benign expression off his face and says: "Madam" (*Minha Senhora*). He pauses and then continues, looking me in the eyes: "you have made a fool of your son, you are making a fool of your son, and you are always going to make a fool of your son."

Three times the word 'fool' resounds in the room where, now, only the doctor and I are present.

The doctor uses an extremely offensive word for 'fool': *pateta*, which is also the name the Walt Disney figure of Goofy has been called in Portuguese. As applied to my son (or to what I am turning my son into) the word *pateta* is redolent of idiocy and silliness. One can be mad and dignified; one can be a fool and loveable (like Goofy himself); one can even be a 'holy' fool; but one cannot be called *pateta* and be deserving of respect.

Despite the shame—even now, 40 years after the incident, it fills me with shame to write down what I have just written—I go to see the people who have recommended the doctor to me and tell them of what has happened. They are serious people. They are good people. They do not believe me. "You must have provoked him," one of them says.

I must have. I must have thought that the doctor and I could 'share' information about my son. I must have forgotten my role. I was 'out of character.'

This happened 40 years ago. Since then, I have never been able to generally trust the psy-chiatric profession again, although I trust a few individual psychiatrists. And I am—again in general—prejudiced against the great array of health workers who hover over my son and with whom I am compelled to come into contact. I think of psychiatrists, psychologists, therapists, social workers, special need teachers and the whole caring industry. Only last year I heard the head of a famous healthcare institution say, and I paraphrase: "Our great assets are the infrastruc-tures and the qualified personnel; for that is what this institution is for: to provide employment to the community."

The person who said this is herself the mother of a child with a disability. I know she did not mean to forget about the 'clients,' but her words show to what point she has internalised a model of care as enterprise. For the health industry, then, my son has become a client. Ben him-self thinks otherwise. Once, writing a Christmas card to his doctor, he asked me for the word that would define their relationship: "What am I to Doctor X?" I suggested a multiple choice between 'friend,' 'patient' and the now usual word 'client.' Inspired perhaps, he wrote: "Best wishes from your 'ill person' Ben." This does not work in English, but the French equivalent would be *ton malade*; in Portuguese, Ben wrote: *o teu doente*.

It is not politically correct for Ben to consider himself an 'ill person'; he is, after all, a person with a now well-known syndrome that is not to be marked negatively. As a matter of fact, when

Ben sees a person whose facial expressions or body image convey disability, he calls out: "Look, mother, a person with disability," but when I ask him if he is 'disabled' (*deficiente*), his answer is clear: "No, I am efficient" (*eficiente*). Which he is.

Yet, during some months around his 20th birthday, in the period after the death of his father, Ben used to say: "I want to be reborn"; "I want to be born like other people"; "I am fed up with this illness"; "I cannot think of people; the persons come not into my head, their faces are enshrined." I must have fed him all these words or his brothers or the people around him. But the use is his even if the grammatical structuring remains arduous. "Repeat so that I may understand," he says sometimes and then repeats, word for word, what had been said to him.

Ben loves words. He collects languages and loves dictionaries, like the Dickens character from *David Copperfield*, Mr Dick, with whom Ben has a lot in common. At night, we read dictionaries as bedtime stories. He stores up long lists of words in different languages, looks for the connections between them and has become, in his own right, a kind of scholar in comparative linguistics. He is also good at structural linguistics, especially phonology, and we have long conversations about the contrastive phonological systems of the Dutch, Portuguese, English, French and German languages. He has difficulty connecting these words into meaningful sentences, however, but tries very hard and writes letters to me in which he explores the connections between words and concepts. Time is a favourite subject. One of the letters reads: "I would like to have more time to think of my things and be calm and serene" (when asked "which things?" the answer was: "my things without a name"); or "the beginning of the past and the end of the future is infinite" (my translation).

There are thousands of Ben's 'letters' around the house, explorations of words, of himself and of others. What I learn from this compulsive linguistic activity is how easy it is to play with language and how difficult to enter Wittgensteinian language games, to use language in context and in contact, to engage with others in word and deed. 'Words about words about words about words' is a game. Living with ourselves and others is vital.

Living with Ben, and witnessing his daily endeavour to navigate reality with his load of words and languages, has given me a tremendous respect for all easygoing, commonsensical exchanges between people: "Hello!" "How are you!" "A nice day, isn't it?" "What a lovely dog," "a coffee please" . . . simple formulae that can be learned by rote, but not "by heart." What connects these and other words to ourselves and to others is an energy that comes from places in the body—heart, lungs, breath, throat. It is in the 'missing link' between articulating sentences and engaging our whole bodies where 'meaning' lies.

It is difficult for Ben to occupy an in-between space (Sibony 2016): between words and bodily feelings, between feelings, words and emotions. But he is good with emotions, although not so much when connected to words carrying meaning. Ben explores sensations with nonsense syllables that are sung, shouted, murmured or whispered in complicity with me, his mother. ("This must not be done," says therapist A, "it may strengthen the symbiotic relationship and stand in the way of Ben's autonomy"; more recently, however, author B says the opposite: symbiotic parents of clients with autism can be useful; they mirror the emotions to the person who lacks mirror-neurons) (Isebaert 2017: 76). Whatever the verdict, it is now possible to embrace Ben, who now also smiles and sometimes expresses sadness instead of anger.

Ben's senses seem developed to the extreme: he hears and sees things that lie outside ordinary human capacity and his reactions to colour, smell and touch are uncanny. He speaks in oxymorons when his observations and feelings trouble him: "I felt a dark contentment," "a nervous serenity," "a white anger" (Ben has a predilection for the word 'serene' which also in Portuguese—*sereno/a*—sounds odd and archaic). Colour is Ben's medium, his language and his love. He defines characters in terms of colours. His mother is red but ruby when she is angry. People who are 'confused'—Ben

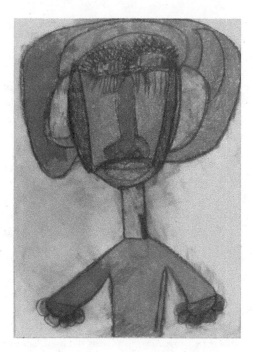

Figure 38.1 Bernardo Mendes Retrato do artista americano Lemmy, 2016

calls vagrants or loners who speak to themselves in the streets 'confused'—are almost always indigo blue. Strong, capable people are usually dark green. Bright yellow and light green are dominant for cheerful people. People who have died are purple, the colour of passion, he claims.

These colours are there for all to see, because Ben is a ferocious painter, making huge portraits of everyone he loves, likes or hears about and especially, of everyone who dies. These portraits all have the same cubist-like features but are in reality large compositions of colour and excel through a strong, professional trace in dry pastels. Ben's paintings have received some attention in alternative art circles. He himself loves exhibition openings: they serve soft drinks and biscuits.

Again, the question is how to speak of Ben's whole person to someone in the health professions? There, Ben is taken up in a world of labels and reduced to bits and pieces according to the questionnaires, diagnosis-charts or multiple-choice measurements that, as follows, only consider the elements already formulated in the questions. One can argue, and I am sure I would listen to the arguments, that in order to provide healthcare for everyone, it is essential to find common denominators for the great variety of people and their conditions. I am also sensitive to the argument of budget and financing that needs planning and diversification according to the degree of care needed for each person and his or her condition. In fact, I am extremely sensitive about the issue of money in healthcare and secretly think that 'money' should be the first item on every programme in medical humanities. And again, I know that the scientific discourse about Ben must include all persons and that research is imperative to relieve their suffering and help their integration. It must of necessity make abstraction of real people.

Alfred Korzybski—who fought abstraction in diagnosis and wanted language to remain close to reality (yes, but what reality? And can we assess reality beyond categories forged by language?)—described abstraction as "'selecting,' 'picking out,' 'separating,' 'summarizing,' 'deducting,' 'removing,' 'omitting,' 'disengaging,' 'taken away,' 'stripping'" (Kodish and Kodish 2011: 67). This is what scientists must do in order to find ways to 'treat' people, even if this implies looking at them through charts and diagnosis, seeing what the instruments of measuring allow them to discover. Can medical humanities, which have been said to explore "the intersection between the Humanities and Medicine in the therapeutic relationship with patients" (ulices.org/projectos-investigacao/narrative-and-medicine.html), provide the space where a focus on diagnosis can be reconciled with a holistic and intuitive view of the patient as a person?

Generally speaking—'generally' again—I am as weary of the Academic Industry as I am of the Health Industry. They may be said to share similar 'assets' and serve analogous purposes. Both fields are equally prone to power games and have the potential for abuse. As is the case of life in general, in both fields, something good can happen and does happen. I am often sceptical of the way the humanities are acclaimed as the potential saviour of medicine—as 'humane-based.' I am then reminded of moments in history where cruelty and love of music or literature go hand-in-hand. In order to improve health care and make it more attuned to the carers and patients, political engagement rather than literature seems to be required. A new way of society is called for, a better way of living together: institutions that prefer patients over bureaucracy. Charles Dickens was perhaps too stringent in opposing "facts to fancy" in his novel *Hard Times* (I call upon anyone to mark a hundred student essays about the opposition between 'facts and fancy' in the novel in order to see my point), but the too strict boundaries that the novel exposes between facts and interpretation, and the apology of the human factor, remain significant.

I see a field like medical humanities as an opportunity to create contexts for new languages

In these contexts, new ways of speaking may happen, less conditioned by the formal requirements of academic publications or the tenets of what is deemed 'scientific.' Rather than a field that may foster the academic preparation of health carers or art students or professionals in the humanities, medical humanities may open a space for what must at all costs be preserved in science, in philosophy and in all human endeavours: that which is particular, personal, ineffable (the "Effaninaeffable/Deep and inscrutable singular Name" as T. S. Eliot has it in his poem 'The Naming of Cats') (Eliot 2001: 2). Medical humanities may allow for both a new thinking and a methodology that come out of a place where words and bodies meet. As Michel Serres (2016: 80) writes, this would be a body "not of concepts, but of singularities, of examples, of events."

It is true that Ben has taught me that, in order to turn away from concepts, one must have the capacity to form concepts and that the word 'example' itself implies conceptualisation. But I know exactly what Michel Serres means. He points towards both thinking 'with' and 'of' the body: "It is starting from the individual, from the object that we are able to think" (ibid.: 341, my translation).

Ben has revolutionised my whole thinking: he forced me to abandon all familiar concepts. ("Can I be a cemetery?" he used to ask in his early concept-forming years. I said no, he couldn't and then discovered a sonnet by Baudelaire (*Les fleurs du mal*, LXXVI: Spleen) saying "*Je suis um cimetière*"). He forced me to reconsider the most common words; he took me into the foreign country of everyday reality.

Through Ben, I learned to trust his present doctor, the psychologist at his Day-Centre, his devoted GP, and the social worker who helps me fill out the never-ending bureaucratic forms. They all have names. Their families have names. Their beloved departed who now live in cemeteries have names. For a name-hungry person like Ben, people hold no secrets. And people who are questioned by Ben must of necessity surrender to his way of seeing the world.

Ben's present doctor has attended to my son for the last 20 years. He is the first to see Ben without me being present and to treat him as an autonomous person. I can very well imagine how Ben speaks to his doctor: each topic brings about new items that in turn must be treated separately to be further developed in subdivisions. I would like to compare Ben's never-ending accounts to a long, winding sentence by Proust or Saramago. But Ben lacks the lightspeed and flexibility of normal (yes, I use the word 'normal') talk. His way of relating has more in common with a computer search, each item leading to a further clarification to the extent where he does not know anymore what the original search was about. "I am enmeshed," says Ben and I wonder at his use of the 'net' metaphor so common when speaking of language: David Copperfield complained that, when he was little, he could see people in bits and pieces but was unable to form a net in which to catch them (Dickens 1996: 29). Wittgenstein's comparison of language "nets" (*Tractatus* 6.341) also comes to mind, and so does Iris Murdoch's novel *Under the Net* (1954), which is an allusion to the philosopher. Ben is enmeshed in the net of language and I suppose this to be the reason why he so obsessively wants to get a grasp on it. This could lead me further and say that Ben is a born-postmodernist. He certainly is a deconstructionist with each word referring to another word without really ever touching ground.

Ben's doctor, however, seems to be able to listen to Ben. When I am called into his office, the doctor knows all about the latest records Ben has bought and the ones he is going to buy; he knows whom Ben is going to visit and who has visited him (and so do all our neighbours . . .). The doctor is a big man, well dressed and groomed and very good at tempering a traditional Portuguese formality with a kind of boyishness. Ben painted his portrait in yellows and bright greens, so everything is said. The doctor has hung Ben's portrait on the walls of his office, amidst other beautiful art works. I trust this doctor (almost) completely. I trust him as much as I am capable of trust. And then, of course, this doctor calls me by my title. He is the first of Ben's psychiatrists to do so.

In Portugal, there is a tradition of addressing everyone who has a University degree by his or her title. Every BA graduate is called 'doctor.' Not to be called by one's title is an offense and many people, including me, hasten to call almost everyone 'doctor' so as not to make a mistake. In the medical world where I have travelled with Ben, I have always been called 'Ben's mother' or just 'madam' (my husband was addressed as 'doctor,' of course). Ben's present doctor addresses me by my title: '*Senhora Doutora*.' He used to be a student of the abusive psychiatrist I referred to earlier and when I told him about the 'goofy' incident, he said something like: "I cannot gauge what happened but I believe you. Yet, I must also tell you that, personally, I have learned a lot from this man."

These words suddenly unblocked my anger. They not only provided me with a new angle with which to evaluate the 'bad doctor in the story,' but they were proof of great courage and integrity on the part of another doctor who had been his pupil. The words nurtured a broader and more nuanced view because they were capable of, momentarily, bringing together, two opposing parties. And it was a third party, 'the third man,' who had been capable of doing this, creating an in-between space where things may be re-valued and, perhaps, transformed.

This, I believe, is what medical humanities are about. They are about inventing a space—inventing by creating—where people from all conditions can meet: doctors, patients, nurses, teachers, humanists, hard scientists, orderlies, authors, artists, children, animals; a place where what is imprecise, cloudy and changing can be spoken of, shown and expressed. It is a world where we can exist as approximate creatures, imperfect, full of contradictions and very much alive. There is place here for everything I have been trying to say: power, ambivalence, growth, trauma, illness, syndrome, language, abuse, paintings, philosophy, love. Especially, however, there is space for movement, for what fuels life.

*

Ben used to scream when he heard the word 'perhaps.' But some weeks ago, he asked me what the expressions 'perhaps,' 'maybe,' 'who knows' mean, offering the three synonyms in a row.

At a loss (as always), I answered that this really meant that something was going to happen in the future, 'soon' and I specify, as I must: July 2018 for a new sweater; a visit to Belgium in 2019; in 2025 a new car; in 2037 my death. I use a very common, imprecise Portuguese word for 'soon,'—'*logo*'—that has the simple function of putting things off to a more convenient time. Ben loves the liquid sound, so I play with the word and repeat it many times, rolling the sound L in repetitive, melodious word play. It creates a moment of hilarity, where we both laugh and at the end Ben usually gives me a kiss: a shy, dry peck on the mouth.

By now, Ben knows as I know that there is no guarantee that these things will 'really' happen at the appointed dates, that each date is subjected to a new 'soon'—the sweater of July 2018 might very well be deferred to August 2018. But in this movement of deferral (Derrida 1972) life happens, people think and speak, health workers nurture and cure, patients wait or die. Ultimately this is going to happen to everyone. As Ben says: "When I am dead my bones will rot in the cemetery." And he once wrote: "What I love to do in my spare time is to visit my father in the cemetery."

Until then we are alive and soon, soon, soon, as Alice Munro says ('Soon' 2005), something will come up: a new person, a new thought, a new word.

This is what I have been able to say, Alan. And I could find no other form than this, a letter. Thank you for thinking of me for your project,

With best wishes

Marijke

References

Baudelaire C. 1961. *Œuvres complètes*. Bibliothèque de la Pléiade. Paris: Gallimard.

Bettelheim B. 1967. *Empty Fortress: Infantile Autism and the Birth of the Self*. London: Free Press.

Derrida J. 1972. *La dissémination*. Paris: Éditions du Seuil.

Dickens C. 1850/1996. *The Personal History of David Copperfield*. With Introduction and Notes by Jeremy Tambling. Harmondsworth: Penguin Books.

Dickens C. 1854. *Hard Times*. Penguin rev. ed. 2003. With Introduction and Notes by Kate Flint. Harmondsworth: Penguin.

Eliot TS. 1939/2001. *Old Possum's Book of Practical Cats*. London: Faber and Faber.

Fernandes, Isabel. "Narrative and Medicine". Available at: www.ulices.org/projectos-investigacao/narrative-and-medicine.html. Last accessed: 1 May 2018.

Fernandes I, et al. 2015. *Creative Dialogues. Narrative and Medicine*. Newcastle: Cambridge Scholars Publishing.

Isebaert L. 2017. *Solution-Focused Cognitive and Systemic Therapy: The Bruges Model*. London: Routledge.

Kodish SP, Kodish BI. 2011 (3rd ed.). *Drive Yourself Sane: Using the Uncommon Sense of General Semantics*. Pasadena, CA: Extensional Publishing.

Munro A. 2005. *Runaway*. London: Chatto & Windus.

Murdoch I. 1954/1960. *Under the Net*. Harmondsworth: Penguin Books.

Serres M. 2016. *Pantopies ou le monde de Michel Serres. De Hermès à Petite Poucette. Entretiens avec Martin Legros et Sven Ortoli*. Paris: Éditions Le Pommier.

Sibony D. 2016. *L'entre-deux. L'origine en partage*. Paris: Points. Éditions du Seuil.

Wing L. 1972. *Autistic Children: A Guide for Parents and Professionals*. New York, NY: A Citadel Press Book.

Wittgenstein L. 1922/1961. *Tractatus Logico-Philosophicus*. DF Pears, BF McGuinness (trans.). London and Henley: Routledge & Kegan Paul.

39

HEALTH HUMANITIES

A democratising future beyond medical humanities

Paul Crawford and Brian Brown

Introduction and background

In this chapter we will describe what we mean by 'health humanities,' a term—and a movement—which we have been promoting over the last decade, and discuss how this extends and develops the traditional concerns of the medical humanities, using examples from our own work.

Historically, the medical humanities movement has led in foregrounding the salience of the arts and humanities to medical education, and has explored how medicine and its work can be inflected by these, for example through the study of the history of medicine, the philosophy of medicine, anatomical drawing, ethics, literature and drama. This is laudable and for many years the medical humanities have been the visible discipline for this kind of work alongside arts in health and expressive arts movements. Yet in the form of our wider public culture, the arts and humanities afford one of the greatest routes towards health, wellbeing, resilience and social connections. Indeed, in many parts of the world, it is as if they are a 'shadow,' informal and not necessarily medically driven 'health and social service.'

It is this wider and more diffuse experience of the arts, humanities and creative activity that has prompted us to consider how the humanities and health can be moved out of medical schools and into the wider health and social care community. Therefore, in response to this more diffuse reality, over the last ten years or so the field of health humanities has developed and been defined and characterised (Crawford 2007; Crawford et al. 2010; Jones et al. 2014; Crawford et al. 2015; Crawford et al. forthcoming). This has provided an alternative vision and platform for a more inclusive, democratised, medical and non-medical application of the arts and humanities to enhance healthcare, health and wellbeing. It is a field that aims to foreground the potential benefits of applied humanities as much as applied arts. In so doing, the field of health humanities subsumes the various unipolar initiatives, for example in arts in health or expressive therapies and the specialist field of medical humanities. For us, the field of health humanities comprises an over-arching, defining and dynamic body of work that incorporates, and is not solely aligned with, these subfields. More than a "terminological shift" (Jones et al. 2014: 6) from 'medical humanities,' it is a superordinate evolution.

In one of our earliest attempts to define this new field, in 2010 we argued for a "more inclusive, outward-facing and applied discipline, embracing interdisciplinarity and engaging with the contributions of those marginalized from the medical humanities" (Crawford et al. 2010: 4). Here, we meant the general public, patients, clients and service users, informal carers, allied health professionals and other members of the workforce in health, social and education settings. We also sought to include the diverse and not-necessarily-professionalised creative practitioners in the arts and humanities. Moreover, we hoped that research in the health humanities would foreground the health and wellbeing experience and cultural capital of wider populations of ordinary people rather than the vested interests of arts and humanities organisations or bodies.

Health humanities champion the application of the arts and humanities in interdisciplinary research, education and social action to inform and transform health and social care, health and wellbeing. It is driven by the needs of the general public and their sense of what does them good. It aims to be inclusive of viewpoints and contributions from within and beyond medicine; value the experiences and resources of the public; explore diverse approaches to achieving, maintaining or recovering quality of life; and strives for demonstrable impacts, not least in providing new evidence and insights for the education or practices of those planning, organising or working for the health of any population.

With the rapid growth of health humanities research units and courses worldwide, spearheaded by the International Health Humanities Network (www.healthhumanities.org), the field is generating substantial funding for programmes of work to influence and shape public health and wellbeing *with and without* medicine. A decentralised, democratic approach is at the heart of the health humanities and this is why the movement is taking off. It has not adopted a medical definition for what it does, and destabilises the kinds of hierarchies of expert knowledge which constrain innovation in applying the arts and humanities for health and wellbeing. It goes beyond the medicalisation of creative practices as is seen in 'Arts on prescription' initiatives. It also transcends the world of individual or even group therapy, where a therapist or leader dispenses therapeutic wisdom, instead seeking to democratise leadership in innovation and application. As such, we have sought to foreground mutuality, equality and parity of contribution as key principles in the health humanities.

In essence, within the health humanities we strongly maintain that not everything for health and wellbeing has to come from professionals or dedicated therapists. Members of the general public can make themselves and others better through many different creative actions and activities. Once basic needs have been met, they are the public's greatest route towards health and wellbeing. They are not there to replace healthcare but to give everyone a better shot at a happier life. We now see a much more democratised recognition that the arts and humanities are as important as blood tests, injections or pills for our wellbeing. You don't need a prescription to go to an arts or drumming group, or join a choir, and yet such activities can bring huge benefits.

But no patient is an island, and health humanities research, not least in our recent programme 'Creative Practice as Mutual Recovery,' has also demonstrated that people with health problems, family carers and health, social care and education professionals can recover health and wellbeing *together* through creative activities. We see so many bad news stories in the press and from academic analysts about health services in crisis (Costa-Font 2017; Hignett et al. 2018). It is not just people with an 'illness' who need to recover; their informal carers also may need some help dealing with the pressure of their work (Horton 2015; Olasoji et al. 2017). That is why we need more shared cultural experiences that bring those people together. Moreover, the value of bringing people together on shared projects towards common goals has recently been highlighted in the UK with a renewed focus on the problems of loneliness (McDaid et al. 2017) and the appointment of a Minister for Loneliness (BBC 2017). Academics studying health, as well as policymakers, are enamoured of the idea that it is good to bring people together, for all kinds of reasons—from enhancing wellbeing and longevity to reducing the financial burden on public services.

In our own case, we were fortunate to gain funding from the UK's Arts and Humanities Research Council in 2010 to initiate the International Health Humanities Network, and there has now been a substantial body of work looking at how communities can recover through collective artistic practice. After all, we all depend on multiple resources. We need medical ones, of course, but not everything in our society that brings us health and wellbeing needs to be directed by medics. Not everything needs a medical model or a medical explanation. Whether you are a doctor, a nurse, an occupational therapist, a patient, a friend or family carer, the arts and humanities are available to you. For example, if you suffer from depression, reading groups can help (Dowrick et al. 2012), as can music (Daykin et al. 2018) and poetry (Fraser 2011). These are just a few of many possible examples. In this way, we hope to bring within the ambit of the health humanities this rich body of literature, practice and experience concerning the beneficial effects of creative and aesthetic activities, especially those that get people together in situations where they all have something to contribute.

The argument can easily be made that maybe these activities are a 'cheap fix,' and enable managers, policymakers and governments to avoid responsibilities that might better be dealt with through collective provision. The empowerment of patients and the desire to reduce clients' reliance on health and social care services has unfortunate associations with neoliberal politics and efforts to make services less accessible (Brown and Baker 2018). However, there is a great deal more to the health humanities than saying 'we've got less resources, so you need to sort yourselves out and leave the medics alone.' It is about saying that there are wonderful resources—resources beyond what medical professionals can provide—and you don't need 'official' permission to access them. We need to get off the hook that medical, scientific knowledge is the only game in town.

What would happen to public wellbeing overnight if people couldn't read, share stories or tell jokes? Or if they couldn't watch films, enjoy theatre, dance, visit museums and galleries? Or sing, play, listen or dance to music? Or engage with the many other crafts, creative sports and activities going on all across this world? Any society would surely and deeply struggle to cope. Our contention within the health humanities is that without the arts and humanities we would be in a really, really bad place.

We now turn to illustrate some of the principles of health humanities through a recent large Arts and Humanities Research Council-funded programme in the UK entitled 'Creative Practice as Mutual Recovery: Connecting Communities for Mental Health and Wellbeing.' This comprised 14 projects involving various creative practices such as photography, storytelling, clay modelling, music and diverse arts activities in adult education, and ran from 2013 to 2018, that we describe in the next section as exemplifying some of the mission of health humanities.

Creative Practice as Mutual Recovery

'Creative Practice as Mutual Recovery' (CPMR) was a highly collaborative study that aimed to examine how creative practice in the arts and humanities could promote the kinds of connectedness and reciprocity that support 'mutual recovery' in terms of mental health and wellbeing. The idea of 'mutual recovery' extends out of the increasingly influential notion of 'recovery' in mental health care—referring to the possibility of achieving a meaningful and more resilient life irrespective of mental health 'symptoms' or disabilities. Typically, however, recovery-based initiatives tend to focus exclusively on people identified as having mental health needs—the service users—and overlook how hard-pressed informal carers and health, social care and education personnel may also need to 'recover' or be 'recovered' in terms of their own mental health and wellbeing. Over the course of our project, in a way typical of the health humanities, we sought to investigate and interrogate just the kind of fake boundaries that are applied to and between different disciplines, professional roles or activities in the creative practices and mental health recovery. Recovery initiatives or arts interventions are typically delivered to groups of clients. We wanted to create something more mutual, so in our creative projects service users, practitioners and informal carers were invited to work together on an equitable, mutualistic or reciprocal basis.

Our central proposition in this project was that creative practice could be a powerful tool for bringing together a range of social actors and communities of practice in the field of mental health, encompassing a diversity of people with mental health needs, informal carers and health, social care and education personnel, to establish and connect communities in a mutual or reciprocal fashion to enhance mental health and wellbeing. Such an approach is congruent with a "new wave of mutuality" marked by "renewed interest in co-operation" (Murray 2012; Brown 2016).

This five-year study added a new dimension to the current health humanities projects supported by the AHRC. Its substantive arts- and humanities-led programme of work packages was complemented by a process of evaluation using measures of mental wellbeing and social connectedness, to provide evidence that can be applied in transformative impacts in policy, provision and practice. At the outset the programme was co-created with people with lived experience of mental health challenges. We did not anticipate quite how our activities would act as a 'beacon,' but as the project progressed additional sub-projects involving yoga, capoeira (a Brazilian dance and martial arts activity), comedy and art gallery workshops joined the programme. As the project came to fruition, links were established with researchers in the arts and humanities, social and health sciences and third and statutory sector organisations supporting people with mental health needs. This will build capacity for the generation of the forms of social and cultural connectedness that are known to facilitate mental health recovery (Tew 2012). The programme of activities funded by the AHRC was won as part of the UK research councils' focus on 'connected communities.' Consistent with this ethos, central themes in this research are the contribution of shared community values and participation in this mutual recovery agenda, and the ways in which self-reliance and resilience can be 'co-produced' to support mental health and wellbeing in community settings. This ambitious, multidisciplinary research programme addresses the AHRC 'Connected Communities' vision through establishing new connections between academic and partner communities in order to enhance participation, prosperity, sustainability, and health and wellbeing.

The overall research question was: *What is the nature, effect and value of creative practice as mutual recovery in advancing connected communities for mental health and wellbeing?*

Research context

Our focus on mental health was prompted by our own backgrounds and expertise, and also by its significance as a major contemporary health problem, as the second greatest financial and social burden after cardiovascular disease (WHO 2005). In this context, the focus on notions of 'recovery' might seem to offer a new paradigm for mental health care that enables those affected to lead interesting, variegated and fulfilling lives despite their symptoms. The idea of 'recovery' is sometimes promoted with appealing allusions to the US civil rights movement, and by reference to its favour with the mental health service user and psychiatric survivor movement in the UK. In its more emancipatory forms, 'recovery' approaches locate the difficulties of those experiencing distress in social contexts, privilege the views of those who suffer, stress the cultivation of resilience and challenge the authority and expertise of traditional providers. This context means that 'recovery' is a contested concept in the field of mental health, with a key debate being whether it should remain a grassroots movement rather than something that is professionally controlled and administered. But either way, what we are seeing is the emergence of a new set of institutions, practices, identities and discourses of 'recovery.' This, as we have discovered ourselves, opens up possibilities of broader conceptualisations of 'recovery.'

Importantly, the notion of recovering a more resilient life and cultivating positive social and cultural connections for mental health and wellbeing through mutual practices and relationships is something that has implications beyond people with mental health conditions or challenges, or experiencing mental health crises. This focus on mutuality, or reciprocity, means that the processes of recovery could have benefits for others involved. This could include those with more general wellbeing needs, informal carers and health, and social care and education personnel (who are often themselves subject to high stress, mental health problems and burnout). Viewing recovery in this reciprocal way opens up new possibilities for examining how recovery for mental health and wellbeing could occur through shared practices within and across these groups or communities, and how creative practice may assist such a mutual process. This relational ontology of recovery is important since it counters currently individualised conceptions of recovery within services and policy, instead seeing it as based around interactional processes, identities and social relationships. 'Mutual recovery' is therefore a very useful term because it instigates a more fully social and deeper understanding of mental health recovery processes, encompasses diverse actors in the field of mental health, and attends to the need to track signs of wellbeing and improvement across this field.

Typically, divisions tend to exist between those with mental health needs, informal carers, health, social care and education personnel and arts practitioners. What our set of creative practice projects sought to explore was the hitherto neglected issue of how these groups can be brought together in and through the co-production of creative capital or resources. This involved areas such as visual arts, music, dance, drama, stories, narratives, histories and philosophies in order to forge stronger connections that can support mental health and wellbeing recovery and advance shared understanding. In community settings—where helpers can be left isolated or facing a heavy burden—there is an increasingly austere, demanding, production-line healthcare system (Crawford and Brown 2011; Crawford et al. 2011); threat looms large; and compassion fatigue is becoming all too common (Rothschild 2006; Gilbert 2009; Crawford et al. 2013). There are mounting concerns about the mental health and wellbeing of informal carers (Pinquart and Sörensen 2003; Konerding et al. 2018), and health, social care and education personnel (Rudow 1999; Edwards et al. 2000) alongside people with mental health difficulties. During the programme, it became clear that this broadening out of 'recovery' should extend to creative practitioners. As various scholars have noted, for example in the case of musicians, this need for recovery can and should be extended to arts practitioners who face challenges with their physical and mental health (Williamon and Thompson 2006; Kreutz et al. 2008; Araújo et al. 2017; Ascenso et al. 2017; Perkins et al. 2017).

In other words, the notion of a clear separation in terms of mental health and wellbeing between people with mental health needs, informal carers, health, social care and education personnel and creative practitioners—such as expressive arts therapists, performers and community arts personnel—has become blurred. It is time to extend beyond a reductive focus on recovery of particular patient groups and conditions and investigate ways that informal carers, health, social care and education personnel and diverse creative practitioners can also be supported to develop wellbeing and resilience *together*.

In summary, this research presented a timely move, congruent with the rise of health humanities, to bring together diverse academic and community partners to share insights, approaches, methods and analytic tools in order to mobilise the concept and develop creative practice as mutual recovery—this, to better connect communities for mental health and wellbeing. It marks a radical shift in vision in approaches to mental health that could transform how people with mental health difficulties, informal carers, health, social care and education personnel and creative practitioners work together and take new opportunities to build egalitarian, appreciative and substantively connected communities—resilient communities of mutual hope, compassion and solidarity.

Findings

Using methods and skills from science, social science and arts and humanities, the CPMR programme found compelling and substantial quantitative and qualitative evidence that diverse and shared creative practices can help people recover mental health and wellbeing as measured through the Warwick Edinburgh Mental Wellbeing Scale (Stewart-Brown et al. 2011) *together*—'mutual recovery'; and increase social connectedness within and between groups of people as measured by Secker et al.'s (2009) social inclusion measure. These can include people with experience of mental difficulties, informal or family carers and health, social care, education and creative practitioners.

While there were many accounts from participants of the enjoyment they derived from the activities and the positive life changes entailed, there were some drawbacks that will inspire future research and developments in practice. For example, clay modelling did not suit everybody due to the nature of clay itself; in the adult community education context, some arts participants preferred either to work alone or without an explicit focus on improving wellbeing; and the extent to which online or digital storytelling can promote mutuality remains uncertain. In addition, despite our attempts to foster mutuality by getting practitioners and service users to work together, professionals' roles sometimes limited or acted as a barrier to their participation in shared creative practice. Indeed, on one occasion the request that practitioner participants should fill the questionnaires in as well as clients was met with bafflement. People with severe mental disorders sometimes struggled to remain engaged without direct mental health professional support. All these aspects are potentially remediable, and highlight where additional work is need or appropriate support might facilitate and shape engagement so as to derive the full benefits.

The CPMR programme proved influential for policy and practice development relevant to social and cultural aspects of mental health and wellbeing. The programme attracted several prestigious awards and nominations, including the music project whose team has achieved the 2016 Arts and Health Award from the Royal Society for Public Health. This signals that health bodies and learned societies are increasingly taking an interest in these kinds of approaches. There were multiple, high-profile and diverse impacts that resulted from the programme's activities in the UK and overseas, delivering accessible creative products available to the public as films, plays, fiction, events, symposia, websites and exhibitions. Importantly, the CPMR programme attracted multiple positive comments from both the public and project participants. These comments are made available in the final showcase report in association with Mental Health Foundation, UK.

To date, the CPMR programme has directly informed training courses for medics, psychiatrists, medical students, midwives, health visitors, therapists, teachers in adult community education/schools/high schools; and the work of community care and health care organisations at a regional, national and international level. It has also led to ongoing arts initiatives in community centres, and an additional AHRC-funded Dementia, Arts and Well-Being Network that adopted a 'mutual recovery' approach to its work.

We made a number of recommendations based on the programme. First, that health, social care, education and arts organisations should consider promoting more shared creative practices to benefit the mental health and wellbeing of all communities that they serve, including practitioners and family carers. In particular, such organisations should determine strategies for how these opportunities can be maximised to enhance their environments in feasible and innovative ways. Second, health, social care, education and arts professionals should consider the benefits of engaging in shared creative practices with their peers, other professionals and non-professionals—including people with mental health difficulties and their informal carers. Finally, that further research is required on how other kinds of creative practice not investigated in this study might promote mutual recovery of mental health and wellbeing.

Through the CPMR project we have been able to foreground a number of features of the health humanities as we see them and as we have tried to promote them over the past decade. First, we have attempted to bring service users, carers and practitioners together in creative activity because we believe that getting people together to work with a common goal has valuable health benefits. This is underscored by recent publicity in the UK about the deleterious effects of loneliness (Richard et al. 2017; BBC 2018). Second, we have sought to integrate the concerns of the health humanities with the rich body of practical knowledge originating in the creative therapies and in creative practice, which has helped to break through the barriers that have often existed between these approaches. Third, we have tried to incorporate informal carers—a massive number of people amounting to seven million in the UK alone (Carers UK 2018)—a group that has not figured prominently in the medical humanities hitherto. Fourth, we have sought to privilege the creative activity rather than the medical aspects of the problem. Thus, rather than select people on the basis of their putative diagnosis, we have included people with a wide variety of problems and symptoms, and also recognised that carers and professionals may have vulnerabilities or sources of distress in their lives too. We have therefore sought independence from the predominantly medical frame that governs much medical humanities and social science work and instead foreground experience, creativity and the aesthetics of the work. In this way we hope to open up new spaces for collaboration, creation and inquiry.

Acknowledgements

We are grateful to the Arts and Humanities Research Council for funding the research described in this chapter: 'Creative Practice as Mutual Recovery: Connecting Communities for Mental Health and Wellbeing' (Grant numbers: AH/K003364/1; AH/J011630/1) and the Dementia, Arts and Well-Being Network (AH/N00650X/1). Our thanks go to our co-investigators on the CPMR programme, Professor Mike Wilson, Professor Susan Hogan, Professor Aaron Williamon and Professor Lydia Lewis, who contributed substantially to the framing of ideas about 'creative practice as mutual recovery' represented and described here and to the additional project leads and teams. Finally, we thank our project partners, supporting organisations and many individuals who offered their support, advice and encouragement for this body of work, not least David Crepaz-Keay, Tony Devaney and Debbie Butler who, from the start, brought important insights as people with experience of mental health difficulties.

References

Araújo L, Wasley D, Perkins R, et al. Fit to perform: An investigation of higher education music students' perceptions attitudes and behaviors toward health. *Frontiers in Psychology*. 2017; 8: 1–19.

Ascenso S, Williamon A, Perkins R. Understanding the psychological wellbeing of professional musicians through the lens of positive psychology. *Psychology of Music*. 2017; 45: 65–81.

Atanasova D, Koteyko N, Brown B, Crawford P. 2017. Representations of mental health and arts participation in the national and local British press, 2007–2015. *Health: An Interdisciplinary Journal for the Social Study of Health, Illness and Medicine*. In press. https://doi.org/10.1177/1363459317708823.

BBC. 2017. Minister for loneliness appointed to continue Jo Cox's work. Available at: www.bbc.co.uk/news/uk-42708507. Last accessed: 3 March 2018.

BBC. 2018. How should we tackle the loneliness epidemic? Available at: www.bbc.co.uk/news/uk-42887932. Last accessed: 17 March 2018.

Brown B. Towards a critical understanding of mutuality in mental health care: Relationships, power and social capital. *Journal of Psychiatric and Mental Health Nursing*. 2015; 22: 829–35.

Brown B. Mutuality in health care: Review, concept analysis and ways forward. *Journal of Clinical Nursing*. 2016; 25: 1464–75.

Brown B. (In press) Digital health humanities. In: S Adolphs, D Knight (eds.) *Routledge Handbook of English Language and Digital Humanities*. London: Routledge.

Brown B, Baker S. The social capitals of recovery in mental health. *Health*. 2018. doi: 10.1177/1363459318800160. [Epub ahead of print].

Brown B, Manning N. Genealogies of recovery: The framing of therapeutic ambitions, *Nursing Philosophy*. 2018; 19: e12195.

Carers UK. 2018. State of caring. Available at: www.carersuk.org/for-professionals/policy/policy-library/state-of-caring-2018-2. Last accessed: 18 May 2019.

Costa-Font J. The national health service at a critical moment: When Brexit means hectic. *Journal of Social Policy*. 2017; 46: 783–95.

Crawford, P. 2007. Health humanities innovation. Paper presented on 28 November 2007. *Knowledge Transfer from Medical Professionals to Industry: An ESRC Business Seminar*. Biocity, Nottingham.

Crawford, P. 2018. Incomprehensibility and mutual recovery, *Performing Psychologies: Imagination, Creativity and Dramas of the Mind*. Nicola Shaughnessy with a neuroscientist, Philip Barnard. London: Bloomsbury Methuen.

Crawford P, Brown B, Tischler V, Baker C. Health humanities: The future of medical humanities? *Mental Health Review Journal*. 2010; 15: 4–10.

Crawford P, Brown B. Fast healthcare: Brief communication, traps and opportunities. *Patient Education & Counselling*. 2011; 82: 3–10.

Crawford P, Gilbert P, Gilbert J, Gale C. The language of compassion. *Taiwan International ESP Journal*. 2011; 3: 1–16.

Crawford P, Hallawell B. Where is the love? *Learning Disabilities Practice*. 2011; 14: 9.

Crawford P, Gilbert P, Gilbert, J et al. The language of compassion in acute mental health care. *Qualitative Health Research*. 2013; 23: 719–27.

Crawford P, Brown B, Baker C, et al. 2015. *Health Humanities*. London: Palgrave.

Crawford P, Brown B, Charise A (eds.) (Forthcoming). *Companion to Health Humanities*. Routledge: London.

Daykin N, Mansfield L, Meads C, et al. What works for wellbeing? A systematic review of wellbeing outcomes for music and singing in adults. *Perspectives in Public Health*. 2018; 138: 39–46.

Dowrick C, Billington J, Robinson J, et al. Get into reading as an intervention for common mental health problems: Exploring catalysts for change. *Medical Humanities*. 2012; 38: 15–20.

Edwards D, Burnard P, Coyle D, et al. Stress and burnout in community mental health nursing: A review of the literature. *Journal of Psychiatric and Mental Health Nursing*. 2000; 7: 7–14.

Fraser D. Mood disorders and poetry: Archaeology of the self. *Journal of Poetry Therapy*. 2011; 24: 105–15.

Gilbert P. 2009. *The Compassionate Mind*. London: Constable.

Hignett S, Lang A, Pickup L, et al. 2018. More holes than cheese: What prevents the delivery of effective, high quality and safe health care in England? *Ergonomics*. 2018; 61: 5–14.

Hogan S, Pink S. 2012. Visualising interior worlds: Interdisciplinary routes to knowing. In: S Pink (ed.) *Advances in Visual Methodology*. London: Sage, 230–48.

Hopper K. Rethinking social recovery in schizophrenia: What a capabilities approach might offer. *Social Science and Medicine*. 2007; 65: 868–79.

Horton R. Caring for adults in the EU: Work–life balance and challenges for EU law. *Journal of Social Welfare and Family Law*. 2015; 37: 356–67.

Jones T, Wear D, Friedman LD (eds.) 2014. *Health Humanities Reader*. New Brunswick, NJ: Rutgers University Press.

Konerding U, Bowen T, Forte P, et al. 2018. Investigating burden of informal caregivers in England, Finland and Greece: An analysis with the short form of the burden scale for family caregivers (BSFC-s). *Aging and Mental Health.* 2018; 22: 280–87.

Kreutz G, Ginsborg J, Williamon A. Music students' health problems and health-promoting behaviors. *Medical Problems of Performing Artists.* 2008; 23: 3–11.

McDaid D, Bauer A, Park A-L. Making the economic case for investing in actions to prevent and/ or tackle loneliness: a systematic review: A briefing paper. September 2017. Personal Social Services Research Unit, London School of Economics. Available at: www.lse.ac.uk/business-and-consultancy/ consulting/assets/documents/making-the-economic-case-for-investing-in-actions-to-prevent-and-or-tackle-loneliness-a-systematic-review.pdf. Last accessed: 18 May 2019.

Murray R. 2012. *The New Wave of Mutuality: Social Innovation and Public Service Reform.* London: Policy Network.

Olasoji M, Maude P, McCauley K. Not sick enough: Experiences of carers of people with mental illness negotiating care for their relatives with mental health services. *Journal of Psychiatric and Mental Health Nursing.* 2017; 24: 403–11.

Pérez Vallejos E, Haslam-Jones E, Pickard D. Creative practices as mutual recovery: Flamenco-Yoga Papales de Trabajo sobre Cultura, *Educacion y Desarollo Humano.* 2018; 14: 80–89.

Perkins R, Ascenso S, Atkins L, et al. Making music for mental health: How group drumming mediates recovery. *Psychology of Well-Being.* 2016; 6: 1–17.

Perkins R, Reid H, Araújo L, et al. Perceived enablers and barriers to optimal health among music students: A qualitative study in the music conservatoire setting. *Frontiers in Psychology.* 2017; 8: 1–15.

Pinquart M, Sörensen S. Differences between caregivers and noncaregivers in psychological health and physical health: A meta-analysis. *Psychology and Aging.* 2003; 18: 250–67.

Richard A, Rohrmann S, Vandeleur CL, et al. Loneliness is adversely associated with physical and mental health and lifestyle factors: Results from a Swiss national survey. *PLoS ONE.* 2017; 12, e0181442.

Rothschild B. 2006. *Help for the Helper: The Psychophysiology of Compassion Fatigue and Vicarious Trauma.* New York, NY: W.W. Norton & Co.

Rudow B. 1999. Stress and burnout in the teaching profession: European studies, issues, and research perspectives. In: AM Huberman (ed.) *Understanding and Preventing Teacher Burnout: A Sourcebook of International Research and Practice.* Cambridge: Cambridge University Press, 38–58.

Secker J, Hacking S, Kent L, et al. Development of a measure of social inclusion for arts and mental health project participants. *Journal of Mental Health.* 2009; 18: 65–72.

Stewart-Brown SL, Platt S. Tennant A, et al. The Warwick-Edinburgh Mental Well-being Scale (WEMWBS): A valid and reliable tool for measuring mental well-being in diverse populations and projects. *Journal of Epidemiology and Community Health.* 2011; 65: A38–A39.

Tew J. Review: Challenging the stigma of mental illness, Patrick Corrigan, David Roe and Hector Tsang. *The British Journal of Social Work.* 2012; 42: 581–83.

Williamon A, Thompson S. Awareness and incidence of health problems among conservatoire students. *Psychology of Music.* 2006; 34: 411–30.

World Health Organisation (WHO). 2005. Preventing chronic diseases: A vital investment. WHO global report. Available at: www.who.int/chp/chronic_disease_report/contents/en. Last accessed: 18 May 2019.

40

DOCTORS NEED SAFE CONFESSIONAL AND CATHARTIC SPACES

What we learned from the research project 'People Talking: Digital Dialogues for Mutual Recovery'

Jon Allard, Michael Wilson and Alan Bleakley

Doctors losing libido

The newly elected (2017) President of the British Medical Association (BMA), Professor Pali Hungin, describes a crisis amongst doctors resulting from structural factors—particularly chronic under-resourcing. The crisis involves exacerbation of doctors' mental health problems—not only in the acute sense such as suicidal ideation, but as a chronic condition of "disillusionment" and "loss of joy" (Hungin 2017), akin to loss of libido. Clare Gerada (2017), former chair of the Royal College of General Practitioners, describes "a profession in distress." Medicine is a profession whose urge to create is deeply frustrated, the aesthetic overridden by the instrumental and functional, the functional a burden where the UK has 2.8 doctors per 1,000 people:

> fewer doctors per head of population than most other countries in the Organisation for Economic Co-operation and Development (OECD) . . . Out of the 33 countries for which the OECD has provided data, the UK ranks 22nd. The only European countries with fewer doctors per head of population are Poland and Slovenia.
>
> *(Moberly 2017)*

In the UK, one in four people generally will suffer a mental health problem at some stage in their lives, making mental health the largest field of disability (23% of all ill health) (HMG DH 2011). While doctors have stressful jobs, and this is a structural problem creating vulnerability to mental health issues, they are reluctant to admit to such problems (Manning 2012). This is a cultural problem—doctors are socialised into a faux invincibility. A 2013 review of the literature on the mental health of UK doctors revealed that: "27% . . . show significant stress . . . (doctors) have a 7% lifetime prevalence of substance misuse . . . (and) a suicide rate that is higher than the general population and significantly higher than other professions" (Howe 2013). Doctors in the UK National Health Service (NHS) may be seen to be in a permanent state of recovery from working within an increasingly dysfunctional system. A 2017 survey revealed a worsening situation from the 2013 review above, where 60% of doctors admitted to some form of ongoing mental illness (eurekadoc 2017). A 2015 report showed that 48% of UK junior doctors who had completed their Foundation Programme and prior to Specialist training planned to leave the NHS (many to work abroad), while in 2011 this figure was only 29% (Campbell 2015). This drain of a talented workforce is a symptom of ever-worsening UK work conditions. While the UK Government claims that more funds are being spent on the NHS than ever before, the fact remains that UK healthcare resourcing is amongst the poorest in post-industrial countries, and, as a consequence, health outcomes for the population are relatively poor when compared with near-neighbours such as the Netherlands, Germany or Belgium (Niemietz 2016).

Survey results noted above offer an overview of doctors' concerns, but nothing of the fine grain of symptoms of overwork and consequent stress. While the pilot study we draw from below has a very small sample of doctors (n=5), and this involved four consultant psychiatrists and one experienced GP and then is open to bias, the data have face validity when considered as a series of case studies (n=1). These doctors' stories reveal fascinating fine-grain aspects to the career work circumstances that might lead to debilitating stress and how such stress may be repressed, denied and sublimated. In short, doctors took the opportunity to confess, and to resist conformist professional identities.

The pilot project

We set up a pilot research project to connect the communities of mental health service users, carers and doctors within a readily accessible digital medium with the aim of promoting 'mutual recovery' (explored below) through storytelling. The medium of digital storytelling is an 'everyday,' or 'available,' art that requires no particular skill or creative ability in narrative (Alexander 2012). This chapter reports on an important slice through that project, a finding whose contours we could not predict. Given the opportunity, doctors in the study readily admitted to vulnerability and sought safe spaces in which to confess and exercise catharsis or expression of otherwise contained emotions with familial overtones.

Following the medical consultation model, our study was, again, case-based with just 13 participants, five of whom were doctors, five service users with mild to moderate mental health symptoms and three carers. From the doctors' stories, we were able to gauge just how much pressure they are under in the current UK National Health Service (NHS) that can be read as a dysfunctional system. While medicine sets out to heal, it is poor at healing itself (Peterkin and Bleakley 2017), as the story fragments considered in this chapter indicate.

Theoretical underpinning to the pilot project

Stories

A story is characterised as having a plot, usually with a crisis or turning point, and real or imaginary characters; after the turning point, unpredictable things may happen (Ricoeur 1984). Stories are produced in a social context, with a teller and an audience, often transmitting normative cultural lore to bind social groups, but also challenging and disrupting social norms through resistance and invention.

Stories are the stuff of clinical encounters (Kleinman 1989; Bleakley 2005). Patients typically tell their stories in fragments where the doctor turns the "chief *concern*" (the patient's own understanding of his or her symptoms) into a medical narrative, a story of the "chief *complaint*" or main symptom, shaped as a standard 'case' and shared with colleagues (Schleifer and Vannatta 2013). In the medical context, telling stories hopefully leads to a successful diagnosis, treatment plan and cure. But doctors often do not listen closely enough to their patients' stories, and interrupt the telling too quickly, so that the patient does not articulate the chief complaint. This can lead to a misdiagnosis or poor care through miscommunication. Often, misdiagnoses do not have serious consequences and may be corrected. However, an estimated 15–20% of medical errors arise through misdiagnoses (discovered at post-mortem) (Sanders 2010).

Importantly, other than in informal contexts, doctors rarely have the opportunity to tell their own stories to each other or to the patients they treat; and almost never to their patients' carers. We identify such 'story blocking' as an untreated symptom of medical culture, where the need for doctors to tell their stories has, in recent years, led to an explosion in medical auto-ethnography (Farrell et al. 2015).

Digital storytelling

The American oral historian Studs Terkel recalled collecting stories from a single mother on a housing project in his native Chicago. As Terkel recorded her testimony, she was busy cooking food for her children who in turn were creating chaos around the apartment. When he was finished and packing away his recording equipment, the woman's children came up to Terkel and insisted on hearing their mother on the tape, so he replayed the interview. The mother, initially embarrassed, soon began to listen intently, finally remarking: "Gee, I never knew that's what I thought."

Digital Storytelling is a nascent form of first-person storytelling, utilising the readily available and accessible new tools of IT multi-media to craft narratives (placed on a customised website) that can be enhanced by visual images. It is a creative form particularly suited to individuals who have never before ventured into the world of 'creativity' or the arts, as a "vernacular creativity" (Burgess 2006). The economy of the form, coupled with the intimacy of the potential use of personal photographs, creates an opportunity for anyone who has a story to share to create a lasting artefact in a relatively simple way, utilising accessible computer software. It is a democratising form, allowing access to wider audiences for voices that are often hidden or unheard.

Mutuality

Collaboration and gendered division of labour were the primary forces behind the success of Ice Age hunting and gathering groups, where small, mobile groups must have adopted "congregation" as a core social value (Pagel 2013). In later agricultural societies, planting and harvesting of crops and domestication of animals required highly co-ordinated effort, with collaboration acting as a higher value than individualism. Pagel (2013) describes a "natural history of human cooperation" in terms of the brain being "wired for culture." Collaborative values are grounded in quality of relationships and intimacy, based on kindness and trust (Sennett 2012). Where free market capitalism and neoliberalism can be seen to have produced rampant individualism and gross inequalities (Stiglitz 2012), so a new wave of commentators has called for social justice based on principles, rituals and politics of local cooperation. Acquiring social capital in the forms of friendship groups, family support, professional support and networking helps to achieve resilience against mental health issues, also reducing stigma (Gele and Harslof 2010; Webber et al. 2014). Doctors suffering stress and burnout primarily need mutuality, or accessible and trustworthy support networks (Peterkin and Bleakley 2017).

Resilience

Comparing today's doctors with previous generations, Clare Gerada (2017) notes that: "resilience is a process, not a personality trait." The context for medical practice has changed radically in a short space of time so that today, "while doctors might work fewer hours, they are often unsupported." Much can be learned about resilience from survivors of natural disasters, accidents, political conflicts and wars (Joseph 2011). Gonzales (2012) describes how supposed forms of resilience developed in the aftermath of trauma may themselves become additional symptoms and remain untreated, and this is particularly the case for consistent, long-term stress of the kind that doctors may suffer. Further, victims may fail to call for help. After the 9/11 attack on the World Trade Center, the Federal Emergency Management Agency made $155 million dollars available for post-trauma counselling, expecting up to a quarter of a million to apply. As Gonzales says: "Just 300 people turned up." Doctors regularly face the traumas of their patients, including mental health issues that may result in domestic violence, self-harm or suicide attempts, and have to soak this up. Such consultations and encounters may re-stimulate doctors' own unresolved psychological issues, sometimes dormant or unconscious until stirred. With psychiatrists as the exception, doctors do not learn how to deal with such transference effects in clinical encounters as part of their medical education, relying instead on what is often a blunt and unsophisticated resilience. While resilience has been positioned at the centre of the UK Government's mental health strategy, focused on supportive communities and ready access to services (HMG DH 2011), it is often forgotten that health professionals are themselves vulnerable and, as noted above, may not only need to develop resilience but also to engage with appropriate therapeutic interventions where resilience collapses, fails to develop or was the wrong initial psychological strategy. Mistakenly, resilience has been assumed amongst the medical profession, where junior doctors are tempered in the furnaces of long and demanding hospital shifts. Such naturalistic encounters cannot be assumed to develop effective psychological health strategies, and are often counter-productive.

Recovery

Joseph (2011) describes "posttraumatic growth" in the wake of trauma following losses such as separation, divorce, illness and bereavement to potentially trauma-inducing events, such as assault, accidents and natural disasters, as illustrating powers of deep recovery (Amering and Schmolke 2009: 215). This supposedly upholds the maxim that what doesn't kill us makes us stronger, where trauma can facilitate "new meaning, purpose and direction in life" (ibid.). Sennett (2012: subtitle) challenges such stoic self-reliance, placing mutuality before individual resilience as the "rituals, pleasures and politics of cooperation," suggesting that properly conceived professional and social support can act as a prophylactic against stress and burnout.

Discovery

Beyond recovery is a horizon of discovery or potential (Peterkin and Bleakley 2017). Arnhild Lauveng (2013) tells of a distressing descent into a schizophrenic condition of hearing voices and having visions in which she was controlled by malevolent forces. Lauveng was regularly hospitalized and treated with drugs, self-harmed and attempted suicide on several occasions. She describes how she overcame symptoms not only to gain resilience but also to flourish and become a clinical psychologist, treating fellow schizophrenics. She moved from recovery to discovery. The current President of the British Medical Association (Hungin 2017), however, notes that while medicine is in an age of 'discovery,' its practitioners are living through a period of 'recovery,' stressed as never before, so that the knowledge fruits of cutting-edge research are spoiled as translation into everyday medicine is frustrated through excessive work pressures.

Key findings

Doctors' concerns

In our project, doctors, patients and carers met productively as 'citizens,' challenging conventional power relationships, while doctors embraced the opportunity to tell their stories, where the personal-confessional genre dominated. Such stories were often cathartic, related to childhood memories or emotionally charged contexts moving beyond sentimental recollection. For doctors, confession goes against the grain of professional veneer, where identity construction is grounded in identification with the norms of medical culture as heroic, masculine and tempered. A classic early product of this is 'empathy decline' and associated 'hardening' of feelings (loss of sensibility and sensitivity) (Bleakley 2014). However, doctors in our study showed acute empathic responses to others' stories of pain, such as this humane response to service users' recollections of being confined in mental hospitals (described by one service user as a "wretched life of misery . . . Within a room with others in pain"):

Story 1 extract

So many of the stories here contain so much pain. I didn't sign up to this project to spend my whole time laughing, but I am surprised by myself at how hard I find it to read through a tale of suffering and then just close the page. I don't really know how to react to it digitally. At work I think I am quite good at responding to difficult narratives but seeing them here is different. Please don't stop writing them if that is what you need or want to say, but seeing them here without a response feels quite harsh . . .

Development of resilience, mutuality, recovery and discovery

Socrates argued that the greatest challenge facing humans is how to control and educate *thumos*, variously translated as 'desire,' 'anger' and 'unbridled emotion' (Plato 2005). Perhaps a major difference between those with mental health issues and those who lead more 'normal' lives is that the latter have developed ways of educating *thumos* or the passions, channelling these in socially acceptable ways. This is an indication of a mature resilience and opens up doors to discovery or more innovative ways of leading a life, challenging habits and conventions.

Two of the doctors in the study wrote stories of having to show resilience within their work in the face of excessive demands within the NHS leading to a build-up of frustration that could spill out in anger. These stories were Socratic—drawing on rhetorical or persuasive argument—where it is hard to disagree with the psychiatrist below that cuts to NHS mental health services in the current climate of austerity are grinding people down. The psychiatrist wins you over because he invites you into his world in personal identification with his own frustration and anger, his *thumos*. He also shows his vulnerability and humanity in the last line, a winning move:

Story 2 extract

I think I need a holiday. I realise that when things get stressful, as they seem now with so few resources and so many expectations, that I look for something or someone to get angry with. It is so easy to scapegoat someone or something so that I can get my frustration out, but often it is unfair or disproportionate. If I was retired I would probably get angry with the neighbour's hedge, but at the moment I get angry with the cuts to mental health services. It is hard to keep things in perspective.

One psychiatrist confessed to a history of depression and recovery:

Story 3 extract

Looking back I was probably depressed in my teenage years but it can be difficult to separate from adolescent angst. I was definitely depressed at University, I think at its worst in the fourth year. I was depressed again in my first year as a doctor. Lack of confidence and feeling out of depth with responsibilities made the tiredness of long hours worse . . . I have been moved to tears when I remember the GP that listened to me for 40 minutes at the end of his surgery when I went to seek help in distress. He must've had a long day too. I am in a much better place now. Much more balance in my life, more confidence, more in control, better at taking care of myself. But now and again I get that lost in the fog feeling. Luckily the journey out seems shorter these days.

Another psychiatrist—writing in the third person, under the name 'Ed'—describes growing up with a disabled sister, where he grounds his development of care and empathy needed as a humane doctor and not just a technician:

Story 4 extract

Ed's 'luck' was his sister Ellie. Ed always explained that she was born early and had brain damage, his family had adopted her as a baby. She was 3 years older than Ed, couldn't speak, or walk and dribbled out of her mouth . . . all the time.

Another story by the same psychiatrist showed movement from resilience to discovery emerging in a story about his mother suffering a stroke:

Story 5 extract

Mum had a stroke last year, but fortunately she seems to have made a good recovery. It affected the part of her brain where she thinks of the reasons not to say things, so she lost her inhibitions for a few weeks. She said 'fuck' quite a lot and before the stroke, she pretty much used to cross herself when she just said 'bloody' or 'blast.' She howled with laughter at anything rude and if I am honest, was mostly a lot more fun than the woman that raised me.

A third psychiatrist wrote about bringing up a daughter severely disabled on the autistic spectrum, and how this had spawned resilience and a sense of discovery:

Story 6 extract

The present challenge for us as Sarah's parents is whether our undying love for her is strong enough to; perhaps, have to let her go to the extent that we are not able to see her very often. She clearly identifies her carers and her new supported care house . . . as her family and her home and our presence, especially at her home, troubles her and confuses her. I do not think she knows what we are there for, now that she is being cared for by other people.

A fourth doctor (GP) wrote poignantly about his grandfather's alcoholism. He identified with his grandfather's good and bad habits, more or less taking him as a roguish role model, having metaphorically known the grandfather 'inside out'—and empathised with his suffering—from medical scrutiny of his death certificate:

Story 7 extract

My Grandfather was a musician and loved jazz. That was before he drank himself to an early grave according to his daughter; my mother. I checked his death certificate recently. Carcinoma of the head of the pancreas. What a horrible way to go. I know that because I am a doctor, I think he would have been proud of that. It would explain the jaundice that's for sure. It seems so unjust now to write him off as an alcoholic. He painted, played the violin, smoked, listened to Oscar Peterson and I am guessing womanised. I like him.

Healing fiction

James Hillman (1984) suggests that the purpose of story is to 'heal' not just persons, but fiction or writing itself. For example, personal-confessional narratives can so easily lapse into self-indulgence, or soap operas—does the genre itself then not need to be 'healed'? In terms of recovery and discovery, the psychiatrist who wrote about his own recovery from depression showed not only a sharing of vulnerability uncommon amongst doctors, but also a 'healing' of the fictional mode of cathartic confession, as the story is not at all narcissistic, and moves beyond confession as catharsis to insight:

Story 8 extract

My busiest week was 120 hours on-call (during which I slept a little) but was working on my feet for 80 of them. I remember feeling cross, that if we were at war I could understand such excessive demands being made of me. I thought the system was trying to break me so that I would never grumble again and just follow orders. The other thing I think makes it worse is feeling everyone else is 'coping fine' adding to your sense of failure and aloneness.

Conclusions and implications

The philosopher Jacques Derrida (1998) challenged the 'explanatory' trope in the history of philosophy or metaphysics that deals with first principles. What if language—the very medium we draw on to offer final explanations—is itself beyond explanation or resists 'closure'? Metaphysics attempts to draw all phenomena into 'presence' or visibility in order to explain them, but what if 'presence' itself is largely an absence? Derrida called this 'the absent present.' The psychologist Andy Clark (2016) describes "a world in which unexpected absences are as perceptually salient as any concrete event"—again, the absence of presence. Perhaps the most telling symptom of mental illness is the inability to adapt to change in the environment (central to which is resilience) including unexpected absences or breaks in routine. This applies just as much to doctors as their patients and the patients' carers.

The absence of presence runs throughout doctors' interactions: patients tell incomplete, fragmentary and sometimes incoherent stories so that the doctor must inhabit the untold story of the patient as much as the told. Central to this are doctors listening to stories in their consulting rooms or clinics where the context of the patient's life constitutes a major absence, and, for various reasons, doctors may not listen well or may focus on inappropriate cues. Finally, doctors' mental health is not supposed to exist and then be discussed or researched. It must exist as the black box of medicine—we see the input and the output in terms of patient care, but we do not see the fine-grain psychological stress of the doctor who retires hurt or contemplates suicide, or turns to alcohol or drugs for solace. These currents are major absent presences in medical culture.

References

Alexander B. 2012. *The New Digital Storytelling: Creating Narratives with New Media.* Santa Barbara, CA: Praeger.

Amering M, Schmolke M. 2009. *Recovery in Mental Health: Reshaping Scientific and Clinical Responsibilities.* Oxford: Wiley-Blackwell.

Bleakley A. Stories as data, data as stories: making sense of narrative inquiry in clinical education. *Medical Education.* 2005; 39: 534–40.

Bleakley A. 2014. *Patient-Centred Medicine in Transition: The Heart of the Matter.* Dordrecht: Springer.

Burgess J. Hearing ordinary voices: cultural studies, vernacular creativity and digital storytelling. *Continuum: Journal of Media & Cultural Studies.* 2006; 20: 201–14.

Campbell D. Almost half of junior doctors reject NHS career after foundation training. *The Guardian.* 5 December 2015. Available at: www.theguardian.com/society/2015/dec/04/almost-half-of-junior-doctors-left-nhs-after-foundation-training. Last accessed: 26 November 2017.

Clark A. 2016. *Surfing Uncertainty: Prediction, Action, and the Embodied Mind.* Oxford: Oxford University Press.

Derrida J. 1998. Corrected ed. *Of Grammatology.* Baltimore, MD: Johns Hopkins University Press.

eurekadoc 2017. Available at: http://eurekadoc.com/how-a-different-kind-of-vision-can-save-you-from-burnout. Last accessed: 26 November 2017.

Farrell L, Bourgeois-Law G, Regehr G, Ajjawi R. Autoethnography: introducing 'I' into medical education research. *Medical Education.* 2015; 49: 974–82.

Gele AA, Harslof I. Types of social capital resources and self-rated health among the Norwegian adult population. *International Journal for Equity in Health.* 2010; 9: 8.

Gerada C. 2017. My prescription for dejected doctors? A reality check. *The Guardian.* 24 November 2017.

Gonzales L. 2012. *Surviving Survival: The Arts and Science of Resilience.* New York, NY: Norton.

Hillman J. 1984, 2nd ed. *Healing Fiction.* Dallas, TX: Spring Publications.

Hungin P. 2017. Foreword to: The changing face of medicine and the role of doctors in the future: Presidential Project 2017. London: British Medical Association (BMA). Available at: www.bma.org.uk/collective-voice/policy-and-research/education-training-and-workforce/changing-face-of-medicine. Last accessed: 26 November 2017.

HMG DH. 2011. No health without mental health (Royal College of Psychiatrists). Available at: www.rcpsych.ac.uk/PDF/No%20Health%20without%20Mental%20Health.pdf. Last accessed: 26 November 2017.

Howe A. 2013. Doctors' health and wellbeing. *BMJ Careers.* 17 September 2013. Available at: http://careers.bmj.com/careers/advice/view-article.html?id=20014522. Last accessed: 26 November 2017.

Joseph S. 2011. *What Doesn't Kill Us: The New Psychology of Posttraumatic Growth.* London: Piatkus.

Kleinman A. 1989. *The Illness Narratives: Suffering, Healing and the Human Condition.* London: Basic Books.

Lauveng, A. 2013. *A Road Back from Schizophrenia: A Memoir*. New York, NY: Skyhorse Publishing.

Manning S. The doctor battling drink and depression will see you now . . . *The Independent on Sunday*. 4 November 2012, 4–5.

Moberly T. UK has fewer doctors per person than most other OECD countries. *BMJ*. 2017; 357: j2940. Available at: www.bmj.com/content/357/bmj.j2940. Last accessed: 6 November 2018.

Niemietz K. 2016. Universal healthcare without the NHS: towards a patient-centred health system. Institute of Economic Affairs. Available at: https://iea.org.uk/publications/universal-healthcare-without-the-nhs. Last accessed: 10 May 2018.

Pagel M. 2013. *Wired for Culture: The Natural History of Human Cooperation*. London: Penguin Books.

Peterkin A, Bleakley A. 2017. *Staying Human During the Foundation Programme and Beyond: How to Thrive After Medical School*. Baton Rouge, FL: CRC Press.

Plato. 2005. *Phaedrus* (Penguin Classics). Harmondsworth: Penguin.

Ricoeur, P. 1984. *Time and Narrative: Volume 1*. London: University of Chicago Press.

Sanders L. 2010. *Diagnosis: Dispatches from the Frontlines of Medical Mysteries*. London: Icon Books.

Schleifer R, Vannatta JB. 2013. *The Chief Concern of Medicine: The Integration of the Medical Humanities and Narrative Knowledge into Medical Practices*. Ann Arbor, MI: University of Michigan Press.

Sennett R. 2012. *Together: The Rituals, Pleasures and Politics of Cooperation*. London: Allen Lane.

Stiglitz JE. 2012. *The Price of Inequality*. London: Allen Lane.

Webber M, Corker E, Hamilton S, et al. Discrimination against people with severe mental illness and their access to social capital: findings from the Viewpoint survey. *Epidemiology and Psychiatric Sciences*. 2014; 23: 155–65.

41

ALL THANKS TO THE WORDS OF A STRANGER

An homage to the UK's National Health Service

Sophie Holloway

Doctor

4:30. Half an hour behind; the clock on the wall ticks on, a constant reminder, a permanent pressure. The bitter, steaming coffee is liquid energy, willing me on. The challenges of the day are dragging me down; the Grim Reaper a constant companion with his heavy looming breath—my all-too-familiar enemy. An image of a patient's face, changed beyond recognition by the cruelty of his sudden death, burned into the back of my eyes. While rewarding, this job is heart-breaking. Still, I move on. There's a waiting room full of patients who need my help, and who wants to see a damaged doctor?

I call the next patient and wait to see what the subsequent ten minutes will bring. The door opens slowly with a squeak that snaps my attention away from the screen displaying an ever-expanding list of emails demanding replies—my very own emergency department. Through the door enters a small, elderly woman; her hunched shoulders and tear-streaked cheeks are mirrored by an uncomfortable knot in the pit of my stomach. The tense atmosphere in my small room turns thicker with emotion. My cracked heart aches a little more at the thought of encountering more tragedy today. Now is the time to put on my well-worn 'doctor's mask'— the protective membrane that prevents my own emotions from spilling out and staining the patient's being.

I meet her eyes and am faced with dark blue pools of sorrow, heartbreak and pain. Without her uttering a word, I knew her worst nightmare had spilled over into reality. She shuffles slowly, already defeated, to take her place at the other side of the desk. A small silence ensues as the woman visibly tenses. In this moment, I want nothing more than to hug this broken human, to physically hold her shattered pieces together, the comfort of human touch letting her know that it's okay; to encourage her to share her pain, to let me in. But something holds me back. A hug would result in that silent unspoken barrier between patient and doctor being crossed. It would be 'unprofessional.' I settle on placing a box of tissues in front of her. She takes one and inhales deeply. She begins to explain how her husband of 50 years had suffered a stroke two days ago, how he was currently in hospital unable to move, how she had nowhere else to turn, nobody else to talk to. Her words come out slowly and carefully—an eggshell vocabulary; one wrong word and she would lose the small amount of composure she had mustered to speak to me.

Leaning forward, I listen to every word. Despite my many years of training, no lecture could teach me how to 'fix' this patient. The best I can offer is my undivided attention, allowing her to voice her worries and concerns in an environment where she will not be judged. Witnessing such pain, that I am powerless to stop, is an uncomfortable feeling for someone who is used to fixing pain with the ease of a signature conjuring a prescription. The only medicine I can give is words and gestures. I try the stock phrases taught to me many moons ago by the actor-patients in medical school—prescriptive, simple, clinical—uttering: "That must be terrible for you"; preventing me from having to delve into my own feelings and worries; preventing me from giving away too much of myself. Hardly feeling adequate, I reach inside for more. There are some situations where is it impossible not to feel, not to give away a small chunk of yourself. This is one of them. Only the most hard-nosed, battle-worn doctor could get away scratch-free from this type of consultation. The small, wrecked figure of the person in front of me deserves a doctor who could take her suffering and feel it with her, to give her some sort of strength to keep her going. And what bigger strength is there than love? I remind her of the fact that although most of her husband's future is uncertain, the one thing he could rely on was her love. I remind her that medicine can be a wonderful thing and that the team at the hospital would work night and day to take care of her husband. The thing he needed most was her just sitting with him, supporting him and caring for him; this was the greatest gift she could give. Her husband was a very lucky man to have someone willing to do this at the toughest point in his life. At this, her small moist eyes threaten once more to leak tears. I hope more than anything that my softly spoken words, meant in the kindest way possible, will give this woman the resilience to walk the tough road ahead.

It pains me, when the time comes, to turn back to my computer and summarise the tragic tale in her notes. The fragile connection I had initially worked so hard to gain was snapped like an elastic band pulled too tight, as if the turn of my chair towards the desk had stretched it that little too far. The sound of talking was replaced by the tapping of the keyboard. So much of my job is paperwork and I resent it greatly. The short ten minutes I'm permitted to dedicate to one patient is simply too little time to complete a consultation, meaning I often have to make a start on the notes while the patient is still there just to check on the veracity of details. I know this is bad medicine, and against all communication skills training, but what am I to do? Typing as fast as my fingers will let me, I finish a brief account of what's happened while it is fresh in my mind. I try to think of an appropriate way to end our sorry meeting. As the lady gathers her things and her thoughts, I promise, a true promise from the bottom of my heart, that I am there for her; anytime she feels it is too much, or needs to talk, my door is open. I insist on her visiting me again next week, not just for her sake, but showing that I am genuinely worried about the welfare of this now vulnerable woman. The privilege of being able to do this and give such continuity of care makes me grateful of my career choice. She nods a small 'thank you doctor' and gets up slowly to leave. I notice she may be standing a little taller, a little less hunched, and I hope this is the impact I have had. This is a problem I cannot fix but if I can make a slight improvement to this patient's mental strength, I feel that I have at least done my job. I am reminded that although the pull of this beloved profession of mine is often heroic glory—to save people's lives performing dramatic complex procedures—it is in fact the small victories lessening suffering that give you the strength to survive in a world of pain, indignity and distress. Small victories stuffed into ten minutes.

Patient

4:30. I'm sitting on yet another uncomfortable NHS chair. The clock ticks behind me and I'm reminded I have somewhere more important to be. My appointment should have been half an hour ago and the guilt only swells inside me with every minute that passes. I clutch another terrible, tasteless tea, my only source of energy for the past few days. The constant bombardment of information and questions is slowly sapping what little reserves I have left. Never have I felt my life flip upside down so quickly, everything I know has been ripped from me; so now I find myself here, in a different, but strangely familiar, NHS waiting room, this time for myself. A huge part of my brain tugs for me to leave, that this is selfish when the person that matters most to me is lying sick in a hospital bed. But I am scared, the most scared I have ever been, and I'm worried I will just stop functioning. I do not have the strength to go on without him by my side. For 50 years we have been side by side, waking up together, cooking together, shopping together, going to sleep next to each other, exchanging tenderness. Now I am lost, having to learn to do all of these things on my own. We were never gifted with children, our friends have been slowly diminishing in number and I have nowhere else to turn. The big gaping hole that is loneliness threatens to swallow me. So I find myself here, in need of someone who will understand and tell me how to carry on.

The sound of my name echoes around the room and it makes me jump from my tired daze. I lift myself onto my creaking legs and walk with heavy steps to my allocated room. As the hours have passed, the harder it has been to even move my ageing body. I open the door with a small squeak. I was expecting a warm, pleasant doctor, ready and willing to listen, but this isn't the sight that greets me. Instead I am faced with a tired, stressed-looking human, so engrossed in her computer screen that she barely notices me entering the room. The room is littered with empty coffee cups and stacks of papers; complete chaos that I worry may reflect the doctor's abilities. She turns to face me and I visibly see her face drop as she catches my eye. I immediately want to turn around. I have made a mistake. I should have listened to that part that is nagging me to leave, now shouting as loud as it can muster. This doctor did not want to see a woman on the verge of defeat with eyes continually brimming with tears. She visibly carries her own suffering and weariness.

The atmosphere in the room is tense, icy, knitted from emotional traces. What happened to the doctor's office as a place of comfort and reassurance—the person who would offer you solutions for your ailments or support for your sagging soul? As I reluctantly take a seat, I meet the eyes of the so-called 'expert.' The look of disappointment has faded from her face and has been replaced by a different expression, one I can't quite figure out, almost as if fighting off emotion. There appears to be a moment of conflict in her eyes and a miniscule movement towards me as if she might hug me, so transient that I question whether it was there at all. A hug is what I need—someone to feel my pain with me and give me the comfort of human touch. Please touch me! My heart lifts for a moment, hoping that this stranger has read my needs, but then collapses as quickly to disappointment as a battered box of tissues is placed in front of me. I can see the sentiment but it's almost laughable that a box of tissues may help soothe the anguish inside. Still, I take one from the box as an invitation that she is prepared to listen, a symbolic gesture at best.

Having to force my words over the lump growing at the back of my throat, I recount how I had found my husband looking odd and unable to speak after breakfast, how I had watched the man I knew so well nearly slip away as the ambulance crew packed him into the back of their van like a delivery service, how I later saw the fear in his eyes as he lay in a hospital bed unable to communicate his needs, life ebbing away. The words I've been so desperate to say surprisingly roll off my tongue without me trying, but with each word I get a small stab of pain in my heart, forcing me to take my time. Leaning towards me, the doctor listens intently, nodding, encouraging me to continue. After what seems like an eternity, I take a breath and await a reply. "That must be terrible for you." It sounds hollow, reverberating around the room; odd, devoid of real feeling, like it has been said too many times to too many people; the words not quite holding the meaning they imply, mechanical. For a moment I am worried that this will be all I get, that this doctor just doesn't care enough about my hurt for her to show an inch of feeling, understanding or sympathy. A bubble of rage rises up from the pit of my stomach, one that's been building for days, but is now threatening to burst free. It's not her fault; I'm angry at life itself for running dry. Just as the vicious flames reach the tip of my tongue, they are extinguished by the word I never expected to be uttered from what I assumed was the cold doctor: 'love.' The one thing I had given to my husband for over 50 years without thinking about its strength and power—reliable, unchanging, necessary, unconditional. We had overcome plenty of challenges in our lives together with the constancy of underlying love keeping us going, and this would be no different. She assured me that my beloved husband was being taken good care of and that I just needed to be with him. It caused relief to wash over me and that triggered gravity-led trails of tears. It was as if a well-hidden lump of emotion that needed to be released had been teased out by the sweet words of this relative stranger. Right then I get what I came here for, a human connection of understanding—someone to share my burden, to share some responsibility.

But then a connection that has burst into flames turns as quickly to cold ash. Simply a turn of the eyes and a transfer of attention leave me feeling alone and abandoned once again. The glaringly bright screen of the computer becomes the doctor's false gaze. I think back to how it was as a child to see a doctor; a grand, pompous doctor in his smart tweed suit who told you what was wrong and what you must do without allowing you even the smallest of sentences in reply. But then, at least I did not have to compete with the Cyclops eye of technology. An eye that is a round silence interrupted only by the dull tapping of a keyboard sits, revolving, in the small room and demands that I wait. Feeling trapped, drained and exhausted, I have no more left to say. What is she typing so furiously? And why now? I take the cue that this conversation is over and begin to gather myself together, in every way imaginable, to face going back to the antiseptic-smelling hospital bay where my loved one is lying alone. Before I leave, the doctor interrupts me. She promises me, and I feel it as wholly genuine, that I am not alone, that her door is open whenever I need it. She insists that I visit her again in a week's time, to tell her how both my husband and I are doing, and to let her know of anything she can help with. I think she is being optimistic about my husband, but this moment means more to me than any prescription, as the unholy cramp of the past few minutes passes.

I feel grateful that a health system can guarantee a free, uninterrupted appointment with a doctor who has the time to really listen, despite the obvious stresses of the job. I will always be able to find someone who will care, and share my hurt, and try her best to make it better. For this I am thankful. We need to be more appreciative of this indiscriminating, wonderful service that really does help the people who need it most. Although I am fully aware of the long, hard road I have in front of me, it gives me strength to know there will always be someone not too far behind ready to catch me if I fall, or fail. I thank the doctor and leave walking that little bit taller, feeling a little less defeated—all thanks to the words of a stranger.

PART VIII

Overview

Celebrating the flaw in the Persian rug

42

NEGOTIATING RESEARCH IN THE MEDICAL HUMANITIES

Maria Athina (Tina) Martimianakis,
Cynthia R. Whitehead and Ayelet Kuper

We open this conclusion, which focuses on research in the medical humanities, by citing once again (see Introduction) Alexis de Tocqueville from the fourth volume of *Democracy in America*:

> There are certain vices and certain virtues that were attached to the constitution of aristocratic nations and that are so contrary to the genius of the new peoples that you cannot introduce those vices and virtues among them . . . They are like two distinct humanities, each of which has its particular advantages and disadvantages, its good and its evil which are its own. So you must be very careful about judging the societies that are being born by the ideas that you have drawn from those that are no longer. That would be unjust, for these societies, differing prodigiously from each other, are not comparable.
>
> *(2010: 1282–83)*

In this passage de Tocqueville cautions readers that judging the cultural makeup of the newly constituted American republic by the standards of European aristocracy is unproductive. There are many reasons for this, the most important being that the purpose of art as a social mechanism shifted from adornment to usefulness as the movement of self-determination took hold in the American colonies. There is much to learn from appreciating this shift. His caution, to avoid unjust comparisons, also applies when thinking about the established methods of the arts and humanities as long-standing traditions in the Western academy. These established traditions are neither naïve nor disinterested movements. De Tocqueville's passage reminds us that the 'aristocratic' versions of the arts and humanities associated with the Greco-Roman civilisations, the Enlightenment, the Renaissance, progress and humanity have been traditionally white Eurocentric male worldviews supporting aesthetics that led to social division—those who could afford to engage with the arts and those who could not. Their function to some extent was to reinforce the superiority of an upper class by rendering vulgar and coarse all who could not claim to be 'classically' schooled. While this political project changed over the years, it is still part of the genetic makeup of the field of medical humanities and any other new field that purports to establish an aesthetic by drawing from what has preceded. As we will argue, being methodologically selective has not erased the tendency towards division in the field of medical humanities. For example, in the Introduction, Bleakley makes a case for democratisation as an aim or function for medical humanities, particularly in health settings where the effects of power are felt as hegemonic and oppressive. However, we know from history and contemporary politics that democracy has a dangerous underbelly. The interests of the vulnerable are not always realised through representational forums that channel the voice of the majority or the more powerful. Given that the topic of our chapter is research, we asked: 'what role should representation, voice, and political projects have in the research agendas of the medical humanities?'

As per de Tocqueville's caution, we deliberately refrain from judging the work included in this volume by any formal measure of truth or aesthetic associated with the particular methods of any discipline. Our own histories and disciplinary backgrounds, in any case, render us an idiosyncratic panel of authors in an emergent field that is best served by the possibility of imagining multiple origin stories—a point to which we return later in this chapter. Instead, we focus on how this collection of work—the *Routledge Handbook of the Medical Humanities*—serves to set up a geography of operations for medical humanities inclusive of the tensions and contestations that inevitably go along with boundary setting. Our goal is to make visible the transactional nature of such boundary setting and invite readers to participate in the field's development by considering the various ways in which research factors into the evolution of the field. Can we call the aim of medical humanities 'democratisation' when the field has yet to develop a method for negotiating differences? What happens axiologically when we set up different territories of function for a field?

Aesthetics and the politics of resistance

Bleakley introduces this volume with a conversation about aesthetics and the politics of resistance. Through his discussion, the arts and humanities are epistemologically positioned as mechanisms of socialisation—political tools that should always be used with purpose and intent. For the arts and humanities to be linked to a democratising project within medicine, proponents must aim explicitly to work towards liberating the profession of its past transgressions, flattening problematic hierarchies that interfere with collaboration and the sharing of expertise, and maintaining a focus on the patient as a person. These aims become an axiology—a moral purpose of sorts—that Bleakley argues (though not all of this book's authors appear to agree) should underpin the practice of medical humanities. Referencing Weiss, he writes: "art can be sterile unless mobilised as a form of resistance and justice." To us, these opening thoughts become a centring focus for considering how research relates to the political projects of the humanities.

Bleakley's Introduction explicitly links aesthetics and power. While such a link might be counter-intuitive to many in the scientistic world of medicine, to speak of aesthetics within the medical humanities is to accept that in medicine there are sensory experiences that conjure up something beyond the ordinary perceptual properties of the bodies, objects, languages and spaces that make up the practice of caring for the ill. Aesthetics can only be constituted through intersubjectivity and art is the medium by which this shared agreement of what counts as 'beauty' is formulated. The authors of this volume propose that the work of rendering something 'beautiful' is a political act, an exercise of power—that it would be dangerous then to assume innocence in the artistic representation of health and illness. How, then, does aesthetics as a method for making meaning afford power to the medical humanities? And what is the role of research in both supporting and problematising this form of meaning-making?

There are, for example, those subjects and objects that the medical humanities help us to see as beautiful, to render acceptable or even desirable, to transform from abnormal to normal. If (as Eichbaum et al. write in Chapter 32) "even the most aggressive and malignant cancers can present themselves as beautiful pictures under a microscope," what cannot be redeemed aesthetically? A researcher might ask, what and who is served by making cancer out to be beautiful? How do subjects and objects become reified? Here the interest would be to understand why it seems that socio-culturally some things in medicine can only be experienced as beautiful, desirable and admirable, like compassion, empathy and altruism, while some others can only be related to as ugly, undesirable and abhorrent, like death and the diseases that stifle youth, vigour, and life's idealised potential. In Chapter 31, for example, Neill describes how medicine historically made much greater use of the sense of smell in medical diagnosis. As medical smells are mostly malodorous and perceived as offensive, their use is declining in the sanitised world of modern medicine. Instead of appreciating them for their medical uses, now professionals must learn to hide their sense of disgust of the malodours of patients.

A values-based research agenda, conscious of the tendencies of the field towards divisiveness, describes, catalogues and historicises these renderings and simultaneously problematises them for their aesthetic properties—the power relations that underpin the meaning-making that inevitably will make some people look, feel and sound normal and others not (see Chapter 8). What a research agenda focused on the aesthetics of health humanities allows us to do is to look into a mirror and appreciate that our capacity to render makes us vulnerable to the rendering of others. It allows aesthetics to be part of a politics for resistance. For medicine this is particularly important because the power to render is amplified through the medical gaze with direct implications for how patients experience their journeys in the health care system—a topic addressed implicitly or explicitly in many of the chapters in this volume, particularly by those authors who employ storytelling in their work.

Chapter 1 establishes the importance of storytelling in this volume, demonstrating that stories, together with aesthetics, are able to transform. Storytelling, perhaps the most political of tools, is a foundational element of the medical humanities. Stories can give voice to the powerless, open the eyes of the powerful or simply render others human. The emotive properties of stories in the medical humanities paint over the sterility of the clinical experience. Stories can anger or frustrate. They can be accusatory or forgiving. They can be a cry for help or a desire to be released from responsibility. Ultimately, they serve to focus attention on the details the storyteller finds important and serve as an invitation to the reader to experience health care through the eyes of another. Like the patient describing her relationship with her doctor, stories are a way to gain insights about one's self:

> I wasn't in love with him, but I had come to depend on him. I was accustomed to taking care of myself and I had let him take care of me. I let him see that I was scared. And when I let him see my fear, I had to see it, too. My own fragility. The stuff I couldn't just power through.
>
> *(Davenport, Chapter 1)*

However, stories can also disempower, colonise and finalise. We see this when we study whose stories are told, by whom and for what purpose. In Chapter 11 Bleakley relives the experience of losing his father to cancer while having to navigate a physician's directive that kept the truth of the severity of his father's illness from him, forcing the family to be complicit in a facade in the name of good health care. In trying to make sense of this experience years later, he writes:

> In other words, the capital of emotional response and grief held within the family comes to be owned and distributed by the medical profession according to its whims, rather than an open and transparent ethical framework. Medicine colonises the voices of patient and family.

The stories we tell in health care, whether or not they are framed as being part of the medical humanities, are a rich source of research data, conveying important functional information that may, in turn, improve the practice of medicine. Shwetz (Chapter 17) highlights, for example, the narratives of the anti-vaccination movement. Given the compelling and complex narrative structures of anti-vaccination, she suggests that health care professionals will only be able to tackle the fear of vaccines by engaging with this narrative complexity. Empirically then, stories are repositories of attitudes, perceptions, opinions and experiences. As we make sense of stories and storytelling in the medical humanities, we have the opportunity to consider a broader political project for health care in our local communities and beyond.

Stories also open or close worlds of possibilities through their power to socialise group members into accepted norms, to transmit accepted ways of being and thinking from one generation to the next, to act as a moral compass. As with *Aesop's Fables*, which are the Western canon's classic moral tales, we find storytelling being used in the medical humanities to signpost a more virtuous path through the problematic landscapes of medicine. Quite a few of the chapters in this book contribute to this genre of tales with moral purpose. Researchers can use these tales to make sense of contemporary healthcare issues. When the research foregrounds power relations, making sense of them can also contribute to social justice imperatives—as long as we remember to interrogate the authoring of the text, its explicit and implicit purposes, and the manifest and latent functions it might have in reproducing socio-political relationships. It is because of the role of storytelling as moral compass that there is an inescapable reproduction of norms. Established critical research methods can help mitigate the reproduction of Western dominance in medical humanities but—as we have noted above—no research method is 'innocent.' As well, we must consider the importance of developing methodologies that fit the circumstances and realities of the medical humanities (a consideration to which we return later in this chapter when we consider the role of expertise).

This book makes a direct link between the medical humanities and social justice imperatives, so it is not surprising that one clear storyline running through this book is the attempt to take on the 'othering' that pervades healthcare practices. Within this volume, authors trouble the othering of people for ways of being that are often stigmatised both in medicine and in many other societal contexts: e.g., for being gay (Chapter 8), for being old (Chapter 15), for being disabled (Chapter 38). Indeed, the use of narrative to counteract stigma in this way has a long tradition in the medical humanities, broadly conceived—think, for example, of the transformative effects of the Broadway production of 'Angels in America' at the height of the AIDS crisis—and has frequently been used as a pedagogical argument for the incorporation of the humanities into health professions curricula. An understanding of how aesthetic and storytelling both contribute to a mechanism of socialisation and to political projects of reform can be achieved empirically through research that studies how metaphors, for example, contribute to a complex social organisation of the clinical space (we discuss this in more detail below) or how stories as confessionals or reflexive exercises can call attention to problematic power relations in our renderings of others (see Chapters 6 and 35). This latter approach entails stepping back and considering how our situated and embodied appreciation of the medical humanities can be contributing to the reproduction of a hegemonic Western aesthetic. There are opportunities to think about how race, culture and class intersect with the politics of aesthetics and storytelling in a globalising world and to contribute to movements that seek to address health disparities and inequities locally and internationally.

The theme of vulnerability that cuts across the contributions to this volume invites researchers to also consider the role of storytelling in exposing the harm done to patients, trainees, and others by the language and metaphors of medicine operationalised in health care contexts.

Piemonte (Chapter 14) examines the effects of medical slang, showing that while it can be emotionally protective for clinicians, it also distances them from the suffering of their seriously ill patients. By attending to these metaphors, Piemonte is able to understand that:

> We need only to get our students to see that medicine is full of people who may be having the crisis of their lives, and who are, simultaneously and absurdly, also just items on a to-do list. Our job is simply to help them recognise this incongruity, to recognise that they participate in a medical system that unconsciously encourages them *not* to see patients as whole people with rich and sometimes tragic lives, but as 'things to do.'

Bleakley, in Chapter 11, similarly tackles medicine's use of language, in this case the dominant metaphors of the body as a machine and medicine as war, calling out these metaphors as maintaining medicine as an imperialistic and authoritarian enterprise which resists democratisation to the detriment of its patients. Lingard and Goldszmidt (Chapter 16), on the other hand, focus on metaphors related to clinical supervision, describing how language can severely limit our understanding of a complex, nuanced task. Clearly there is room and utility in adopting research practices within medical humanities that can make sense of language practices in health care contexts.

The medical humanities as a geography of operations have also focused on material aspects of care, attempting to reset medicine's moral compass by showcasing non-linguistic medical practices that wound, that cause suffering, and that prevent healing; see, for example, Martin's (Chapter 25) troubling of the armour-like masks that medical professionals put on when adopting the doctor *persona*. Still others move beyond problematic practices to focus on their effects, including O'Mahony's (Chapter 9) faulting of medicine (drawing on Ivan Illich's legacy) for causing "cultural iatrogenesis," turning suffering into pain and medicalising death; and Wong's (Chapter 10) reconstruction of the practices of medicine—within medical education—as an amusement park for medical student gamification. Still others foreground the alternative, virtuous path: in both Davenport's (Chapter 1) description of her emotional connection to her equally suffering physician and Holloway's (Chapter 41) poignant telling of an encounter from the perspectives of both the doctor and the patient, virtue and healing (if not health) come to be through moments of interaction between two human beings. In all of these, if only implicitly (we are, after all, meant to be reading these texts, these stories, and learning from them), the medical humanities become a way to socialise practitioners and learners into ways of thinking, speaking and being that are more beneficial for patients. Research can support this process both by creating evidence for the role of the medical humanities as an educational practice in development of expertise (see Chapter 3) and in using the products of medical humanities pedagogy as data.

The politics of expertise: competing for authority in medical humanities

An orientation that links stories with the establishment of moral direction makes sense for a field still positioning itself as legitimate within the medical realm, for it is often argued that in medicine, everything taught to and done by the health professional must be done in service of the patient. So what does it mean for physician identity if having the opportunity to enjoy, appreciate and/or criticise the arts and humanities while being in the practice of medicine improves the care of patients? Should this knowledge not therefore be claimed to be the purview of a health professional? If not, then what should the links be "between an enterprise dedicated to the inculcation of human values and an enterprise dedicated to the exploration of human values" (Jones and Wear, Chapter 5)? And who has the expertise to study and answer this important question?

When a field—such as the medical humanities—is organising, the potential for partial uptake of methodological traditions affords exciting opportunities to scholars who are freed to introduce new (or perhaps just different) approaches of inquiry to support the socio-political operations of the developing knowledge base. 'New' or 'different' of course do not automatically equate with 'better,' and—not surprisingly—the issue of who is authorised to judge quality is a topic explicitly and implicitly reflected in this book.

Measuring quality is an essential part of establishing a field's boundaries in the Bordieuvian sense, as it establishes the rules by which membership in the field can be claimed and by which the field's rewards, responsibilities and resources are distributed. This issue is taken up by Jones and Wear (Chapter 5) who raise the question of who should be considered an 'expert' in the field of medical humanities, for without 'recognised' experts (and of course an associated body of expertise), how will this epistemic field earn a bona fide seat in the academy? Jones and Wear take issue with claims to authority and voice in the field by individuals who are not qualified with recognisable expertise in the "theories and methods of the arts and humanities disciplines" for it devalues the quality and legitimacy of the field. They observe that:

> where clinical expertise and disciplinary knowledge unquestionably matter in health-care education and practice (you wouldn't seek out an historian or a physical therapist if you needed a hysterectomy), when it comes to the arts and humanities, expertise and credentialing seem to matter very little or not at all.

They also distinguish between consuming the products of the arts and humanities and the activity of an expert who studies to understand how these objects have come to be defined and what effects they have in the world—the difference between appreciating an artefact and understanding how the artefact has come to be. Who is 'expert' is a fundamental question that has significant material effects in an epistemic field, the most important being agenda setting. The expert has the authority to define, at and for a given point in time, the 'right' way for both generating and appreciating the aesthetics of medical practice.

This distinction is not unlike that made by Mathieu Albert in his work about the field of medical education (another hybrid, highly contested field). Albert (2004) speaks about knowledge and meaning-making in medical education as happening on a continuum. One pole represents claims of legitimacy from scientists who would like to produce knowledge for other scientists (production for producers) while maintaining control of the field, deciding on what questions are worth researching and continuing to use and apply the methodologies and markers of rigour in which they were trained in other disciplines. On the other side of the spectrum sit those who claim that the field of medical education should produce knowledge for physicians (production for users). At this pole, scientists and clinicians share the authority and legitimacy to decide which questions are worth answering. Having read this volume, we have come to appreciate that using established methods from arts and humanities disciplines as the legitimate measures for assessing the quality of those forms of knowledge-making being applied in, or growing out of, the field of medical humanities will undoubtedly obfuscate important ways of knowing by drawing attention away from the details of the local, contingent and experiential to some other theorised and abstracted concept of 'right,' which may be peripheral to the practice of medicine.

Referring again to an example provided by Jones and Wear (Chapter 5):

> Simply asking surgery residents to respond to a question about a painting such as: "What do you see?" or about a poem, such as: "What do you think?", is neither train- ing nor educating. The response to such questions in a humanities classroom would be more questions: What does the painting or poem mean? How can you make an argument for its meanings? What are the specific elements in the painting or images in the poem to support them?

Whether explicitly said or not, by virtue of the publication of this volume, we can argue that the notion that the field requires formalisation to the degree suggested by Jones and Wear is still contested. There are many exemplars in this volume of authors, some not credentialled in the humanities, who reference or demonstrate in their writing the importance and application of the humanities gaze in the work and life of a health professional (we discuss this further in the section on the role of stories). Others, such as Crawford and Brown in Chapter 39, reject altogether the need to adopt a pre-existing structure for how to think about or apply teachings from the arts and humanities. They go so far as to reject the reified aesthetics of illness and suf- fering foregrounded as artefacts in the medical/health humanities. To make this rejection clearer they stringently adopt the term 'health humanities' as a "decentralised, democratic approach" which "destabilises the kinds of hierarchies of expert knowledge which constrain innovation in applying the arts and humanities for health and wellbeing."

Those who feel aligned with or part of the 'field' of medical humanities may very well decide that it will stay in this liminal space of becoming; a state where gazing at a painting to 'see' is perceived as valuable to local constituents because of the specific meaning-making it affords the doctor. In these simple exercises, then, we come to appreciate that there is a proximal association to both the arts and humanities disciplines and the practice of medicine that contemporary medical humanities enjoy. There is reason and rationale for this. 'What do you see?' is not a simple question when asked of a physician. Evoking the medical gaze epitomises the power a physician has in decreeing what is 'health' and what is 'illness,' what is 'normal' and what is 'anomaly,' and what is life and what is death. It is the power of this gaze that is being mitigated when a physician is told to look at a painting and describe what they see. It is the voice of evidence that is muffled when a physician is asked what they think about a poem. 'What do you see?' and 'what do you think?' are exercises in learning to un-see through the biomedical gaze, or at least to be able to take off that gaze and take in the personal and the subjective. There is no right answer to the question of what you see when you look at a painting or what a poem means to you. For this reason, asking such things of physicians can become interventions that aim to counter the effects of a culture of objectification and aspired certainty.

What, then, should the field's knowledge base be? Should we be thinking of it as a binary of two poles fighting for control over a spectrum of activities, or is it more productive to consider how to protect the field's geography as a contested space, a space for tensions to sprout, a space where there are multiple forms of knowledge that contradict and challenge each other? Is it a space for drawing attention to moral dilemmas, for making visible the power relations inherent in aesthetics? It struck us that the term 'negotiation,' so common in the critical social science disciplines in which we work, appears only once in the book, where (in Chapter 18) Cotterrell presents a cautionary tale of humanism as governmentality. That chapter, written in the first per- son, in the voice of the artist, briefly alludes to negotiation as a tool for maintaining a respectful openness while striving for intersubjectivity:

Aware of my limitations, I always opted for negotiation, frequently attempted to engender empathy and occasionally tried to build enough ambiguity to encourage an opponent to experience the same uncertainty, ensuring that I would never be a risk to the world.

To strive "never to be a risk to the world" through negotiation is to open one's boundaries to deliberation. So should the purpose of the medical humanities be to "contest" and create uncertainty within a field, such as medicine, which valorises certainty? This idea has been reviewed extensively in the Introduction. We return to it again in the conclusion as we contemplate its implications for research.

A researcher would consider the alignment of ontology with axiology, epistemology and methodology. Is the ontological position of the medical humanities, then, that there should not be an ontological position—or a postmodern relativism—but rather an appreciation that the very notion of ontology runs counter to the desire to maintain a fluid and dynamic negotiation of objects, concepts and subjects that seem to constitute medical humanities at this point in time (as represented in the compilation of this volume)? We see, for example, the two main social imperatives argued for in this volume, to strive to democratise and to fight for social justice, as being a product of a process of resistance to formalisation. Democracy is about competition for voice and representation—it is a collective vision for individuation. Social justice is a pull away from this individuation to an integrative desire for social consciousness—a desire to curb powerful groups to allow those with less power to develop voice. What we are suggesting is that, by setting them side by side, there is the potential for a democratic vision to learn from the tension of co-existing with a social justice movement in a way that moves away from the ideational and aspirational to the socio-political realm where the practice of medicine happens. For example, Wellbery (Chapter 37) calls for the medical humanities to adopt a social justice orientation as a way to escape the "questionable exclusions of empathy," contending that "fostering social empathy might counteract the implicit and explicit biases of individual empathy." She argues that stories (and the learning of empathy) must strive to shift the medical gaze for single interactions to operating "within a framework of institutional values that support the pursuit of social justice on a larger scale" and that the medical humanities can help medicine achieve this new orientation because they "represent the general through the particular, and thus model empathy's full potential by providing an opportunity to extrapolate from concrete experience to its broader contexts."

The research project of the medical humanities then cannot be merely documentary or revisionary. It cannot focus only on the philosophical or on the science behind the pedagogy of expression and representation. The research project of the medical humanities is by necessity as much about undoing what we know as it is about painting a landscape of contemporary socio-political and cultural practices. As Bleakley notes in the Introduction, "medical or health humanities is a work in (or as) progress." It is for this reason then that only reaching to old, well-worn, methodologies is risky. It is too comfortable for the space that medical humanities seem to want to occupy. The process then hinges on negotiation (that is the word we know but there might be other words which we are not aware of that connote a process of dynamic becoming that is openly transactional). It is a process of negotiating differences to reach a temporary intersubjectivity. We agree with Bleakley and others in this volume that such a process needs an axiology that directs transactions towards mutual gain. We have discussed how values are transmitted informally through the storytelling that cuts across medical humanities practices. It also happens formally through the medical humanities as educational practice.

The medical humanities as educational practice

If the research project of the medical humanities is about negotiating differences, foregrounding socio-political practices and questioning certainties, what then is its educational project? While this volume is neither a textbook nor a manual for educators, the descriptions of curriculum and pedagogy embedded in a number of chapters hint at similar goals arising in that realm as well. In Chapter 23 Ramaswamy and Ramaswamy vividly describe using 'Theatre of the Oppressed' with medical students across India to

> enable the body to be free and to open the mind to new sensations, leading to a heightened awareness of our feelings. An important element in these workshops is fun. Students experience a sense of aliveness that amazes them and rediscover a part of themselves that had been sidelined and lost in the mad rush of everyday routine. This discovery always leads to a feeling of liberation and great power.

Liberatory pedagogy of this kind, when successful, helps flatten hierarchies, instilling orientations that are often intended to be in line with one or both of the competing social imperatives (democratisation and social justice) we see running through this volume. Those same radical alignments are embedded in the ontology and history of the body-mapping techniques Costanzo describes using in Chapter 30. However, those literally and figuratively messy techniques are, in her account, limited to wellness workshops—to regions of the parallel curriculum that are tolerated but not mainstream, that are intended to inform learners' personal lives rather than their health-related knowledge. For her formal course, aimed both at "students on a pre-med path" and those wanting to learn more about the discipline of Anthropology, Costanzo maintains her criticality, including her focus on embodiment, but takes a more traditional pedagogical approach to teaching anthropological theories intertwined with health-related themes. Mentioning in passing that she co-teaches this course with a physician, she side-steps the contested theoretical/epistemic question (as above) of who should be allowed to teach about the medical gaze—and also the material/socio-political question of whose voice carries perceived legitimacy to the varied members of her student audience.

While these authors use pedagogical techniques that have been explicitly developed to inculcate learners with an orientation to freedom and advocacy, other educational designs described in this volume use less obviously activist-oriented means to achieve the same ends. The explicit goal of most curricula that carry an association with medical humanities is that they contribute to the training of caring, compassionate, informed physicians who will do better by their patients (Chapter 3). Reid and Levine (Chapter 34) outline their experience of using online learning technology to rethink the possibilities for their medical humanities course. While technology is often associated in the medical humanities literature with objectivist notions of technoscience, with standardisation, and with a production (vs growth) model of education, Reid and Levine make use of the affordances of their Massive Open Online Course (MOOC) to create an intentionally democratising forum in which individual learners draw on their enormously wide-ranging lived experiences to affectively and dialogically teach their professors and each other. In addition, through bringing a "more interdisciplinary and embodied" view from the global south to MOOC participants around the world, they were able to foreground "how this trans-disciplinary space of Medical Humanities might be understood as both a local project, with local actors, agendas and perspectives, and as part of a broader global effort to bring together fields of experience and knowledge that have historically been forced apart." Through this combination of dialogue, lived experience, the local and the global, a potentially oppressive technology is turned into a pedagogical tool both for democratisation and for teaching for social justice. To support this effort, we see an emergent research agenda focused on validating the effectiveness of medical humanities educational interventions and documenting what effects this training has on physician expertise and the care of patients, particularly those patients who are constituted as most vulnerable.

Conclusion: towards an aesthetics of praxis

We have vested a tremendous amount of moral and socio-political responsibility in the medical humanities to divest medicine of all that is problematic. In this concluding chapter we have thus come full circle in our quest to seek connections between rational thinking, aesthetics, and human progress—topics that are implicated in what we have come to appreciate as knowledge, research and pedagogy within the contemporary medical humanities.

Whether the authors come to it through research or through education, the orientation towards social justice that permeates so many of this book's chapters is not intended to be primarily theoretical but rather to inform praxis. This gives research a particular kind of agenda because, as we have argued, it is not solely in service of knowledge production but also anchored in the needs of patients and their health care providers. For example, Ramaswamy and Ramaswamy (Chapter 23) argue that the medical humanities help health professionals to reconnect with "the core values in medicine by reconstituting the practice of medicine in a relational matrix," where "the doctor, patient and caregiver as collaborators" are "in the project of creating wellness for communities." Kumagai and Naidu (Chapter 6) argue for a critical perspective to underpin the rehumanising project of the medical humanities wherein the "the object of knowledge and the goal of learning" is less about content and more about "ways of knowing and acting in the world." They label this orientation (after Paulo Freire) 'critical consciousness,' and describe it as "awareness of Self, Other, and the World, as well as an awareness of social injustice and a commitment to act to address injustice." This activist political orientation invites researchers to study the shifts in priorities, to create the evidence for resistance and transformation, and to document the historical materiality of the stories and language that have created the intersubjectivity for these movements. It also argues for the equal importance of non-Western ways of thinking, of knowing, and of using stories in the transformation of health care—an area in which we as white Western scholars are inevitably underinformed but which we recognise to be underrepresented within the field.

We started this chapter with a reminder that research has its own geo-political terrain, a highly contested terrain that is also undergoing transformation. Donovan and de Leeuw (Chapter 7) echo this assertion, arguing that "the arts and humanities help to show that health disparities result from subtle engagements and inactions that are situated in diverse geographies." The social is thus extended to the global, and medicine's project of healing is expanded to include an appreciation of the geo-politics that affect the access to health that patients experience before they even enter the realm of the clinic. And yet the global needs to be translated to the local and specific in order to be enacted in the everyday. This includes an appreciation of the histories and axiological underpinnings of specific research (and educational) practices and, as we have argued, entails opening up a deliberate space for new methodologies and ontologies. The borders of the contested field of the medical humanities are being continually reconfigured through negotiations of space, place, time and aesthetics. Research is both implicated in and complicated by this shifting topography, and (as the contents of this book illustrate) it has not yet played a central role in the medical humanities literature for a variety of historical and epistemological reasons. Given the multiplicity of origin stories for the medical humanities, it is impossible to imagine them coalescing into a single research agenda. However, in writing this conclusion we have proposed a number of possible research questions which we have tried to align with the field's current preoccupations. We hope that these are useful to the many scientists, clinicians and practitioners of the medical humanities as they negotiate the boundaries of its research in the future.

References

Albert M. Understanding the debate on medical education research: A sociological perspective. *Academic Medicine.* 2004; 79: 948–54.

de Tocqueville A. 2010. *Democracy in America.* Historical-Critical Edition of *De la démocratie en Amérique.* Edited by Eduardo Nolla. Indianapolis, IN: Liberty Fund. (xxi–1569).

INDEX

Page numbers in *italics* denote a figure, **bold** a table, n an endnote

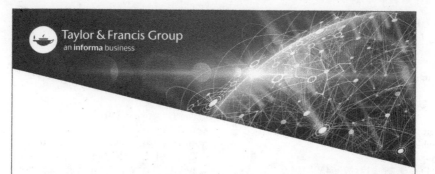